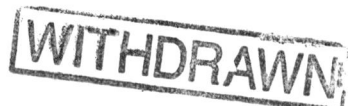

The Evidence Base for Diabetes Care

The Evidence Base for Diabetes Care

Edited by

R. Williams
Nuffield Institue for Health, University of Leeds, Leeds, UK

W. Herman
Department of Internal Medicine, University of Michigan, Ann Arbor, USA

A.-L. Kinmonth
Department of Public Health and Primary Care, Institute of Public Health, Cambridge, UK

N. J. Wareham
Department of Public Health and Primary Care, Institute of Public Health, Cambridge, UK

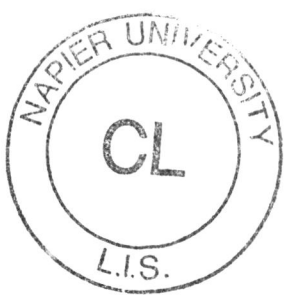

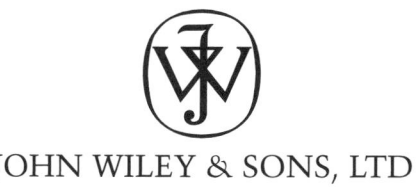

JOHN WILEY & SONS, LTD

Copyright © 2002 by John Wiley & Sons, Ltd,
The Atrium, Southern Gate, Chichester,
West Sussex PO19 8SQ, England

Telephone   (+44) 1243 779777

Email (for orders and customer service enquiries): cs-books@wiley.co.uk
Visit our Home Page on www.wileyeurope.com or www.wiley.com

This publication is designed to provide accurate and authoriative information in regard to the
subject matter covered. It is sold on the understanding that the Publisher is not engaged in
rendering professional services. If professional advice or other expert assistance is required, the
services of a competent professional should be sought.

Other Wiley Editorial Offices

John Wiley & Sons, Inc., 111 River Street, Hoboken, NJ 07030, USA

Jossey-Bass, 989 Market Street, San Francisco, CA 94103-1741, USA

Wiley-VCH Verlag GmbH, Boschstr. 12, D-69469 Weinheim, Germany

John Wiley & Sons Australia Ltd, 33 Park Road, Milton, Queensland 4064, Australia

John Wiley & Sons (Asia) Pte Ltd, 2 Clementi Loop #02-01, Jin Xing Distripark,
Singapore 129809

John Wiley & Sons (Canada) Ltd, 22 Worcester Road, Etobicoke, Ontario, Canada M9W 1L1

British Library Cataloguing in Publication Data

A catalogue record for this book is available from the British Library

ISBN 0 471 98876 6

Typeset in 10/12pt Times Roman by Footnote Graphics, Warminster, Wiltshire
Printed and bound in Great Britain by Antony Rowe Ltd, Chippenham, Wilts.
This book is printed on acid-free paper responsibly manufactured from sustainable forestry in
which at least two trees are planted for each one used for paper production.

Contents

Contributors List

AMANDA ADLER — *Diabetes Trials Unit, Radcliffe Infirmary, Woodstock Road, Oxford OX2 6EH, UK*

ELIZABETH BARRETT-CONNOR — *Department of Family and Preventive Medicine, University of California, San Diego, 9500 Gilman Drive, La Jolla, CA 92093-0607, USA*

THOMAS BUCHANAN — *Medicine, Obstetrics and Gynaecology, and Physiology and Biophysics, USC Keck School of Medicine, 6602 General Hospital, 1200 N States Street, Los Angeles, CA 90089-9317, USA*

AMAN CHUGH — *1500 East Medical Center Drive, Division of Cardiology, Level B1, Ann Arbor, Michigan 48109, USA*

MAX DE COURTEN — *Office of the WHO Representative for South Pacific, PO Box 113, Suva, Fiji Islands*

KIM EAGLE — *University Hospital, 1500 E Medical Center Drive, 3910 Taubman Center, Box 0366, Ann Arbor, MI 48109-0366, USA*

MICHAEL ENGELGAU — *Division of Diabetes Translation Mailstop K-10, 477 Buford Highway NE, Atlanta, GA 30341-3724, USA*

EVA FELDMAN — *Department of Neurology, University of Michigan Health System, 4414 Kresge III, Box 0588, 200 Zina Pritcher Place, Ann Arbor, MI 48109, USA*

LINDA FRIED — *Renal Section, VA Pittsburgh Healthcare System, 4N167 University Drive, Pittsburgh, PA 15213, USA*

BRIAN FRIER — *Department of Diabetes, Royal Infirmary of Edinburgh, Edinburgh EH3 9YW, Scotland, UK*

JOHN FULLER — *Department of Epidemiology and Public Health, University College London, 1-19 Torrington Place, London WC1E 6BT, UK*

EDWIN GALE — *Medical School Unit, Southmead Hospital, Bristol BS10 5NB, UK*

MICHAEL G. GOLDSTEIN — *Clinical Education and Research, Bayer Institute for Health Care Communication, 400 Morgan Lane, West Haven, CT 06516, USA*

SIMON GRIFFIN — *Department of Public Health and Primary Care, University of Cambridge, Institute of Public Health, University Forvie Site, Robinson Way, Cambridge CB2 2SR, UK*

SARA GROSSI — *Department of Oral Biology, State University of New York at Buffalo, 135 Foster Hall, Buffalo, NY 14214, USA*

ALLEN HAMDAN — *110 Francis Street, Suite 5B, Boston MA 02215, USA*

RICHARD HAMMAN — *Department of Preventive Medicine and Biometrics, Box B-119, 4200 East Ninth Avenue, Denver, CO 80262, USA*

WILLIAM HERMAN — *Department of Internal Medicine and Epidemiology, 1500 East Medical Center Drive, 3920 Taubman Center, Box 0345, Ann Arbor, MI 48109, USA*

SUSAN HICKENBOTTOM — *Department of Neurology, University of Michigan Health System, 1914 Taubman Center, Box 0316, 1500 E Medical Center Drive, Ann Arbor, MI 48109, USA*

R. JOHN JARRETT — *45 Bishopsthorpe Road, London SE26 4PA, UK*

T. MARK JOHNSON — *Bert M. Glaser National Retina Institute, 901 Dulaney Valley Road, Suite 200 Baltimore, MD 21204, USA*

ANN-LOUISE KINMONTH — *General Practice and Primary Care Research Unit, Dept. of Public Health & Primary Care, Institute of Public Health, University Forvie Site, Robinson Way, Cambridge CB2 2SR, UK*

RON KURTZ — *Department of Ophthalomolgy, University of California, Irvine Dept. of Opthalmology, 118 Med Surge I, Irvine, CA 92697-4375, USA*

WILLIAM LEDOUX — *Health Research Scientist, VA Puget Sound, MS 151, 1660 S Columbia Way, Seattle, WA 98108, USA*

THERESA MARTEAU — *Guy's, King's and St Thomas's Medical School, Kings College, Guy's Campus, London Bridge, London SE1 9RT, UK*

DAVID MCCANCE — *Regional Centre for Endocrinology and Diabetes, Royal Victoria Hospital, Belfast BT12 6BA, Northern Ireland, UK*

RAJENDRA MEHTA — *Department of Internal Medicine, Division of Cardiology, Veterans Hospital, 1215 Fuller Road 111A, 7E Ann Arbor, MI 48105, USA*

K. M. VENKAT NARAYAN — *Division of Diabetes Translation, Mailstop K-10, 477 Buford Highway NE, Atlanta, GA 30341-3724, USA*

AKINLOLU OJO — *Department of Internal Medicine, University of Michigan Health System, 3914 E Taubman Center, Box 0364, 1500 E Medical Center Drive, Ann Arbor, MI 48109-0364, USA*

STEVE O'RAHILLY — *Department of Medicine and Clinical Biochemistry, Box 157, Addenbrooke's Hospital, Cambridge CB2 2QQ, UK*

TREVOR ORCHARD — *Department of Epidemiology, Graduate School of Public Health, University of Pittsburgh, Diabetes and Lipid Research, 3512 Fifth Avenue, Pittsburgh, PA 15213, USA*

DAVID PENCHEON — *Eastern Region Public Health Observatory, Institute of Public Health, University Forvie Site, Robinson Way, Cambridge CB2 2SR, UK*

FRANK B. POMPOSELLI JR — *Division of Vascular Surgery, Department of Surgery, Beth Israel Deaconess Medical Center, Harvard Medical School, Boston, Massachusetts, USA*

GAYLE REIBER — *Department of Health Services and Epidemiology, Univeristy of Washington, VA Research Career Scientist, VA Fuget Sound Health Care System (152), 1660 South Columbian Way, Seattle, WA 98108, USA*

URBAN ROSENQVIST — *Department of Public Health Uppsala Science Park, S-751 853, Uppsala, Sweden*

DEBRA ROTER   *Department of Health Policy and Management, John Hopkins School of Public Health, 624 N Broadway, Rm 750, Baltimore, MD 21205, USA*

KEN SHAW   *Queen Alexandra Hospital, Cosham, Portsmouth PO6 3LY, UK*

DAVID SIMMONS   *Department of Rural Health, University of Melbourne, Snepparton 3632, PO Box 6500, Victoria, Australia*

ZACHARY SIMMONS   *Division of Neurology, Penn State College of Medicine, M.S. Hershey Medical Center, Hershey, PA 17033, USA*

JAY S. SKYLER   *Division of Endocrinology, Diabetes and Metabolism, University of Miami, Chairman, NIDDK Type 1 Diabetes TrialNet, 1450 NW 10th Avenue – Suite 3061, Miami, Florida 33136, USA*

GEORGE TAYLOR   *Department of Cardiology, Restorative Sciences and Endodontics, The University of Michigan School of Dentistry, 1011 N University, Ann Arbor, MI 48109-1078, USA*

JAAKKO   *Diabetes and Genetic Epidemiology Unit, Department*
TUOMILEHTO   *of Epidemiology and Health Promotion, National Public Health Institute, Department of Public Health, University of Helsinki, Mannerheimintie 166, 00300 Helsinki, Finland*

NICHOLAS J.   *Department of Public Health and Primary Care, Institute*
WAREHAM   *of Public Health, University Forvie Site, Robinson Way, Cambridge CB2 2SR, UK*

NICOLE WEDICK   *Department of Family and Preventive Medicine, University of California, San Diego, 9500 Gilman Drive, La Jolla, CA 92093-0607, USA*

RHYS WILLIAMS   *Nuffield Institute for Health, University of Leeds, 71-75 Clarendon Road, Leeds LS2 9PL, UK*

DEBORAH   *Division of Epidemiology, Department of Family and*
WINGARD   *Preventive Medicine, University of California, San Diego, 9500 Gilman Drive, La Jolla, CA 92093-0607, USA*

JOHN WRIGHT   *Bradford Royal Infirmary, Bradford BD9 6RJ, UK*

1

The Evidence Base for Diabetes Care

RHYS WILLIAMS, WILLIAM HERMAN, ANN-LOUISE
KINMONTH AND NICHOLAS J. WAREHAM
Nuffield Institute for Health, Leeds LS2 9PL, UK

DIABETES

Diabetes is increasingly common throughout the world. Its prevalence is well over 5% in many developed countries[1], and is rising in the USA[2-5], the UK[6], and, most strikingly, in developing countries[7-10] and among indigenous peoples[11,12]. Although most of this rise is the result of an increased incidence and, probably, an increased detection of type 2 diabetes, type 1 diabetes is also increasing in frequency, particularly in young children[13]. An earlier age of onset for type 2 diabetes is also reported, with diagnosis now occurring in children and adolescents[15-17].

For people with diabetes, whether type 1 or type 2, the disorder can have a profound influence on all aspects of life and can affect most organs of the body. In the current absence of a 'cure', it is present for life. In addition, family members, friends and work colleagues are all closely involved in living with the disorder. The long-term effects of diabetes result from its vascular complications; the microvascular complications of retinopathy, neuropathy and nephropathy, and the macrovascular complications of cardiovascular disease, cerebrovascular disease and peripheral vascular disease. Without intervention these may produce visual impairment, lower limb ulceration and gangrene, renal failure and premature and sudden death.

Diabetes is thus an increasingly important health and economic issue for those who have the disorder, those who provide them with health care and those who fund and plan the provision of that care. A complex set of decisions taken by individuals and organisations determines how health care is delivered to people with diabetes. Historically such decisions have been taken in a rather

The Evidence Base for Diabetes Care. Edited by R. Williams, W. Herman, A.-L. Kinmonth and N. J. Wareham.
© 2002 John Wiley & Sons, Ltd

unsystematic manner, leading to variation in the quality of care, the persistence of practices for which there is little evidence and the slow introduction of new interventions that have been demonstrated to be effective. The increasing appreciation throughout the health care industry of the need for decisions to be based on sound evidence is not driven by one party alone. For patients, practices and health care planners alike, it represents an opportunity to shape the delivery of care on the basis of evidence of effectiveness. This is particularly relevant to a disorder such as diabetes. This book is devoted to providing the evidence base on which policy decisions should rest.

The past 20 years have seen considerable progress in producing evidence to support treatments aimed at reducing the risk of diabetes and its complications. Two landmark trials deserve particular notice. The Diabetes Control and Complications Trial (DCCT) in people with type 1 diabetes showed that microvascular complications can be reduced by 30–50% through intensive control of blood glucose[18]. These findings have recently been paralleled in people with type 2 diabetes, by the UK Prospective Diabetes Study (UKPDS)[19], which also demonstrated the crucial importance of effective blood pressure control. These major trials have addressed some of the issues in diabetes care, but other trials and non-experimental forms of evidence have become available for different aspects of diabetes prevention and care. This book describes that evidence, in order to act as a basis for health care decisions in the future, and to demonstrate the areas in which further evidence is needed to underpin health care delivery.

'EVIDENCE-BASED PRACTICE' AND THE EVIDENCE BASE FOR PRACTICE

'Evidence-based medicine' and 'evidence-based practice' may be new terms but they are not new concepts. What is new is the judgement of what constitutes evidence firm enough to justify continuing current practice or to support changes in practice. There is an increasing recognition that, in the face of an enormous quantity of published evidence of variable quality, health care practitioners need help and guidance as to how they can best access this evidence and which parts of it are of sufficiently high quality to be of use to them. This book sets out to examine critically the evidence that is currently available in the field of diabetes prevention and care, and to present it in an accessible form to assist in bridging the gap between evidence and action. The potential of 'evidence-based practice' to contribute to the prevention of disease, its early identification and effective treatment presents a challenge which this book tries, in a small part, to meet.

The term 'evidence-based practice' is preferable to the narrower, but more widely used, term 'evidence-based medicine'. The former emphasises

the importance of health professionals other than doctors and the importance of health-related activities other than those most obviously associated
with physicians. In defining evidence-based practice, three components are
essential:

- the determination, whenever possible, to base decisions on evidence accumulated through research;
- use of the *best possible* evidence available at the time the decision needs to
  be made; and
- use of the evidence most appropriate to a particular patient or population.

The first two of these components have been incorporated into the definition
offered by Sackett *et al.*[20] that evidence-based medicine (or practice) is 'the
conscientious, explicit and judicious use of current best evidence in making
decisions about the care of patients.' We would widen that definition to
include people who are not yet patients and who, if prevention is effective,
may never become patients. Thus we include prevention as well as care, cure
and rehabilitation.

Gray[21] has commented that health care decisions have, in the past, been
based largely on professional values and the availability of resources. He terms
this 'opinion-based decision making'. The widespread advocacy of introducing
research-based evidence into this process is a relatively recent phenomenon.
Although this process will make more effective use of scarce resources, it is
important to realise that increasing the extent to which practice is based on
research will not necessarily reduce the level of resources. Evidence-based
care is not necessarily cheaper care.

We have chosen to call this book *The Evidence Base for Diabetes Care* to
emphasise, from the outset, that it is a commentary on the extent to which
aspects of diabetes prevention and care can or cannot be based on high-quality
evidence. It is not intended to be a textbook of how to care for people with
diabetes. Although it refers to clinical guidelines, it is not a collection of
evidence-based guidelines.

EVIDENCE-BASED DIABETES PRACTICE

Diabetes is a particularly good example of the potential for evidence-based
practice. There are at least four reasons for this (see Box 1.1).

First, individuals with diabetes are leaders among those with a chronic
disease in their involvement in self-care and, more recently, the development
of health services. There is a tremendous potential for using the influence of
the patient to change care for the better. Most diabetes care is based on long-
term behavioural change. Such change will not take place unless the affected
person is willing and assisted to make these changes. What better way is there

---

Box 1.1. The potential of diabetes for evidence-based practice

- The person with diabetes is central to the management of the condition.
- There is a considerable quantity of high-quality evidence available.
- The worldwide prevalence and impact of diabetes is increasing at a dramatic rate.
- Diabetes care is multidisciplinary – evidence-based *practice* is important rather than the narrower evidence-based *medicine*.

---

of encouraging evidence-based practice than to provide a summary of the evidence on which their care is based to patients themselves?

Second, there is high-quality evidence available relevant to diabetes prevention and care which needs to be translated into practice. As with other fields, however, there is also evidence which is not of such high quality, and areas for which little evidence exists at all.

Third, the increasing prevalence of diabetes and its public health importance, particularly in developing countries, is a major impetus for a review of the evidence base for practice.

Fourth, diabetes care is multidisciplinary. The person with diabetes and, in most instances, the family, are at the centre of all diabetes health care activities but it is also recognised that, to be successful, diabetes care needs to involve the co-operation and collaboration of many practitioners – nurses, dieticians, podiatrists, psychologists and doctors. Thus diabetes care is a particularly striking example of evidence-based practice as opposed to evidence-based medicine.

THE LIMITS OF EVIDENCE-BASED PRACTICE

While strongly advocating the advantages of evidence-based practice, some potential disadvantages need to be recognised. These are that:

- the evidence we need is not always available;
- the evidence that is available is not always accessible; and
- the evidence that is accessible is not always of the highest quality.

Lack of available evidence is not merely a result of the necessary studies not yet having been carried out. One of the 'credibility gaps' developing between the advocates of evidence-based practice and professionals engaged in day-to-day patient care is that studies which faithfully reflect the clinical and behavioural complexities of individual patients not only have not yet been done but are unlikely *ever* to be done. Many clinicians, it has been said, 'struggle to apply the results of studies that do not seem that relevant to their daily practice'[22]. Randomised controlled trials have a number of strong points, but the ready generalisation of their results to 'real life' clinical situations is not one of them, for example due to the selection of participants, and the often unusually high quality of care offered.

Too strong an emphasis on the need for evidence to support practice can easily be translated into an unwillingness to do *anything* which is not based on evidence. Thus the positive message of evidence-based practice can, if taken to extremes, become a form of 'evidence-based paralysis' which acts to the detriment of patient and population.

Inaccessible evidence, even of the highest quality, is of no use to the practitioner. There are several current initiatives which make evidence more accessible and provide assessments of its quality. These include the Cochrane Collaboration[23,24], 'Effective Healthcare Bulletins'[e.g. 25] and a clutch of new journals (such as *Evidence-based Medicine*). Whether or not these initiatives, or others like them, will have beneficial effects on the health outcomes of individuals or populations is hard to determine.

EFFICACY, EFFECTIVENESS, EFFICIENCY, ACCEPTABILITY AND APPROPRIATENESS

Studies in health services or health systems research frequently use terms such as efficacy, effectiveness and efficiency. 'Efficacy' is defined by Last[26] as the extent to which a specific intervention produces a beneficial result *under ideal conditions*. 'Effectiveness', on the other hand, is the extent to which the intervention does what it is intended to do 'in the field'[27] or 'in the real world'. Randomised controlled trials tend to focus on efficacy although, when analysed 'by intention to treat', come at least part of the way towards the assessment of effectiveness.

'Efficiency' is an economic concept defined as 'the ratio of what is produced to the resources put in'[28]. In other words, what resources are used in achieving a given unit of output. Holland[29] includes effectiveness and efficiency in his definition of health care evaluation – 'the formal determination of the effectiveness, efficiency and acceptability' of an intervention. 'Acceptability' he describes as an aspect of health care' which, if overlooked, may make even effective and efficient interventions 'fail to reach the stated objective if the population refuses to utilise it'[28]. Most studies and texts which do address acceptability seem to view this only from the point of view of the recipients of health care. Acceptability to the practitioner is also a consideration – acceptable in relation to their day-to-day activities but also, in a broader sense, to their views of the ethical stance and ethos of their profession.

'Appropriateness' is not synonymous with 'acceptability' but conveys the rather different elements of being suitable in relation to the location in which care is delivered, the needs of the patient at that time, and practicable in relation to the ability of the patient to understand and act upon the advice or treatment given.

SOME OTHER TERMS EXPLAINED

Throughout this book, various other epidemiological terms have been used to describe risk in the context of a clinical trial. These can be summarised as follows in relation to a trial which randomises subjects to two groups – an intervention group and a control group. Imagine, for the sake of simplicity, two dichotomous outcomes – cure and non-cure, for example.

	Outcome		
	Alive	Dead	
Experimental group	A	B	A + B
Control group	C	D	C + D

Then the following rates can be defined:

Experimental event rate (EER)	=	B/(A + B)
Control event rate (CER)	=	D/(C + D)
Absolute risk reduction (ARR)	=	CER – EER
Relative risk reduction (RRR)	=	(CER – EER)/CER
Number needed to treat (NNT)	=	1/ARR

Analogous calculations can be performed in relation to adverse effects[29].

	Adverse effect		
	Absent	Present	
Experimental group	A	B	A + B
Control group	C	D	C + D

Experimental (adverse) event rate (E(A)ER)	=	B/(A + B)
Control (adverse) event rate (C(A)ER)	=	D/(C + D)
Absolute risk of adverse events	=	E(A)ER – C(A)ER
Relative risk of adverse events	=	(E(A)ER – C(A)ER)/C(A)ER
Number treated for one adverse event	=	1/Absolute risk of adverse event

Both relative and absolute risk have their place but, in order to understand relative measures, knowledge of what they are relative *to* is needed. For example, a relative risk reduction of 50% could mean going from an absolute risk of 1% to 0.5%, or from 20% or 10%. However, the absolute risk reductions, which in this case would be 0.5% and 10%, demonstrate markedly different benefits. Authors have been encouraged to include absolute measures, when available, with or without their relative equivalents.

THE HIERARCHY OF EVIDENCE

There are several suggested hierarchies for grading evidence. Examples of two of these are that used by the US Task Force on Preventive Health Care[30] and that suggested by Chalmers[31]. The US Task Force template distinguishes between the strength of a recommendation and the quality of the evidence (see Box 1.2). Chalmers' hierarchy ranks the source of evidence in a similar fashion to the second component of the US Task Force's template (see Box 1.3).

Our intention here is to clarify and comment on a field of evidence, and as editors we developed a modified version of the US Task Force's ratings. Our modification is shown in Box 1.4, and authors have been encouraged to use this approach. However, where authors have chosen a different way to summarise the evidence, we have respected their approach.

[Box 1.4 about here]

Box 1.2. template for assessing recommendations and evidence[30]

Strength of the recommendation
- There is good evidence to support the use of the procedure
- There is fair evidence to support the use of the procedure
- There is poor evidence to support the use of the procedure
- There is fair evidence to reject the procedure
- There is good evidence to support the rejection of the procedure

Quality of the evidence
- (I)   Evidence obtained from at least one properly randomised controlled trial
- (II-1) Evidence obtained from well-designed controlled trials without randomisation
- (II-2) Evidence obtained from well-designed cohort or case-controlled analytical studies, preferably from more than one centre or research group
- (II-3) Evidence obtained from multiple timed series with or without intervention, or from dramatic results in uncontrolled experiments
- (III) Opinions of respected authorities based on clinical experience, descriptive studies or reports of expert committees

---

Box 1.3. Hierarchy of evidence advocated by Chalmers[31]

Highest –   Meta-analysis of randomised controlled trials
    –   Randomised controlled trials
    –   Non-randomised controlled trials
    –   Cohort studies
    –   Case control studies
    –   Case series
Lowest –   Case reports

Box 1.4. Our modification of the US Task Force's ratings

Strength of recommendations
- There is good evidence of effectiveness/benefit
- There is fair evidence of effectiveness/benefit
- There is poor evidence of effectiveness/benefit
- There is fair evidence of lack of effectiveness or lack of benefit
- There is good evidence of lack of effectiveness or lack of benefit

HOW TO USE THIS BOOK

The chapters in this book are arranged to reflect the chronology of diabetes. They start with considerations of definition and classification, proceed through prevention of the condition itself, the prevention of complications and then the organisation of care. When appropriate, there are separate chapters for type 1 and type 2 diabetes, for example in relation to prevention. When the same principles apply to both, as for the treatment of established complications, they are combined in a single chapter.

We have brought together potentially contrasting views of the evidence – views of clinicians, on the one hand, and epidemiologists on the other. This is intended to bring out the different perspectives of practice and research at the level of the individual and the population. In many cases, authors have been able to organise their literature searches according to Cochrane Collaboration principles[23] and the results of these searches, for randomised controlled trials (RCTs) are systematically presented in tables. In the chapters dealing with the prevention and treatment of established complications we have asked teams (rather than individual authors) to contribute, since the span of topics is so wide. Throughout this book authors have been asked to clarify and comment upon the evidence in each of their topic areas and to highlight what remains to be resolved by future research. We hope that this book will be useful to policy makers as a guide to what is already known, to patients and their representatives to allow them to establish whether their care includes all interventions known to be effective, and to those responsible for planning future research to identify major areas of uncertainty.

REFERENCES

1. King H, Rewers M (1993) Global estimates for prevalence of diabetes mellitus and impaired glucose tolerance in adults. WHO Ad Hoc Diabetes Reporting Group. *Diab. Care*; **16**: 157–177.
2. Wetterhall SF, Olson DR, DeStefano F, Stevenson JM, Ford ES, German RR, Will JC, Newman JM, Sepe SJ, Vinicor F (1992) Trends in diabetes and diabetic complications, 1980–1987. *Diab. Care*; **15**: 960–967.
3. Harris MI, Flegal KM, Cowie CC, Eberhardt MS, Goldstein DE, Little RR, Wiedmeyer H-M, Byrd-Holt DD (1998) Prevalence of diabetes, impaired fasting glucose, and impaired glucose tolerance in US adults. The Third National Health and Nutrition Examination Survey, 1988–1994. *Diab. Care*; **21**: 518–524.
4. Anon. (1997) Trends in the prevalence and incidence of self-reported diabetes mellitus–United States, 1980–1994. *M.M.W.R.* **46**: 1014–1018.
5. Leibson CL, Obrien PC, Atkinson E, Palumbo PJ, Melton LJ (1997) Relative contributions of incidence and survival to increasing prevalence of adult-onset diabetes mellitus – a population-based study. *Am. J. Epidemiol.* **146**: 12–22.
6. Gatling W, Budd S, Walters D, Mullee MA, Goddard JR, Hill RD (1998) Evidence of an increasing prevalence of diagnosed diabetes mellitus in the Poole area from 1983 to 1996. *Diabet. Med.* **15**: 1015–1021.
7. Hodge AM, Dowse GK, Gareeboo H, Tuomilehto J, Alberti KG, Zimmet PZ (1996) Incidence, increasing prevalence, and predictors of change in obesity and fat distribution over five years in the rapidly developing population of Mauritius. *Int. J. Obes. Relat. Metab. Disord.* **20**: 137–146.
8. Hodge AM, Dowse GK, Zimmet PZ, Collins VR (1995) Prevalence and secular trends in obesity in Pacific and Indian Ocean island populations. *Obes. Res.* **3**: Suppl 2: 77s–87s.
9. King H, Rewers M (1993) Diabetes in adults is now a Third World problem. World Health Organization Ad Hoc Diabetes Reporting Group. *Ethn. Dis.* **3**: Suppl, S67–74.
10. Dabelea D, Hanson RL, Bennett PH, Roumain J, Knowler WC, Pettitt DJ, (1998) Increasing prevalence of Type II diabetes in American Indian children. *Diabetologia* **41**: 904–910.
11. Bennett PH, Knowler WC (1979) Increasing prevalence of diabetes in the Pima (American) Indians over a ten-year period. In: International Congress Series No. 500. Diabetes 1979. Amsterdam, Excerpta Medica, 507–511.
12. Daniel M, Rowley KG, McDermott R, Mylvaganam A, O'Dea K (1999) Diabetes incidence in an Australian Aboriginal population. *Diab. Care* **22**: 1993–1998.
13. Kitagawa T, Owada M, Urakami T, Tajima N (1994) Epidemiology of type 1 (insulin-dependent) and type 2 (non-insulin-dependent) diabetes mellitus in Japanese children. *Diabetes Res. Clin. Pract.* **24**: Suppl: S7–13.
14. Pinhas-Hamiel O, Dolan LM, Daniels SR, Standiford D, Khoury PR, Zeitler P (1996) Increased incidence of non-insulin-dependent diabetes mellitus among adolescents. *J. Pediatr.* **128**: 608–615.

15. Rosenbloom AL, Joe JR, Young RS, Winter WE (1999) Emerging epidemic of type 2 diabetes in youth. *Diab. Care* **22**: 345–354.
16. Glaser NS, Jones KL (1998) Non-insulin dependent diabetes mellitus in Mexican–American children. *West. J. Med.* **168**: 11–16.
17. Kitagawa T, Owada M, Urakami T, Yamauchi K (1998) Increased incidence of non-insulin dependent diabetes mellitus among Japanese schoolchildren correlates with an increased intake of animal protein and fat. *Clin. Pediatr. (Phila.)* **37**: 111–115.
18. The Diabetes Control and Complications Research Group. (1993) The effect of intensive treatment of diabetes on the development and progression of long-term complications in insulin-dependent diabetes mellitus. *N. Engl. J. Med.* **329**: 977–986.
19. UK Prospective Diabetes Study Group (1998) Intensive blood-glucose control with sulphonylureas or insulin compared with conventional treatment and risk of complications in patients with Type 2 diabetes (UKPDS 33). *Lancet* **352**: 837–853.
20. Sackett DI, Rosenberg WMC, Gray JAM, Haynes RB, Richardson WS (1996) Evidence-based medicine: what it is and what it isn't. It's about integrating individual clinical expertise and the best external evidence. *Brit. Med. J.* **312**: 71–72.
21. Gray JAM (1997) Evidence-based healthcare. In: *Evidence-based Healthcare: How to Make Health Policy and Management Decisions*, ed. JAM Gray, Edinburgh: Churchill-Livingstone.
22. Knottnerus JA, Dinant GJ (1997) Medicine based evidence, a prerequisite for evidence based practice. *Brit. Med. J.* **315**: 1109–1110.
23. Chalmers I, Sackett D, Silagy C (1997) The Cochrane Collaboration. In: *Non-random Reflections on Health Services Research: On the 25th Anniversary of Archie Cochrane's 'Effectiveness and efficiency'*, eds A Maynard and I Chalmers. London: BMJ Publishing Group.
24. (1997) The Cochrane Library. BMJ Publishing Group' 1997 (Issue 4).
25. Effective health care: the treatment of depression in primary care. No. 5 in the series 'Effectiveness bulletins'. Leeds, 1993.
26. Last JM (1983) *A Dictionary of Epidemiology*. Oxford Medical Publications, Oxford: Oxford University Press.
27. Cochrane AL (1971) Effectiveness and efficiency: random reflections on health services. The Rock Carling Fellowship 1971. The Nuffield Provincial Hospitals Trust, 1972.
28. Holland WW (1983) Concepts and meaning in evaluation of health care. In: *Evaluation of Health Care*, ed. WW Holland. Oxford: Oxford Medical Publications.
29. Bjerre LM, LeLorier J (2000) Expressing the magnitude of adverse effects in case-control studies: the number of patients needed to be treated for one additional patient to be harmed. *Brit. Med. J.* **320**: 503–506.
30. Report of the US Preventive Service Task Force (1989) Guide to clinical preventive services. An assessment of the effectiveness of 169 interventions. Baltimore: Williams and Wilkins.
31. Chalmers TC, Celano P, Sacks HS, Smith H Jr. (1983) Bias in treatment assignment in controlled clinical trials. *N. Engl .J. Med.* **309**: 1358–1361.

Part I

EVIDENCE-BASED DEFINITION AND CLASSIFICATION

2

Classification of Diabetes

MAX DE COURTEN

International Diabetes Institute, Victoria 3162, Australia

EVOLUTION OF THE CLASSIFICATION OF DIABETES

Over 2000 years ago two Indian physicians, Charaka and Sushruta[1] were the first to recognise that diabetes is not a single disorder. Throughout history renowned scientists and physicians such as Galen, Avicenna, Paracelcus and Maimonides have made reference to diabetes[2]. During the eighteenth and nineteenth centuries a less clinically symptomatic variety of the disorder was again noted. It was identified by heavy glycosuria, often detected in later life and commonly associated with overweight rather than wasting. Under the present classification this would be regarded as type 2 diabetes.

A huge step forward in understanding the aetiology of diabetes was achieved through the experiments by Josef von Mering and Oskar Minkowski which led to the theory of pancreatic diabetes and were published as 'Diabetes Mellitus After Extirpation of the Pancreas' in 1889. The discovery was made after removing the pancreas from a dog which, although it survived the experiment, began urinating on the laboratory floor. Minkowski tested the dog's urine for glucose, as he did with clinic patients with polyuria, and found a high glucose content. This discovery inspired their work relating to the isolation of insulin from the pancreas for use in the therapy of diabetes, for which Banting and Best won the Nobel Prize in 1921.

In 1936, Harold Himsworth[3] proposed that there were at least two clinical types of diabetes, insulin-sensitive and insulin-insensitive. He suggested that insulin-sensitive diabetics were insulin deficient and required exogenous insulin to survive, while the other group did not require insulin. This observation was based on clinical evidence, as at that time no assays were available for the measurement of insulin. The Australian scientist, Joseph Bornstein, who developed the first bioassay for insulin and was eventually awarded a Nobel Prize, initially gained little recognition for his work until he went to work in

The Evidence Base for Diabetes Care. Edited by R. Williams, W. Herman, A.-L. Kinmonth and N. J. Wareham.
© 2002 John Wiley & Sons, Ltd

London with Robin Lawrence[4]. Following the development of the bioassay for insulin and its measurement in individuals with diabetes, it became increasingly apparent that there were at least two major distinct forms of diabetes. With the help of the assay, these were now not only separable on the basis of age at diabetes onset, but also by the levels of endogenous insulin. The difference in age at onset led to the use of the terms 'juvenile-onset' and 'maturity-onset' diabetes which was thought to be largely consistent with their observed treatment differences described as insulin-dependent diabetes mellitus (IDDM) and non-insulin dependent diabetes mellitus (NIDDM).

EVOLUTION IN DIAGNOSTIC CRITERIA FOR DIABETES

The question of diagnostic criteria for type 1 diabetes does not usually give risk to much debate because of its clear acute-onset phenotype, and the logical link between aetiology (lack of insulin) and treatment modality. However, the recognition of a non-insulin-dependent form of diabetes, in which there was a much less clear distinction between normality and disease, created a need for diagnostic criteria. Classification with only the help of symptoms and clinical signs was soon regarded as unsatisfactory. Another major impetus for the development of diagnostic criteria was the recognition that the absence of standardisation was an obstacle to epidemiological and clinical research.

In 1964, the World Health Organisation (WHO) convened an Expert Committee on Diabetes Mellitus which attempted to provide a universal classification of the diabetes syndrome. But it was not until 1980 that an international accepted classification was established.

Two international work groups, the National Diabetes Data Group (NDDG) of the National Institutes of Health, USA in 1979[5], and the World Health Organisation (WHO) Expert Committee on Diabetes in 1980[6] proposed and published similar criteria for diagnosis and classification. They both recognised that diabetes was an aetiologically and clinically heterogeneous group of disorders with hyperglycaemia shared in common.

The NDDG/WHO classification system incorporated data from research conducted during the previous decades and set the path for unifying nomen-clature, diagnostic criteria and requirements such as the amount of oral glucose load used. The inclusion of impaired glucose tolerance (IGT) into the diabetes classification followed the recognition that a zone of diagnostic uncertainty existed in the oral glucose tolerance test (OGTT) between what was clearly normal glucose tolerance and diabetes.

However, controversy continued around the criteria, and minor changes to the classification took place in 1985, letting the WHO slightly modify its criteria to coincide more with the NDDG values, whereas NDDG later modified the diagnostic requirements by dropping the intermediate sample during the OGTT, to be identical with the WHO recommendations. With the 1985

WHO Study Group classification[7], a number of clinical classes of diabetes were agreed upon, which included the major two as insulin-dependent diabetes mellitus (IDDM) and non-insulin dependent diabetes mellitus (NIDDM). The terms type 1 and type 2 diabetes were omitted in the 1985 revision and Malnutrition-related Diabetes Mellitus (MRDM) was introduced as a new class. The other important classes were retained from the 1980 document as Other Types and Impaired Glucose Tolerance (IGT) as well as Gestational Diabetes Mellitus (GDM). These classifications were widely accepted for the next decade and represented a compromise between a clinically and an aetiologically based system. This had the advantage that cases where the specific cause or aetiology was unknown could still be classified according to their clinical presentation.

Recent changes to the classification of diabetes

Data from genetic, epidemiological and aetiologic studies continued to accumulate throughout the 1980s and 1990s, and the understanding of the aetiology and pathogenesis of diabetes improved. With the application of universal criteria for diagnosis and standardised testing procedures, estimation of the global burden of diabetes became possible[8].

Nevertheless, calls continued to revisit the NDDG and WHO recommendations to further fulfil the aims set out by the NDDG in 1979 in order to take into account the dynamic phasic nature of diabetes[9]. Advances such as the use of immunological markers of the type 1 diabetes process suggested that the clinical classification of diabetes into IDDM and NIDDM was unsatisfactory. Equally, age of diabetes onset was increasingly regarded as a confounding factor in the classification, rather than its basis. Frequently clinicians observed autoimmune forms of diabetes among adults and diabetes with features of NIDDM in adolescents. In addition, many adult patients with NIDDM were well controlled for several years with diet and oral hypoglycaemic agents but needed insulin later in the course of their disease. At a time when auto-antibody measurement was not available, it would have remained uncertain if these patients had type 2 with a progressive insulin insufficiency or if they had slowly progressing type 1 diabetes. With the help of the immune markers many patients previously classified as type 2 were then reclassified as having type 1 diabetes[10]. As an indicator of this transitional time, terms such as type 1½ entered the literature.

A thought-provoking attempt at keeping staging of glucose intolerance separate from (sub-) classification according to aetiological type was proposed by Kuzuya and Matsuda for a new classification of diabetes mellitus[11]. Their concept sought to separate the criteria related to aetiology and those related to the degree of deficiency of insulin or insulin action and to define each patient on the basis of these two criteria. This concept was taken on by the American

Diabetes Association's expert group, which has convened since 1995 to review the literature and determine what changes to the classification were necessary. WHO also convened a Consultation in December 1996 to consider the issues and examine the available data, and a provisional report was published in 1998[12], which was adopted with minor modifications in 1999[13].

This latest classification is based on stages of glucose tolerance with a complementary sub-classification according to the aetiological type. Diabetes mellitus is defined as a group of metabolic diseases characterised by hyperglycaemia resulting from defects in insulin secretion, insulin action, or both. Common to all types of diabetes mellitus is chronic hyperglycaemia, which is associated with long-term damage, dysfunction and failure of various organs, especially the eyes, kidneys, nerves, heart and blood vessels.
Hyperglycaemia can be sub-categorised regardless of the underlying cause, into:

- Insulin required for survival (includes the former IDDM).
- Insulin required for control – i.e. for metabolic control, not for survival (includes the former insulin treated NIDDM).
- Not insulin requiring, i.e. treatment by non-pharmacological methods or drugs other than insulin (includes NIDDM on diet alone /or combined with oral agents).
- Impaired Glucose Tolerance (IGT) and/or impaired fasting glycaemia (IFG).
- Normal glucose tolerance.

In this new classification, stages reflecting the various degrees of hyperglycaemia are set across the disease processes which may lead to diabetes mellitus in an individual (Figure 2.1). In all circumstances it should now be possible to categorise each individual with diabetes mellitus according to clinical stage. The stage of glycaemia may change over time depending on the extent of the underlying disease processes, and impact of therapeutic glucose control. The presence of hyperglycaemia is not an essential consequence of the underlying disease process because in certain situations this may not have progressed far enough to cause high levels of blood glucose. Reframing the classification in terms of aetiology allows identification of the defect or process which leads to diabetes. For instance, the presence of islet cell antibodies makes it likely that a person has the type 1 autoimmune process even at a time when they are normoglycaemic. In contrast to type 1 and type 3 diabetes (Other Specific Types) there are still few sensitive or highly specific indicators of the type 2 process at present, although these are likely to become apparent as aetiological research progresses.

The possibility that individuals may change over time across glycaemic stages in both directions reflects the observation that in some individuals with diabetes, adequate glycaemic control can be achieved with weight reduction, exercise and/or oral agents. These individuals, therefore, do not require insulin

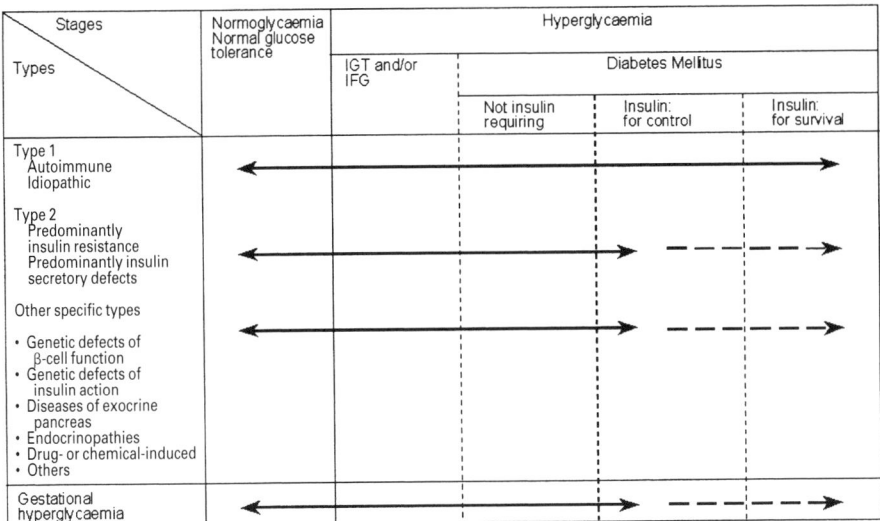

Figure 2.1. Disorders of glycaemia: aetiological types and stages. Reproduced from, Definition Diagnosis and Classification of Diabetes Mellitus and its Complications[13].

and may even revert from having diabetic glucose values to IGT or normoglycaemia. Other individuals require insulin for adequate glycaemic control but can survive without it. These individuals, by definition, have some residual insulin secretion. Individuals with extensive beta-cell destruction, and therefore no residual insulin secretion, require insulin for survival which could result from any type of diabetes. Table 2.1 shows the classification of glycaemic disorders.

Gestational hyperglycaemia

Both the WHO and ADA committees agreed to adopt a common aetiological classification and share unified terminology. They suggested that the terms 'insulin-dependent diabetes mellitus' and 'non-insulin-dependent diabetes mellitus' and their acronyms 'IDDM' and 'NIDDM' should be eliminated, and that type 1 and type 2 be reintroduced with an emphasis on using arabic rather than roman numerals. The aetiological type named type 1 includes the majority of cases which are primarily due to pancreatic islet beta-cell destruction and are prone to ketoacidosis. This sub-type also includes cases attributable to an autoimmune process, as well as those prone to ketoacidosis in which beta-cell destruction is of uncertain aetiology (idiopathic). Forms of beta-cell destruction or failure where specific causes can be identified are now classified as Other Specific Types.

Table 2.1. Aetiological classification of disorders of glycaemia.

Type 1 *(Beta cell destruction)*
  Autoimmune
    Clinically rapidly progressive
    Clinically slowly progressive
  Idiopathic

Type 2 (*Ranging from predominantly insulin resistance to a predominantly secretory defect with or without insulin resistance*)

Other specific types
• Genetic defects of beta cell function eg MODY 1-3, mtDNA
• Genetic defects in insulin action e.g. type A insulin resistance
• Diseases of the exocrine pancreas
• Endocrinopathies
• Drug- or chemical-induced
• Infectious e.g. congenital rubella
• Uncommon forms of immune-mediated diabetes e.g. "stiff man" syndrome
• Other genetic syndromes, sometimes associated with diabetes

Gestational hyperglycaemia

Type 2 includes the common major form of diabetes which results from defects in insulin secretion, almost always with a major contribution from insulin resistance.

The former class of 'Malnutrition-related Diabetes Mellitus' (MRDM) was deleted, because the evidence that diabetes can be caused by malnutrition or protein deficiency *per se* was not convincing. Its subtype of Protein-deficient Pancreatic Diabetes (PDPD or PDDM) was considered as a malnutrition modulated or modified form of diabetes mellitus. The other former subtype of MRDM, Fibrocalculous Pancreatic Diabetes (FCPD), was classified as a disease of the exocrine pancreas, which may lead to diabetes mellitus and assigned to type 3 (Other Specific Types).

The class 'Impaired Glucose Tolerance' was classified as a stage of impaired glucose regulation, since it can be observed in any hyperglycaemic disorder, and is itself not diabetes.

A clinical stage of Impaired Fasting Glycaemia was introduced to classify individuals who have fasting glucose values above the normal range, but below those diagnostic of diabetes. Gestational Diabetes Mellitus (GDM) corresponding to diabetes type 4, was defined as carbohydrate intolerance of variable severity with onset or first recognition during pregnancy. The definition applies irrespective of whether or not insulin is used for treatment or whether the condition persists after pregnancy. It does not exclude the possibility that unrecognised glucose intolerance may have antedated or begun concomitantly with the pregnancy. After pregnancy ends, the woman has to be reclassified, either into diabetes mellitus, IGT or normal glucose tolerance. Unfortunately, the question of the best diagnostic criteria for GDM is the major area where the

ADA and WHO recommendations have not been able to come to a consensus. The WHO recommendations for GDM have remained the same since 1985. They suggest that an OGTT should be performed after overnight fasting (8–14 hours) using a 75 g glucose load, with plasma glucose measured at two hours (2 h). Pregnant women who meet WHO criteria for diabetes or IGT should be classified as having GDM. They suggest that at least six weeks post-pregnancy, a woman should be reclassified based on the results of 75 g load OGTT. Major issues such as the inclusion in the definition of GDM of women with glucose values which would have led to them being classified as IGT had they not been pregnant are not discussed in the WHO document. The controversies concerning the definition of Gestational Diabetes are discussed in full in Chapter 10.

CURRENT CRITERIA FOR DIAGNOSIS OF DIABETES MELLITUS

Diabetes has been linked to a number of other conditions including hypertension, obesity, dislipidaemia and coronary heart disease, and also to environmental factors such as physical activity and nutrition. To complicate the picture further, several genetic factors are thought to play a significant role in the predisposition to diabetes and its complications. With so many factors involved in the aetiology of this disease or disease group, it is not surprising that a single biomedical test, such as blood glucose, has not produced a definitive and precise threshold for diagnosis or prediction of the disease and its complications. As discussed above, throughout the history of diabetes classification various methods and cut-off values were employed as diagnostic of diabetes until the desire to conduct international comparisons encouraged the development of standardised diagnostic criteria. Such an approach has obvious merits for epidemiological studies, but can present the clinician with difficulties when considering individual patients.

Both the ADA[14] and WHO[13] recommended the following changes to the criteria which were used since 1985 (Table 2.2):

- The fasting plasma glucose (FPG) threshold for the diabetes category was lowered from 7.8 to 7.0 mmol/l.
- Impaired fasting glycaemia (FPG 6.1–6.9 mmol/l) was introduced as a new category of intermediate glucose metabolism (named impaired fasting glucose by the ADA). The term IFG was originally coined by Charles *et al.*[15] with a fasting plasma glucose level between 6.1 mmol/l and <7.8 mmol/l. The ADA, and subsequently the WHO, altered the upper end to correspond to the new lower diagnostic criteria for diabetes. The fasting glucose concentration of 6.1 mmol/l has been chosen as the upper limit of 'normal'.

Table 2.2. Values for diagnosis* of diabetes and other categories of hyperglycaemia

	Glucose concentration, mmol/l			
	Plasma		Whole blood	
	Venous	Capillary	Venous	Capillary
Diabetes mellitus:				
Fasting				
or	≥7.0	≥7.0	≥6.1	≥6.1
2 h post glucose load	≥11.1	≥12.2	≥10.0	≥11.1
Impaired Glucose Tolerance:				
Fasting concentration				
and	<7.0	<7.0	<6.1	<6.1
2 h post glucose load	≥7.8 and	≥8.9 and	≥6.7 and	≥7.8 and
	<11.1	<12.2	<10.0	<11.1
Impaired Fasting Glucose:				
Fasting	≥6.1 and	≥6.1 and	≥5.6 and	≥5.6 and
	<7.0	<7.0	<6.1	<6.1
2 h (if measured)	<7.8	<8.9	<6.7	<7.8

*Note that both ADA and WHO state that diabetes can only be diagnosed in an individual when these
diagnostic values are confirmed on another day.

Blood glucose measurements show considerable day-to-day variability and
therefore it is recommended that diabetes only be diagnosed when two
abnormal values have been found for tests conducted on separate days. This
recommendation is based on concerns about the potential implications of the
disease label to an individual. Duplicate testing reduces the probability of
attributing the label in error. However, the evidence base for the diagnostic
threshold, the studies relating blood glucose to risk of retinopathy, are all based
on single OGTTs. Adding a requirement for duplicate testing is, in effect,
equivalent to raising the diagnostic threshold for a single test.

EVIDENCE BASE FOR DIAGNOSTIC THRESHOLDS

BIMODAL GLUCOSE DISTRIBUTION AS A DETERMINANT OF DIAGNOSTIC THRESHOLD

The 2 h cut-point originates from the shape of the distribution of 2 h glucose in
various populations and the shape of the risk curve relating 2 h glucose to
the microvascular complications of diabetes. In certain high risk populations,
11.1 mmol/l was found to the point separating two components of the bimodal
population distribution of 2 h PG values[16,17,18]. In addition, in several studies,
the prevalence of diabetes-related microvascular disease was found to sharply
increase above 2 h PG levels of around 11.1 mmol/l and similarly at fasting
plasma glucose levels of 7.8 mmol/l[19].

Based on the chosen 2 h PG thresholds of 11.1 mmol/l and 7.8 mmol/l FPG, an enormous body of clinical and epidemiological data was then collected. Newer data in lower risk populations did not demonstrate bimodality. In these populations, glucose values were more normally distributed, making it difficult to identify a threshold separating those individuals who are at substantially increased risk for some adverse outcomes caused by diabetes from those who are not[20,21]. It has been suggested that the phenomenon of bimodality is only apparent in certain high prevalence populations because of statistical power[22].

Table 2.3 contains the results of various studies which are cited to have blood glucose values following a bimodal distribution and the antimodal cut-points within those populations. It is evident from these studies that the cut-points

Table 2.3. Antimodal cut-points of FPG and/or 2 h PG distributions in different populations.

Population	Gender	Age	No.	FPG	2 h PG	Mean
Pima Indians[23]	Both	>24 years	960	9.3	12.6	12.6
Nauruans[24]	Male	20–29	69		200 (11.1)	12.6
		30–39 years	42		282 (15.7)	13.6 ≥30
		40–49	46		282 (15.7)	
		50+	38		200 (11.1)	
	Female	20–29	95		200 (11.1)	
		30–39	40		251 (13.9)	
		40–49	43		224 (12.4)	
		50+	47		224 (12.4)	
Samoa[25]	Male	35–44	56		208 (11.6)	10.4
		45–54	76		185 (10.3)	
		55+	65		158 (8.8)	
	Female	35–44	82		179 (9.9)	
		45–54	89		167 (9.3)	
		55+	100		216 (12.0)	
Mexican Americans[26]	Both	25–34	248		307 (17.1)	13.9
		35–44	208		231 (12.8)	12.5 ≥35
		45–54	194		224 (12.4)	
		55–64	171		218 (12.1)	
Egyptians[27]	Both	>19 years	1018	129 (7.2)	207 (11.5)	11.5
Kiribati[28]	Both	30–39	504		12.7	13.1
		40–49	363		13.1	
		50+	232		13.9	
Wanigela[29]	Both	25–34	265		10.4	12.1
		35–44	219		14.9	
		45–54	95		9.4	
		55+	73		13.5	
Wanigela[29]	Both	25–34	299	7.5		7.4
		35–44	244	7.3		
		45–54	113	7.3		
		55+	82	7.7		

vary by age, gender and ethnic group, indicating the difficulty of selecting a single diagnostic value to be used internationally.

LONG-TERM DIABETES COMPLICATIONS AS USED FOR DEFINING DIABETES THRESHOLDS

Diabetes mellitus is characterised by hyperglycaemia, which is associated with long-term damage, dysfunction and failure of various organs. Several studies[30,31] have confirmed relationships between hyperglycaemia and the risk of developing such micro- and macrovascular complications as retinopathy, neuropathy, nephropathy and cardiovascular disease. However, many have compared the rates of each condition in subjects already classified according to the diagnostic criteria as having diabetes or not. Few studies consider whether the current diagnostic glucose levels represent the best level for predicting an increased risk of such complications, and no formal statistical threshold for any complication has been consistently demonstrated.

The relationships of FPG and 2 h PG with the development of retinopathy were evaluated in a study undertaken in the Pima Indian population over a wide range of plasma glucose cutpoints[23]. Both variables were similarly associated with retinopathy, indicating that by this criterion, each could work equally well for diagnosing diabetes. The authors concluded that both measures were equivalent in terms of the properties previously used to justify diagnostic criteria. These findings were confirmed in a similar study in Egypt, in which the FPG and 2 h PG were each strongly and equally well associated with retinopathy[27]. For both the FPG and the 2 h PG, the prevalence of retinopathy was markedly higher above the point of intersection of the two components of the bimodal frequency distribution (7.2 mmol/l and 2 h PG 11.5 mmol/l).

Using Receiver Operating Characteristic (ROC) curves, it is possible to determine the value of a diagnostic test which provides maximum sensitivity and specificity for predicting the occurrence of a given complication associated with diabetes[32]. A ROC curve is a graphical representation of the relationship between sensitivity and specificity for any diagnostic test. It is constructed by plotting the true positive rate (sensitivity of the test) against the false positive rate (1 − specificity) for a series of possible thresholds. Such values have been calculated for the Pima Indian population in relation to retinopathy, and the optimum cut-off values among those over 24 years of age were 7.2 mmol/l for a fasting plasma glucose test and 13.0 mmol/l for a 2 h postload glucose test. These values differ from the cut-off values suggested as diagnostic of diabetes from the bimodal distribution of blood glucose results, particularly for the fasting value. The use of ROC analyses for predicting nephropathy among the Pima population indicated that the various measures of hyperglycaemia were poor at predicting this complication. No study has reported ROC curves for glucose values predicting cardiovascular disease.

EVIDENCE FOR MATCHING THE FPG THRESHOLD WITH THE 2 H PG THRESHOLD

One part of the justification for lowering the fasting glucose diagnostic threshold is to identify the same percentage of the population as identified by the 2 h cut-point. This implies that the 2 h cut-point is the criterion that best identifies individuals at risk of developing complications as a result of hyperglycaemia. However, in many populations the tests identify different individuals[33,34,35].

The 1985 WHO criteria selected the fasting and 2 h cut-offs on estimates of the thresholds for microvascular disease. After reviewing the statistical relation between the FPG distribution and 2 h PG distribution, it became evident that these criteria effectively defined diabetes by the 2 h PG alone because the fasting and 2 h cut-point values were not equivalent at those levels. Almost all individuals with FPG greater than or equal to 7.8 mmol/l have 2 h PG levels of 11.1 mmol/l or above when given an OGTT. On the other hand, only about one-quarter of those with 2 h PG exceeding 11.1 mmol/l (and without previously known diabetes) have FPG greater than 7.8 mmol/l[36]. Thus, the cut-point of FPG 7.8 mmol/l defined a greater degree of hyperglycaemia in comparison to the cut-point of 2 h PG 11.1 mmol/l. Understandingly, this discrepancy is undesirable, and therefore the ADA Expert Committee investigated cut-point values for both tests which reflect a similar degree of hyperglycaemia and risk of adverse outcomes.

The decision to change the diagnostic cut-point for the FPG to 7.0 mmol/l was based on the belief that the cut-points for the FPG and 2 h PG should diagnose similar conditions, given the equivalence of the FPG and the 2 h PG in their associations with vascular complications. Based on the populations considered, the summary estimate for the FPG cut-point was chosen at the upper end of the equivalence estimates as the FPG of 7.0 mmol/l is slightly higher than most of the investigated cut-points which would give the same prevalence of diabetes at the criterion of 2 h PG 11.1 mmol/l. Therefore the committee noted that slightly fewer people will be diagnosed with diabetes if the new FPG criterion is used alone than if either the FPG or the OGTT is used and interpreted by the previous WHO and NDDG criteria. This acknowledgement was confirmed by numerous studies showing that an equivalence of prevalence has not yet been achieved with the revised FPG cut-point.

Reviewing the history and science behind the diagnostic criteria shows the tension between the need for international consensus and evidence of heterogeneity in ideal diagnostic levels in different populations. There are large differences in the prevalence of the major forms of diabetes, their determinants and the associated complications among various ethnic groups worldwide. However, studies conducted in only a few single ethnic groups have been considered as evidence for the development of international diagnostic criteria. In particular, the work on Pima Indians has been used extensively to predict at what glycaemic level the risk of developing diabetic complications increases. The Pima Indians have the highest rate of diabetes in the world[37], they develop diabetes at a younger age than other groups[38] and their blood glucose measurements show a bimodal distribution which may not be apparent in all populations[39]. Generalising the data from this specific population to other ethnic groups may not be ideal.

IMPAIRED GLUCOSE TOLERANCE (IGT) AND IMPAIRED FASTING GLYCAEMIA (IFG) AS NEW RISK-FACTOR CATEGORIES FOR DIABETES

In the previous classification of diabetes, Impaired Glucose Tolerance was included as a separate class of diabetes. This meant that until 1980, people with a 2 h post-glucose load plasma glucose level between 7.8 mmo/l to 11 mmol/l were diagnosed with diabetes. It is now categorised together with IFG as a stage in the natural history of disordered carbohydrate metabolism with higher than normal fasting (IFG) or 2 h post-oral glucose load (IGT) glucose levels not reaching diabetic thresholds (see Table 2.2). As such, IGT and IFG were regarded in the absence of pregnancy (where they contribute to the class of gestational diabetes) not as clinical entities in their own right but as risk factors for future diabetes and cardiovascular disease[40]. This new categorisation rescued them from being assigned to a disease that could restrict life insurance and certain jobs and other social penalties in some countries. IGT or IFG can be observed as intermediate stages in any of the disease processes listed in Figure 2.1 under the assumption that persons within this stage are at higher risk than the general population for diabetes[41]. Individuals with IGT have a raised risk of macrovascular disease[42,43] as IGT is associated with other known CVD risk factors including hypertension, dyslipidaemia and central obesity[12]. The diagnosis of these risk categories, therefore, may have important prognostic implications, particularly in otherwise healthy, ambulatory individuals.

Numerous population-based studies have calculated the risk of progression from IGT to diabetes. Two reviews[44,45] including 15 different populations from Europe, the USA, India, Africa and the Pacific island of Nauru, reported an annual rate of development of diabetes varying from 2% to 14%. Not surprisingly, the risk was highest in those populations with a high background prevalence of diabetes. Data on IFG are still scarce, but in two studies there was an annual conversion rate to diabetes of 1% in middle-aged French civil servants[46], and 6% in a high-prevalence population in Mauritius[47].

Underlying this concept of progression from an intermediate risk state is the assumption that there are three separate glycaemic states: normoglycaemia, diabetic hyperglycaemia and in between the two a non-diabetic hyperglycaemia, which confer different level of risk for developing diabetes-related complications. However, across the glucose spectrum in the few longitudinal studies of the natural history of increasing glucose intolerance and development of diabetes related complications, no clear threshold has been observed. Indeed, the relationships are curvilinear. In addition, the development of diabetes complications seems to be related both to the duration and degree of glycaemic exposure. Little attention has been paid to the relationship between these two variables, mainly because determination of exposure duration requires sophisticated metabolic surveillance systems. Hence, rarely are comparisons made between individuals with moderate levels of hyperglycaemia for extended periods and individuals with high levels over short time frames.

WHAT IS THE BEST DIAGNOSTIC TEST?

ASSESSMENT OF DIABETES-RELATED SYMPTOMS

The clinical diagnosis of diabetes is often prompted by symptoms such as polyuria and polydipsia, recurrent infections, unexplained weight loss and, in severe cases, drowsiness and coma. In such cases a single blood glucose determination in excess of the diagnostic values indicated in Figure 2.2 (black zone) establishes the diagnosis. Figure 2.2 also defines levels of blood glucose below which a diagnosis of diabetes is unlikely in non-pregnant individuals. These criteria are unchanged from the 1985 WHO report[7]. For clinical purposes, an OGTT to establish diagnostic status need only be considered if casual blood glucose values lie in the uncertain range (i.e. between the levels that establish or exclude diabetes) and fasting blood glucose levels are below those which establish the diagnosis of diabetes.

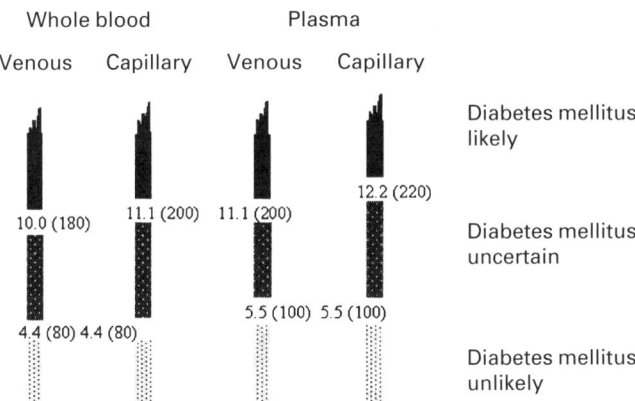

Figure 2.2. Unstandardised (casual, random) blood glucose values in the diagnosis of diabetes in mmol/l (mg/dl). Taken from the 1999 WHO Study Group Report[13].

However, data from population-based studies show that symptoms of hyper-glycaemia (such as thirst and polyuria) have a poor sensitivity and specificity for diabetes[48]. Therefore, it is not recommended that symptoms form part of the screening process, although it remains good clinical practice to look for diabetes in someone presenting with typical symptoms of hyperglycaemia.

URINE GLUCOSE MEASUREMENT

Perhaps the first diagnostic test for diabetes was described in ancient China with the observation that ants were attracted to the urine of persons with diabetes. The London physician Thomas Willis (1621–1675) noted that diabetic urine tasted 'wondrous sweet' and in 1766 another Englishman, Matthew Dobson, demonstrated the chemical presence of sugar in diabetic urine and observed that serum from diabetics was sweet-tasting. By the 1840s, such chemical tests as Fehling's were developed for sugar in urine. Benedict's urine test was described in 1911 and for many decades remained the mainstay for assessing control of diabetes.

Urine glucose measurement, though cheap and convenient, has inadequate sensitivity[49], and therefore, for more accurate and reliable diagnostic tests the blood-based assessment of hyperglycaemia is relied upon. Evidence concern-ing the sensitivity and specificity of non-blood tests is considered in full in Chapter 8 on screening.

BLOOD-BASED ASSESSMENT OF HYPERGLYCAEMIA

Random blood glucose

Few studies have examined the properties of random blood glucose (measured by reflectance meter in both studies) in relation to other means of diabetes testing (Table 2.4). In these two studies an OGTT was performed in the whole population irrespective of the random glucose value obtained. In order to achieve a sensitivity of 80–90%, the specificity of a random glucose determina-tion seems to be significantly lower than that of fasting glucose. Furthermore, WHO 1985 criteria (in which the fasting plasma threshold was 7.8 mmol/l) were used as the gold standard in both studies, but if current criteria were applied, performance of the test is likely to be slightly worse. People who are diabetic only on the new, lower fasting value (and who have a non-diabetic 2 h value) are more likely to have normal random blood glucose values.

Blood glucose meters and whole blood glucose determination

Blood glucose meters have often been used as part of screening programmes for diabetes. However, the precision of these meters is limited, and it is

Table 2.4. The performance of a random whole blood glucose determination in comparison to an OGTT.

Engelgau *et al.*[50]

At sensitivity of 90%*:	Median specificity 48–52% (according to age group)
At specificity of 90%:	Median sensitivity 49–52%
Optimal:	Median sensitivity 73–76%
Median specificity 76–78%	

Qiao *et al.*[51]

Cut-off 5.8 mmol/l	Sensitivity 63%, specificity 85%**
Cut-off 5.2 mmol/l	Sensitivity 78%, specificity 62%**

*The cut-off value of random whole blood glucose for a sensitivity of 90% was 4.4-6.7, depending on age and post-prandial period.
**Sensitivities and specificities were worse in women than men at all thresholds.

generally recommended that the diagnosis of diabetes is made on laboratory measurements of glucose. Even for the initial screening test, laboratory testing is preferred, and meters should only be considered if they are the only way of providing a screening service to a given population or individual. If meters are used, their imprecision, and the possibility of a false negative result, should be considered when interpreting the results. The accuracy of glucose results measured by glucose meters may be low, with only 35–83% of readings being within ±10% of the adjusted laboratory plasma glucose values[52,53]. The evidence on which the diagnostic thresholds are based comes from studies using laboratory plasma glucose measurements. The thresholds for other types of blood samples (e.g. whole blood in Table 2.1) equivalent to the threshold given for the plasma values have been calculated as being about 10% lower than in plasma. However, formal comparisons in large populations have not been published, and these values may not be as reliable as the plasma thresholds.

ORAL GLUCOSE TOLERANCE TEST

The oral glucose tolerance test (OGTT) has for many years been the accepted standard for the diagnosis of diabetes. It is, however, time consuming and inconvenient requiring considerable preparation. Many would therefore regard it as unsuitable for widespread use among people with risk factors for diabetes. Unless conducted in the inpatient setting, the recent dietary intake and duration of the pre-test fast cannot be standardised in the way the protocol demands, and these factors can affect the results[54,55]. Paired OGTTs performed two to six weeks apart have shown that among people who are diagnosed as having diabetes in an initial OGTT, 95% of values in the second OGTT lie within ±20% of the initial fasting glucose and ±36% of the initial 2 h glucose[56].

It is recommended that the OGTT should be administered in the morning after at least three days of unrestricted diet (greater than 150 g of carbohydrate daily) and usual physical activity. A reasonable carbohydrate containing meal (30–50 g) should be consumed on the evening before the test. The test should be preceded by an overnight fast of 8–14 hours, during which water may be drunk. Smoking should not be permitted during the test. The presence of factors that influence interpretation of the results of the test should be recorded (e.g. medications, inactivity, infection, etc.).

There is also little published evidence supporting the appropriate glucose amount. These are currently 75 g anhydrose glucose for adults and 1.75 g of glucose per kg body weight, up to a total of 75 g of glucose for children. The origin of these recommendations is a mid-Atlantic compromise between the 50 g and 100 g used in Europe and the USA before international standardisation. When glucose monohydrate is used, the corresponding amount is 82.5 g, which may give rise to confusion and another potential source of measurement error.

Fasting blood glucose measurement

The ADA Expert Committee recommended using the fasting glucose alone as a diagnostic criterion, thus simplifying fieldwork and reducing the burden on participants. The WHO, by contrast, recommended retention of the OGTT.

A new intermediate group of individuals whose glucose levels, although not meeting criteria for diabetes, are too high to be considered normal was established based on fasting blood glucose measurement and called impaired fasting glucose. Although this is conceptually similar to the definition of IGT based on intermediate 2 h PG values, the thresholds chosen were not selected to be comparable along the considerations underlying the agreement on the diagnostic FPG threshold for diabetes (see above). Table 2.1 shows that the range of glucose values between the lower and upper 2 h cut-offs for IGT is constant across the different biological specimen categories at 3.3 mmol/l. However, the range for the fasting glucose cut-points for IFG is 0.9 mmol/l in plasma and 0.5 mmol/l in whole blood. As the definition of IGT is broader, it is likely that IGT will identify more people as having impaired glucose homeostasis than IFG.

When both tests, FPG and 2 h PG, are applied on the same individual a 3×3 table emerges to classify their glucose intolerance status (Table 2.5).

Fasting versus oral glucose tolerance testing

The ADA diabetes classification document has received a lot of attention, with its recommendations to perform diabetes diagnosis generally with fasting plasma glucose alone. This was a deviation from the 1985 WHO recommendations and not completely followed by the new WHO statement which supported the retention of the OGTT unless circumstances prevented it from being performed. Furthermore, the WHO retained the recommendation for epidemiological studies to restrict diabetes screening to the 2 h post-OGTT value in situations where the fasting state of the participants cannot be assured.

In a situation of partial overlap of the distributions of fasting and 2 h diabetes values in a population, any algorithm utilising several tests in parallel (such as scoring individuals using their fasting and 2 h glucose values for classification by whichever meets the diabetes criterion) will yield increased numbers. Table 2.5 shows how different criteria used together would classify patients with different blood glucose levels, and how changing thresholds would affect glucose intolerance groups.

There is complete agreement in classifying individuals at either extreme of the glucose distribution (the grey shaded areas in Table 2.5). However, for individuals with a FPG between 6.1 and 7.8 mmol/l and a 2 h glucose between 7.8 and 11.1 mmol/l, how they are classified depends on the criteria used. This discordance between the classification systems means that if either criterion was used alone, it would inevitably identify different groups of individuals. This will also impact on incidence and prevalence rates. A number of recent studies have shown that using FPG would result in the misclassification of a significant proportion of people with diabetes (when defined according to the 2 h level)[57–67]. It is likely that all these people are at risk of diabetes-related complications; in other words they can be considered as being genuinely diabetic and therefore the OGTT may be necessary to exclude diabetes in anyone with a positive screening blood test. Approximately 35% of all people with newly diagnosed diabetes still have a normal fasting glucose, whereas 15–20% have a normal 2 h value. This distribution differs between men and women, with women being more commonly diagnosed on the basis of the 2 h glucose level[68]. This is also

Table 2.5. Diagnostic category of individuals with different glucose cut-off levels according to WHO (1985), ADA (1997) and WHO (1998) classification criteria.

		2 h plasma glucose (mmol/l)		
		<7.8	7.8–11.1	≥11.1
Fasting plasma glucose (mmol/l)	<6.1	N N N	IGT IGT IGT	D D D
	6.1–7.0	N IFG IFG	IGT IFG + IGT IFG + IGT	D D D
	7.0–7.8	N D D	IGT D D	D D D
	≥7.8	D D D	D D D	D D D

reflected in the observation that IGT seems to occur more often in women than elevated but not yet diabetic fasting glucose levels (IFG), which was seen more frequently in men in the Finnish study of the Botnia population[69].

HbA$_{1c}$ as a diagnostic test

Glycosylated haemoglobin (HbA$_{1c}$) is attractive both as a screening and diagnostic test, because it is simple, requires no preparation of the patient, and directly relates to treatment targets. Furthermore, its relationship to retinopathy in population studies is as close as that of fasting or 2 h post-load blood glucose[23]. In addition, data from a large prospective population study identified HbA$_{1c}$ as a good predictor of excess mortality observed in diabetic men and as a continuously distributed risk factor through the whole male study population[70].

Cross-sectional comparisons of HbA$_{1c}$ values as indicators of long-term hyperglycaemia with 2hPG are always limited by which is chosen in the comparison as the standard[27].

Both the ADA and WHO suggested that HbA$_{1c}$ should not be used for the diagnosis of diabetes at this stage, although some studies have shown that the frequency distributions for HbA$_{1c}$ have characteristics similar to those of the FPG and the 2 h PG. Also in these studies the likelihood of having or developing microvascular disease rises sharply with increasing HbA$_{1c}$ levels, making it possible to identify a threshold level. Furthermore, in type 2 diabetes HbA$_{1c}$ is increasingly the measurement of choice in monitoring treatment, and decisions on when and how to implement therapy are often made on the basis of HbA$_{1c}$. These observations have led some experts to recommend HbA$_{1c}$ measurement as a diagnostic test[71] and the Japanese Diabetes Association has already included HbA$_{1c}$ in its diagnostic classification.

However, the measurement of HbA$_{1c}$ is not yet standardised around the world, and so it is not currently possible to produce diagnostic thresholds that would be valid in all laboratories.

Importance of reliable diabetes tests

The impact of a diagnosis of diabetes on an individual can be dramatic. Once this chronic disease is diagnosed, significant behavioural changes are often recommended which can impact not only on the person with diabetes but also on those who live with them. The ability to gain approval for health insurance and employment in some societies may be affected. The psychological burden associated with the diagnosis of a chronic disease for which a cure has not yet been satisfactorily developed may be significant. Given the implications of diagnosis, if a single set of diagnostic criteria is to be employed internationally the diagnostic cut-off values should be highly specific or identify as few false positives as possible. The difficulty then is that among those individuals who are more vulnerable to complications the criteria would have low sensitivity (ability to identify true cases) and therefore may not offer an acceptable level of clinical care. Of course, in an ideal world a diagnostic test would be both highly sensitive and specific, but in diabetes this is not the case. Most clinical tests identify those who are clearly positive or negative and some that appear in between the two, thus making the selection of a diagnostic cut-off value an arbitrary decision. If a value is chosen that identifies as many true cases as possible there will also be an increase in the number of false positives, and vice versa. The pertinence of any chosen diagnostic cut-off value is therefore related to the reliability and validity of the diagnostic test.

CONCLUSIONS

Diabetes mellitus is a complex of diseases sharing raised blood glucose levels that lead to short- and long-term complications.

The causative factors for diabetes are diverse and range from infections to single-gene defects with complex environmental and biological interactions probably predominant.

Scientific progress and better understanding of diabetes had led to a classification expanding from describing a single disease state to distinguishing at least four different types of diabetes mellitus. This number of overall sub-types may not be expanded in future because the classification allows newly described specific types of diabetes with a distinct aetiology to be moved out of the type 2 class (a largely aetiologically insufficiently understood class of DM) to type 3 (other specific types).

The classification of diabetes into different types is driven by differing needs, including aetiological research and clinical practice. The old descriptive age-of-onset classes gave way to a treatment-related classification, which has in turn been superseeded by a system based on aetiology. Type 4 diabetes (Gestational Diabetes Mellitus) is still the exception, as the basis for classification is the common context rather than aetiology.

The diagnostic criteria for diabetes are based on the common characteristic of hyperglycaemia. Achievements in accuracy and methodological standardisation of internationally accepted testing procedures have resulted in the widespread application of two diagnostic tests; fasting blood glucose determination and measurement of blood glucose two hours after an oral glucose tolerance test. In the near future, a third marker of hyperglycaemia, HbA_{1c}, is likely to be added to this list.

The acceptance of a diagnostic standard across the various aetiologic sub-types of DM has resulted in considerable progress in describing the epidemiology of diabetes. With improved characterisations of diabetic phenotypes across many populations and sub-groups (such as the elderly), it is apparent that the threshold distinguishing normal and abnormal blood glucose levels may not be universal. If this observation is correct, it is a major challenge to diagnostic uniformity, and several important diabetes studies have already elected to apply their own criteria in parallel with standard international ones[72].

REFERENCES

1. Major RM (1954) *A History of Medicine*. Oxford: Blackwell . p. 67.
2. Zimmet P (1997) The challenge of diabetes – diagnosis, classification, 'Coca-colonization', and the diabetes epidemic. In Fischer EP, Moller G (eds) *The Medical Challenge Complex Traits*. Munchen: Piper, pp. 55-110.
3. Himsworth HP (1936) Diabetes mellitus: its differentiation into insulin-sensitive and insulin-insensitive types. *Lancet* **1**: 117–20.
4. Bornstein J, Lawrence RD (1951) Plasma insulin in human diabetes mellitus. *Br. Med. J.* **2**: 1541–4.
5. National Diabetes Data Group (1979) Classification and diagnosis of diabetes mellitus and other categories of glucose intolerance. *Diabetes* **28**: 1039–57.
6. World Health Organization (1980) Expert Committee on Diabetes Mellitus, Second Report. Geneva: WHO.
7. World Health Organization (1985) Diabetes Mellitus: Report of a WHO Study Group. Technical Report Series No. 727. Geneva: WHO.
8. King H, Rewers M (1993) Global estimates for prevalence of diabetes mellitus and impaired glucose tolerance in adults. *Diabetes Care* **16**: 157–177.
9. Abourizk N, Dunn J (1990) Types of diabetes according to National Diabetes Data Group Classification. Limited applicability and need to revisit. *Diabetes Care* **13**: 1120–1123.
10. Turner R, Stratton I, Horton V, Manley S, Zimmet P, Mackay IR, Shattock M, Bottazzo GF, Holman R: UKPDS 25: autoantibodies to islet-cell cytoplasm and glutamic acid decarboxylase for prediction of insulin requirement in type 2 diabetes. UK Prospective Diabetes Study Group. *Lancet* **350**: 1288–1293.
11. Kuzuya T, Matsuda A (1997) Classification of diabetes on the basis of etiologies versus degree of insulin deficiency. *Diabetes Care* **20**: 219–220.
12. Alberti KGMM, Zimmet PZ for the WHO Consultation (1998) Definition, diagnosis and classification of diabetes mellitus and its complications. Part 1: Diagnosis and classification of diabetes mellitus. Provisional report of a WHO Consultation. *Diab. Med.* **15**: 539–553.
13. World Health Organization (1999) Definition, Diagnosis and Classification of Diabetes Mellitus and its Complications – Part 1: Diagnosis and Classification of Diabetes Mellitus. Geneva: WHO.
14. American Diabetes Association (1997) Report of the expert committee on the diagnosis and classification of diabetes mellitus. *Diabetes Care* **20**: 1183–1197.
15. Charles MA, Fontbonne A, Thibult N, Warnet JM, Rosselin GE, Eschwege E (1991) Risk factors for NIDDM in white population: Paris Prospective Study. *Diabetes* **40**: 796–799
16. Raper LR, Balkau B, Taylor R, Milne B, Collins V, Zimmet P (1983) Plasma glucose distributions in two pacific populations: the bimodality phenomenon. *Tohoku. J. Exp. Med.* **141 Suppl**: 199–206.

17. Flock EV, Bennett PH, Savage PJ, Webner CJ, Howard BV, Rushforth NB, Miller M (1979) Bimodality of glycosylated hemoglobin distribution in Pima Indians: relationship to fasting hyperglycemia. *Diabetes* **28**: 984–989.

18. Zimmet P, Whitehouse S (1978) Bimodality of fasting and two–hour glucose tolerance distributions in a Micronesian population. *Diabetes* **27**: 793–800.

19. Rushforth NB, Miller M, Bennett PH (1979) Fasting and two-hour post-load glucose levels for the diagnosis of diabetes. The relationship between glucose levels and complications of diabetes in the Pima Indians. *Diabetologia* **16**: 373–379.

20. Friedlander Y, Kark JD, Kidron M, Bar-On H (1995) Univariate and bivariate admixture analyses of serum glucose and glycated hemoglobin distributions in a Jerusalem population sample. *Hum Biol.* **67**: 151–170.

21. Cohen P, Dix D (1984) The oral glucose tolerance test: an objective method of interpretation. *Acta Diabetol. Lat.* **21**: 181–189.

22. Omar MA, Seedat MA, Dyer RB, Motala AA, Knight LT, Becker PJ (1994) South African Indians show a high prevalence of NIDDM and bimodality in plasma glucose distribution patterns. *Diabetes Care* **17**: 70–73

23. McCance DR, Hanson RL, Charles M, Jacobsson LTH, Pettitt DJ, Bennett PH, Knowler WC (1994) Comparison of test for glycated haemoglobin and fasting and two hour plasma glucose concentrations as diagnostic methods for diabetes. *British Medical Journal* **308**: 1323–1328

24. Zimmet P, Whitehouse S (1978) Bimodality of fasting and two-hour glucose tolerance distributions in a Micronesian population. *Diabetes* **27**: 793–800

25. Raper LR, Taylor R, Zimmet P, Milne B, Balkau B (1984) Bimodality in glucose tolerance distributions in the urban polynesian population of Western Samoa. *Diab. Res.* **1**: 19–26

26. Rosenthal M, McMahan CA, Stern MP, Eifler CW, Haffner SM, Hazuda HP, Franco LJ (1985) Evidence of bimodality of two hour plasma glucose concentrations in Mexican Americans: Results from the San Antonio heart study. *J. Chron. Dis.* **38**: 5–16.

27. Engelgau MM, Thompson TJ, Herman WH, Boyle JP, Aubert RE, Kenny SJ, Badran A, Sous ES, Ali MA (1997) Comparison of fasting and 2-hour glucose and HbA$_{1c}$ levels for diagnosing diabetes. *Diab. Care* **20**: 785–791

28. Loo SG, Dowse GK, Finch C, Zimmet P (1993) Bimodality analysis of frequency distributions of 2-hour plasma glucose concentrations in the urban micronesian population of Kiribati. *Journal of Diabetes and Its Complications* **7**: 73–80

29. Dowse GK, Spark RA, Mavo B, Hodge AM, Erasmus RT, Gwalimu M, Knight LT, Koki G, Zimmet PZ (1994) Extraordinary prevalence of non-insulin-dependent diabetes mellitus and bimodal plasma glucose distribution in the Wanigela people of Papua New Guinea. *Med. J. Aust.* **160**: 767–774

30. Collins V, Dowse G, Finch C, Zimmet P, Linnane A (1989) Prevalence and risk factors for micro- and macroalbuminuria in diabetic subjects and entire population of Nauru. *Diabetes* **38**: 1602–1610.

31. Collins V, Dowse G, Plehwe W, Imo T, Toelupe P, Taylor H, Zimmet P (1995) High prevalence of diabetic retinopathy and nephropathy in Polynesians of Western Samoa. *Diabetes Care* **18**: 1140-1149.

32. Smith PJ, Thompson TJ, Engelgau MM, Herman WH (1996) A generalized linear model for analysing receiver operating characteristic curves. *Stat. Med.* **15**: 323–333. (published erratum appears in *Stat. Med.* (1997) **16**: 1299)

33. DECODE Study Group on behalf of the European Diabetes Epidemiology Study Group (1998) Will new diagnostic criteria for diabetes mellitus change phenotype

of patients with diabetes? Reanalysis of European epidemiological data. *Brit. Med. J.* **317**: 371–375.

34. The DECODE study group. European Diabetes Epidemiology Group (1999) Is fasting glucose sufficient to define diabetes? Epidemiological data from 20 European studies. Diabetes Epidemiology: Collaborative analysis of Diagnostic Criteria in Europe. *Diabetologia* **42**: 647–654.

35. The DECODE study group. European Diabetes Epidemiology Group (1999) Consequences of the new diagnostic criteria for diabetes in older men and women. DECODE Study (Diabetes Epidemiology: Collaborative Analysis of Diagnostic Criteria in Europe). *Diabetes Care* **22**: 1667–1671.

36. Harris MI, Hadden WC, Knowler WC, Bennett PH (1987) Prevalence of diabetes and impaired glucose tolerance and plasma glucose levels in the US population aged 20–74 yr. *Diabetes* **36**: 523–534.

37. Knowler W, Bennett P, Hamman R, Miller M (1978) Diabetes incidence and prevalence in Pima Indians: A 19-fold greater incidence than in Rochester, Minnesota. *Am. J. Epidemiol.* **108**: 497–504.

38. Knowler W, Pettitt D, Saad M, Bennett P (1990) Diabetes mellitus in the Pima Indians: incidence, risk factors and pathogenesis. *Diab. Metabol. Rev.* **6**: 1-27.

39. Rushforth N, Bennett P, Steinberg A, Burch T, Miller M (1971) Diabetes in the Pima Indians. Evidence of bimodality in glucose tolerance distributions. *Diabetes* **20**: 756–765.

40. Fuller JH, Shipley MJ, Rose G, Jarrett RJ, Keen H (1980) Coronary heart disease risk and impaired glucose tolerance: the Whitehall Study. *Lancet* **i**: 1373-1376

41. Harris MI, Zimmet P (1992) Classification of diabetes mellitus and other catergories of glucose intolerance. In Alberti K, DeFronzo RA, Keen H, Zimmet P (eds) *International Textbook of Diabetes Mellitus*. John Wiley & Sons, pp. 3–18.

42. Harris MI (1989) Impaired glucose tolerance in the US population. *Diabetes Care* **12**: 464–474.

43. Harris M, Zimmet P (1997) Classification of diabetes mellitus and other categories of glucose intolerance. In Alberti K, Zimmet P, DeFronzo R, Keen H (eds) *International Textbook of Diabetes Mellitus – Second Edition*. Chichester: John Wiley and Sons, pp. 9–23.

44. Alberti K (1996) Impaired glucose tolerance – Fact or fiction. *Diab. Med.* **13**: 6–8.

45. Edelstein S, Knowler W, Bain R, Andres R, Barrett-Connor E, Dowse G, Haffner S, Muller D, Collins V (1997) Predictors of progression from impaired glucose tolerance to NIDDM: An analysis of six prospective studies. *Diabetes* **46**: 701–10.

46. Charles M, Fontbonne A, Thibult N, Warnet J-M, Rosselin G, Eschwege E (1991) Risk factors for NIDDM in white population. Paris Prospective Study. *Diabetes* **40**: 796–799.

47. Shaw J, Zimmet P, de Courten M, et al. Impaired fasting glucose or impaired glucose tolerance. What best predicts future diabetes in Mauritius? *Diabetes Care* **22**: 399–402.

48. Welborn TA, Reid CM, Marriott G (1997) Australian diabetes screening study: impaired glucose tolerance and non-insulin-dependent diabetes mellitus. *Metabolism* **46 (Suppl 1)**: 35–9.

49. Davies MJ, Williams DR, Metcalfe J, Day JL (1993) Community screening for non-insulin-dependent diabetes mellitus: self-testing for post-prandial glycosuria. *Q. J. Med.* **86**: 677–84.

50. Engelgau MM, Thompson TJ, Smith PJ, Herman WH, Aubert RE, Gunter EW, Wetterhall SF, Sous ES, Ali MA (1995) Screening for diabetes mellitus in adults. The utility of random capillary blood glucose measurements. *Diabetes Care* **18**: 463–466

51. Qiao Q, Keinanen-Kiukaanniemi S, Rajala U, Uusimaki A, Kivela SL (1995) Random capillary whole blood glucose test as a screening test for diabetes mellitus in a middle-aged population. *Scand. J. Clin. Lab. Invest.* **55**: 3–8.
52. Chan JC, Wong RY, Cheung CK, Lam P, Chow CC, Yeung VT, Kan EC, Loo KM, Mong MY, Cockram CS (1997) Accuracy, precision and user-acceptability of self blood glucose monitoring machines. *Diabetes Res. Clin. Pract.* **36**: 91-104.
53. Poirier JY, Le Prieur N, Campion L, Guilhem I, Allannic H, Maugendre D (1998) Clinical and statistical evaluation of self-monitoring blood glucose meters. *Diabetes Care* **21**: 1919–24.
54. Kanan W, Bijlani RL, Sachdeva U, Mahapatra SC, Shah P, Karmarkar MG (1998) Glycaemic and isulinaemic responses to natural foods, frozen foods and their laboratory equivalents. *Indian J. Physiol. Pharmacol.* **42**: 81–89
55. Sermer M, Maylor CD, Gare DJ, Kenshole AB, Ritchie JW, Farine D, Cohen HR, McArthur K, Holzapfel S, Biringer A (1994) Impact of time since last meal on the gestational glucose challenge test. The Toronto Tri-Hospital Gestational Diabetes Project. *Am. J. Obstet. Gynecol.* **171**: 607–616
56. Mooy JM, Gootenhuis PA, de Vries H, Kostense PJ, Popp-Snijders C, Bouter LM, Heine RJ (1996) Intra-individual variation of glucose, specific insulin and proinsulin concentrations measured by two oral glucose tolerance tests in general Caucasian population: The Hoorn Study. *Diabetologia* **39**: 298–305.
57. Harris MI, Eastman RC, Cowie CC, Flegal KM, Eberhardt MS (1997) Comparison of diabetes diagnostic categories in the US population according to 1997 American Diabetes Association and 1980–85 World Health Organisation diagnostic criteria. *Diabetes Care* **20**: 1859–1862.
58. de Vegt F, Dekker JM, Stehouwer CD, Nijpels G, Bouter LM, Heine RJ (1998) The 1997 American Diabetes Association criteria versus the 1985 World Health Organization criteria for the diagnosis of abnormal glucose tolerance: poor agreement in the Hoorn Study. *Diabetes Care* **21**: 1686-90.
59. Wahl PW, Savage PJ, Psaty BM, Orchard TJ, Robbins JA, Tracy RP (1998) Diabetes in older adults: comparison of 1997 American Diabetes Association classification of diabetes mellitus with 1985 WHO classification. *Lancet* **352**: 1012–1015.
60. Chang CJ, Wui JS, Lu FH, Lee HL, Yang YC, Wen MJ (1998) Fasting plasma glucose in screening for diabetes in the Taiwanese population. *Diabetes Care* **21**: 1856–1860.
61. Gimeno SG, Ferreira SR, Franco LJ, Iunes M (1998) Comparison of glucose tolerance categories according to World Health Organization and American Diabetes Association diagnostic criteria in a population-based study in Brazil. The Japanese–Brazilian Diabetes Study Group. *Diabetes Care* **21**: 1889–92.
62. Shaw JE, Zimmet PZ, de Courten M, Dowse GK, Chitson P, Gareeboo H, Hemraj F, Fareeed D, Tuomilehto J, Alberti K (1999) Impaired fasting glucose or impaired glucose tolerance: what best predicts future diabetes? *Diabetes Care* **22**: 399–402.
63. Wiener K, Roberts NB: The relative merits of haemoglobin A_{1c} and fasting plasma glucose as first-line diagnostic tests for diabetes mellitus in non-pregnant subjects. *Diab. Med.* **15**: 558–563.
64. Gomez-Perez FJ, Aguilar-Salinas CA, Lopez-Alvarenga JC, Perez-Jauregui J, Guillen-Pineda LE, Rull JA (1998) Lack of agreement between the World Health Organisation category of impaired glucose tolerance and the American Diabetes Association category of impaired fasting glucose. *Diabetes Care* **21**: 1886–1888.
65. Balkau B, Eschwege E, Tichet J, Marre M, DESIR Study Group (1997) Proposed criteria for the diagnosis of diabetes: Evidence from a French epidemiological study (DESIR). *Diabetes & Metabolism* **23**: 428–434.

66. Cordido F, Muniz J, Rodriguez IL, Beiras AC (1999) New diagnostic criteria for diabetes and mortality in older adults. *Lancet* **353**: 69–70.
67. Ko, GTC, Woo J, Chan JCN, Cockram CS (1998) Use of the 1997 American Diabetes Association diagnostic criteria for diabetes in a Hong Kong chinese population. *Diabetes Care* **21**: 2094–2097
68. Williams J, Zimmet P, de Courten M, Shaw J, Chitson P, Tuomilehto J, Alberti G (in press) Gender differences in impaired fasting glycaemia and impaired glucose tolerance. Does sex matter? *Diabetes Care*.
69. Tripathy D, Carlsson M, Almgren P, Isomaa B, Taskinen M, Tuomi T, Groop L (2000) Insulin secretion and insulin sensitivity in relation to glucose tolerance: lessons from the Botnia study. *Diabetes* **49**: 975–980
70. Khaw KT, Wareham N, Luben R, Bingham S, Oakes S, Welch A, Day N (2001) Glycated haemoglobin, diabetes, and mortality in men in Norfolk cohort of european prospective investigation of cancer and nutrition (EPIC-Norfolk). *British Medical Journal* **322**: 15–18.
71. Peters AL, Davidson MB, Schriger DL, Hasselblad V, the Meta-analysis Research Group on the Diagnosis of Diabetes Using Glycated Hemoglobin Levels (1996) A clinical approach for the diagnosis of diabetes mellitus: an analysis using glycated hemoglobin levels. *JAMA* **276**: 1246–1252
72. UK Prospective Diabetes Study (UKPDS) Group (1998) Intensive blood-glucose control with sulphonylureas or insulin compared with conventional treatment and risk of complications in patients with type 2 diabetes (UKPDS 33). *Lancet* **352**: 837–853.

3

Evidence-based Definition and Classification: A Commentary

STEVE O'RAHILLY

Addenbrooke's Hospital, Cambridge CB2 2QQ, UK

DIABETES CLASSIFICATION: BEYOND STAMP COLLECTING

Humans appear to have a powerful instinct to classify. In part this may spring from a purely intellectual and aesthetic requirement to create some sort of order from the bewildering chaos of observable natural phenomena. This inbuilt taxonomic imperative is likely, however, to have more utilitarian roots. To be able to manipulate the natural world to improves one's comfort and/or survival, one needs to understand its nature. The classification of natural phenomena into related groups is an essential first step towards this compre- hension. Given the powerful threat represented by illness, it is not surprising that the classification and reclassification of disease has been a continued obsession of the healing professions since their earliest recorded history. In Chapter 2, Max de Courten provides a balanced and thorough account of how we have reached the currently accepted glycaemic criteria for the *diagnosis* of diabetes mellitus, and its *classification* into sub-types. In this short comment- ary I will concentrate entirely on the latter concept. In fact, I believe that the two terms italicised above are, in essence, tautologous. I would argue that the term *definition* is more appropriate for what is in essence a committee's prag- matic choice of a point on a glycaemic continuum, and that we should reserve the term *diagnosis* for occasions when we have more insight into the nature of a particular disease process.

WHAT IS THE PURPOSE OF CLASSIFICATION IN DIABETES?

To the practising clinician, the ability to classify a sub-type of diabetes is relevant if it provides information regarding the likely natural history of disease

The Evidence Base for Diabetes Care. Edited by R. Williams, W. Herman, A.-L. Kinmonth and N. J. Wareham.
© 2002 John Wiley & Sons, Ltd

and/or its response to therapy which is more accurate than if that distinction had not been made. To the diabetes researcher, accurate classification is essential, as discovering the aetiological factors for a type of diabetes will be much more difficult if we have, through our ignorance, inadvertently lumped together several conditions that have substantially different aetiologies. Currently, the most telling examples of the clinical importance of such distinctions are provided by conditions listed under the 'other specific types' heading in the current WHO/ADA classification. Individually, these conditions are not common but, together, they may represent perhaps 5% of any diabetic clinic population, and are therefore directly relevant to millions of people worldwide. Thus, there are now compelling clinical reasons for clinicians, once they have defined someone as having diabetes mellitus, to do their best to try and make a diagnosis (or classify, if you prefer). The clinical reasons for doing so include the following:

1. *Better prediction of the rate of progression of metabolic abnormality.* Patients with glucokinase deficient diabetes (MODY2) tend to have very stable modest levels of hyperglycaemia throughout life[1] and, if this disorder is unrecognised, may be inappropriately treated with insulin for prolonged periods. Other forms of MODY associated with HNF mutations, in contrast, lead to progressive beta cell failure and the need for insulin treatment[2]. The label of MODY, however, if given to a patient in whom type 1 diabetes is detected before complete insulinopaenia has occurred, can be highly dangerous.

2. *Associated organ dysfunction directly resulting from the aetiological agent.* In many of the 'specific types' of diabetes the aetiological agent/s, be they genetic or environmental, will often have direct deleterious effects on other organs and or systems. These can result in serious unrecognised morbidity unless their presence is actively sought, or they can be inappropriately dismissed as somehow 'secondary' to the diabetic state.

The best-recognised examples are the hepatic dysfunction, arthritis and hypogonadism of haemochromatosis and the exocrine pancreatic failure and malabsorption of chronic pancreatitis. Patients whose diabetes results from a primary disorder of insulin action commonly have severe polycystic ovarian syndrome and the skin lesion acanthosis nigricans[3]. Patients with partial lipodystrophy may go unrecognised for prolonged periods and often have severe hypertriglyceridaemia[4]. Mitochondrial diabetes may be accompanied by undiagnosed sensorineural deafness, and other endocrine dysfunctions such as hypothyroidism and hypoparathyroidism can be present[5]. Patients with HNF1b mutations frequently have renal dysfunction that is unrelated to diabetic nephropathy[6].

3. *Increased risk of associated diseases.* The best example of this is type 1 diabetes where the immunogenetic background of patients renders them susceptible to the development of other organ-specific autoimmune disorders such as hypothyroidism, coeliac disease, pernicious anaemia etc. Knowledge

that a specific subset of diabetic patients has a particularly increased risk of these other diseases could allow screening programmes for these conditions to be better targeted.

4. *Response to therapy.* A powerful argument of the 'diagnostic nihilist' is that, irrespective of the cause of diabetes, we have only a limited range of antihyperglycaemic therapies and we have done a pretty good job by trying these empirically in our patients. To a large extent this remains true, but a broader range of treatments is likely to become available in future. There are already examples of situations where specific sub-types of diabetes have particular responses to certain drugs. Thus, recent evidence suggests that patients with HNF4a mutations (MODY3) are hypersensitive to the effects of sulphonylureas and may develop severe hypoglycaemia in response to them[7]. Patients with some lipodystrophic forms of diabetes may benefit from thiazolidinediones, and leptin also appears to be a promising agent for these subjects[8].

5. *Risks to family members.* Patients with diabetes frequently ask about risks to family members. If a specific genetic sub-type is diagnosed, then precise risk estimates can be given, and screening applied where appropriate.

HOW WILL THIS ULTIMATELY APPLY TO COMMONER FORMS OF DIABETES?

TYPE 2 DIABETES

Representing as it does the majority of people with diabetes worldwide, type 2 diabetes is unfortunately the least satisfactory of the classifications. This reflects the fact that there are likely to be many aetiological and pathophysiological routes to developing a condition of sustained, survivable hyperglycaemia. How are we likely to make progress in further dissecting this large group into clinically relevant aetiological subgroups?

1. *Further definition of specific types.* It is possible that, lurking among the type 2 diabetic population, are a number of as yet unrecognised single-gene syndromes. As the genetic effort to identify such monogenic diseases intensifies, some such conditions will emerge[9]. While they may be important, they are unlikely to represent a large proportion of people with what we currently call type 2 diabetes.

2. *Classification on pathophysiology.* As we gain more insight into the pathophysiological features of type 2 diabetes, we may achieve a meaningful definition of sub-phenotypes that may prove useful. For many years researchers have sub-grouped subjects into those predominantly characterised by insulin secretory dysfunction versus those with insulin resistance. This will continue to be useful but, unfortunately, interpretation is often difficult because of the

effect that disease progression, whatever its initial aetiology, has on beta-cell function. Newer insights into sub-phenotypes may come from new technology, e.g. measurement of intramyocellular triacylglycerol[10], serum adiponectin[11] etc.

3. *Role for polygenic determinants.* The great promise of polygenics has yet to be fulfilled. However, there are signs of life. Thus, a frameshift mutation in an immune signalling protein, NOD2, has recently been found in ~6% of patients with Crohn's disease versus ~2% of controls[12]. Presumably such subjects will now be studied intensively for differences in their natural history and response to treatment compared to Crohn's patients who do not have this mutation. An intronic polymorphism in the calpain 10 gene has been hailed as the first type 2 diabetes polygene[13]. However, the situation is complex, with inconsistent findings in other studies[14] and no clear mechanism of action as yet being defined. A common polymorphism in PPARγ appears to reduce the risk of type 2 diabetes[15]. The search is continuing and more polymorphic variants contributing susceptibility to type 2 diabetes will undoubtedly be found.

4. *Gene–environment interaction.* The role of non-genetic effects in producing type 2 diabetes should not be underestimated. Undoubtedly, dietary factors and physical inactivity play a role[16]. There is increasing realisation that they will interact with particular genotypes. Thus we have recently demonstrated an interaction between dietary fat type and the common PPARγ polymorphism with the beneficial effects of a high unsaturated/saturated fat intake in terms of adiposity and fasting insulin being confined to those with the PPARγ Ala12 genotype[17].

5. *Need for a multidimensional classification.* In the future, we may not simply be able to use a pithy, but meaningless, phrase to 'classify' a patient's diabetes. We may need to classify an individual according to the genotypes at particular loci and incorporate quantitative measure of risk factors such as diet and level of physical activity. This may be demanding but should lead to individualised therapy, not only with drugs but also with specific diet and exercise prescriptions.

TYPE 1 DIABETES

The relevance of further sub-classifying type 1 diabetes may appear less immediately apparent than for type 2. After all, once total beta-cell destruction has occurred then insulin replacement therapy will have to be used irrespective of the cause. However, certain genetic sub-types may be at much higher risk of other autoimmune diseases or complications, for example, and the identification of these at an early stage would be highly relevant. The real importance of sub-phenotyping in type 1 diabetes will be in the research effort to identify at risk and presymptomatic individuals and to intervene in their autoimmune process using therapies that are directed at their particular disease processes. This is still a long way off, but vigorous efforts are underway[18].

CONCLUSIONS

Diabetes mellitus is no more a diagnosis than is 'anaemia' or 'hypercalcaemia'. We are making considerable progress in the definition of the more readily identifiable sub-types of diabetes, and the immediate clinical relevance of defining these sub-types accurately is becoming clear. Making better sense of the disorders that we currently classify as type 1 and type 2 diabetes will be more challenging, but the recognition of phenotypic subtypes within these broad classifications will be an essential step toward the identification of aetiological factors, both genetic and environmental. Continued attempts to improve the classification of diabetes is more than a stamp-collecting exercise. Philately may get us somewhere.

REFERENCES

1. Owen K, Hattersley AT (2001) Maturity-onset diabetes of the young: from clinical description to molecular characterization. *Best Pract. Res. Clin. Endocrinol. Metab.* **15**: 309–23. Review.
2. Fajans SS, Bell GI, Polonsky KS (2001) Molecular mechanisms and clinical pathophysiology of maturity diabetes of the young. *N. Engl. J. Med.* **27 345**: 971–80. Review.
3. O'Rahilly S, Moller DE (1992) Insulin receptor mutations in syndromes of insulin resistance. *Clin. Endocrinol.* **36**: 121–132.
4. Jackson SN, Howlett TA, McNally PG, O'Rahilly S, Trembath RC (1997) Dunnigan–Kobberling Syndrome: an autosomal dominant form of partial lipodystrophy. *Q. J. Medicine* **90**: 27–36.
5. Barrett TG (2001) Mitochondrial diabetes, DIDMOAD and other inherited diabetic syndromes. *Best Pract. Res. Clin. Endocrinol. Metab.* **15**: 325–43. Review.
6. Pontoglio M (2000) Hepatocyte nuclear factor 1, a transcription factor at the crossroads of homeostasis. *J. Am. Soc. Nephrol.* **11 Suppl 16**: S140–3.
7. Pearson ER, Liddell WG, Shepherd M, Corrall RJ, Hattersley AT (2000) Sensitivity to sulphonylureas in patients with hepatocyte nuclear alpha gene mutations. Evidence for pharmacogenetics in diabetes. *Diabet. Med.* **17**: 543–5.
8. Arioglu E, Duncan-Morin J, Sebring N, Rother KI, Gottlieb N, Lieberman J. et al. (2000). Efficacy and safety of troglitazone in the treatment of lipodystrophy syndromes. *Ann. Intern. Med.* **133**: 263–74.
9. Barroso I, Gurnell M, Crowley VEF, Agostini M, Schwabe JW, Soos MA et al. (1999) Dominant-negative mutations in human PPARγ are associated with severe insulin resistance, diabetes mellitus and hypertension. *Nature* **402**: 880–3.
10. Szczepaniak LS, Babcock EE, Schick F, Dobbins RL, Garg A, Burns DK. McGarry JD, Stein DT (1999) Measurement of intracellular triglyceride stores by H spectroscopy: validation in vivo. *Am. J. Physiol.* **276**: E977–89.

11. Yamauchi T, Kamoni J, Waki H, Terauchi Y, Kubota N, Hara K et al. (2001) The fat-derived hormone adiponectin reverses insulin resistance associated with lipoatrophy and obesity. *Nat. Med.* **7**: 941–6.
12. Ogura Y, Bonen DK, Inohara N, Nicolae DL, Chen FF, Ramos R et al. A (2001) A frameshift mutation in NOD2 associated with susceptibility to Crohn's disease. *Nature* **411**: 603–6.
13. Horikawa Y, Oda N, Cox NJ, Li X, Orho-Melander M, Hara M et al. (2000) Genetic variation in the gene encoding calapin-10 is associated with diabetes mellitus. *Nat. Genet.* **26**: 163–75.
14. Evans JC, Frayling TM, Cassell PG, Saker PJ, Hitman GA, Walker M et al. (2001) Association of the calpain-10 gene with type 2 diabetes mellitus in the United Kingdom. *Am. J. Hum. Gen.* **69**: 544–52.
15. Alshuler D, Hirschorn JN, Klannemark M, Lindgren CM, Vohl MC, Nemesh J et al. (2000) The common PPAR gamma Pro12Ala polymorphism is associated with decreased risk of type 2 diabetes. *Nat. Genet.* **26**: 76–80.
16. Tuomilehto J, Lindstrom J, Eriksson JG, Valle TT, Hamalainen H, Ilanne-Parikka P et al. (2001) Prevention of type 2 diabetes mellitus by changes in lifestyle among subjects with impaired glucose tolerance. *N. Engl. J. Med.* **344**: 1 390–2.
17. Luan J, Browne PO, Harding A-H, Halsall DJ, O'Rahilly S, Chatterjee VKK, Wareham NJ (2001) Evidence for gene-nutrient interaction at the PPAR gamma locus. *Diabetes* **50**: 686–689.
18. Todd JA (1999) From genome to aetiology in a multifactorial disease, type 1 diabetes. *Bioessays* **21**: 164–74.

Part II

PREVENTION OF DIABETES

4

Prevention of Type 1 Diabetes

University of Miami, Florida 33136, USA

Type 1 diabetes is characterized by immune-mediated pancreatic islet ß-cell destruction, absolute insulin deficiency, and thus dependence on insulin therapy for the preservation of life[1]. The type 1 diabetes disease process involves (1) a genetic predisposition, conferred principally by 'diabetogenic' genes in the major histocompatibility complex (MHC) on the short arm of chromosome 6; (2) non-genetic (environmental) factors that appear to act as triggers in genetically susceptible people; and (3) activation of immune mechanisms targeted against pancreatic islet ß-cells. The initial immune response engenders secondary and tertiary responses which collectively result in impairment of ß-cell function, progressive destruction of ß-cells, and consequent development of type 1 diabetes. The process is insidious and may evolve over many years, with the overt expression of clinical symptoms becoming apparent only when most ß-cells have been destroyed. Yet, even at disease onset, 10–20% of ß-cells remain. Improvement in their function accounts for the 'honeymoon' period often seen during the first years after onset of type 1 diabetes.

Over the last two decades, much investigation has been directed at interdicting the type 1 diabetes disease process, both during the stage of evolution of the disease and at the time of disease onset[2–14]. The goal of intervention prior to disease onset is to arrest immune destruction and thus delay or prevent clinical disease. The goal of intervention at disease onset is to halt the destruction of ß-cells, perhaps allowing residual ß-cells to recover function, thus lessening the severity of clinical manifestations.

Studies aimed at delay or prevention of clinical type 1 diabetes are critically dependent on the ability to identify individuals at risk of the disease. Although family members of patients with type 1 diabetes have a 10- to 20-fold increased risk compared to the general population, amongst newly diagnosed patients with type 1 diabetes only 10–15% have a relative known to have the disease[15]. Thus, efforts have been directed at identifying potential risk markers both in

The Evidence Base for Diabetes Care. Edited by R. Williams, W. Herman, A.-L. Kinmonth and N. J. Wareham.
© 2002 John Wiley & Sons, Ltd

relatives and, to a lesser extent, in the general population. Because case finding is easier among relatives (due to their 10- to 20-fold increased risk), most intervention studies aimed at disease prevention have focused on relatives. All evidence suggests that the type 1 disease process is the same in sporadic non-familial cases[16,17] as it is in relatives[18,19].

Although studies in animal models have used degree of insulitis as a histo-pathological indicator of the type 1 diabetes disease process, histological studies in human beings are very limited[20]. Thus, ß-cell function (insulin secretion), measured by assessing C-peptide response (either basal or more likely, in response to a provocative challenge) has been used to evaluate interventions in new-onset type 1 diabetes[21], while the evolution from prediabetes to overt hyperglycemia has been used in trials prior to disease onset.

This chapter will review evidence concerning interventions designed to interdict the type 1 diabetes disease process. To facilitate the discussion, the evolution of the disease can be divided into a number of stages, depicted in Figure 4.1, through which individuals progress. Interruption of the sequence at any stage is likely to be important[13]. The stages are: (1) genetic susceptibility, modulated by genetic protection, identified by finding of susceptibility genes without dominant protective genes; (2) initiation of autoimmunity, presumably by an environmental trigger, with a cellular immune response leading to immune-mediated islet infiltration (insulitis), with the stage identified by the presence of circulating autoantibodies; (3) impairment of ß-cell function resulting in loss of first-phase insulin response (FPIR) during an intravenous

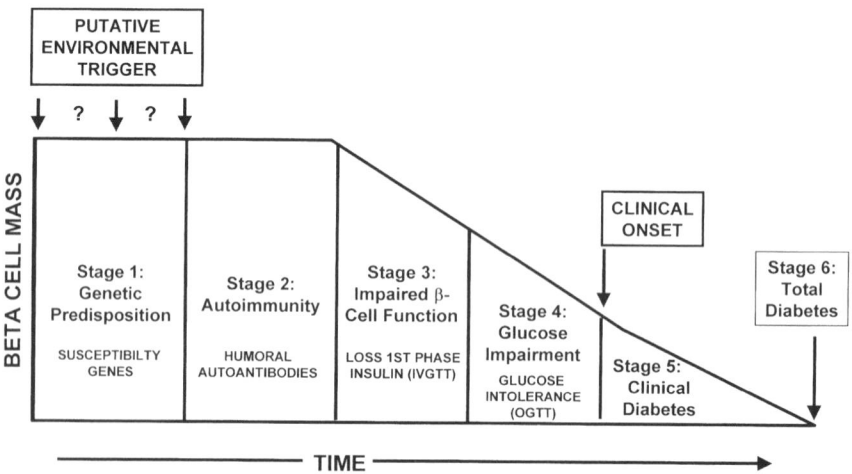

Figure 4.1.

glucose tolerance test (IVGTT); (4) impaired glucose tolerance (IGT) and/or impaired fasting glucose (IFG), but without overt diabetes; (5) clinical onset of type 1 diabetes; (6) 'total' diabetes with loss of all ß-cell function and mass (evidenced by lack of any C-peptide response to provocative challenge).

RISK IDENTIFICATION

The identification of individuals at risk of type 1 diabetes, the ability to predict disease development, is crucial for studies of disease prevention. In family members, testing for autoantibodies (i.e. identification at stage 2) is usually used, and in this circumstance genetic testing is of limited value. On the other hand, genetic testing may be useful for identifying individuals in the general population or in infant relatives for prospective follow-up for the appearance of autoantibodies or for recruitment into trials aimed at prevention of initiation of autoimmunity. Indeed, there are several studies underway involving screening of newborns or infants for genetic markers[22–26] with the goal of following these subjects (with or without intervention) for the appearance of autoimmunity. In addition, there are studies following offspring of diabetic parents for the appearance of autoimmunity[27].

GENETICS

About 40–50% of genetic predisposition to type 1 diabetes is conferred by genes on the short arm of chromosome 6, either within or in close proximity to the class II human leukocyte antigen (HLA) region of the MHC. At least 16 other loci have been suggested to be involved, with the largest contribution (about 10% of the genetic predisposition) being accounted for by the flanking region of the insulin gene on chromosome 11[28,29].

The relationship between type 1 diabetes and specific HLA region alleles is complex. There is a strong positive relationship with HLA-DR3 and DR4 and a strong negative relationship with DR2. Indeed, more than 90% of Caucasians with type 1 diabetes are HLA-DR3 and/or DR4. There is an even stronger relationship of type 1 diabetes when DQ loci (DQα and DQß) are considered together with DR loci so that the predisposition to type 1 diabetes in Caucasians is with DR3,DQB1*0201 and DR4,DQB1*0302, with the strongest association being the DQα DQß combination DQA1*0501-DQB1* 0302. Other DQ alleles confer protection from type 1 diabetes; DQA1*0201-DQB1*0602 provides protection even in the presence of DQ susceptibility alleles[30], suggesting that protection is dominant over susceptibility.

To date, for the purposes of most studies of type 1 diabetes prevention, genetic attention has focused solely on the HLA region genes. The other loci have been ignored. The studies of infants have screened for high-risk alleles, and some intervention studies have excluded individuals with protective HLA alleles[31,32].

AUTOANTIBODIES

A number of circulating autoantibodies to islet cell markers may be detected at diagnosis of type 1 diabetes. Indeed, current classification of diabetes uses the presence of autoantibodies to define type 1 diabetes or autoimmune diabetes (the exception being those individuals prone to ketoacidosis but without antibodies, classified as type 1 idiopathic)[33]. The autoantibodies include cytoplasmic islet cell antibodies (ICA), insulin autoantibodies (IAA), and antibodies directed against glutamic acid decarboxylase (GAD) and islet tyrosine phosphatases IA-2 and IA-2ß[34]. (The antibodies to IA-2 include the antibody ICA-512 directed at a component of IA-2, while the antibodies to IA-2ß include one directed against an insulin granule membrane protein, phogrin [phosphatase homologue of granules from rat insulinoma]).

The first antibody to be identified was ICA using a classical immuno-fluorescence assay[35]. Although the presence of ICA has been shown to be predictive of type 1 diabetes[16–19], and although the addition of IAA can improve prediction[36], it has become clear that ICA alone is not a reliable predictor of diabetes[37]. Moreover, it has been demonstrated that prediction is greatly improved by using a combination of autoantibodies to ICA, insulin, GAD, IA-2 and perhaps IA-2ß[27,34,38–40]. Nonetheless, accurate assessment of the risk of type 1 diabetes in siblings is complicated, as not all those with four autoantibodies progress[41]. In the circumstance of infants of diabetic mothers, one needs to be cautious during the first year of life that transient maternally acquired antibodies are not present[42]. A strategy has been proposed for distinguishing these as maternal in nature[42].

METABOLIC CHANGES

In people destined to have type 1 diabetes, a progressive metabolic defect can be demonstrated, measured as a decline in ß-cell function detected by a decrease in early first-phase insulin release (FPIR) during an intravenous glucose tolerance test (IVGTT)[43–45]. Standardized procedures have been agreed upon, so that the test is done uniformly throughout the world[46]. Decrease of FPIR correlates strongly with other risk factors, such as autoantibodies, and the combined use of autoantibodies and FPIR response permits more accurate risk quantification[47,48]. For example, the Childhood Diabetes in Finland Study assessed whether it is clinically relevant to classify siblings of children with recent-onset type 1 diabetes mellitus into various stages of preclinical diabetes[49]. A total of 758 siblings were graded using two classification systems, based on number of autoantibodies and FPIR. There was a greater risk of progression and a shorter time to diagnosis of diabetes in those with more antibodies, particularly with loss of FPIR[49]. In the Diabetes Prevention Trial – Type 1 (DPT-1), low FPIR in ICA-positive relatives was projected to be indicative of a risk of type 1 diabetes of 50% over five years and 60% of subjects so identified actually progressed to diabetes[32].

Metabolic testing with evaluation of FPIR can be used to identify the subgroup of individuals with elevated levels of autoantibodies who are at the greatest risk of relatively rapid progression to diabetes. Nonetheless, individuals with multiple islet autoantibodies in whom FPIR is intact have an increased risk for development of diabetes, although this may be delayed for 10–20 years after first detection of autoantibodies.

SUMMARY

In summary, risk identification for prediction of type 1 diabetes is possible. Such risk assessment may be accomplished using a combination of genetic, immunological (autoantibodies), and metabolic (FPIR, glucose tolerance) parameters both in relatives of patients with type 1 diabetes and in the general population.

INTERRUPTION OF THE TYPE 1 DIABETES DISEASE PROCESS

Given that type 1 diabetes is an immunologically mediated disease, a number of immune intervention strategies have been proposed to interdict the disease process. The scientific basis for all the intervention strategies tested in human beings has been well established in animal models. In particular, there have been extensive studies in the NOD (non-obese diabetic) mouse and the BB (Biobreeding) rat, two models of spontaneous type 1 diabetes[8,50,51]. Most animal studies have been aimed at disease prevention. In contrast, the first human studies were initiated at the time of clinical diagnosis[2–13]. This was done to ensure that the subjects participating in clinical investigations clearly had disease. Yet, the trade-off is that by the time of disease onset most ß-cell function has been lost, making the demonstration of successful intervention more difficult. In fact, it is quite possible that interventions which might be successful if applied early in the disease process would fail to show effectiveness when tested so late in the course of the disease. Appreciation of this dilemma, coupled with better predictors of disease development, has led to some controlled trials designed to test interventions that might delay or prevent the development of clinical hyperglycemia. However, interventions used in these otherwise healthy individuals must be confined to ones with a very favourable safety profile.

STUDIES IN NEWLY DIAGNOSED DIABETES

Several interventions have been evaluated in individuals with newly diagnosed type 1 diabetes, in an attempt to interdict the disease process and preserve ß-cell function. Interpretation of these has been complicated by a number of factors. Early studies often used 'remission' as an outcome, based on cessation of insulin therapy or very low doses of insulin. In fact, there was even a recommended definition of remission promulgated[52]. Yet, most recent investigations have focused more on preservation of C-peptide as a biochemical marker of ß-cell function[2]. Moreover, it has come to be appreciated that more intensive insulin therapy and/or better maintenance of glycaemic control results in better preservation of ß-cell function[53–56]. Of these, probably the best data come from the Diabetes Control and Complications Trial (DCCT)[56]. Individuals who entered the DCCT with high residual ß-cell function (stimulated C-peptide levels of 0.2-0.5 pmol/ml) (n=303) and who were randomized to intensive therapy to maintain normoglycemia, showed a significantly slower decline in stimulated C-peptide levels than did those randomized to conventional therapy[56]. As a consequence of these observations, aggressive glycaemic control with intensive insulin therapy is important for preservation of endogenous ß-cell function in patients with type 1 diabetes. Current strategy involves maintaining insulin therapy at the highest dose that does not induce hypoglycaemia. Moreover, this precludes use of remission characterized by cessation of insulin therapy or reduction of insulin dose as an end-point in clinical trials. The current approach, used by most investigators in the field, and consistent with the recommendations of the Immunology of Diabetes Society[57], is to use C-peptide response to evaluate ß-cell function.

A wide variety of interventions has been considered, and many have been tested in small pilot studies or in clinical trials[2–13]. In this chapter, discussion will generally be confined to those interventions that have been tested in randomized, controlled clinical trials.

Cyclosporine. Cyclosporine has been studied in new onset diabetes in several randomized trials, as well as a number of open trials[58–67]. Two of these – the Canadian/European Study[60] and the French Cyclosporine Study[58] – were large multicentre randomized controlled trials with sufficient subjects (188 and 122 subjects, respectively) to draw meaningful conclusions. These (as well as the other smaller studies) have demonstrated that cyclosporine results in either better preservation of ß-cell function and/or greater likelihood of remission than that seen in placebo or historical control patients. Although at least one study suggested that there was a sustained beneficial effect after discontinuation of cyclosporine[66], the authors concluded that the magnitude and duration of that benefit do not appear sufficient to justify cyclosporine treatment in clinical practice. This is particularly the case given the potential of nephrotoxicity with cyclosporine usage[68,69]. The toxicity of cyclosporine is such that it cannot safely be considered in new-onset type 1 diabetes. Cyclosporine studies included the first two large-scale randomized controlled trials of immune intervention in type 1 diabetes. Moreover, they were important in that they convincingly demonstrated that the type 1 diabetes disease process could be impacted by immune intervention, thus fulfilling the criteria that human type 1 diabetes is an immune-mediated disease.

Azathioprine. Azathioprine has been studied in several small randomized trials in new onset diabetes, either alone or in combination with glucocorticoids[70–73]. As with cyclosporine, in some – but not all – of the studies, subjects treated with azathioprine had more insulin-free 'remissions', lower insulin requirement, and higher glucagon stimulated C-peptide levels. One exception was a study in children aged 2–20. Azathioprine may result in severe leukopenia (but this can be avoided with careful monitoring and dose titration) and there is an unquantified concern about oncogenic potential. As a consequence of fears about potential toxicity, there were no further studies of azathioprine in type 1 diabetes.

Nicotinamide. Nicotinamide has been used in many studies in new onset diabetes[74–90]. Results of individual studies have been mixed, with some showing marginal beneficial effects of nicotinamide and others being without effect. To collectively examine the potential effects of nicotinamide, a meta-analysis of the first 10 of these studies has been reported[91]. The 10 randomized controlled trials (five of which involved placebo) conducted in recent-onset diabetes and included in the meta-analysis involved a total of 211 nicotinamide-treated patients. One year after diagnosis, baseline C-peptide was significantly higher in nicotinamide-treated patients compared with control patients (0.73 ± 0.65 versus 0.32 ± 0.56 ng/ml, p < 0.005). Moreover, the statistical difference remained when the analysis was confined to the five placebo-controlled trials. This combined analysis suggests a therapeutic effect of nicotinamide in preserving residual ß-cell function when given at diabetes diagnosis in addition to insulin. Adverse effects of nicotinamide were minimal. Thus, it is surprising that there has not been much apparent use of nicotinamide in new onset diabetes, although it is being studied in a large prevention trial, as discussed below.

BCG vaccine. Vaccination with BCG (bacillus Calmette-Guerin strain of Mycobacterium bovis) has been studied in new-onset diabetes. A pilot trial in

17 subjects appeared promising, in that it led to transient 'clinical remission'[92]. However, three randomized controlled trials (involving a total of 192 subjects) of BCG in new-onset diabetes failed to demonstrate a beneficial effect after one to two years[93-95]. Although this would apparently put to rest the notion of using the BCG vaccine, unfortunately these studies may suffer from each being too small and thus too under-powered to firmly conclude that there was no effect.

Linomide. Linomide (quinoline-3-carboxamide) is a synthetic immuno-modulator which results in complete protection from insulitis and diabetes in NOD mice[96]. The effects of linomide on insulin needs and ß-cell function were evaluated in a one-year study in 63 subjects (randomized 2:1 linomide and placebo) with recent onset diabetes[97]. In the linomide group, both insulin dose and HbA_{1c} were lower, and there was a trend for higher C-peptide values. In a post-hoc sub-group analysis performed in 40 patients (25 from the linomide group and 15 from the placebo group) who still had detectable residual ß-cell function at entry, linomide was associated with higher C-peptide values. The authors felt that these results support further studies to define the effects of linomide in type 1 diabetes. Unfortunately, the manufacturer withdrew linomide from further study due to side-effects in other (non-diabetes) trials. A similar drug, leflunomide, has been marketed for the treatment of rheumatoid arthritis, but has not been evaluated for potential effects in type 1 diabetes.

Insulin. As noted earlier, several studies have suggested that early and more aggressive insulin treatment may result in preservation of ß-cell function, better metabolic control, and/or a prolonged honeymoon period[53-56]. As a consequence, at least two studies were specifically designed to evaluate the effects of vigorous insulin therapy on preservation of ß-cell function in recent-onset diabetes. In a study from Tampa, 26 adolescent subjects were random-ized either to conventional insulin therapy or to a two-week course of intra-venous insulin delivered via an artificial pancreas to maintain blood glucose levels in the low normal range[98]. During the two-week intervention, the experimental-therapy group received four times more insulin than the con-ventionally treated group. Subsequently, both groups were treated similarly. The experimental group had better preservation of ß-cell function (meal stimulated C-peptide levels) and lower HbA_{1c} levels for at least one year after randomization. A study from Munich sought to clarify whether the beneficial effect seen in the Tampa study was a consequence of the intensification of therapy or the route of insulin administration (intravenous)[99]. To that end, 10 subjects with newly diagnosed diabetes were randomized to either a two-week high-dose intravenous insulin infusion or intensive insulin therapy with four injections per day. By the third week, both groups were treated similarly with intensive insulin therapy and were followed for one year. Changes in stimulated C-peptide concentrations between months 0 and 12 were not significant in either group, suggesting that both therapies were effective in preserving ß-cell function.

Oral insulin. Oral administration of insulin to young NOD mice decreases insulitis and delays the onset of diabetes[100–102]. This is consistent with the immunological concept of 'oral tolerance'[103], which suggests that antigens administered by the oral route favour the generation of the T-helper-2 (Th2) and T-helper-3 (Th3) subsets of CD4+ T-cells and the 'type 2' and 'type 3' cytokines they respectively produce, cytokines which inhibit the T-helper-1 (Th1) and 'type 1' cytokine mediated ß-cell destruction which leads to type 1 diabetes. That these regulatory cells have been generated was shown by the fact that co-transfer of spleen cells from animals treated with oral insulin prevents adoptive transfer of diabetes[100,103]. The idea of using oral insulin to slow the destructive processes in human type 1 diabetes is appealing, since oral insulin has no metabolic effects, and the safety of the insulin molecule in human beings is well established. Three randomized controlled trials (involving a total of 418 subjects) have evaluated oral insulin in new-onset diabetes[104–106]. Unfortunately, oral insulin did not modify the rate of decline of ß-cell function, although one study claimed potential beneficial effects using post-hoc analyses.

Heat-shock protein peptide. The 60 kDa heat-shock protein (hsp60) is thought to be one of the target self antigens involved in the ß-cell destruction which leads to type 1 diabetes[107]. An immunomodulatory peptide from hsp60, p277, arrests ß-cell destruction and maintains insulin production in newly diabetic NOD mice[108]. In a small randomized controlled trial in 35 subjects with diabetes diagnosed within six months, the treated group showed better preservation of C-peptide at 10 months, suggesting a potential beneficial effect[109]. These results support further studies to define the effects of hsp60, p277 in type 1 diabetes.

Anti-CD3 monoclonal antibody. Studies in mouse models of type 1 diabetes have shown that non-FcR binding anti-CD3 monoclonal antibody can prevent development of insulitis and hyperglycaemia and can even reverse diabetes, and appear to induce a state of tolerance to diabetes[110–112]. A non-FcR binding anti-CD3 monoclonal antibody [hOKT3g1(Ala-Ala)] was studied in a randomized controlled phase I/II trial in 24 subjects with new-onset type 1 diabetes[113,114]. Treatment involved a 14-day course of the antibody in escalating doses for four days followed by full dose (45 ug/kg/d) for 10 days. The treated group showed improved glycaemic control and better preservation of C-peptide (in response to a mixed meal) at 12 months, with the suggestion that the treatment effect was maintained at 18 months as well. Thus, this very small study suggested a beneficial effect, leading to the conclusion that this therapy warrants further evaluation in larger randomized controlled trials.

Studies in Individuals at High Risk of Type 1 Diabetes

In addition to attempts to interdict the disease process and preserve ß-cell function in newly diagnosed type 1 diabetes, studies have been initiated to try to delay or prevent the clinical onset of type 1 diabetes. Although a number of immunosuppressive drugs (e.g. azathioprine or cyclosporine) have been considered and some even given to a few individuals[115–118], these were not really evaluated in a disciplined way. More recently, large-scale multicentre randomized controlled clinical trials have been initiated to evaluate nicotin-amide, parenteral insulin, oral insulin and the elimination of cows' milk from infant feeding.

Nicotinamide. Nicotinamide has been used in prediabetes. No effect was seen in one tiny pilot study[119]. In two others, subjects given nicotinamide appeared to fare better than untreated historical control subjects[120]. In another study, insulin secretion seemed better preserved in six treated subjects than in seven control subjects[121].

The largest nicotinamide study to date emanates from Auckland, New Zealand[122]. In this study, during the period 1988–91, school children aged 5–8 (with no immediate family history of diabetes) were randomized by school to receive ICA testing. A total of 33 658 children were offered testing: 20 195 accepted and 13 463 declined. Of those tested, 185 were ICA positive. Of these, 173 were treated with nicotinamide (maximum dose 1.5 g/day) on the basis of either ICA levels of ≥10 JDF units and first phase insulin release < 25th percentile of normal, or those with ICA >20 JDF units. Another 48 335 children were neither screened nor treated, and served as controls. They were followed for 7.1 years. The rate of development of diabetes was $7.14/10^5$ per year in the nicotinamide treated group versus $16.07/10^5$ per year in the comparison group. The rate in those who refused testing was $18.48/10^5$ per year. After age adjustment, the tested group had a rate of diabetes of 41% (20–85 95% confidence interval) of the other groups combined, which is significant (p = 0.008). When an intention to treat analysis was performed by combining the treated group with those who refused testing, the rate of diabetes was less than in the comparison group, but the difference did not reach statistical significance. No adverse effects were seen in treated subjects.

Two large multicentre randomized, double-masked, controlled clinical trials have been initiated to evaluate the effects of nicotinamide in high-risk rela-tives of individuals with type 1 diabetes. These are the German (Deutsch) Nicotinamide Diabetes Intervention Study (DENIS) and the European Nicotinamide Diabetes Intervention Trial (ENDIT).

In DENIS, individuals at high risk for developing type 1 diabetes within three years were identified by screening siblings (aged 3–12) of patients with diabetes for the presence of high titre ICA[123]. Subjects (n = 55 were randomized into placebo and high-dose nicotinamide-slow release (1.2 g/m^2/day) groups and followed in a controlled clinical trial using a sequential design. Rates of diabetes onset were similar in both groups throughout the observation period (maximum 3.8 years, median 2.1 years). The authors assert that the sequential design provides a 10% probability of a type II error against a reduction of the cumulative diabetes incidence at three years from 30 to 6% by nicotinamide. The trial was terminated when the second sequential interim analysis after the eleventh case of diabetes showed that the trial had failed to detect a reduction of the cumulative diabetes incidence at three years from 30 to 6% (p = 0.97). The data do not exclude the possibility of a weaker, but potentially meaningful, risk reduction in this cohort, or a major clinical effect of nicotinamide in individuals with less risk of progression to type 1 diabetes than those studied.

ENDIT is a prospective, placebo-controlled double-blind trial, in ICA-positive, first-degree relatives, aged 5–40 years, of an individual who developed type 1 diabetes under the age of 20 years, and who are themselves positive for ICA[47,48]. Untreated subjects with these enrolment criteria have a projected risk of type 1 diabetes of 40% over a five-year period. Subjects (n = 528) were randomized into placebo and high-dose nicotinamide (1.3 g/m^2/day) groups to determine if a 35% reduction in incidence of type 1 diabetes can be achieved during five years of treatment. ENDIT is an international study conducted in 20 countries. More than 35000 first-degree relatives were screened. Masked comparisons are performed at six-month intervals by a review committee, with study completion projected for 2002.

Insulin. Insulin has been shown to delay the development of diabetes and insulitis in animal models of spontaneous diabetes (BB rats and NOD mice)[126–132]. In human beings, several pilot studies of insulin use in high-risk relatives of individuals with type 1 diabetes were conducted, two of which have been reported in detail. In one pilot study, from Boston, insulin was offered to 12 subjects, five of whom accepted and seven declined, and served as a comparison group[133]. In this study, insulin therapy consisted of five days of continuous intravenous insulin every nine months, coupled with twice daily subcutaneous insulin. Life table analysis suggested that this treatment may delay the appearance of diabetes.

In another pilot study, from Munich (the Schwabing Insulin Prophylaxis Trial), there were 14 high-risk first-degree relatives of people with type 1 diabetes randomized to either experimental treatment or a control group[134,135]. In the experimental treatment group, intravenous insulin was given by continuous infusion for seven days, followed by daily injections for six months.

Intravenous insulin infusions were repeated every 12 months. In the treatment group three of the seven individuals (follow-up from time of eligibility: 2.3 to 7.1 years) and in the control group six of the seven untreated individuals (1.7 to 7.1 years) developed clinical diabetes. Life table analysis showed that clinical onset of type 1 diabetes was delayed in experimental subjects compared with control subjects (diabetes-free survival: 5.0 ± 0.9 years versus 2.3 ± 0.7 years; $p < 0.03$).

The preliminary results from these pilot studies suggest that in high-risk relatives insulin has the potential to delay or prevent the development of overt diabetes. It was also appreciated that insulin is ß-cell specific, does not have generalized effects on the immune system, has well understood effects on people, and has known side-effects that are controllable. This led to the Diabetes Prevention Trial of Type 1 Diabetes (DPT-1), a randomized, controlled, multicentre clinical trial, conducted throughout the USA and Canada to test whether intervention with insulin can delay the appearance of overt clinical diabetes[136]. DPT-1 screened and analyzed 84 228 samples from relatives of patients with type 1 diabetes for islet cell antibodies (ICA), and found 3152 (3.73%) relatives who were ICA positive on initial testing. Of these, 2103 (67%) underwent staging to quantify risk of type 1 diabetes, and 372 relatives progressed in their staging evaluations to be classified as having a risk projection for type 1 diabetes of greater than 50%. A total of 339 participants were randomized either to the intervention group or to the close observation group. The experimental intervention group received parenteral insulin – both annual intravenous insulin infusions and twice-daily low-dose subcutaneous insulin injections (0.25 units per kg per day). An oral glucose tolerance test was performed every six months; the diagnosis of diabetes was confirmed by a second test. The median duration of follow-up was 3.7 years. Diabetes was diagnosed in 139 participants – 69 in the intervention group and 70 in the close observation group. The average proportion of participants who progressed to diabetes was 15.1% per year in the intervention group and 14.6% per year in the close observation group. The cumulative incidence of diabetes in the intervention group was virtually the same as in the observation group. Thus, insulin in the dose and regimen used did not delay or prevent the development of type 1 diabetes. However, most participants diagnosed with diabetes were asymptomatic at the time of diagnosis.

Oral insulin. As noted earlier, oral administration of insulin[100–101] or insulin B-chain[102] to young NOD mice decreases insulitis and delays the onset of diabetes. Moreover, spleen cells from animals treated with oral insulin prevent adoptive transfer of diabetes[100,103]. Therefore, DPT-1 also included a protocol testing whether oral insulin (7.5 mg/day) can delay the appearance of overt clinical diabetes. In this randomized, placebo-controlled, double-masked, multicentre clinical trial, nearly 100 000 relatives have been screened to identify and randomize 350 to 360 relatives classified as having a risk projection for type 1 diabetes of 26–50% over five years. The trial will complete enrolment in 2002 and will follow subjects for two years thereafter.

In addition to oral insulin, nasal insulin may also lead to tolerance. Two studies are currently examining its effects. One is a double-blind, placebo-controlled, pilot crossover study in Melbourne, Australia – the Intranasal insulin trial (INIT)[137]. That study, amongst first-degree relatives, is examining the effects of intranasal insulin on surrogate markers – autoantibodies and T-cell proliferative and cytokine responses to relevant antigens. The other – the Diabetes Prediction and Prevention (DIPP) Project – is a study being conducted in Turku, Finland among newborns from the general population (i.e. without relatives with diabetes) with high-risk genotypes for type 1 diabetes[138].

Milk proteins. In some epidemiological and case-control studies, it has been suggested that there is a reciprocal relationship between infant breast-feeding and subsequent development of type 1 diabetes[139,140]. It has been proposed that breast-feeding may be a surrogate for the absence of consumption of cow milk proteins (CMP)[140]. These highly controversial hypotheses are supported by one meta-analysis[140], but challenged in another as being confounded by bias[141]. In Finland, a small prospective study suggests that exclusive breast-feeding reduces the risk of diabetes development[142]. On the other hand, a prospective study in the USA, using appearance of antibodies as the end-point, failed to find a relationship[143]. Another Finnish cohort of high-risk newborns found that short duration of breast-feeding, together with early introduction of cow milk proteins, led to increased appearance of islet auto-antibodies[144].

In spite of the controversy, the notion has been developed that consumption of CMP, particularly during a 'critical window of vulnerability' early in life, may lead to the initiation of the immunologic attack against pancreatic islet β-cells and increase susceptibility to type 1 diabetes[145]. Others argue that the issue really relates to the immune function of the mucosal barrier[146]. The champions of the cows' milk hypothesis cite an array of evidence in support of the CMP hypothesis – epidemiologic data, disease rates in animal models, humoral and cellular immune markers directed against CMP in patients with new-onset type 1 diabetes, and identification of a peptide sequence on bovine serum albumin (BSA) with homology to sequence on the islet cell protein ICA-69 (or p69) ('molecular mimicry')[145]. To test the hypothesis, a multi-national randomized prospective trial, TRIGR (Trial to Reduce Incidence of Diabetes in Genetically at Risk), has been initiated to determine whether the frequency of type 1 diabetes can be reduced by preventing exposure to CMP during early life[147]. This randomized prospective trial may screen 6000 infants who have a parent or sibling with type 1 diabetes to identify 2000 newborns who will be followed for 10 years for the development of type 1 diabetes. For eight months they will receive either a conventional CMP formula or a formula in which there has been replacement of CMP with casein hydrolysate. This would be a 'true' primary prevention strategy.

SUMMARY

In individuals with new-onset type 1 diabetes mellitus, two large randomized controlled trials with adequate power to answer the question of preservation of ß-cell function have been conducted, both with cyclosporine, both demonstrating positive effect (Evidence Level I). Unfortunately, the side-effects result in a risk:benefit ratio that precludes the use of this intervention. Also, in new-onset type 1 diabetes, a meta-analysis has been performed that demonstrates a small beneficial effect of nicotinamide on C-peptide (Evidence Level I). Unfortunately, because of the relatively small magnitude of the effect, this intervention has not been widely used. A subset analysis from the Diabetes Control and Complications Trial – of individuals who entered with high residual ß-cell function and were randomized to intensive therapy– showed a slower decline in stimulated C-peptide than those randomized to conventional therapy (Evidence Level II). Although this demonstrated that aggressive glycaemic control can preserve ß-cell function (as well as many other beneficial effects), this approach is not as widely used as it should be. None of the other studies described above – completed or underway – will be able to provide Level I or Level II evidence.

In the prevention of diabetes, the only large randomized controlled trial to be completed is the DPT-1 parenteral insulin study, which convincingly showed that insulin – in the dose and manner used in that study – was without beneficial effect in delaying or preventing type 1 diabetes (Evidence Level 1A). The DPT-1 oral insulin study and the ENDIT study are sufficiently powered and enrolled to expect that their outcome will be at Evidence Level 1A, but the results are as yet unknown. The TRIGR study, if it completes enrolment and follow-up, also has the potential of providing Level 1A evidence. None of the other studies described above – completed or underway – will be able to provide Level I or Level II evidence.

REFERENCES

1. Atkinson MA, Maclaren NK (1994) The pathogenesis of insulin dependent diabetes mellitus. *New England Journal of Medicine* **331**: 1428–1436.
2. Skyler JS (1987) Immune intervention studies in insulin-dependent diabetes mellitus. *Diabetes Metabolism Reviews* **3**: 1017–1035.
3. Pozzilli P (1988) Immunotherapy in type 1 diabetes. *Diabetic Medicine* **5**: 734–738.
4. Harrison LC, Campbell IL, Colman PG, Chosich N, Kay TWH, Tait BD,

Bartholomeusz RK, DeAizpurua HJ, Joseph JL, Chu S, Kielczynski WE (1990) Type 1 diabetes: immunology and immunotherapy. *Advances in Endocrinology & Metabolism* 1: 35–94.

5. Andreani D, DiMario U, Pozzilli P (1991) Prediction, prevention, and early intervention in insulin dependent diabetes. *Diabetes Metabolism Reviews* 7: 61–77.
6. Skyler JS, Marks JB (1993) Immune intervention in type 1 diabetes mellitus. *Diabetes Reviews* 1: 15–42.
7. Pozzilli P, Kolb H, Ilkova HM (eds) (1993) New trends for prevention and immunotherapy of insulin dependent diabetes mellitus. *Diabetes Metabolism Reviews* 9: 237–348.
8. Bach JF (1994) Insulin-dependent diabetes mellitus as an autoimmune disease. *Endocrine Reviews* 15: 516–542.
9. Gale EA, Bingley PJ(1997) Can we prevent IDDM? *Diabetes Care* 17: 339–344.
10. Slover RH, Eisenbarth GS (1997) Prevention of type I diabetes and recurrent-cell destruction of transplanted islets. *Endocrine Reviews* 18: 241–258.
11. Rabinovitch A, Skyler JS (1998) Prevention of type 1 diabetes. *Medical Clinics of North America* 82: 739–755.
12. Pozzilli P (1998) Prevention of insulin-dependent diabetes mellitus 1998. *Diabetes Metabolism Reviews* 14: 69–84.
13. Schatz DA, Krischer JP, Skyler JS (1999) Now is the time to prevent type 1 diabetes. *Journal of Clinical Endocrinology and Metabolism* 85: 495–498.
14. Becker DJ, LaPorte RE, Libman I, Pietropaolo M, Dosch H-M (1999) Prevention of type 1 diabetes: is now the time? *Journal of Clinical Endocrinology and Metabolism* 85: 498–506.
15. Gardner SG, Bingley PJ, Sawtell PA, Weeks S, Gale EAM (1997) Rising incidence of insulin dependent diabetes in children aged under 5 years in the Oxford region: time trend analysis. *BMJ* 315: 713–717.
16. Schatz D, Krischer J, Horne G, Riley W, Spillar R, Silverstein J, Winter W, Muir A, Derovanesian D, Shah S, Vadheim CM, Rotter JI, Maclaren NK (1994) Islet cell antibodies predict insulin-dependent diabetes in United States school age children as powerfully as in unaffected relatives. *Journal of Clinical Investigation* 93: 2403–7.
17. Bingley PJ, Bonifacio E, Williams AJK,Genovese S, Bottazzo GF, Gale EAM (1997) Prediction of IDDM in the general population: strategies based on combinations of autoantibody markers. *Diabetes* 46: 1701–1710.
18. Riley WJ, Maclaren NK, Krischer J, Spillar RP, Silverstein JH, Schatz DA, Schwartz S, Malone J, Shah S, Vadheim C *et al.* (1990) A prospective study of the development of diabetes in relatives of patients with insulin-dependent diabetes. *New England Journal of Medicine* 323: 1167–1172.
19. Bingley PJ, Christie MR, Bonifacio E, Bonfanti R, Shattock M, Fonte MT, Bottazzo GF, Gale EA (1994) Combined analysis of autoantibodies improves prediction of IDDM in islet cell antibody-positive relatives. *Diabetes* 43(11) 1304–1310.
20. Imagawa A, Hanafusa T, Tamura S, Moriwaki M, Itoh N, Yamamoto K, Iwahashi H, Yamagata K, Waguri M, Nanmo T, Uno S, Nakajima H, Namba M, Kawata S, Miyagawa JI, Matsuzawa Y (2001) Pancreatic biopsy as a procedure for detecting *in situ* autoimmune phenomena in type 1 diabetes: close correlation between serological markers and histological evidence of cellular autoimmunity. *Diabetes* 50: 1269–1273.
21. Kolb H, Gale EA (2001) Does partial preservation of residual beta-cell function justify immune intervention in recent onset type I diabetes? *Diabetologia* 44: 1349–1353.

22. Rewers M, Bugawan TL, Norris JM, Blair A, Beaty B, Hoffman M, McDuffie RS, Hamman RF, Klingensmith G, Eisenbarth GS, Erlich HA (1996) Newborn screening for HLA markers associated with IDDM: Diabetes Autoimmunity Study in the Young (DAISY). *Diabetologia* **39**: 807–812.
23. Nejentsev S, Sjoroos M, Soukka T, Knip M, Simell O, Lovgren T, Ilonen J (1999) Population-based genetic screening for the estimation of type 1 diabetes mellitus risk in Finland: selective genotyping of markers in the HLA-DQB1, HLA-DQA1 and HLA-DRB1 loci. *Diabetic Medicine* **16**: 985–992.
24. Kupila A, Muona P, Simell T, Arvilommi P, Savolainen H, Hamalainen AM, Korhonen S, Kimpimaki T, Sjoroos M, Ilonen J, Knip M, Simell O (2001) Juvenile diabetes research foundation centre for the prevention of type 1 diabetes in finland. Feasibility of genetic and immunological prediction of type 1 diabetes in a population-based birth cohort. *Diabetologia* **44**: 290–297.
25. Ronningen KS (1997) Genetics in the prediction of insulin-dependent diabetes mellitus: from theory to practice. *Annals of Medicine* **29**: 387–392.
26. Schatz D, Muir A, Fuller K, Atkinson M, Crockett S, Hsiang H, Winter B, Ellis T, Taylor K, Saites C, Dukes M, Fang Q, Clare-Salzler M, She JX (2000) Prospective assessment in newborns for diabetes autoimmunity (PANDA): a newborn diabetes screening program in the general population of Florida. *Diabetes* **49**(Suppl 1): A67.
27. Ziegler AG, Hummel M, Schenker M, Bonifacio E (1999) Autoantibody appearance and risk for development of childhood diabetes in offspring of parents with type 1 diabetes: the 2-year analysis of the German BABYDIAB Study. *Diabetes* **48**: 460–468.
28. Todd JA, Farrall M (1997) Panning for gold: genomewide scanning in type 1 diabetes. *Diabetes Reviews* **5**: 284–291.
29. Pugliese A (1999) Unraveling the genetics of insulin-dependent type 1A diabetes: the search must go on. *Diabetes Reviews* **7**: 39–54.
30. Pugliese A, Gianani R, Moromisato R, Awdeh ZL, Alper CA, Erlich HA, Jackson RA, Eisenbarth GS (1995) HLA DQB1*0602 is associated with dominant protection from diabetes even among islet cell antibody positive first degree relatives of patients with insulin-dependent diabetes. *Diabetes* **44**: 608–613.
31. Greenbaum CJ, Schatz DA, Cuthbertson D, Zeidler A, Eisenbarth GS, Krischer JP, for the DPT-1 Study Group (2000) Islet cell antibody positive relatives with human leukocyte antigen DQA1*0102, DQB1*0602: identification by the diabetes prevention trial-1. *Journal of Clinical Endocrinology and Metabolism* **85**: 1255–1260.
32. Diabetes Prevention Trial – Type 1 (DPT-1). Study Group. Protocol. Available at https://www. moffitt.usf.edu/sec/dpt1.
33. American Diabetes Association Expert Committee on the Diagnosis and Classification of Diabetes Mellitus (1997) Report of the rxpert committee on the diagnosis and classification of diabetes mellitus. *Diabetes Care* **20**: 1183–1197.
34. Verge CF, Stenger D, Bonifacio E, Colman PG, Pilcher C, Bingley PJ, Eisenbarth GS (1998) Combined use of autoantibodies (IA-2ab, Gadab, IAA, ICA) in type 1 diabetes: combinatorial islet autoantibody workshop. *Diabetes* **47**: 1857–1866.
35. Bottazzo GF, Florin-Christensen A, Doniach D (1974) Islet-cell antibodies in diabetes mellitus with autoimmune polyendocrine deficiencies. *Lancet* **2**: 1279–1283.
36. Krischer JP, Schatz D, Riley WJ, Spillar RP, Silverstein JH, Schwartz S, Malone J, Shah S, Vadheim CM, Rotter JI, Maclaren NK (1993) Insulin and islet cell autoantibodies as time-dependent covariates in the development of insulin-dependent diabetes: a prospective study in relatives. *Journal of Clinical Endocrinology and Metabolism* **77**: 743–749.

37. Gardner SG, Gale EA, Williams AJ, Gillespie KM, Lawrence KE, Bottazzo GF, Bingley PJ (1999) Progression to diabetes in relatives with islet autoantibodies. Is it inevitable? *Diabetes Care* **22**: 2049–2054.
38. Verge CF, Gianani R, Kawasaki E, Yu L, Pietropaolo M, Jackson RA, Chase HP, Eisenbarth GS (1996) Prediction of type I diabetes in first-degree relatives using a combination of insulin, GAD, and ICA512bdc/IA-2 autoantibodies. *Diabetes* **45**: 926–933.
39. Maclaren N, Lan M, Coutant R, Schatz D, Silverstein J, Muir A, Clare-Salzer M, She JX, Malone J, Crockett S, Schwartz S, Quattrin T, DeSilva M, Vander Vegt P, Notkins A, Krischer J (1999) Only multiple autoantibodies to islet cells (ICA), insulin, GAD65, IA-2 and IA-2beta predict immune-mediated (Type 1) diabetes in relatives. *Journal of Autoimmunity* **12**: 279–287.
40. Krischer JP, Cuthbertson D, Yu L, Orban T, Maclaren NK, Jackson R, Winter WE, Schatz DA, Palmer JP, Eisenbarth GS, and the DPT-1 Study Group. Screening Strategies for the Identification of Multiple Antibody Positive Individuals. *Journal of Clinical Endocrinology and Metabolism*. In Press.
41. Kulmala P, Savola K, Petersen JS, Vahasalo P, Karjalainen J, Lopponen T, Dyrberg T, Akerblom HK, Knip M (1998) Prediction of insulin-dependent diabetes mellitus in siblings of children with diabetes. A population-based study. The Childhood Diabetes in Finland Study Group. *Journal of Clinical Investigation* **101**: 327–336.
42. Naserke HE, Bonifacio E, Ziegler AG (2001) Prevalence, characteristics and diabetes risk associated with transient maternally acquired islet antibodies and persistent islet antibodies in offspring of parents with type 1 diabetes. *Journal of Clinical Endocrinology and Metabolism* **86**: 4826–4833.
43. Srikanta S, Ganda OP, Gleason RE, Jackson RA, Soeldner JS, Eisenbarth GS (1984) Pre-type 1 diabetes. Linear loss of beta cell response to intravenous glucose. *Diabetes* **33**: 717–20.
44. Chase HP, Garg SK, Butler-Simon N, Klingensmith G, Norris L, Ruskey CT, O'Brien D (1991) Prediction of the course of pre-type 1 diabetes. *Journal of Pediatrics* **118**: 838–841.
45. Bohmer KP, Kolb H, Kuglin B, Zielasek J, Hubinger A, Lampeter EF, Weber B, Kolb-Bachofen V, Jastram HU, Bertrams J, Gries FA (1994) Linear loss of insulin secretory capacity during the last six months preceding IDDM. *Diabetes Care* **17**: 138–141.
46. Bingley PJ, Colman P, Eisenbarth GS, Jackson RA, McCulloch DK, Riley WJ, Gale EA (1992) Standardization of IVGTT to predict IDDM. *Diabetes Care* **15**: 1313–1316.
47. Bingley PJ (1996) Interactions of age, islet cell antibodies, insulin autoantibodies, and first-phase insulin response in predicting risk of progression to IDDM in ICA+ relatives: the ICARUS data set. Islet Cell Antibody Register Users Study. *Diabetes* **45**: 1720–1728.
48. Chase HP, Cuthbertson D, Dolan LM, Kaufman F, Krischer JP, Schatz DA, White N, Wilson DM, Wolfsdorf J (2001) The DPT-1 study group: first-phase insulin release during the intravenous glucose tolerance as a risk factor for type 1 diabetes. *Journal of Pediatrics* **138**: 244–249.
49. Mrena S, Savola K, Kulmala P, Akerblom HK, Knip M, and the Childhood Diabetes in Finland Study Group (1999) Staging of preclinical type 1 diabetes in siblings of affected children. *Pediatrics* **104**: 925–930.
50. Atkinson MA, Leiter EH (1999) The NOD mouse model of type 1 diabetes: as good as it gets? *Nature Medicine* **5**: 601–604.

51. Greiner DL, Rossini AA, Mordes JP (2001) Translating data from animal models into methods for preventing human autoimmune diabetes mellitus: *caveat emptor* and *primum non* nocere. *Clinical Immunology* **100**: 134–143.

52. Kolb H, Bach JF, Eisenbarth GS, Harrison LC, Maclaren NK, Pozzilli P, Skyler J, Stiller CR (1989) Criteria for immune trials in type I diabetes. *Lancet* **2**: 686.

53. Mirouze J, Selam JL, Pham TC, Mendoza E, Orsetti A (1978) Sustained insulin induced remissions of juvenile diabetes by means of an external artificial pancreas. *Diabetologia* **14**: 223–227.

54. Madsbad S, Krarup T, Faber OK, Binder C, Regeur L (1982) The transient effect of strict glycemic control on ß cell function in newly diagnosed type I (insulin-dependent) diabetic patients. *Diabetologia* **22**: 16–20.

55. Perlman K, Ehrlich RM, Filler RM, Albisser AM (1984) Sustained normoglycemia in newly diagnosed type 1 diabetic subjects: short-term effects and one-year follow-up. *Diabetes* **33**: 995–1001.

56. Effect of intensive therapy on residual ß-cell function in patients with type 1 diabetes in the diabetes control and complications trial: a randomized, controlled trial. The Diabetes Control and Complications Trial Research Group (1998) *Annals of Internal Medicine* **128**: 517–523.

57. Immunology of Diabetes Society. Draft guidelines for intervention trials in subjects with newly-diagnosed type 1 diabetes. www.idsoc.org/Draft_Guidelines.html

58. Feutren G, Papoz L, Assan R, Vialettes B, Karsenty G, Vexiau P, DuRostu H, Rodier M, Sirmai J, Lallemand A, Bach JF, for the Cyclosporin/Diabetes French Study Group (1986) Cyclosporin increases the rate and length of remissions in insulin dependent diabetes of recent onset: results of a multicentre double-blind trial. *Lancet* **ii**: 119–124.

59. Bach JF, Feutren G, Boitard C (1989) Immunoprevention of insulin-dependent diabetes by cyclosporin. In Andreani D, Kolb H, Pozzilli P (Eds) *Immunotherapy of Type 1 Diabetes.* Chichester: John Wiley & Sons, pp. 125–136.

60. The Canadian-European Randomized Control Trial Group (1988) Cyclosporin-induced remission of IDDM after early intervention: association of 1 year of cyclosporin treatment with enhanced insulin secretion. *Diabetes* **37**: 1574–1582.

61. Martin S, Schernthaner G, Nerup J, Gries FA, Koivisto VA, Dupre J, Standl E, Hamet P, McArthur R, Tan MH, Dawson K, Mehta AE, Van Vliet S, von Graffenried B, Stiller C, Kolb H (1991) Follow-up of cyclosporin a treatment in type 1 (insulin dependent) diabetes mellitus: lack of long-term effects. *Diabetologia* **34**: 429–434.

62. Chase HP, Butler-Simon N, Garg SK, Hayward A, Klingensmith GJ, Hamman RF, O'Brien D (1990) Cyclosporin A for the treatment of new-onset insulin-dependent diabetes mellitus. *Pediatrics* **85**: 241–245.

63. Skyler JS, Rabinovitch A, Miami Cyclosporine Diabetes Study Group (1992) Cyclosporine in recent onset type 1 diabetes mellitus: effects on islet beta-cell function. *Journal of Diabetes and Its Complications* **6**: 77–88.

64. Bougneres PF, Carel JC, Castano L, Boitard C, Gardin JP, Landais P, Hors J, Mihatsch MJ, Paillard M, Chaussain JL, Bach JF (1988) Factors associated with early remission of type 1 diabetes in children treated with cyclosporine. *New England Journal of Medicine* **318**: 663–670.

65. Bougneres PF, Landais P, Boisson C, Carel JC, Frament N, Boitard C, Chaussain JL, Bach JF (1990) Limited duration of remission of insulin dependency in children with recent overt type 1 diabetes treated with low-dose cyclosporine. *Diabetes* **39**: 1264–1272.

66. De Filippo G, Carel JC, Boitard C, Bougnères PF (1996) Long-term results of early cyclosporin therapy in juvenile IDDM. *Diabetes* **45**: 101–104.
67. Jenner M, Bradish G, Stiller C, Atkison P, for the London Diabetes Study Group (1992) Cyclosporine: a treatment of young children with newly-diagnosed type 1 (insulin dependent) diabetes mellitus. *Diabetologia* **35**: 884–888.
68. Parving HH, Tarnow L, Nielsen FS, Rossing P, Mandrup-Poulsen T, Osterby R, Nerup J (1999) Cyclosporine nephrotoxicity in type 1 diabetic patients. A 7-year follow-up study. *Diabetes Care* **22**: 478–483.
69. Assan R, Timsit J, Feutren G, Bougneres P, Czernichow P, Hannedouche T, Boitard C, Noel LH, Mihatsch MJ, Bach JF (1994) The kidney in cyclosporin A-treated diabetic patients: a long-term clinicopathological study. *Clinical Nephrology* **41**: 41–49.
70. Harrison LC, Colman PG, Dean B, Baxter R, Martin FIR (1985) Increase in remission rate in newly diagnosed type 1 diabetic subjects treated with azathioprine. *Diabetes* **34**: 1306–1308.
71. Cook JJ, Hudson I, Harrison LC, Dean B, Colman PG, Werther GA, Warne GL, Court JM (1989) A double-blind controlled trial of azathioprine in children with newly-diagnosed type 1 diabetes. *Diabetes* **38**: 779–783.
72. Silverstein J, Maclaren N, Riley W, Spillar R, Radjenovic D, Johnson S (1988) Immunosuppression with azathioprine and prednisone in recent onset insulin-dependent diabetes mellitus. *New England Journal of Medicine* **319**: 599–604.
73. Silverstein J, Maclaren N, Riley W, Radjenovic D, Spillar R (1990) Double blind trial with azathioprine and steroids in newly-diagnosed IDD. *Diabetes* **39**(Suppl 1): 294A.
74. Vague P, Viallettes B, Lassman-Vague V, Vallo JJ (1987) Nicotinamide may extend remission phase in insulin dependent diabetes. *Lancet* **i**: 619–620.
75. Mendola G, Casamitgana R, Gomis R (1989) Effects of nicotinamide therapy upon beta-cell function in newly diagnosed type 1 (insulin-dependent) diabetes mellitus patients. *Diabetologia* **32**: 160–162.
76. Pozilli P, Visalli N, Ghirlanda G, Manna R, Andreani D (1989) Nicotinamide increases c-peptide secretion in patients with recent onset type 1 diabetes. *Diabetic Medicine* **6**: 568–572.
77. Chase HP, Butler-Simon N, Garg S, McDuffie M, Hoops SL, O'Brien D (1990) A trial of nicotinamide in newly diagnosed patients with type 1 (insulin-dependent) diabetes mellitus. *Diabetologia* **33**: 444–446.
78. Viallettes B, Picq R, du Rostu M, Charbonnel B, Rodier M, Mirouze J, Vexiau P, Passa Ph, Pehuet M, Elgrably F, Vague P (1990) A preliminary multicentre study of the treatment of recently diagnosed type 1 diabetes by combination nicotinamide-cyclosporin therapy. *Diabetic Medicine* **7**: 731–735.
79. Lewis MC, Canafx DM, Sprafka JM, Barbosa JJ (1992) Double-blind randomized trial of nicotinasmide on early onset diabetes. *Diabetes Care* **15**: 121–123.
80. Ilkova H, Gorpe U, Kadioglu P, Ozyazar M, Bagriacik N (1991) Nicotinamide in type 1 diabetes of recent-onset: a double-blind placebo controlled trial. *Diabetologia* **34**(Suppl 2): A179.
81. Guastamacchia E, Ciampolillo A, Lollino G, Caragiulo L, De Robertis O, Lattanzi V, Giorgino R (1992) Effetto della terapia con nicotinamide sull'induzione della durata della remissione clinica in diabetici tipo 1 all'esordio sottoposti a terapia insulinica ottimizzata mediante microinfusore. *Il Diabete* **4**(Suppl 1): 210.
82. Gonzalez-Clemente JM, Munoz A, Fernandez-Usac E (1992) Desferrioxamine and nicotinamide in newly diagnosed type 1 diabetes: a randomized double-blind placebo controlled trial. *Diabetologia* **35**(Suppl 1): A202.

83. Paskova M, Ikao I, Trozova D, Bono P (1992) Nicotinamide in children with newly diagnosed type 1 diabetes mellitus. *Diabetologia* **35**(Suppl 1): A203.
84. Pozzilli P, Visalli N, Boccuni ML, Baroni MG, Buzzetti R, Fioriti E, Signore A, Cavallo MG, Andreani D, Lucentini L, Crino A, Cicconetti CA, Teodonio C, Amoretti R, Pisano L, Pennafina MG, Santopadre G, Marozzi G, Multari G, Campea L, Suppa MA, De Mattia GC, Cassone-Faldetta M, Perrone F, Greco A, Ghirlanda G, The IMDIAB Study Group (1994) Randomized trial comparing nicotinamide and nicotinamide plus cyclosporin in recent onset insulin-dependent diabetes (IMDIAB 1). *Diabetic Medicine* **11**: 98–104.
85. Pozzilli P, Visalli N, Boccuni ML, Baroni MG, Buzzetti R, Fioriti E, Signore A, Cavallo MG, Andreani D, Lucentini L, Matteoli MC, Crino A, Cicconetti CA, Teodonio C, Amoretti R, Pisano L, Pennafina MG, Santopadre G, Marozzi G, Multari G, Campea L, Suppa MA, De Mattia GC, Cassone-Faldetta M, Marietta G, Perrone F, Greco A, Ghirlanda G (1994) Combination of nicotinamide and steroid versus nicotinamide in recent-onset IDDM. The IMDIAB II Study. *Diabetes Care* **17**: 897–900.
86. Taboga C, Tonutti L, Noacco C (1994) Residual beta-cell activity and insulin requirements in insulin-dependent diabetic patients treated from the beginning with high doses of nicotinamide. A two-year follow-up. *Recenti Progressi in Medicina* **85**: 513–516.
87. Pozzilli P, Visalli N, Signore A, Baroni MG, Buzzetti R, Cavallo MG, Boccuni ML, Fava D, Gragnoli C, Andreani D, Lucentini L, Matteoli MC, Crino A, Cicconetti CA, Teodonio C, Paci F, Amoretti R, Pisano L, Pennafina MG, Santopadre G, Marozzi G, Multari G, Suppa MA, Campea L, De Mattia GC, Cassone-Faldetta M, Marietta G, Perrone F, Greco AV, Ghirlanda G, The IMDIAB Study Group (1995) Double-blind trial of nicotinamide in recent-onset IDDM (the IMDIAB III study). *Diabetologia* **38**: 848–852.
88. Satman I, Dinccag N, Karsidag K, Ozer E, Altuntas Y, Yilmaz MT (1995) The effect of nicotinamide in recent-onset type 1 diabetes regarding the level of beta cell reserve. *Klinik Gelisim* **8**: 3882–3886.
89. Visalli N, Cavallo MG, Signore A, Baroni MG, Buzzetti R, Fioriti E, Mesturino C, Fiori R, Lucentini L, Matteoli MC, Crino A, Corbi S, Spera S, Teodonio C, Paci F, Amoretti R, Pisano L, Suraci C, Multari G, Sulli N, Cervoni M, De Mattia G, Faldetta MR, Boscherini B, Bitti MLM, Marietta G, Ferrazzoli F, Bizzarri C, Pitocco D, Ghirlanda G, Pozzilli P, The IMDIAB Study Group(1999) A multi-centre randomized trial of two different doses of nicotinamide in patients with recent-onset type 1 diabetes (the IMDIAB VI). *Diabetes Metabolism Research and Reviews* **15**: 181–185.
90. Vidal J, Fernandez-Balsells M, Sesmilo G, Aguilera E, Casamitjana R, Gomis R, Conget I (2000) Effects of nicotinamide and intravenous insulin therapy in newly diagnosed type 1 diabetes. *Diabetes Care* **23**: 360–364.
91. Pozzilli P, Browne PD, Kolb H (1996) Meta-analysis of nicotinamide treatment in patients with recent-onset IDDM. The Nicotinamide Trialists. *Diabetes Care* **19**: 1357–1363.
92. Shehadeh N, Calcinaro F, Bradley BJ, Bruchlim I, Vardi P, Lafferty K (1994) Effects of adjuvant therapy on development of diabetes in mouse and man. *Lancet* **343**: 706–707.
93. Pozzilli P on behalf of the IMDIAB Group (1997) BCG vaccine in insulin-dependent diabetes mellitus. IMDIAB Group. *Lancet* **349**: 1520–1521.
94. Elliott JF, Marlin KL, Couch RM (1998) Effect of bacille Calmette–Guérin

vaccination on C-peptide secretion in children newly diagnosed with IDDM. *Diabetes Care* **21**: 1691–1693.

95. Allen HF, Klingensmith GJ, Jensen P, Simoes E, Hayward A, Chase HP (1999) Effect of Bacillus Calmette–Guerin vaccination on new-onset type 1 diabetes. A randomized clinical study. *Diabetes Care* **22**: 1703–1707.

96. Gross D, Sidi H, Weiss L, Kalland T, Rosenmann E, Slavin S (1994) Prevention of diabetes mellitus in non-obese diabetic mice by linomide, a novel immunomodulating drug. *Diabetologia* **37**: 1195–1201.

97. Coutant R, Landais P, Rosilio M, Johnsen C, Lahlou N, Chatelain P, Carel JC, Ludvigsson J, Boitard C, Bougneres PF (1998) Low dose linomide in Type I juvenile diabetes of recent onset: a randomised placebo-controlled double blind trial. *Diabetologia* **41**: 1040–1046.

98. Shah SC, Malone JI, Simpson NE (1989) A randomized trial of intensive insulin therapy in newly diagnosed type 1 insulin-dependent diabetes mellitus. *New England Journal of Medicine* **320**: 550–554.

99. Schnell O, Eisfelder B, Standl E, Ziegler AG (1997) High-dose intravenous insulin infusion versus intensive insulin treatment in newly diagnosed IDDM. *Diabetes* **46**: 1607–1611.

100. Zhang ZJ, Davidson LE, Eisenbarth G, Weiner HL (1991) Suppression of diabetes in NOD mice by oral administration of porcine insulin. *Proceedings of the National Academy of Sciences USA* **88**: 10252–10256.

101. Bergerot I, Fabien N, Maguer V, Thivolet C (1994) Oral administration of human insulin to NOD mice generates CD4[+] T cells that suppress adoptive transfer of diabetes. *Journal of Autoimmunity* **7**: 655–663.

102. Polanski M, Melican NS, Zhang J, Weiner HL (1997) Oral administration of the immunodominant B-chain of insulin reduces diabetes in a co-transfer model of diabetes in the NOD mouse and is associated with a switch from Th1 to Th2 cytokines. *Journal of Autoimmunity* **10**: 339–346.

103. Weiner HL (1997) Oral tolerance for the treatment of autoimmune diseases. *Annual Review of Medicine* **48**: 341–351.

104. Pozzilli P, Pitocco D, Visalli N, Cavallo MG, Buzzetti R, Crino A, Spera S, Suraci C, Multari G, Cervoni M, Manca Bitti ML, Matteoli MC, Marietti G, Ferrazzoli F, Cassone Faldetta MR, Giordano C, Sbriglia M, Sarugeri E, Ghirlanda G (2000) No effect of oral insulin on residual beta-cell function in recent-onset type I diabetes (the IMDIAB VII). IMDIAB Group. *Diabetologia* **43**: 1000–1004.

105. Chaillous L, Lefevre H, Thivolet C, Boitard C, Lahlou N, Atlan-Gepner C, Bouhanick B, Mogenet A, Nicolino M, Carel JC, Lecomte P, Marechaud R, Bougneres P, Charbonnel B, Sai P (2000) Oral insulin administration and residual beta-cell function in recent-onset type 1 diabetes: a multicentre randomised controlled trial. Diabete Insuline Orale group. *Lancet* **356**: 545–549.

106. Krischer J, Ten S, Marker J, Coutant R, Kukreja A, Zhang Ch, Zhong S, Raskin P, Bode B, Vargas A, Rogers D, Schatz D, Deeb L, Marks J, Schwartz S, Malone J, Rapaport R, Zeidler A, Maclaren N (2001_ Endogenous insulin retention by oral insulin in newly diagnosed antibody positive type-1 diabetes. *Diabetes* **50**(Suppl 2): Abstract 180-OR.

107. Elias D, Markovits D, Reshef T, Van der Zee R, Cohen IR (1990) Induction and therapy of autoimmune diabetes in the non-obese diabetic (NOD/LT) mouse by a 65-kDa heat shock protein. *Proceedings of the National Academy of Sciences USA* **87**: 1576–1580.

108. Elias D, Reshef T, Birk OS, Van der Zee R, Walker MD, Cohen IR (1991) Vaccination against autoimmune mouse diabetes with a T-cell epitope of the

human 65 kDa heat shock protein. *Proceedings of the National Academy of Sciences USA* **88**: 3088–3091.

109. Raz I, Elias D, Avron A, Tamir M, Metzger M, Cohen IR (2001 ß-cell function in new-onset type 1 diabetes and immunomodulation with a heat-shock protein peptide (DiaPep277): a randomised, double-blind, phase II trial. *Lancet* **358**: 1749–1753.

110. Herold KC, Bluestone JA, Montag AG, Parihar A, Wiegner A, Gress RE, Hirsch R (1992) Prevention of autoimmune diabetes with nonactivating anti-CD3 monoclonal antibody. *Diabetes* **41**: 385–391.

111. Chatenoud L, Thevet E, Primo J, Bach J-F (1994) Anti-CD3 antibody induces long-term remission of overt autoimmunity in nonobese diabetic mice. *Proceedings of the National Academy of Sciences USA* **91**: 123–127.

112. Chatenoud L, Primo J, Bach J-F (1997) CD3 antibody-induced self tolerance in overtly diabetic NOD mice. *Journal of Immunology* **158**: 2947–2954.

113. Herold KC, Hagopian W, Auger J, Poumain-Ruiz E, Taylor L, Febres G, Harlan D, Bluestone JA (2001_ Treatment with anti-CD3 monoclonal antibody hOKT3_1(Ala-Ala) improves glycemic control during the first year of type 1 diabetes mellitus. *Diabetes* **50**(Suppl 2): Abstract 138-OR.

114. Herold KC, Hagopian W, Auger J, Poumain-Ruiz E, Taylor L, Donaldson D, Gitelman SE, Harlan D, Xu D, Zivin RA, Bluestone JA (2002) Anti-CD3 monoclonal antibody in new onset type 1 diabetes mellitus. *New Eng. J. Med.* **346**: 1692–1698.

115. Riley WJ, Maclaren NK, Spillar R (1986) Reversal of deteriorating glucose tolerance with azathioprine in prediabetes. *Transplantation Proceedings* **18**: 819–822.

116. Levy-Marchal C, Czernichow P, Quiniou MC, Sachs M, Bach JF (1984) Cyclosporin administration reversed abnormalities in a prediabetic child. *Diabetes* **33**(Suppl 1): 183A.

117. Rakotoambinina B, Timsit J, Deschamps I, Laborde K, Jos J, Boitard C, Assan R, Robert JJ (1995) Cyclosporin A does not delay insulin dependency in asymptomatic IDDM patients. *Diabetes Care* **18**: 1487–1490.

118. Carel JC, Boitard C, Eisenbarth G, Bach JF, Bougnères PF (1996) Cyclosporine delays but does not prevent clinical onset in glucose intolerant pre-type 1 diabetic children. *Journal of Autoimmunity* **9**: 739–745.

119. Dumont-Herskowitz R, Jackson RA, Soeldner JS, Eisenbarth GS (1989) Pilot trial to prevent type 1 diabetes: progression to overt IDDM despite oral nicotinamide. *Journal of Autoimmunity* **2**: 733–737.

120. Elliott RB, Chase HP (1991) Prevention or delay of type 1 (insulin-dependent) diabetes mellitus in children using nicotinamide. *Diabetologia* **34**: 362–365.

121. Manna R, Migliore A, Martin LS, Ferrara E, Ponte E, Marietti G, Scuderi F, Cristiano G, Ghirlanda G, Gambassi G (1992) Nicotinamide treatment in subjects at high risk of developing IDDM improves insulin secretion. *British Journal of Clinical Practice* **46**: 177–179.

122. Elliott RB, Pilcher CC, Fergusson DM, Stewart AW (1996) A population-based strategy to prevent insulin-dependent diabetes using nicotinamide. *Journal of Pediatric Endocrinology and Metabolism* **9**: 501–509.

123. Lampeter EF, Klinghammer A, Scherbaum WA, Heinze E, Haastert B, Giani G, Kolb H (1998) The Deutsche Nicotinamide Intervention Study: an attempt to prevent type 1 diabetes. DENIS Group. *Diabetes* **47**: 980–984.

124. Gale EA, Bingley PJ (1994) Can we prevent IDDM? *Diabetes Care* **17**: 339–344.

125. Gale EA (1996) Theory and practice of nicotinamide trials in pre-type 1 diabetes. *Journal of Pediatric Endocrinology and Metabolism* **9**: 375–379.

126. Gotfredsen GF, Buschard K, Frandsen EK (1985) Reduction of diabetes incidence of BB wistar rats by early prophylactic insulin treatment of diabetes-prone animals. *Diabetologia* **28**: 933–935.

127. Like AA (1989) Morphology and mechanisms of autoimmune diabetes as revealed by studies of the BB/Wor rat. In Hanahan D, McDevitt HO, Cahill GJ (eds) *Perspectives on the Molecular Biology and Immunology of the Pancreatic Beta Cell.* Cold Spring Harbor, Current Communications in Molecular Biology, pp. 81–91.

128. Like AA (1986) Insulin injections prevent diabetes (DB) in BioBreeding/Worcester (BB/W) rats. *Diabetes* **136**: 3254–3258.

129. Vlahos WD, Seemayer TA, Yale JF (1991) Diabetes prevention in BB rats by inhibition of endogenous insulin secretion. *Metabolism* **40**: 825–829.

130. Gottlieb PA, Handler ES, Appel MC, Greiner DL, Mordes JP, Rossini AA (1991) Insulin treatment prevent diabetes mellitus but not thyroiditis in RT6-depleted diabetes resistant BB/Wor rats. *Diabetologia* **34**: 296–300.

131. Atkinson MA, Maclaren NK, Luchetta R (1990) Insulitis and insulin dependent diabetes in NOD mice reduced by prophylactic insulin therapy. *Diabetes* **39**: 933–937.

132. Bowman MA, Campbell L, Darrow BL, Ellis TM, Suresh A, Atkinson MA (1996) Immunological and metabolic effects of prophylactic insulin therapy in the NOD-scid/scid adoptive transfer model of IDDM. *Diabetes* **45**: 205–208.

133. Keller RJ, Eisenbarth GS, Jackson RA (1993) Insulin prophylaxis in individuals at high risk of type 1 diabetes. *Lancet* **341**: 927–928.

134. Ziegler A, Bachmann W, Rabl W (1993) Prophylactic insulin treatment in relatives at high risk for type 1 diabetes. *Diabetes Metabolism Reviews* **9**: 289–293.

135. Füchtenbusch M, Rabl W, Grassl B, Bachmann W, Standl E, Ziegler AG (1998) Delay of type I diabetes in high-risk, first-degree relatives by parenteral antigen administration: the Schwabing Insulin Prophylaxis Pilot Trial. *Diabetologia* **41**: 536–541.

136. Diabetes Prevention Trial – Type 1 (DPT-1) Study Group (2002) Effects of Insulin in Relatives of Patients with Type 1 Diabetes Mellitus. *New Eng. J. Med.* **346**: 1685–1691.

137. Harrison LC, Honeyman MC, Steele C, Wright M, Gellert SA, Colman PG (1999) Intranasal insulin trial (INIT) in preclinical type 1 diabetes. *Diabetes* **48**(Suppl 1): A206.

138. Kimpimaki T, Kupila A, Hamalainen AM, Kukko M, Kulmala P, Savola K, Simell T, Keskinen P, Ilonen J, Simell O, Knip M (2001) The first signs of beta-cell autoimmunity appear in infancy in genetically susceptible children from the general population: the Finnish Type 1 Diabetes Prediction and Prevention Study. *Journal of Clinical Endocrinology and Metabolism* **86**: 4782–4788.

139. Borch-Johnsen K, Joner G, Mandrup-Paulsen T, Christy M, Zachan-Christiansen B, Kastrup K, Nerup J (1984) Relationship between breastfeeding and incidence rates of insulin dependent diabetes mellitus. *Lancet* **2**: 1083–1086.

140. Gerstein H (1994) Cows' milk exposure and type 1 diabetes mellitus. *Diabetes Care* **17**: 13–19.

141. Norris JM, Scott FW (1996) A meta-analysis of infant diet and insulin-dependent diabetes mellitus: do biases play a role? *Epidemiology* **7**: 87–92.

142. Virtanen SM, Rasanen L, Aro A, Lindstrom J, Sippola H, Lounamaa R, Toivanen L, Tuomilehto J, Akerblom HK, Childhood Diabetes in Finland Study Group (1991) Infant Feeding in Finnish Children <7 Yr of Age with Newly Diagnosed IDDM. *Diabetes Care* **14**: 415–417.

143. Norris JM, Beaty B, Klingensmith G, Yu Liping, Hoffman M, Chase HP, Erlich HA, Hamman RF, Eisenbarth GS, Rewers M (1996) Lack of association between early exposure to cow's milk protein and beta-cell autoimmunity. Diabetes Autoimmunity Study in the Young (DAISY). *JAMA* **276**: 609–614.
144. Kimpimaki T, Erkkola M, Korhonen S, Kupila A, Virtanen SM, Ilonen J, Simell O, Knip M (2001) Short-term exclusive breastfeeding predisposes young children with increased genetic risk of type I diabetes to progressive beta-cell autoimmunity. *Diabetologia* **44**: 63–69.
145. Akerblom HK, Savilahti E, Saukkonen TT, Paganus A, Virtanen SM, Teramo K, Knip M, Ilonen J, Reijonen H, Karjalainen J, Vaarala O, Reunanen A (1993) The case for elimination of cows' milk in early infancy in prevention of type 1 diabetes: the Finnish experience. *Diabetes Metabolism Reviews* **9**: 269–278.
146. Harrison LC, Honeyman MC (1999) Cows' milk and type 1 diabetes: the real debate is about mucosal immune function. *Diabetes* **48**: 1501–1507.
147. Paronen J, Knip M, Savilahti E, Virtanen SM, Ilonen J, Akerblom HK, Vaarala O (2000) Effect of cows' milk exposure and maternal type 1 diabetes on cellular and humoral immunization to dietary insulin in infants at genetic risk for type 1 diabetes. Finnish Trial to Reduce IDDM in the Genetically at Risk Study Group. *Diabetes* **49**: 1657–1665.

5

Can Bombing the Immune System Achieve Lasting Peace in the Pancreas? A Commentary

EDWIN A.M. GALE
Southmead Hospital, Bristol BS10 5NB, UK

PREAMBLE

Prevention of type 1 diabetes currently resides at around the same level as peace on earth: eminently desirable, theoretically possible, not as yet demonstrated. Jay Skyler has ably summarised the evidence that β-cell function can be influenced by therapies introduced at the time of diagnosis of type ` diabetes. The immune intervention most convincingly shown to prolong β-cell function following diagnosis is cyclosporine, but its effects are usually transient and the risk of nephrotoxicity disqualifies it from further consideration. Nicotinamide is not known to affect immune function, but animal studies suggest that it can help β-cells to survive in a hostile environment. Its effects in humans following diagnosis are measurable, but clinically unimportant. The most evidence-based means of preserving β-cell function after diagnosis would be the introduction of intensified insulin therapy from the time of diagnosis. The Diabetes Control and Complications Trial demonstrated reciprocal benefit in those with high residual β-cell cell function – intensified therapy protects endogenous insulin secretion, and endogenous insulin secretion permits better control with less hypoglycaemia[1]. These effects may extend for six year following diagnosis, but it is doubtful whether lasting β-cell survival can be achieved beyond this point[2].

Clinicians are sometimes accused of spending more time speculating about the possible benefits of untried therapies than in implementing what is already known. There is certainly reluctance to attempt strict glucose control in those newly diagnosed, partly based on a reasonable wish not to add to the burden of diabetes at this early stage of the disease. The culture of diabetes care varies more between countries than the reader of a text on evidence-based medicine might imagine, but there is something quintessentially British about the desire not to provoke anxiety about future unpleasantness until the opportunity of doing anything useful to prevent it has lapsed. Further investigation of the feasibility, costs and benefits of early aggressive insulin therapy from diagnosis would clearly be justified. It is also clear that trials of immune intervention need to be carefully standardised for glucose control – a powerful reason for insisting on blinded trials wherever feasible in this situation.

The important message from all this is that useful numbers of β-cell are present in many new-onset patients, that it is possible to influence their survival over a matter of years, and that this has the potential to reduce both the risk of long-term complications and the fear of hypoglycaemia. These observations cannot be ignored, and provide justification for a variety of immune interventions currently planned or in trial, as described in Chapter 4. They do not, however, offer a means of disease prevention.

IS DISEASE PREVENTION POSSIBLE?

Although β-cell function can be preserved and extended beyond the time of diagnosis, there is little realistic hope of restoring normal metabolic function at this stage of the disease. it is therefore logical to attempt β-cell rescue at an earlier stage when the β-cell mass is largely intact. Work done over the past 25 years has transformed our understanding of the sequence of events culminating in immune-mediated β-cell failure, but the average diabetes specialist is still in the position of a nephrologist unable to identify renal dysfunction until his patients present for dialysis. Some 90–95% of children with type 1 diabetes have (HLA) human leukocyte antigen genotypes conferring susceptibility to the disease, but only around 5% of those with the highest risk combination will develop diabetes in childhood. Prospective studies have shown that islet autoantibodies typically appear within the first three years of life[3], although this should not be taken as dogma, and the influence of maternal age upon risk of diabetes in the offspring strongly suggests that prenatal influences may also have a part to play[4]. Single islet autoantibodies have little prognostic significance, but a mature humoral immune response involving multiple epitopes of more than one islet antigen is now taken to presage almost inevitable progression to diabetes, even after decades have elapsed[5]. Siblings of a child with diabetes are some 15 times more likely to develop diabetes that those with no family history, and there is a corresponding boost in the prognostic significance of gene and antibody markers in this high-risk population. Family members therefore provide a convenient, accessible and highly motivated group for trials of new therapies.

Against the background of this information, intervention can be considered at three levels: before detectable abnormalities are present (*primary intervention*); after development of immune markers of progression but before the onset of hyperglycaemia (*secondary prevention*); and after presentation with overt hyperglycaemia (*tertiary prevention*). Primary prevention should be offered as early in life as possible; in practice from soon after birth. For the reasons given above, children born to a family affected by diabetes, especially those who carry high-risk HLA genotypes, are most appropriate for trial interventions. Safety is the major criterion for any form of primary prevention, since this will inevitably have to be offered to many who would not in any case have developed the disease.

The safest and most rational form of primary prevention would be modification of environmental determinants of disease. Leading candidates in type 1 diabetes are viruses and infant nutrition. The congenital rubella syndrome is sometimes cited as evidence that a virus can cause type 1 diabetes, and that type 1 diabetes can be prevented by routine rubella vaccination. It is, however, far from certain that children with this syndrome have typical type 1 diabetes, and some clearly have an insulin-resistant form of the disease. Associations between enteroviral exposure *in utero* and subsequent development of diabetes in the child[6,7] raise the possibility that women might at some future date be vaccinated against a range of viruses, but the evidence base for such an intervention is far from established. The alternative environmental explanation, that exposure to cows' milk at an early stage of development might be diabetogenic, remains controversial[8]. The hypothesis is, however, susceptible to experimental testing, and a major multinational trial known as TRIGR (Trial to Reduce IDDM in the Genetically at Risk) is currently underway[9]. More direct forms of immune intervention in the newborn would appear unjustified at our present level of understanding of the disease process, although various forms of vaccination are under consideration.

Secondary prevention is based on prediction by means of circulating islet autoantibodies. The major trials described by Dr Skyler, DPT-1 (parenteral and oral insulin) and ENDIT (nicotinamide), were both based on the traditional islet cell antibodies (ICA) assay, and have confirmed its value as a predictive tool. Two developments, recognition of the predictive power of autoantibody combinations, and introduction of low volume radiobinding assays capable of automation, have advanced the field since then[10]. ENDIT, for example, screened >40 000 first-degree relatives in order to recruit 552 to a five-year placebo-controlled trial of high-dose nicotinamide. Reliance on ICA as the primary screening method meant inclusion of a proportion of lower-risk individuals who subsequently proved to carry no additional antibodies. In contrast, the vast majority of individuals with multiple autoantibodies will eventually develop diabetes[5], and the increased efficiency of screening is such that two trials the size of ENDIT could have been mounted from the same screening population[11].

ENDIT and DPT-1 have demonstrated the feasibility of large-scale controlled trials in antibody-positive first-degree relatives, but the logistics of these trials are on a continental scale, meaning that choice of one intervention might well delay the opportunity to test another by several years. Development of surrogate markers would help to overcome the scale and duration of trials based on progression to diabetes, but the development of cellular markers for this purpose is still in its infancy. For these reasons the current preferred strategy is to pilot interventions after diagnosis as a means of screening out those most suitable for use in major trials of secondary intervention[2].

WHERE NEXT?

It is logical to believe that improved understanding of disease will point the way to prevention. Happily for us, this is not always necessary. James Lind prevented scurvy with lime juice, Edward Jenner prevented smallpox by vaccination, and John Snow halted a cholera epidemic by removing the handle of the water pump in Broad Street, and all three advances were based on shrewd observation rather than scientific hypothesis.

A reasoned approach to the prevention of type 1 diabetes might, however, follow a series of steps as follows:

• What is the natural history of the disease process?
• Are there confirmed aetiological factors in the environment?
• At what stage of development are these operative?
• What are the markers of disease progression?
• What mechanisms are involved in the target organ?
• How might these be forestalled or interrupted?

Despite the massive literature that has accumulated around each of these issues, any critical assessment of the evidence rapidly reveals large holes and major uncertainties in this logical sequence. For example, a medical missionary from Mars with a remit to prevent type 1 diabetes would probably take one look at the 350-fold variation in incidence on our planet and ask what happens if you move people from the same ethnic background from one environment to another? No serious large-scale effort has ever been made to investigate this fundamental question, because that is not the way we conduct science. Conversely, hundreds of millions of dollars have been spent on investigation of diabetes in the non-obese diabetic (NOD) mouse in much the same spirit as Edward Mallory tackled Mount Everest – 'because it is there'. It might be assumed that everything possible is known about the natural history of the disease process in the human model of diabetes, but textbook accounts, faithfully reflected in the introductory paragraphs of articles in high impact scientific journals, typically present a simplified and misleading impression of the disease. Aside from the fact that the phenotype of the disease is changing, and that there is therefore no constant relationship between genotype and phenotype, such accounts typically present type 1 diabetes as a childhood disease. This is at best a half-truth, since at least 50% of cases present in adult life[13] and, depending upon definition, the proportion of adult cases of immune-mediated disease may be much higher than this. A combination of genuine methodological difficulty and semantic confusion has meant that little consensus exists concerning the frequency and definition of immune-mediated diabetes in later life.

There are other fundamental questions to ask. Is the development of childhood diabetes an either-or process? Or does presentation in childhood simply represent acceleration of a slow-burn disease process that is prevalent in the adult population? The rise of childhood type 1 diabetes can be traced back to the middle of the twentieth century, which showed an average annual increase of 2–4% over much of this period[14,15]. An increase of this magnitude in genetically stable populations strongly suggests that environmental influences are important. My own bias is to believe that a more permissive environment drives earlier onset of the disease, a concept I refer to as the 'spring harvest' hypothesis. In this view, 'prevention' of the disease means putting a historical trend into reverse, thus pushing disease onset back into later life where its psychosocial and pathological consequences are likely to prove less devastating[16].

In the interim, cautious trial of immune intervention therapy at diagnosis, as described in Chapter 4, seems fully justified. Induction of mucosal tolerance currently seems the safest and most logical form of intervention, since it attempts to re-educate the immune system rather than to override it[17]. Unfortunately, this form of intervention has proved to be disappointing, possibly because it has been used too late in the disease process. Other, more aggressive forms of immune intervention hold out some promise, but may prove to offer little more than a stay of execution. The human immune system is currently much smarter than we are, and it seems wisest to hesitate before lobbing bombs as it with limited insight into the possible consequences this may have.

REFERENCES

1. Diabetes Control and Complications Trial Research Group (1998). Effect of intensive therapy on residual β-cell function in patients with type 1 diabetes in the Diabetes Control and Complications Trial. *Annals of Internal Medicine* **128**: 517–523.

2. Kolb H, Gale EAM (2001) Does partial preservation of residual beta-cell function justify immune intervention in recent onset type 1 diabetes? *Diabetologia* **44**: 1349–1353.
3. Ziegler A-G, Hummel M, Schenker M, Bonifacio E (1999) Autoantibody appearance and risk for development of childhood diabetes in offspring of parents with type 1 diabetes. *Diabetes* **48**: 460–468.
4. Stene LC, Magnus P, Lie RT, Søvik O, Joner G (2001) Maternal and paternal age at delivery, birth order, and risk of childhood onset type 1 diabetes. *British Medical Journal* **323**: 369–371.
5. Gardner SG, Gale EAM, Williams AJK, Gillespie KM, Lawrence KM, Bottazzo GF, Bingley PJ (1999) Progression to diabetes in relatives with islet autoantibodies: is it inevitable? *Diabetes Care* **22**: 2049–2054.
6. Graves PM, Norris JM, Pallansch MA, Gerling IC, Rewers M (1997) The role of enteroviral infections in the development of IDDM. Limitations of current approaches. *Diabetes* **46**: 161–168.
7. Viskari HR, Koskela P, Lonnrot M, Luonuansuu S, Reunanen A, Baer M, *et al.* (2000) Can enterovirus infections explain the increasing incidence of type 1 diabetes? *Diabetes Care* **23**: 414–415.
8. Harrison LC, Honeyman MC (1999) Cows' milk and type 1 diabetes. The real debate is about mucosal immune function. *Diabetes* **48**: 1501–1507.
9. Hämäläinen A-M, Ronkainen MS, Åkerblom HK, Knip M and the Finnish TRIGR Study Group (2000) Post-natal elimination of transplacentally acquired disease-associated antibodies in infants born to families with type 1 diabetes. *Journal of Clinical Endocrinology and Metabolism* **85**: 4249–4253.
10. Bingley PJ, Bonifacio E, Gale EAM (1999) Predicting type 1 diabetes. In Marshall SM, Home PD, Rizza RA (eds) *The Diabetes Annual*, Volume 12. Elsevier, New York, p. 1–20.
11. Bingley PJ, Williams AJK, Gale EAM (1999) Optimized autoantibody based risk assessment in family members: implications for future intervention trials. *Diabetes Care* **22**: 1796–1801.
12. Karvonen M, Viik-Kajander M, Moltchanova E, Libman IM, LaPorte RE, Tuomilchto J (2000) Incidence of childhood type 1 diabetes worldwide. *Diabetes Care* **23**: 1516–1526.
13. Onkamo P, Vaananen S, Karvonen M, Tuomilchto J (1999) Worldwide increase in incidence of Type I diabetes – the analysis of the date on published incidence trends. *Diabetologia* **42**: 1395–1403.
14. EURODIAB ACE Study Group (2000) Variation and trends in incidence of childhood diabetes in Europe. *Lancet* **355**: 873–876.
15. Gale EAM (2002) The rise of childhood type 1 diabetes in the twentieth century. *Diabetes* (in press).
16. Gale EAM (2002) A missing link in the hygiene hypothesis? *Diabetologia* **45**: 588–594.
17. Gale EAM (2000) Oral tolerance and autoimmune diabetes – will hope triumph over experience? *Lancet* **356**: 526–527.

6

Prevention of Type 2 diabetes

RICHARD F. HAMMAN

University of Colorado School of Medicine, Denver, Colorado, USA

INTRODUCTION

Eliot P. Joslin, founder of the Joslin Clinic in Boston, Massachusetts, may have been the first to propose primary prevention of what is now classified as type 2 diabetes. In 1921 he wrote:

A real headway against the ravages of a disease begins with its prevention rather than its treatment. Prevention implies a knowledge of the predisposing agency. Overweight is a predisposition to diabetes. The individual overweight is at least twice, and at some ages forty times, as liable to the disease. For the prevention of more than half of the cases of diabetes in this country, no radical undernutrition is necessary; the individual is simply asked to maintain the weight of his average fellow man. Diabetes, therefore, is largely a penalty of obesity, and the greater the obesity, the more likely is Nature to enforce it. Granted there is one person in a thousand who has some inherent peculiarity of the metabolism which has led to obesity, but there are 999 for whom being fat implies too much food or too little exercise, or both combined.[1]

Reproduced with permission

Since that time, substantial research has confirmed and extended these observations. In addition to the role of obesity as a major risk factor, studies aimed at understanding the basic pathogenesis and physiology have led us closer to an understanding of the interacting pathways leading to type 2 diabetes mellitus. It has become clearer in the past two years that interventions aimed at reversing these steps can succeed in optimal circumstances (efficacious interventions) due to the completion of three randomized trials of diabetes pre-

The Evidence Base for Diabetes Care. Edited by R. Williams, W. Herman, A.-L. Kinmonth and N. J. Wareham.
© 2002 John Wiley & Sons, Ltd

vention. However, much work remains to understand how to intervene in an effective and efficient way to prevent diabetes in large numbers of people.

Most of the work reviewed here focuses on interventions aimed at individuals, to alter lifestyle and to reduce the metabolic derangements now known to be part of the pathways to disease. Less work has been done on broader social and psychological determinants, yet it may be that primary prevention will require a combination of both individual and societal approaches to be successful. In a later section, the limited attempts to change the environment of schools, churches and communities is reviewed.

There have been a number of summaries of the primary prevention of type 2 diabetes, previously called non-insulin dependent diabetes mellitus (NIDDM), which serve as a background for this review[2-16]. Here, the focus is on studies that attempt to prevent the onset of type 2 diabetes through lifestyle modification, reduction in obesity or through pharmacological means. Studies that attempt to understand the subsequent development of complications of diabetes after onset, even if detected during an asymptomatic stage, are not included here but are dealt with in Chapter 9. Chapter 8 deals with the evidence surrounding the early detection of type 2 diabetes through screening.

RATIONALE FOR THE PREVENTION OF TYPE 2 DIABETES

Several observations align to indicate the increasing need to prevent type 2 diabetes, rather than simply treat it, once established. Chapter 1 has mentioned the increasing prevalence and incidence, excess mortality and limited effectiveness of interventions. In addition to these, diabetes, and particularly type 2 diabetes, incurs high health care costs.

Estimates of costs vary depending on the methods used[17], but from $60[18] to $100 billion[19] in health care costs were spent on diabetes in the USA in 1995, which is variously estimated to be 6–17% of all health care costs. The majority of health care costs for diabetes are spent in developed countries, whereas estimates suggest that the majority of disability-adjusted life years (DALYs) are lost in developing countries, where limited health care budgets are available to deal with the problems of diabetes[18]. Recent studies from US health maintenance organizations (HMOs) have shown approximately two-fold increases in medical care expenses within the first year after diagnosis[20], with the highest expenses being incurred for hospitalizations due to coronary heart disease (CHD) and end-stage renal disease[21] (ESRD).

Eastman *et al.*[22] have estimated that primary prevention of type 2 diabetes, given reasonable assumptions, could be cost-effective, and within the range of other primary prevention activities currently undertaken[23] if there were efficacious interventions available. It is the purpose of this chapter to review relevant data to determine if such interventions exist.

REQUIREMENTS TO PREVENT A CHRONIC DISEASE

As is further developed in Chapter 8 in relation to screening, several pieces of knowledge must be available in order to know if it is possible to prevent any chronic disorder, including diabetes. These include a knowledge of the natural history of diabetes (with a reasonably long pre-clinical phase of the natural history), an effective and simple screening test or tests for a high-risk state, and effective interventions that, if applied earlier in the pre-clinical phase, would prevent or delay the onset of the disease.

The pre-clinical stages of the development of type 2 diabetes are well known. For many years it has been shown that glucose levels become elevated prior to the development of diabetes. This stage of the natural history has been called 'chemical diabetes', IGT[24,25], or most recently IFG[26]. However, when fasting glucose begins to rise, this may be a pathophysiologically later stage than is IGT, which usually has elevations of post-challenge glucose as the first detectable change. The use of IFG has only recently been studied, and a full understanding of its prognostic implications are not understood. Nonetheless, impairment of glucose regulation at levels which are lower than used for diagnosis increases the risk of subsequent diabetes from five- to eight-fold[27]. Thus, there is at least one pre-clinical stage for intervention prior to the development of diabetes.

Two major questions need to be answered: (1) Are there efficacious and effective interventions to prevent (or delay) the onset of diabetes? and (2) Does treatment at the time of early diagnosis reduce complications as much or perhaps more than waiting until the time of usual clinical intervention? This chapter will summarize the available clinical trials and observational studies relevant to the first question. The second question is dealt with in Chapter 8.

SELECTION CRITERIA FOR STUDIES

Studies are included if they were either randomized controlled trials (RCTs) or community-based trials, or if they were large, prospective epidemiological studies of sufficient rigor and generalizability to be useful. Some of the historically important studies in diabetes prevention do not meet these criteria for quality but they are mentioned for completeness, with comments about their design or conduct. The numerous clinical, ecological, cross-sectional and retrospective studies that have been conducted have been largely omitted, unless they provide the only evidence bearing on an issue.

Studies were identified through computerized searches of several databases, including Medline, CINAHL, Health Plan, PsycLIT, Helmis, Cochrane Collaboration and Best Evidence. Standard MESH terms were often only partially successful in identifying relevant articles, which were primarily found through a combination of searching published reference lists and contacts with investigators. Unpublished prevention trials were sought through contacts with researchers, although none were found that had been completed but not published. Trials in progress are included in a later section of this chapter. Classification of evidence used in this chapter is shown in Table 6.1, which is based on the US Preventive Service Task Force Criteria[28] for individual studies, and NHLBI (National Heart, Lung and Blood Institute of the NIH) evidence criteria[29] for overall recommendations.

DEFINITION OF TYPE 2 DIABETES MELLITUS

The studies reviewed here use a variety of criteria to define type 2 diabetes. This is inevitable, given the long time period included. It was not possible to identify consistent criteria for all studies. However, the 1985 WHO criteria[24] were used as a reference when possible since the majority of modern studies used them. In prevention trials, the development of any clinical diagnosis of diabetes or measured hyperglycemia meeting defined criteria was usually the outcome of the trial.

No studies published to date have tested for autoimmune markers that would identify subjects developing type 1 diabetes. Since over 90% of people developing diabetes over the age of 50 years will have type 2 diabetes[30], this is a minor limitation. However, proper diagnosis of the etiological type of diabetes as an outcome will become increasingly important in trials in the future, since specific interventions aimed at defined metabolic and immunological pathways will increasingly be tested.

NATURAL HISTORY AND RISK FACTORS FOR TYPE 2 DIABETES

Primary prevention of diabetes requires a thorough knowledge of the natural history of the development of glucose intolerance and risk factors. Once these have been established from observational studies, it is at least theoretically possible that interventions aimed at any of the factors could reduce diabetes risk. A number of recent reviews of risk factors exist[8,31-39], and are summarized in Table 6.2 for individual level risk factors, that is, those that operate on or within a person. This table does not include group-, societal-, or population-level risk factors such as Westernization, commercialization of the food supply, increased motorized transport, television and computer time replacing group and individual activity and interaction, and changes in social mores which alter individual factors over large numbers of people simultaneously.

The information about possible genes related to or causing type 2 diabetes is not included here, since, in the short term, gene-based interventions are unlikely to be available. In the longer term, such approaches may prove feasible and may facilitate a more targeted prevention strategy. Table 6.2 does

Table 6.1. Summary of criteria to evaluate individual studies (1) and overall recommendations (2).

1	U.S. Preventive Service Task Force Criteria[28] (modified by author)
Ia	Properly randomized controlled trials
Ib	Randomized, but with departures from best methods (sequential, date of birth, etc.); conduct otherwise acceptable
Ic	As Ib, but conduct not adequate (high dropout rate (30+%), lack of blinding, etc.)
II-1	Well-designed controlled trials without randomization
II-2	Well-designed cohort or case-control analytic studies, preferably from more than one center or research group; multiple time series with or without intervention
II-2b	Less rigorously conducted observational studies; high dropout rates, etc.
II-3	Dramatic results in uncontrolled experiments; opinions of respected authorities, based on clinical experience
III	Descriptive studies and case reports, or reports of expert committees

2		NHLBI criteria for overall recommendations[29]
A	RCTs* – rich body of data	Evidence is from endpoints of well-designed RCTS (or trials that depart only minimally from randomization) that provide a consistent pattern of findings in the population for which the recommendation is made. Requires substantial numbers of studies involving substantial numbers of subjects
B	RCTs* – limited body of data	Evidence is from endpoints of intervention studies that include only a limited number of RCTs, post-hoc or subgroup analysis of RCTs, or meta-analysis of RCTs. Category B pertains when few RCTs exist, they are small in size, and the trial results are somewhat inconsistent, or the trials were undertaken in a population that differs from the target population of the recommendation
C	Non-randomized trials, observational studies	Evidence is from outcomes of uncontrolled or nonrandomized trials or from observational studies
D	Panel consensus judgment	Expert judgment is based on the panel's synthesis of evidence from experimental research described in the literature and/or derived from the consensus of panel members based on clinical experience or knowledge that does not meet the above criteria. This category is used only in cases where the provision of some guidance was deemed valuable but an adequately compelling clinical literature addressing the subject of the recommendation was deemed insufficient to justify placement in one of the other categories (A-C)

* RCT = randomized controlled trial

not indicate that there may be important heterogeneity of risk, between genders for example, or between populations. Such heterogeneity has been suggested[40,41] and must be taken into account when designing interventions, especially across different population groups.

PREVENTION OF TYPE 2 DIABETES

Interventions have been targeted at altering a number of behavioral factors including obesity, dietary intake and physical activity. Obesity, of course, should be considered the result of behavioral, genetic and physiological factors and not simply behavioral. Pharmacological interventions have primarily used hypoglycemic or anti-hyperglycemic medication to reverse insulin resistance (biguanides, thiazolidenediones), failure of insulin secretion (sulfonylureas), or glycemic excursions (alpha-glucosidase inhibitors). Trials have attempted to alter glucose metabolism using metal supplementation (magnesium, chromium) or antioxidants (beta-carotene, vitamin E). Trials that have used

Table 6.2. Summary of established and possible* individual level risk factors for type 2 diabetes mellitus

Demographic variables	Obesity-related variables
Older age	Higher total adiposity
Male gender	Central fat distribution
Ethnic group	Intra-abdominal fat
Family history of diabetes	Longer duration of obesity
Maternal history of diabetes	Weight gain

Physiological variables	Reproductive variables
High glucose level (fasting and post-challenge)	Diabetes during pregnancy
Low insulin secretion	*Higher parity*
Insulin resistance syndrome (low HDL-C, high triglycerides, hypertension, fibrinolytic defects, glucose intolerance)	*Lack of breast-feeding*

	Dietary variables
Low magnesium level	High caloric intake
Low chromium level	*High total and saturated fat intake*
High plasma non-esterified fatty acids	*Low alcohol intake*
Low sex hormone binding globulin	*Low fiber intake*
Low physical activity	*High glycemic index foods*
Cigarette smoking	*Low Vitamin D intake*
	Low magnesium intake
	Low potassium intake
	Low polyunsaturated fatty acid intake
	Low vegetable fat intake
	Low wholegrain intake

*Variables in italics are not firmly established – differing amounts of evidence exist to support them, although the balance of observational data favors them at this time

pharmacological interventions to reverse obesity include a wider range of anti-obesity agents, since obesity is one of the common pathways through which diabetes develops. Each of these approaches is reviewed below.

Combined lifestyle

Table 6.3 summarizes the intervention studies that have attempted to prevent type 2 diabetes using a combination of lifestyle interventions. These typically include dietary intervention of various types together with increased physical activity. The intensity of the intervention for either component has often varied substantially. Inclusion criteria have also been variable, with most studies using people without diabetes. A small number have included some people classified as having diabetes by older, more sensitive criteria. These would probably now be classified predominantly as IGT or IFG by current criteria.

Several diabetes-related end-points have been studied, including glucose tolerance testing with various criteria, infusion tests and fasting glucose levels. Studies have been included that examine these multiple end-points, since they may inform future trial designs. In each section, RCTs of varying rigor are included by the year in which they were first published, followed by non-randomized interventions. Then, in the case of physical activity and diet, the evidence from prospective observational studies is summarized.

RCTs

Following a community screening program in Uppsala, Sweden, Cederholm[42] identified 51 people with glucose intolerance classified by 1980 WHO criteria[25]. He was able to sequentially randomize 43 of these to a diet and physical activity regimen for six months (n = 25) or to no advice or treatment (n = 18). After six months, the intervention group was 2.2 times (CI 0.8–5.6) more likely to have normal glucose tolerance than the controls. Inverting this relative risk for consistency with other prevention studies, subjects were 0.67 times (CI 0.43–1.05) times as likely to remain abnormal, given the intervention. The absolute risk reduction (ARR) was 25.8/100, or a 33.2% risk reduction (% RR).There were significant, though small, decreases in glucose area under the OGTT curve, systolic BP, BMI, cholesterol and triglycerides compared to the controls.

Among the 13 people who remained glucose-intolerant at six months, 10 took 1.25 mg a day of glipizide for an additional six months, and four returned to normal glucose tolerance. Since control subjects were not retested at 12 months, it is impossible to determine if this improvement was due to the drug, or simply to further follow-up and continuation of the diet and physical activity programme. Lack of follow-up of the controls means that the drug intervention is an unblinded and uncontrolled observation which is not

Table 6.3. Combined lifestyle Interventions in the primary prevention of type 2 diabetes mellitus and related abnormalities.

Author, Reference, evidence code	Population	Intervention	Results	Comments
Combined lifestyle interventions – randomized controlled trials (RCTs)				
Cederholm 1985[42] 1b	**Uppsala, Sweden** 53 subjects aged 47–54 years with glucose intolerance by 1980 WHO criteria: follow-up 6 months. Outcome: diabetes	**Diet + exercise (N = 25):** lower sugar, fat, calories; at 6 months with abnormal OGTT, given glipizide (N = 10). **Control (N = 18):** no advice or therapy	**Diet + exercise: (RR) = 0.67** (0.43–1.05)¹ ARR = 25.8/100 PY to remain glucose-intolerant on OGTT at 6 months versus control. Decrease in glucose AUC, relative BMI, chol., TGs and SBP (p <0.01). **Glipizide:** 4/10 became normal in additional 4–6 months; no control data	Glipizide given to 10/13 persons who did not normalize OGTT at 6 months, but no controls were followed, so these data are not interpretable. Unmasked sequential randomization; no multivariate analysis
Nilsson, *et al.* 1992[43] 1b	**Dalby, Sweden** 63 subjects aged 56 yrs with hyperinsulinemia (≥75th percentile on OGTT): follow-up 1 yr. Outcome: glucose	**Diet + exercise (N = 31):** walking, cycling, gardening. Diet was low-fat, high-fiber, lower calorie. **Control (N = 32)** No intervention	**Diet + exercise:** lost 2.2 kg weight, no changes in F or 2 hr glucose level; insulin and C-peptide levels decreased significantly from baseline. **Control:** increases in glucose levels, no change in weight, insulin or C-peptide. Lipid changes similar in both groups.	12 subjects had IGT – changes similar in all subjects, no apparent improvement in glucose levels. Allocation not masked. Groups small, only one year of follow-up. Dropout rate was 9%
Page *et al.* 1992[44] 1a	**Oxford feasibility study** 31 subjects aged 18–60 years. $\bar{x}$ = 40 years. Two abnormal CIGMA tests not diabetic or normal at baseline; follow-up 2 yrs. Outcome: Glucose	**Diet + exercise (N = 23):** low fat, sugar, increase exercise (20′ × 3 per week); weight loss to BMI <25) for 6 months actively, then told to continue for up to 24 months. **Control (N = 8):** no advice	**Diet + exercise:** No change in F glucose at 6, 24 months. One BMI unit weight loss in each group at 6 months, no change overall at 2 years. Significant decrease in SBP and $V0_{2 \, max}$ at 6 months, not maintained at 2 years	Intention to treat presented. 4/18 lifestyle subjects were noncompliant and 5 dropped out within 6 months. Intensity of intervention limited. Randomization schedule not said to be masked. CIGMA not directly comparable to oral IGT.
Singh *et al.* 1993[46] 1b	**Indian Diet Heart Study** Moradabad, India 621 volunteers aged 21–68 yrs. $\bar{x}$ =48 yrs. Follow-up 24 weeks. Outcome: glucose	**Diet + exercise: (N = 310):** moderately intensive intervention of low-fat, high fruit and vegetable diet plus exercise. **Control (N = 311)** limited advice	**Diet + exercise:** lost 3.6 kg weight; F glucose decreased significantly (−1.16 mmol/L). BP and lipids improved. No OGTT done. Changes were greatest in those making most lifestyle change. **Control:** Lost 1.4 kg weight; no	Randomization by card: single blind to physician. Intention to treat analysis. Subjects not very overweight at baseline (BMI $\bar{x}$ = 24, range 21–28). No long-term follow-up. 104/621 with diabetes at baseline by non-WHO criteria (fasting whole blood

Table 6.3. contd.

Study	Intervention	Results	Comments
Katzel et al. 1995[45,47] Ic	**Baltimore, MD** 170 males aged 46–80 years x̄ = 61 yrs randomized to 3 groups, follow-up 9–12 months. Outcome: IGT	**Weight loss:** decreased IGT prevalence from 57% to 41%. F and 2 hr glucose, F insulin and insulin AUC decreased (p <0.001). Lipids and BP improved in weight loss versus control. **Exercise:** IGT prevalence stable (47% versus 49% pre-post); glucose levels and AUC increased in exercise group, but 2 h insulin area decreased. BP did not change versus controls. TG decreased, but prevalence of CVD risk profiles did not. **Control:** IGT increased from 44% to 67% (p = 0.06 versus weight loss) and all glucose and insulin parameters increased	change in F glucose (−0.04 mmol/L) Healthy subjects with negative stress or thallium ETT. Allocation masking and randomization method not stated. Less than one year of follow-up. Not blinded. Lipid changes in exercise group were completely due to weight loss, not exercise. Fewer changes in older men than younger ones. Diet and exercise groups were evaluated at ~10 months, controls at ~1 year. Dropouts = 33% in weight loss, 31% in exercise and control groups. No differences between baseline values of dropouts and continuing subjects
	Weight loss (N = 73): intensive behavioral education. **Exercise** (N = 71): endurance training aimed at increasing V0$_{2max}$. **Control** (N = 26): limited education		glucose >6.1 mmol/L and 2 hr >7.7 mmol/L) – probably includes many subjects with IGT rather than diabetes
Hellenius et al. 1995[48,49] Ic	**Sollentuna, Sweden** 157 healthy men aged 35–60 (x̄ = 46) years randomized to four groups, follow-up 6 months. Outcome: glucose	**Diet:** no weight loss. **Exercise:** −0.3 BMI unit weight loss, lower F insulin and insulin AUC. **Diet + exercise:** −0.6 BMI unit weight loss, lower F insulin and insulin AUC. 6–8% increase in F glucose, no significant change in OGTT, no differences between groups. Higher IGF binding protein-1 in all intervention groups, but greatest in D+E, suggesting improved insulin resistance and secretion	No multivariate analysis, no mention of dropouts or compliance. Intervention was done by physicians and dietitians, early in trial. Not clear how much reinforcement given. No masking of allocation or statement of blinding
	Diet (N = 40): lower calorie, fat, alcohol. **Exercise** (N = 39): aerobic, 30–45 minutes 2–3 times per week to 60–80% of heart rate. **Diet + exercise** (N = 39): both diet and exercise. **Control** (N = 39): no intervention		
Coleman et al. 1995[50] Ic	**Fitness after 45, Baltimore, MD USA** 99 men aged x̄ = 60 years, randomized 12-month follow-up; analyzed like nonrandomized study	**Weight loss:** IGT RR = 0.3 (0.10–0.91)[1] among normals at entry; 25–28% decrease in OGTT glucose and insulin areas, 20% decrease in fasting insulin levels. 21% increase in hyperglycemic clamp M value (more insulin	52% dropout rate in weight loss group, 42% in controls; no blinding. 15 NGT in weight loss group, 9 in control at baseline. Analysis is like nonrandomized study
	Weight loss (N = 73): 3 months on American Heart Association Step 1 diet, then 9 months hypocaloric diet. **Weight maintenance** (N = 26): 12 months of AHA Step		

Table 6.3. contd.

Reference	Study	Intervention	Results	Comments
	due to dropouts. Outcome: IGT	1 maintenance diet	sensitive) in 8 subjects. **Weight maintenance:** 32% increase in OGTT glucose area; no changes in insulin levels or areas	
Anderssen *et al.* 1996[52,53] Ib	**Oslo Diet and Exercise Study (ODES), Norway** 219 subjects (198 men, 21 women) aged 40 years in unmasked, randomized 2 × 2 factorial design, follow-up at one year. Outcome: glucose	**Diet** (N = 55): reduced calorie, low fat in 3 sessions. **Exercise** (N = 54): supervised 3 × per week to 60–80% of peak heart rate. **Diet + exercise** (N = 67): both diet and exercise. **Control** (N = 43): no intervention	**Diet:** −1.63 BMI unit weight loss; decreased FPG, 1 hr insulin. **Exercise:** −0.65 BMI unit weight loss; decreased 1 hr insulin, no change in FPG versus control. **Diet + exercise:** −2.2 BMI unit weight loss, decreased FPG, insulin, increased VO_{2max} versus control	BMI >24, DBP 86–99 mmHg, unmasked study, allocation not said to be blinded. Dropouts 4.6% in 1 year – highest in exercise group (9.3%). Groups similar at entry. No multivariate adjustment for minor differences; no note of IGT or DM status
Torjesen *et al.* 1997[54], Anderssen *et al.* 1998[53] Ib	**Oslo Diet and Exercise Study (ODES), Norway** As above	As above	**Diet:** −1.3 BMI unit weight loss; decreased HOMA-R, fasting C-peptide, proinsulin, TGs, mean BP, increased HDL-C. **Exercise:** −0.3 BMI unit weight loss; decreased mean BP, increased HDL-C, lower HOMA-R (p = 0.18). **Diet + exercise:** −3.7 BMI unit weight loss; decreased HOMA-R, FPG, 1 hour glucose, mean BP, TGs, increased HDL-C. **Control:** +0.4 BMI unit weight gain No change in PAI-1 in any group	Note differences to previous report of same subjects for amount of weight loss. Changes in HOMA-B (insulin secretion) inconsistent. Change in BMI correlated with change in HOMA-R in diet group, but not in exercise or diet + exercise groups. Later paper[53] shows that change in waist circumference post-intervention was the most important determinant of changes in glucose and insulin levels, independent of fitness. Also predicted change in hemostatic variables (euglobulin clot lysis time, factor VII)
Pan *et al.* 1997[55] Ib	**DaQing IGT and Diabetes Study, China** 577 over-25-year-olds with IGT by WHO criteria, randomized by clinic, followed for 6 years. Outcome: diabetes	**Diet** (N = 130): lower fat, alcohol, higher vegetables; weight loss in those with BMI ≥25. **Exercise** (N = 141): increase by 1 unit/day (local scale). **Diet + exercise** (N = 126). **Control** (N = 133): information only	**Diet:** 10.0/1000 PY RR* = 0.69 (p = 0.028), ARR = 5.7/1000 PY. **Exercise:** 8.3/1000 PY RR* = 0.54 (p = 0.000), ARR = 7.4/1000 PY. **Diet + exercise:** 9.6/1000 PY RR* = 0.58 (p = 0.001), ARR = 6.1/1000 PY. **Control:** 15.7/1000 PY RR* = 1.0 * adjusted for FPG, BMI at baseline	Randomized by clinic; 8.1% dropout in 6 years. Similar results in lean and obese subjects. No blinding; allocation not masked, since by clinic

Table 6.3. contd.

Dyson *et al.* 1997[56,280] Ib	**Fasting Hyperglycemia Study (FHS) II** (Lifestyle) UK and France; 227 persons aged 30–65 ($\bar{x}$ = 50 yrs); factorial design with sulfonylurea; follow-up 1 year. Outcome: diabetes	**Basic lifestyle** (N = 116); **Reinforced lifestyle** (N = 111): low-fat diet, increased fiber, hypocaloric if BMI ≥22; aerobic physical activity given once a year in basic group, and every 3 months in reinforced group	**Basic:** 1.5 kg weight loss at 3 months, no change at 1 year; no changes in percentage with diabetes, glucose intolerance, or high BP. **Reinforced:** weight loss similar to basic group; no changes in percentage with diabetes, glucose intolerance or high BP; fitness, insulin sensitivity, TGs significantly improved	Dropouts 18% in reinforced advice, 7% in basic advice at 1 year. Randomization schedule not masked
Wing *et al.* 1998[59] Ic	**Pittsburgh, PA, USA** 154 overweight nondiabetics aged 40–55 years ($\bar{x}$ = 46) with 1 + diabetic parent; follow-up up to 2 years. 72/154 with IGT at baseline. Outcome: diabetes	**Diet** (N = 37): low fat, low calorie. **Exercise** (N = 37): 1500 Kcal/wk moderate exercise. **Diet + exercise** (N = 40): combination of other interventions. **Control** (N = 40): written material	**6 months:** decreases in F glucose, F insulin in D and D+E groups; also in lipids, BP. **12 months:** No change in F glucose between groups, though weight loss maintained in D, D+E at 60% and 72% of 6 month levels. **24 months:** Control 7% with diabetes: **D:** 30.3%; **E:** 14%; **D + E:** 15.6%. FPG, OGTT, weight loss did not differ between groups. In multivariate model, −4.5 kg weight loss (4.5% of initial weight) predicted RR of 0.696 (0.526–0.865) for type 2 DM among NGT; RR = 0.744 (0.592–0.897) among IGT subjects. No differences in type 2 diabetes between intervention groups, once weight loss accounted for	Groups similar at baseline. Dropouts: 6 months, 15%; 12 months, 22%; 24 months, 16%. Class attendance averaged only 27% in last 18 months. Little change in diet or exercise at 24 months between groups. Much of the cohort not exposed to intervention during the last 18 months. Not blinded; allocation not said to be masked. Intention to treat analysis used on persons attending follow-up
Narayan *et al.* 1998[60] Ic	**Pima Indians, AZ, USA** 95 overweight nondiabetic subjects aged 25–54 years ($\bar{x}$ = 33.5), follow-up 1 year; pilot study. Outcome: glucose	**Action** (N = 48): diet and exercise advice without weight loss goals. **Pride** (N = 47): Pima culture, limited diet and activity information. Observational control (N = 22)	**Action:** 29% with 2 h glucose ≥7.8 mM/L; BMI (+0.9), BP, 2 h glucose (+1.3mM) and insulin (+8.8 pM) increased more than Pride. **Pride:** 11% with 2 h glucose ≥7.8 mM/L; decreased waist circumference; no increase in 2 h glucose (0.0), less increase in fasting and 2 h insulin (+3.2 pM), BMI (+0.5). **Observational control:** intermediate weight gain and glucose changes between two intervention groups	Class-based diet and exercise lifestyle intervention not effective; focus on cultural approaches and barriers to participation may be more successful. Blinded outcomes, intention to treat analysis; poor compliance with interventions (17–25% attendance at classes), but very low dropout rates for 6, 12 month evaluations (2–3%)

Table 6.3. contd.

Reference	Study	Intervention	Results	Comments
Weinstock *et al.* 1998[62] Ic	**Syracuse, NY, USA** 45 nondiabetic obese women aged x̄ = 43 years, with BMI x̄ = 35, followed for up to 2 years. Outcome: glucose	**Diet** (N = 15): Very low calorie (925 Kcal/d) increasing to 1500 Kcal/d by week 22. **Diet + aerobic exercise** (N = 14): Step aerobics 40 min/week. **Diet + resistance exercise** (N = 16): 40 min/week on large muscle groups	Nonsignificant decrease in F and AUC glucose. No difference between groups. Significantly lower F and AUC insulin to week 44 in all groups, so insulin sensitivity likely increased. F insulin rose in persons followed to week 44–96 weeks with only slight weight regain. Significant decreases in diastolic BP were equal across groups	**All groups treated: no control:** no additive effect of diet with either type of exercise, perhaps due to use of very low calorie diets for rapid weight loss. No important effect on glucose levels: no data presented on percentage with IGT. 20% dropout at 44 weeks; 51% at 96 weeks. Allocation not masked
Simkin-Silverman, *et al.* 1998[63] Kuller, *et al.* 2001[64]	**Women's Healthy Lifestyle Project.** Pittsburgh. PA, USA 535 premenopausal women aged 44–50 years (x̄ = 47): follow-up at 54 months. Outcome: glucose	**Lifestyle** (N = 253): lower fat, saturated fat, increased physical activity. **Control** (N = 236): assessment only	**Lifestyle:** −3.0 kg at 18 months, −0.1 kg at 54 months; F glucose +1.6 mg/dl (0.09 mmol/L); lower LDL-C, chol., and SBP; lower waist/hip ratio, TGs, and DBP at 6 months, did not persist at 18 or 54 months. **Control:** gained +2.4 kg at 54 months; F glucose +3.3 mg/dl (0.18 mmol/L)	5% dropouts at 54 months, dropouts similar except for higher BMI at entry (26.3 versus 25). Masking of allocation not noted. No OGTT conducted; diabetes rates not reported
Bergenstal *et al.* 1998[67] Ic	**Community Diabetes Prevention Project (CDPP),** Minnesota, USA 418 community-dwelling nondiabetic persons aged x̄ = 46 years; follow-up 2 yrs; in progress. Outcome: diabetes	**Intervention** (N = 209): diet, exercise, stress management yearly. **Standard** (N = 209) no intervention	RR = 1.0 (0.38–2.80) for diabetes progression (3.5% in each group); no changes in risk factors for insulin resistance at two years between groups	Low-intensity intervention with 2 meetings per year, monthly phone calls, newsletters. Details of randomization and blinding not given
Eriksson *et al.* 1999[68]; Tuomilehto 2001[69] Ia	**Diabetes Prevention Study (DPS)** Finland: 5 centers. 522 men and women aged x̄ = 55 years. BMI = 31, WHO IGT × 2: follow-up 3.2 years. Outcome: diabetes by WHO criteria	**Intervention** (N = 265): diet, exercise, weight loss in 7 sessions in year 1, then 4 times per year. **Control** (N = 257): annual information	Lifestyle incidence rate = 3.2/100 PY versus control = 7.8/100 PY. HR = 0.4 (0.3–0.7) for incident diabetes. ARR = 4.6/100 PY; 58% reduction	Achieved 4.2 kg weight loss in intervention group. Persons with best compliance to lifestyle change had greatest reduction in incidence
DPP Research Group 2001[70-72] Ia	**Diabetes Prevention Program (DPP)** 27 US centers. 3234 men	**Intensive lifestyle** (N = 1079): 16 session curriculum on diet, activity.	Lifestyle incidence rate = 4.8/100 PY versus placebo = 11.0/100 PY; 58% reduction in incidence; similar in both	Achieved 5.6 kg weight loss in lifestyle versus 0.1 kg in placebo groups. Suggestion of greater reduction in

Table 6.3. contd.

	and women; 45% noncaucasian; aged x̄ = 51 years, BMI = 34; follow-up 2.8 years. Outcome: diabetes by ADA criteria	weight loss; at least monthly contact with coach. **Placebo** (N = 1082): annual meeting with written material on lifestyle	genders, all ethnic groups, all ages; ARR = 6.2/100 PY	persons >60 years (71%); NNT = 6.9 to prevent one case
Lifestyle Intervention Studies (non-randomized)				
O'Dea 1984[73] II-3	**Traditional lifestyle in Australian Aborigines, Darby, W. Australia** Pre-post analysis of 14 urban-living subjects, x̄ = 54 years; 7-week intervention. Outcome: diabetes	**Urban diet (pre):** 50% carbohydrate, 40% fat, 10% protein. Subjects hunted/gathered all food in bush for 7 weeks. **Bush diet (post):** approx. 33% carbohydrate, 13% fat, 54% protein	**Diabetes** (N = 10): Average weight loss 1.2 kg/week (−8.1 kg total); decreased F glucose and insulin (p <0.001), glucose AUC by 37%, TGs by −2.87 mmol/L (p <0.001), incremental insulin response improved 72%; 7/10 nondiabetic by ADA fasting criteria; 3/10 became IGT, 0/10 became normal by WHO criteria. **Normal** (N = 4): average weight loss −5.8 kg: glucose AUC lower (p <0.05), no change in F glucose, insulin; decreased TGs	Greater changes in fasting than post-challenge glucose and insulin among persons with diabetes
Eriksson and Lindgarde 1991[57] II-1	**Malmö feasibility study** 217 men aged 47–49 with IGT, follow-up at 6 years. Outcome: diabetes	**Diet and exercise:** (N = 181); **Control:** IGT (N = 79); **Control:** NGT (N = 114)	**Diet + exercise:** significant weight loss, mostly maintained for 6 years; 6-year incidence of diabetes: 10.6/100 PY RR = 0.49 (0.25–0.97), ARR = 10.8/100 PY. **Control:** no weight loss; 6-year incidence of diabetes: 21.4/100 PY	Not randomized: subjects self-selected the intervention or control groups, though 95% of those invited agreed initially. Few details of intervention content or intensity. No blinding. Dropouts 29% in control, 11% in diet + exercise group
Eriksson and Lindgarde 1998[77] II-1	**Malmö feasibility study** 6956 subjects aged 47–49 at baseline, follow-up 12 years for mortality. Outcome: mortality	**Diet and exercise** (IGT, N = 288); **Control:** (IGT, N = 135); Normal (NGT, N = 6389); diabetes (N = 144)	All cause mortality RR = 0.49 (0.27–0.96), ARR = 7.5/1000 PY in IGT intervention group versus IGT controls, adjusted for BMI, smoking, SBP, cholesterol, and 2 h glucose at baseline. Mortality not different from NGT subjects in intervened subjects. Mortality highest in persons with diabetes at baseline	Not randomized. IGT intervention group ~90% compliant with diet and exercise at 6 years. Minimal baseline differences in major mortality and diabetes risk factors between nonrandomized groups. Follow-up completeness not stated for mortality; likely very high

Table 6.3. contd.

Visanathan *et al.* 1997[78] Ramachandran *et al.* 1999[79] II-2b	**Primary Prevention Diabetes Program, Madras, India** 262 persons with family history of diabetes, followed for at least 4 years, pre-post analysis. Outcome: diabetes	**Diet:** High-carbohydrate, low-fat (20%). **Exercise:** primarily 30 minutes per day walking	Persons who increased weight (versus lost weight or kept stable weight) were 5.1 (2.6–13.9) times more likely to develop diabetes, adjusted for baseline glucose and gender. Second analysis of similar smaller subset[119] found persons with normal OGTT more likely to exercise, and have less psychological stress than persons with diabetes at follow-up. No effect of diet compliance	Everyone had intervention in pre-post design. No estimate of dropouts. No blinding. Nested case-control designs

[1] Calculated from data available in the paper, not by the authors. AUC = area under the curve for glucose (AUC glucose) or insulin (AUC insulin); BP = blood pressure; TG = triglycerides; ARR = absolute risk reduction (if not present, data were insufficient to calculate); NNT = number needed to treat.

interpretable. This study adds limited information to the diet and physical activity knowledge, suggesting that short-term intervention with weight loss and modest increases in activity may help normalize glucose tolerance. Because of the short follow-up period and small sample size, it is not clear from this study whether such improvements can be maintained over longer periods.

A one-year intensive lifestyle intervention was conducted in people identified as hyperinsulinemic in Dalby, Sweden by Nilsson and co-workers[43]. Sixty-three hyperinsulinemic people (upper 25th percentile of insulin sum on OGTT) were randomly allocated to passive or active intervention, consisting of lower fat, higher fiber, lower calorie diets and increased physical activity, focused on walking, cycling and gardening. After one year, subjects in the active intervention group had lost 2.2 kg compared to 0.1 kg in the control group, and they had lower insulin and C-peptide levels than in the control group, with no changes in glucose tolerance. Subjects with IGT (n = 12) had similar results to those with normal glucose tolerance. The authors interpreted the fall in insulin and C-peptide as an improvement in insulin resistance. Limited changes in cardiovascular risk factors occurred, with only a small increase in HDL-C, and no change in triglyceride level.

A lifestyle intervention pilot study was completed in Oxford, the UK by Page and co-workers[44]. Thirty-one subjects with two abnormal but not diabetic CIGMA (glucose infusion) tests were randomly allocated to healthy living advice or to the control group in a 3:1 ratio. Intervention subjects were given active lifestyle advice (low fat, high carbohydrate and fiber advice, weight loss to <BMI 25 if obese; increased physical activity (20 minutes, three times per week)). Evaluations were done at six months, when active intervention was stopped, and again at two years.

At six months, there were small but significant increases in VO_{2max} and improvements in systolic BP, but there was no weight loss, and weight was the same in both groups. No changes occurred in fasting glucose levels at six months, and levels had increased in both groups at 24 months. At two years, cholesterol levels had declined similarly in both groups, but there were no other important changes. Compliance, even at six months, was only fair, with 6 out of 31 withdrawing from the study, most in the active intervention group. These results show the difficulty in obtaining weight loss or changes in end-points with limited interventions for lifestyle. They are also consistent with the short-term results of Katzel et al.[45], reviewed later in this chapter, who found that physical activity improvement, in the absence of weight loss, did not result in changes in glucose tolerance over six months.

Singh and colleagues conducted a 24-week diet and physical activity intervention in Moradabad, India to reduce cardiovascular risk factors[46]. They randomly allocated 310 volunteer subjects to intensive diet (low fat, high fruit and vegetable intake) and 311 to simpler written advice (controls) in a single blind design. Randomization used a simple card-based system which could be subject to investigator bias, though groups were reasonably similar at baseline. After 16 weeks, the intensive diet group was asked to increase its activity levels until evaluation at 24 weeks. While diabetes prevention was not the primary goal of this cardiovascular intervention, fasting glucose levels were measured and found to decrease significantly at 24 weeks in the intervention (-1.16 mmol/l or -21 mg/dl) compared with control (-0.04 mmol/l or -1 mg/dl) groups. Concomitantly there was a 3.6 kg weight loss in the intervention group versus only 1.4 kg loss among controls (p <0.05). The average weight was only 65 kg at study entry, however. BMI was not calculated. These data are from short-term follow-up but suggest that intensive lifestyle interventions (greater than those which were attempted in the Oxford pilot study[44]) did have short-term effects, even in people who were relatively non-obese at entry.

Investigators in Baltimore, Maryland conducted an RCT of weight loss versus endurance exercise training interventions (without an observed control group) in middle-aged and older males[45,47]. They recruited 170 healthy men (with no prior diagnoses of diabetes or heart disease, on no medication, with negative exercise stress tests) who were aged 61 years on average. The weight loss group lost an average of 9.5 kg and the prevalence of IGT dropped from 57% to 41% compared to increases in IGT in the control group (44% to 67%). IGT prevalence in the exercise group (who did not lose weight on average) was stable (47% versus 49% pre- to post-intervention). There were also significant decreases in glucose and insulin areas in the weight loss group, whereas only post-load insulin area decreased in the exercise group. There were several methodological problems, however. Drop-outs were over 30% in all groups; no mention was made of the development of diabetes; and no blinding was noted.

This study indicates that weight loss, rather than intensive physical activity, may have a greater impact on diabetes related variables, at least over the short term. Even in the physical activity group, those people with reduction in lipid levels had concomitant weight loss. Older men had less weight loss and other improvements than did younger men, suggesting that interventions in older subjects may be less productive.

A six-month RCT of diet and physical activity was conducted in healthy men (age 35-60, $\bar{x}$ = 46 years) in primary care centers in Sollentuna, Sweden by Hellenius and colleagues[48,49]. Four groups of 39–40 subjects were formed (diet, exercise, both and neither) and dietary advice on weight loss, lower fat and alcohol and higher carbohydrate intake was given over two weeks. Physical activity was increased to two or three times per week, to 60–80% of heart rate, through walking, jogging or other aerobic exercises. Controls had no intervention.

Fasting glucose increased by 6–8% in all groups, and there were no significant changes in OGTT results. Insulin levels at fasting and during the OGTT were lower in the physical activity and diet plus physical activity groups, and

IGF-binding protein-1 (a marker for improved insulin resistance and secretion) was increased in all intervention groups, most markedly in the diet plus physical activity group. Weight loss occurred only in these same groups, but not in the diet only group and changes were small at six months (−0.3 to −0.6 BMI units). Methodological limitations included a limited intensity intervention, lack of blinding, no mention of drop-outs (it is uncertain if this was analyzed as intention to treat), and there was no multivariate analysis to account for small imbalances at baseline. This limited intervention suggests some improvement in insulin resistance with physical activity and small amounts of weight loss[49], but no change in glucose tolerance over the six-month time period.

Colman and co-workers studied the effects of weight loss over one year in middle-aged sedentary men in Baltimore, Maryland[50]. They randomized men to two groups, 73 to a hypocaloric diet to induce weight loss, and 26 men to weight maintenance. Due to high drop-out rates over the intervention (52% in the weight loss group, and 42% in controls) this study is more like a non-randomized study, but provides useful physiological insights. Men who were available for analysis in the weight loss group decreased fasting and post-challenge glucose levels and area under the glucose tolerance curve (AUCg), fasting and post-challenge insulin levels, and had a lower prevalence of IGT. Control men increased their prevalence of IGT, and the AUCg, without changes in insulin levels or areas. In eight men who underwent a hyperglycemic clamp protocol before and after weight loss, insulin sensitivity increased significantly. The strongest correlate of improved glucose area after OGTT was reduction in waist circumference, which correlated with intra-abdominal fat mass.

The Oslo Diet and Exercise Study (ODES) was a randomized one-year 2 × 2 factorial intervention among overweight people (BMI >24) identified from continuing screening of 40-year-old people in Oslo, Norway[51,52]. A low-fat, low-calorie diet and a physical activity program three times per week at 60–80% of peak heart rate were used individually or combined. There were 219 subjects randomized.

The diet intervention resulted in a 1.63 BMI unit weight loss and lower fasting glucose and one hour post 75 g OGTT insulin levels. The physical activity group lost less weight (−0.65 BMI unit on average), and decreased only the 1 h post-load insulin level, without any change in fasting or post-challenge glucose. The combined intervention group had the largest weight loss, along with decreased fasting and post-load glucose and insulin levels. There was no mention of the development of diabetes or IGT. While the study was not blinded, there were only 4.6% drop-outs over one year (highest in the exercise group: 9.3%). As in other reports[44,45], glucose levels appear to be minimally affected in the presence of increased physical activity without weight loss.

A later paper from this study[53] showed that a post intervention change in waist circumference (as a marker for intra-abdominal fat deposits) was the most important determinant of change in glucose and insulin levels, independent of fitness. It also predicted change in hemostatic variables (euglobine clot lysis time, factor VII). There were discrepancies in the reported amount of weight loss in the initial[51,52] (e.g. −1.63 BMI units) and later publications[53,54] (−1.3 BMI units) from this study, which were not accounted for by the authors.

Pan and colleagues identified 577 people with IGT from among 110 660 men and women screened in DaQing, in northern China[55]. Subjects were randomized using their primary care clinic (i.e. all subjects in a clinic received the same intervention) to a factorial design of diet, physical activity, diet plus physical activity or control. The intervention encouraged fewer simple sugars and less alcohol consumption, more vegetable intake, and if BMI was ≥25, weight loss to ≤23 kg/m2. Physical activity advice was aimed at increasing walking or running by at least one unit on an arbitrary scale of activities, and both interventions were conducted through individual and group sessions at a frequency starting weekly, and decreasing to quarterly over the six-year follow-up period. Glucose tolerance was systematically tested every two years, and people with interim symptoms or elevations of fasting glucose were tested as required. Repeat testing by OGTT confirmed diabetes.

Compared with the control group who were given only limited written advice about diabetes and IGT, all intervention groups significantly decreased their incidence of diabetes over the six years. Reductions in diabetes incidence ranged from 31–46% across the groups in adjusted models to account for baseline BMI and fasting glucose. The absolute risk reduction ranged from 5.7–6.1 out of 100 person-years across the intervention groups. Analysis by clinic, which was the original unit of randomization, showed similar results, and reductions in incidence rates were also comparable in both lean and overweight groups. Of interest, the diet plus physical activity group appeared to be no more effective than either diet or physical activity alone, though cross-over effects (e.g. changes in diet in the physical activity group) would have been difficult to detect given the assessment tools used.

These results provide reasonably convincing data that a lifestyle intervention can delay or prevent diabetes. The study does have limitations, largely due to the limited resources available. It was difficult to determine the size of, and compliance with, the actual lifestyle changes made by individuals. No blinding was used in the evaluation of diet or physical activity, so some amount of reporting bias is likely in the assessment of lifestyle change, though the primary end-point is unlikely to be biased by the lack of blinding. Similarly, group-based randomization, necessary due to logistical constraints in performing the intervention, is less rigorous than individual randomization, but appears to have resulted in similar groups at baseline, and a reasonably consistent intervention effect was seen across clinics.

Several strengths of the study should be noted. The drop-out (8.6% in six years) and mortality (1.9% in six years) rates were low. Follow-up was consistent across all groups, and the intervention was developed to be applied in a country with limited resources. The authors estimate that 980 000 new cases of diabetes per year will occur in China in the twenty-first century, so feasible and effective interventions such as this are crucial to reduce the burden of disease.

The Fasting Hyperglycemia Study (FHS II) was designed to identify high-risk subjects for lifestyle and sulfonylurea (glicazide) prevention therapy[56]. Two elevated fasting glucose levels (5.5–<7.8 mmol/l) two weeks apart, in people aged 30–65 years ($\bar{x}$ = 50 yrs) were used to define people with IFG. People with a history of GDM, a first-degree relative with NIDDM, moderate obesity or a history of hyperglycemia or glycosuria were identified via general practitioners in three English and two French centers. There were 227 subjects with IFG, of whom 223 had an OGTT (37% were normal, 37% had IGT (by WHO criteria), and 26% had NIDDM (by WHO criteria)). These 227 subjects were randomized to a factorial lifestyle or sulfonylurea (glicazide) intervention. In the lifestyle portion of the FHS, subjects were randomly allocated to basic (n = 116) or reinforced healthy living advice (n = 111). Basic advice included weight loss (if BMI > 25) and increased physical activity, which was not reinforced. In the reinforced lifestyle group, a low-fat, higher fibre diet was individually prescribed. Subjects with a BMI > 22 were given a detailed calorie-restricted diet for weight loss, and increased activity in the form of swimming, cycling, brisk walking, etc. was recommended, with increasing frequency to five or six times per week.

There was an average 1.5 kg weight loss in both groups, with maximum weight loss at three months, and return to near baseline at one year. In 93 of the 227 who had one year fitness assessments which allowed VO_{2max} to be calculated, there was a small but significant improvement in the reinforced group compared to the basic group, but high drop-out rates made it difficult to determine overall changes. There were no differences at one year in the proportion with diabetes, fasting or 2 h glucose levels or BP between the groups, nor any changes within group from baseline. There was a significant small increase in insulin sensitivity by Continuous Infusion of Glucose with Model Assessment (CIGMA) assessment in the reinforced group, with no changes on the basic advice group. Small changes in total and LDL-cholesterol occurred similarly in both groups.

There were 12% withdrawals overall, though 18% withdrew from the reinforced group and only 7% from the basic group. It appears that relatively small lifestyle changes were induced in this group of volunteers over one year, and these were insufficient to alter glucose tolerance or weight. Whether this is an adequate test of alterations in lifestyle is not clear from an efficacy point of view. However, it does represent a level of intervention that can be accomplished within the constraints of most health care systems. Unfortunately, at this level of lifestyle change, no improvements were realized. It is interesting to note that Eriksson and Lindgarde (over six years)[57] and Bourn (two years, uncontrolled)[58] showed greater changes and impact on glucose tolerance than did this study.

Wing and colleagues conducted a two-year randomized intervention among overweight non-diabetic subjects with a family history of diabetes[59]. Of these 154, 72 had IGT at baseline. They were randomized to one of four interventions: control (literature only), diet (low-calorie, low-fat), physical activity (moderate walking to 1500 Kcal/week) or both diet and physical activity. The intervention groups received intensive group sessions early and refresher sessions throughout the period, although participation dropped to only 27% in the last 18 months and weight regain occurred.

Maximum weight loss occurred at six months, and decreases in fasting glucose and insulin levels were seen in the diet and diet plus physical activity groups. By 12 months, there were no changes in fasting glucose levels between groups, though weight loss was maintained in 60% of diet intervention subjects, and 72% of diet plus physical activity subjects. At two years there were no significant differences between groups, with the control group having the lowest overall incidence of diabetes (7%). When the groups were pooled, modest weight loss (-4.5 kg, which equaled 4.5% of initial weight) predicted a reduction in diabetes incidence. The relative risk (RR) was 0.696 (CI 0.526–0.865) among people with normal glucose tolerance at entry, and a RR of 0.744 (CI 0.592–0.897) among those with IGT. Similar reductions were seen in all groups, with the primary predictors of diabetes incidence being IGT at baseline (higher risk) and weight loss (lower risk). No additional effect of improvement in VO_{2max} was seen.

The authors concluded that the three lifestyle approaches differed in their initial effectiveness but not in their long-term impact, such that baseline glucose and weight had returned to or exceeded baseline levels. However, the finding that modest weight loss in the entire group reduced the incidence of diabetes is very important. It is consistent with the findings from Malmö[57] and other studies[46,51,52] that weight loss, though perhaps not physical activity alone[45], can reduce the development of diabetes, and that the degree of weight loss does not have to be large. However, weight loss has not been found to be consistently associated with improvements in glucose levels or diabetes incidence[43,44,48]. The reasons for these discrepancies remain uncertain but may be related to the magnitude of the initial weight loss, the failure to maintain weight loss, or the degree of initial hyperglycemia.

Pima Indians have the highest prevalence and incidence of type 2 diabetes in the world. To better understand potentially useful interventions in this population, a pilot RCT was undertaken to compare two approaches[60]. Pima 'Action' involved typical structured activity and diet advice, given through classes and individual sessions. Pima 'Pride' was self-directed instruction in Pima history and culture, with limited written instructions on diet and physical activity. Ninety-five obese men and women aged 25–54 years with 2 h OGTT glucose levels < 7.8 mmol/l were randomly allocated to these interventions and evaluated at six and 12 months for changes in diet and physical activity, glucose tolerance, weight and insulin levels.

To the authors' surprise, the 'Pride' group had less worsening of BMI (+0.5 unit), glucose intolerance (11% >7.8 mmol/l at 2 h post-challenge), and 2 h insulin (+3.2 pM) than the 'Action' group (BMI +0.9 units, 29% >7.8 mmol/l glucose at 2 h, +8.8 pM 2 h insulin). The observational group of 23 persons who declined randomization had increases in these variables that were intermediate between the two intervention groups. The authors felt that the 'Action' approach might be culturally less relevant than the 'Pride' approach, though they cautioned that the small differences may have been due to participation bias, rather than the specifics of the interventions themselves.

These results, while disappointing in the context of diabetes prevention among the Pima Indians, identify several important lessons for future interventions, especially in high-risk minority populations. Cultural values may not be adequately addressed by typical classroom-based lifestyle interventions, and numerous individual barriers must be overcome (transportation, need for child care, alcohol-related problems, etc.). This pilot trial had several strengths, including randomization, blinding of outcome assessment and intention to treat analysis, but it was hampered by very poor compliance with all interventions (17–25% attendance at sessions), which was an outcome of the pilot, in and of itself. Weight loss and increases in physical activity present real lifestyle challenges, and are likely to be substantially more difficult in minority populations[61].

In an attempt to determine if insulin resistance could be reduced for longer periods than the majority of prior studies, Weinstock *et al.* performed a 48-week supervised diet and physical activity programme then followed non-diabetic obese women with largely normal glucose tolerance up to 96 weeks[62]. Subjects were randomly allocated to a very low calorie diet (n = 15) alone, or to diet plus either aerobic (n = 14) or resistance exercise (n = 16). No subjects were untreated, since the goal was to determine the effects of added physical activity of different types on insulin resistance.

Rapid weight loss (average of 13.8 kg) was seen at 16 weeks in all groups, and was largely maintained up to 44 weeks in people who attended. There were non-significant decreases in fasting glucose and the area under the OGTT glucose curve (AUC) in all groups. Insulin resistance was improved in all groups, as seen by decreases in fasting insulin levels (61.8% of baseline) and AUC insulin to week 44. Following cessation of the intervention, fasting insulin levels rose to week 96 with only slight weight gain. Surprisingly, there were no additive effects of the physical activity compared with diet alone; however, the use of very low calorie diets with rapid weight loss in all groups appears to have been the primary effect. Unfortunately, drop-out rates were high, with 20% lost at 44 weeks, but 51% at 96 weeks. No data were presented on IGT, but the failure to lower glucose levels post-intervention is surprising, given the significant weight loss.

The high drop-out rate at longer follow-up times makes interpretation difficult. At face value, the results imply that addition of physical activity (aerobic or resistance) added nothing to improvements in insulin sensitivity induced by weight loss, that none of the interventions were helpful in lowering glucose levels, and that improvements in insulin sensitivity seen over the first 44 weeks were easily reversible with little weight gain. This may have been due to the inclusion of primarily women with normal glucose tolerance, though no subgroup analyses were presented to explore the effects of baseline levels of glucose tolerance.

The Women's Healthy Lifestyle Project was aimed at prevention of weight gain and increases in total and LDL cholesterol as healthy women experienced the menopause[63,64] through a combination of dietary changes and increased physical activity (walking, aerobics, dancing, etc.). After 18 months of follow-up, Simkin-Silverman and colleagues[63] found significant decreases in weight, waist hip ratio, blood pressure, lipids and fasting glucose levels. Significant weight loss (-3.0 kg at 18 months) (n = 236) was maintained through a combination of behavioral techniques and incentives compared to the assessment-only control group (n = 253), as were cholesterol and systolic BP decreases. By 54 months[64], weight had returned to baseline levels for the lifestyle group, but controls had gained 2.4 kg. Fasting glucose was less statistically significantly lower in the lifestyle than in the control group, though both had small elevations in levels (lifestyle: +1.6 mg/dL (0.09 mmol/L) from baseline; control: +3.3 mg/dl (0.18 mmol/L). No OGTT was conducted and no comments were made about the incidence of clinical diabetes, which would be unlikely given the age and good health of participants. Thus, this intervention provides data that weight gain can be minimized through middle age with positive effects on cardiovascular risk factors common to the insulin resistance syndrome. However, the impact on glucose levels *per se* among non-diabetics was very small.

Bergenstal and colleagues have undertaken a community-based approach to preventing glucose intolerance in Minnesota[65]. They have randomly allocated 418 subjects to standard and intervention groups. Intervention participants attended two meetings per year focusing on nutrition, physical activity and stress, with monthly calls from nutrition students for encouragement, along with a quarterly newsletter and annual individual counseling. The 418 subjects at entry included 3% with diabetes and 4% with IGT. The remainder had normal glucose tolerance[66].

After two years of follow-up, there were no differences in progression to diabetes or changes in fasting glucose levels between the groups[67]. The study is currently completing four years of follow-up. While the low-intensity community-based intervention was designed to be of low cost, it appears that it may not be effective in reducing glucose intolerance or making important changes in cardiovascular risk parameters, at least over the two years reported to date. Given the relatively small changes seen in more intensive interventions, this result may not be surprising.

The aim of the Finnish Diabetes Prevention Study (DPS) was to determine if an intensive diet and physical activity intervention could delay or prevent type 2 diabetes and worsening of cardiovascular risk factors among people with IGT[68]. A total of 522 overweight people at five centers with IGT on two OGTTs were randomized to either a control or an unmasked intervention group. The mean age was 55 years, BMI was 31, and 67% were women. Seven sessions were held with a nutritionist in the first year, followed with quarterly visits thereafter. The aim of the intervention was to reduce weight by 5% or more and reduce saturated fat intake to less than 30% of energy consumed, while increasing dietary fiber and physical activity. The control group received limited annual diet and physical activity advice.

One year results were reported for the first 212 participants who were randomized[68], and the final report has recently been published[69]. During the average follow-up period of 3.2 years, 86 subjects developed diabetes – 27 in the intervention group (incidence rate of 3.2/100 person-years) and 59 in the control group (7.8/100 person-years). The lifestyle intervention reduced the incidence of diabetes by 58% (Cox adjusted hazard ratio = 0.4, 0.3–0.7, ARR = 4.6/100 person-years). Those who were more successful in achieving the lifestyle goals had lower incidence of diabetes than those who were less successful. On average, the intervention group lost 4.2 kg, while the control group lost 0.8 kg. The authors noted that this modest weight loss led to substantial reductions in diabetes incidence, and that among subjects who lost at least 5% of their initial weight, the risk reduction was even greater. Thus, the overall results are somewhat conservative as an estimate of the relationship between weight loss and reduction of diabetes incidence. Among subjects who did not meet the weight loss goal, but did meet the exercise goal (> 4 hours/week), diabetes was also reduced significantly, even after adjustment for baseline BMI (adjusted hazard ratio = 0.3, 0.1–0.7). This suggests that increased activity has an independent effect on diabetes incidence, however, it is not clear whether the weight loss that did occur in this group was also accounted for in the adjustment. These results are very important in showing, in a well-conducted RCT, that modest weight loss achieved through diet changes and increases in activity can result in substantial reduction in diabetes incidence.

The Diabetes Prevention Program (DPP) was a multicenter primary prevention study among people with IGT[70]. The 27 clinical centers screened over 158 000 people and conducted over 30 000 OGTTs to identify people with IGT and a fasting glucose level from 95–125 mg/dl (5.3–6.9 mmol/L). The trial included 3234 people randomized to three intervention groups, each with just over 1000 subjects per group. There was an unmasked intensive lifestyle group, aimed at reduction of body weight by 7% or more and increased moderate physical activity (usually brisk walking) to at least 150 minutes per week. This was accomplished using an intensive 16-session curriculum, followed by contact weekly or every two weeks and reinforcement, with a toolbox of retention and relapse approaches. The two pharmacological arms (metformin and placebo) are discussed later. The primary end-point was clinical or OGTT diabetes, confirmed by at least two tests, using ADA criteria. Intervention groups were well balanced at baseline with respect to a number of risk factors. The average age of participants was 50.6 years, 68% were women, average BMI was 34.0, and 69% of participants reported a first-degree family history of diabetes[71]. In May of 2002, after an average of 2.8 years of follow-up, the data monitoring board found evidence of significant and substantial effectiveness of both interventions, and terminated the DPP about one year early[72]. The intensive lifestyle intervention reduced the incidence of diabetes by 58%, from an average annual incidence of 11/100 person-years in the placebo group to 4.8/100 person-years in the lifestyle group (crude absolute risk reduction, or ARR = 6.2/100 person-years). This effect was consistent across all subgroups examined, including persons of all racial/ethnic groups, both genders and all ages, including subjects over 60 years of age, where the estimated reduction was 71%. Persons in the lifestyle group lost an average of 5.6 kg of weight compared to 0.1 kg in the placebo group, and 74% met physical activity goals at the end of the core curriculum. No information is currently available from the DPP to understand the relative roles of changes in dietary intake and composition, increased activity and resulting weight loss on reduced diabetes incidence.

Taken together with the Finnish[69] and Chinese[55] results, it now appears established from well-conducted RCTs that lifestyle changes resulting in modest weight loss (5–7% of body weight) through dietary change and increased activity result in the substantial delay or prevention of diabetes over relatively short periods (three to six years) of intervention. Since both the Finnish and US prevention trials were of relatively short duration, it remains uncertain how long the reduced incidence of diabetes can be maintained. The DaQing study suggests that delay of diabetes for up to six years is possible. Even a delay of three years, on average, should have major impacts on long-term complications.

Table 6.3 shows that there are now 17 RCTs testing combined lifestyle interventions that used various diabetes relevant end-points. Of these, seven used diabetes itself, two used IGT and the remaining eight studies used glucose levels with or without measurements of insulin or insulin resistance syndrome (IRS) components (e.g. blood pressure, triglycerides, HDL cholesterol).

Seven studies provide evidence that lifestyle changes reduce diabetes[42,55,59,69,72] or IGT[45,50] risk, whereas two do not[56,67]. These latter two studies had the least intensive interventions. At present, with evidence from China[55], and the recent completion of the Finnish DPS[69] and the DPP[72] in the USA, it appears that type 2 diabetes may be delayed or prevented. Additional analysis of these RCTs is required to understand the duration of the effects, the costs and the cost-effectiveness of the interventions, but the efficacy of lifestyle change leading to weight loss as a method to prevent diabetes is established.

Studies which explored glucose and IRS outcomes were more variable. Three studies that achieved some weight loss had lower levels of glucose and IRS markers (insulin[51], BP[46] or both[69]). An additional three studies with weight loss had improvements in IRS components without changes in glucose levels[43,62,63]. Of the three studies that achieved no weight loss, no change in fasting glucose levels occurred[44,48,60], though two did show improvements in IRS variables[44,48].

Thus, the majority of these studies reported improvements in the IRS syndrome but, without weight loss, most did not find lowered glucose levels. It is not possible to discern from the data presented whether this is due to the mixture of baseline glucose levels in the study groups, though it is tempting to postulate that within the normal range, minimal glucose changes are likely to occur. Thus, studies of high proportions of people with normal glucose levels might not be expected to detect much change, whereas IRS variables that are commonly elevated (e.g. insulin and blood pressure) may be more sensitive to the interventions.

Clinical studies (non-randomized)

Non-randomized interventions can also add useful information to the knowledge of prevention. Studies below include those that used both individual- and community-based approaches.

Odea conducted a pre-post evaluation of 14 Australian Aborigines (10 with diabetes, four normal) who lived in an urban environment and were willing to return to a hunter-gatherer lifestyle in their ancestral homelands for seven weeks[73]. After metabolic evaluation, the subjects and study team travelled into remote northwestern Australia and ate nothing that they did not hunt or gather directly for most of the period. Two environments (one inland and one coastal) provided some variation in intake. On average, 64% of energy intake was from animal sources. It was very low in fat (13%), with approximately 33% carbohydrate and 54% protein. This represented a marked change from the pre-test urban diets, which averaged 50% carbohydrate, 40% fat and 10% protein.

Once in the bush, only about 1200 Kcal/person/day was ingested, resulting in an average loss of 1.2 kg/week (total −8.1 kg) in subjects with diabetes. Upon return to an urban setting, metabolic measurements were repeated. Marked improvements in fasting glucose and insulin levels of the 10 people with diabetes were noted, with significant but smaller changes in post-challenge values.

Using current ADA criteria[26], seven out of 10 became non-diabetic during the bush period. By WHO criteria[24], none became normal, three tested IGT and seven remained diabetic, due to the greater reliance of WHO criteria on post-challenge values. This small study provides powerful evidence that the effects of Westernized urban lifestyle can be partially reversed, and that such a lifestyle contains deleterious elements which markedly worsen glucose tolerance.

Similar cross-sectional findings in Pima Indians living a more traditional lifestyle (in rural Mexico) also support these observations[74]. These simple but elegant studies suggest that such interventions can effectively reverse the trend toward greater energy consumption among indigenous populations.

Eriksson and colleagues[75] conducted community screening of 6956 47–49-year-old men in Malmö, Sweden, starting in 1974. One hundred and eighty-one men with IGT (by pre-WHO criteria) were non-randomly enrolled in a lifestyle intervention at one clinic site, and 79 other men with IGT were not enrolled but were followed, along with a randomly selected normal control group (n = 114). At the six-year follow-up, 161 out of the 181 men with IGT in the intervention group were retested (89%), as were 56 out of 79 non-intervened men (70%), and 114 of the normal controls.

Intervention consisted of unspecified dietary advice and increased physical activity conducted either in groups or individually. There were improvements in VO_{2max} , lowered body weight, BP and serum triglycerides, greatest at one year, but maintained over the six years. Among people in the IGT group without intervention, 21.4% met criteria for diabetes (> 6.7 mmol/l fasting and/or > 11.1 mmol/l at two hours), whereas only 10.6% had diabetes in the intervention group (RR = 0.49 (CI 0.25–0.97)). Subjects who lost the most weight and improved oxygen uptake the most had the greatest improvements in glucose levels. These results were further explored in another report[76] which showed that, in addition to forced vital capacity (as a correlate of fitness), insulin resistance (higher 2 h insulin level) and lower insulin secretion (40 minute insulin increment during the OGTT) predicted diabetes independently among people with normal glucose tolerance.

A 12-year mortality follow-up of this cohort has also been recently published[77]. Mortality among the IGT intervention group was lower than in the non-intervention group (RR = 0.47 (CI 0.24–0.88; ARR = 7.45/1000)), and was the same as for people with normal glucose tolerance. Even though baseline levels of glucose, BMI, lipids and insulin were very similar between the intervention and control groups, the failure to randomize subjects could have introduced important behavioral or other selection bias which might account for the lowered incidence of diabetes and mortality in the intervened group. However, the non-random design may have contributed to long-term adherence. This study suggests that long-term interventions for prevention can be maintained in this population, and gave early support to the concept that lifestyle changes might prevent diabetes and improve long-term mortality.

Ramachandran and colleagues in Madras, India undertook a clinic-based primary prevention programme among subjects who were recruited because one or both parents had diabetes[78,79]. They recruited over 1200 offspring and began a primary intervention program aimed at diet change, weight loss, and increased physical activity (primarily walking). They have reported two analyses of subsets of these subjects[78,79]. In the first analysis, they noted that, among 262 subjects with an average of eight years in the program (and a minimum of four years), weight gain was a strong predictor of subsequent diabetes (OR = 5.1 (CI 2.6–13.9)[78].

In a subsequent analysis, they explored the influence of specific components of the prevention program[79]. They analyzed 187 of the 220 subjects enrolled in a later phase of the program who had at least two years of follow-up (average of 6.8 years), a non-diabetic OGTT at baseline and a repeat OGTT which was either normal by WHO criteria or showed type 2 diabetes. A nested case-control analysis examined the likelihood of continued participation in the diet and physical activity programs, and measures of psychological stress, along with family history, weight reduction, age and gender.

Both participation in physical activity (primarily walking for 30 minutes per day) during the programme (OR = 0.41, (CI 0.19–0.87) and less psychological stress were seen in people who did not develop diabetes. No effect was seen for dietary adherence to a high-carbohydrate, high-fiber, low-fat (20%) diet or, in this subset, for weight loss or family history (comparing two parents with diabetes to one parent with diabetes, since everyone had a family history). The nested retrospective design has important limitations, since diet and physical activity adherence and measures of stress were collected only at the last examination rather than prospectively, making them subject to potential recall bias. It is also not clear whether the subjects were aware of their OGTT results at the time of the interview.

These studies, while non-randomized and with weaker designs, were done in the context of intervention programs which may be feasible in developing countries. They suggest, but do not prove, that such primary prevention interventions may be beneficial.

Other non-randomized clinical studies are not reviewed here due to severe methodological limitations[80].

Community-based studies of lifestyle change

A different approach to diabetes prevention has been attempted in small numbers of studies in adults and children. These studies have focused on community-, church- or school-based interventions aimed at improving cardio-vascular (CV) and diabetes risk factors. Such studies are difficult to evaluate using the usual RCT paradigm since randomization is often not feasible or is not at the individual level (e.g. schools or classrooms may be the unit of randomization, and the number of randomization units are often small). Limited individual assessments may be available. Often the goals include increased knowledge and behavioral change, as well as sustainability of the intervention in addition to changes in physiological parameters. They are briefly reviewed here, since community-based interventions may be the most economically feasible, if they can be shown to be effective.

Adults

Ramaiya *et al.* reported a six-year follow-up of a community health education program among a Hindu Indian subcommunity from Dar Es Salaam, Tanzania[81]. Using a pre-post design, this program resulted in a decrease in diabetes prevalence from 11.8% to 8.2%, and IGT prevalence was said to decrease from 26.5% to 10%. Small significant reductions in fasting and 2 h glucose levels, lipids, BP and weight were noted, along with an increase in physical activity. The senior author has indicated that only the abstract has been published and no follow-up has been continued (George Alberti, University of Newcastle, UK, personal communication). Because published details are limited, it is not clear whether this community intervention, which superficially appears successful, was due to selection and non-response bias, regression to the mean, or to a real effect. If the results are true, it would lend strong support to the idea that community-based diabetes interventions in developing countries can work.

Simmons *et al.* developed a risk factor reduction program for Independent Samoans (from the former Western Samoa) at high risk of type 2 diabetes living in Auckland, New Zealand[82]. A church-based intervention was developed in two churches over two years. The intervention subjects had diabetes awareness sessions, physical activity groups, nutrition education and cooking demonstrations. The control church members, disappointed at having to wait for the intervention, had lower participation in glucose tolerance testing, and started a physical activity group which did not continue.

Over two years, subjects attending the intervention church had no weight gain (compared with +3.1 kg on average in the control group), a decreased waist circumference, and increased knowledge about diabetes and nutrition. Self-reported intake of high-fat foods was lower after the intervention, and the majority of respondents felt it had been useful to them. The intervention church continued the physical activity and nutrition program on a self-sustained basis. It appears that this type of intervention had some success in preventing weight gain (though it did not achieve weight loss).

Due to the non-response at the second evaluation (20% intervention, 25% control) it is possible that response bias 'caused' the effects seen. Since no glucose tolerance testing was done at follow-up, the actual impact on diabetes and glucose intolerance is unknown. Given these limitations, the primary lesson may be that it is possible to motivate social groups to learn more about diabetes prevention, to increase their knowledge and to sustain some of the activities after investigators depart. The program was extended to nine other churches after the completion of this pilot study, largely by community members themselves.

Children

Several studies have attempted to increase knowledge and awareness of diabetes and risk factors in children. These include a small hospital-based health education program[83] and more extensive school-based interventions for fourth grade[84] (aged ~9 years), and fifth grade (aged ~10 years) Mexican American students[85]. While each of these found some pre- to post-intervention improvements in knowledge and reported behavior, the failure to use controls or any random assignment, lack of direct observations of behavior (in contrast to self-reported behavior), as well as the short duration and small numbers of subjects limits the interpretability and utility of the findings.

Other studies have not focused specifically on diabetes, but on risk factors such as physical activity and obesity in children. A large cardiovascular primary prevention project in elementary schools had few of the deficiencies of smaller pilot studies. The Child and Adolescent Trial for Cardiovascular Health (CATCH) randomized 56 intervention and 40 control schools[86]. Outcomes were assessed using a pre-post design. Over 5100 initially third grade students (~8 years of age) from ethnically diverse backgrounds in state schools located in California, Louisiana, Minnesota and Texas participated in a third-grade to fifth-grade intervention including school food service modifications, enhanced physical education (PE), and classroom health curricula.

In intervention school lunches, the percentage of energy intake from fat fell more than in control school lunches. Physical activity intensity increased in PE classes in the intervention schools compared with the control schools. Self-reported daily energy intake from fat among students in the intervention schools was significantly reduced by small amounts (from 32.7% to 30.3% of energy from fat) compared with that among students in the control schools (from 32.6% to 32.2%) ($p < 0.001$).

Intervention school pupils reported significantly more daily vigorous activity than controls (58.6 minutes versus 46.5 minutes of activity). However, body size, BP and cholesterol measures did not differ significantly between treatment groups. Thus, some important evidence of changes in school lunch content and self-reported behavior occurred, although over the three-year period no weight loss or prevention of weight gain occurred. The CATCH intervention is now being implemented in many of the schools in Texas, as well as in other regions, and its dissemination and sustainability are being studied. Another shorter-term CVD prevention activity in schools has also been reported, with some success in decreasing cholesterol, and small decreases in body fat compared to non-intervened children[87].

Two randomized trials of school-based interventions to reduce obesity suggest that schools may be an effective place to counter obesity trends in the USA[88,89]. The 'Planet Health' intervention randomized 10 schools from four communities to intervention or control status in Boston[88]. Gortmaker and colleagues used an extensive interdisciplinary curricular approach focused on improving activity and dietary behaviors of all pupils in grades 6 and 7 (aged ~11–12 years), without specifically targeting obese children. Curricular relevance to other school objectives was used to gain school acceptance of this intensive intervention.

Obesity prevalence declined in intervention schools from 23.6% to 20.3% compared to increases in control schools from 21.5% to 23.7% . The effect was significant for girls, though not for boys, where larger decreases were seen in control schools. Of interest was that television viewing time was reduced to a greater extent and there was less increase in estimated energy intake as well as an increase in fruit and vegetable intake reported in intervention schools. The decreased television viewing time significantly predicted the weight loss among girls, and was similar across ethnic groups.

The second trial, aimed in this intervention at reducing television viewing time, validated these findings[89]. In this study, the natural age-related increases in BMI and skin-folds were significantly lower in intervention than control children, and television watching and video game playing was reduced significantly over six months with no change in reported activity or diet.

These studies stand out as positive examples of an otherwise largely negative set of community-based studies aimed at reduction of body fatness[90]. The limited evidence available suggests that community-based lifestyle approaches may be more useful in changing behavior early in life. They require substantial resources to implement, and are often difficult to evaluate. Of interest are the observations that reduced television watching, at least in the USA, may be an important pathway to reduced obesity rates. Future studies should be done on larger populations over longer time periods to assure that such interventions are effective. Such studies should receive high priority given the rapid increases in diabetes and obesity risks that are occurring across the age span.

Physical activity

Physical activity is one of the primary determinants of energy balance and obesity. It is also one of the factors that has undergone recent decreases in developing countries around the world. The potential for the prevention of diabetes by increases in physical activity has been attractive for many years[1]. Physiological studies have shown that physical activity increases insulin sensitivity and reduces insulin secretion, which may be the primary conduit through which most behavioral risk factors travel to increase diabetes risk. They can be reversed by inactivity[91].

Physical activity has also been shown to reduce obesity and central fat distribution in short-term clinical studies[91]. As physical activity patterns in free living populations are complex, so is the assessment of physical activity in epidemiological studies[91]. Many have used questionnaires to assess leisure-time physical activity, which in many urban populations is the primary determinant of differences in energy expenditure between individuals. This is not the case in rural populations, where a more comprehensive evaluation of work activities is required[92,93]. More exact measures are needed to account for all components of total energy expenditure (including resting metabolic rate and the thermic effect of food), but these are not feasible in large populations over extended periods of time[91]. A number of review papers[91,93-98] and an NIH consensus statement[99] have summarized prior work on physical activity.

RCTs

No RCTs were identified which included increased physical activity versus none, without dietary changes or intended weight loss. Combination interventions to induce weight loss and maintain it with increased activity have become the standard approach. This section will, therefore, focus on prospective observational studies exploring diabetes and related end-points. These have the advantage of longer follow-up than most clinical trials and they cover the range of activities and intensities that occur in everyday life. They have the significant disadvantage of lack of randomization with attendant selection bias, such that persons who report higher levels of activity often have several concomitant behaviors (e.g. healthy diet, absence of smoking) that may also improve health.

Prospective observational epidemiological studies

Table 6.4 summarizes the published prospective epidemiological studies of physical activity and development of type 2 diabetes. In each case, the adjustment variables are noted, but less detail is given about individual studies than in Table 6.3 since they provide somewhat weaker evidence for prevention than RCTs. This is primarily true because any one factor cannot be varied independently of others which may also be associated with altered risk.

In the case of physical activity, people who engage in greater amounts of activity may themselves select other healthy behaviors which are incompletely measured and adjusted for (e.g. less cigarette smoking or altered diet). There may also be a genetic component to physical activity, either based on spontaneous activity[100] or clustering of other genetic factors which facilitate activity[101]. Analyses of twin studies have shown contradictory results concerning associations between physical activity and glucose levels, with one showing a strong genetic effect[101], while the other did not[102]. Regardless of this concern, prospective studies still provide some of the strongest data suggesting that higher levels of physical activity may protect against type 2 diabetes.

One of the earliest studies to explore the role of physical activity was published by Medalie and colleagues from the Israeli Ischemic Heart Disease Project[103]. They did not show detailed results, but noted no association of five-year clinical diabetes incidence with reported measures of physical activity.

In contrast, most other studies have found beneficial effects. For example, the Nurses Health Study followed over 87 000 nurses in the USA for eight years. The first report[104] found that at least weekly vigorous activity was associated with a lower risk of self-reported diabetes (RR = 0.83, CI 0.74–0.93; ARR = 8.8/10 000 person-years) . A recent report utilized interim measures of reported activity, rather than a single baseline measure, and explored the type and amount of activity more thoroughly[105]. There was a graded decrease in diabetes incidence over eight years with increasing metabolic equivalent (MET) levels (1 MET is equivalent to 3.5 ml of oxygen utilization per kilogram body weight per minute), which was consistent among nurses whose only form of physical activity was walking. This provides important evidence that feasible levels of increased activity may result in lower diabetes incidence rates.

Fifteen-year follow-up of University of Pennsylvania male alumni was reported by Helmrich *et al.*[106]. In a widely quoted result, each 500 Kcal increase in leisure time activity was associated with a RR for diabetes of 0.94 (CI 0.90–0.98; ARR = 1.6/10 000 person-years), with the largest reductions in people doing vigorous activity at baseline (RR = 0.69; ARR = 7.5/10 000 person-years). Whether the leisure time recall instrument is capable of such fine distinctions remains an open question, since other studies have not found that such small increments result in reductions in diabetes risk[107].

In a two-year follow-up study of residents of Malta, Schranz *et al.*[108] reported that moderate to high *total* physical activity (not just leisure time) reduced the risk of diabetes among people with normal OGTTs (RR = 0.53; ARR = 2.4/100 person-years) but not among those with IGT. Similar effects were seen when stratified by obesity and positive family history.

Self-reported diabetes was studied in a nested case-control design among a cohort of Iowa women by Kaye and co-workers[109]. They found that over a two-year period the age-adjusted odds ratio for medium versus low reported physical activity was 0.7 (CI 0.5-0.9) and for women reporting high levels of activity it was 0.5 (CI 0.4–0.7) . The overall incidence of diabetes in this cohort was about 1% at two years. BMI, waist–hip ratio and education were also independently associated with diabetes. Once obesity measures were adjusted for, there was no longer an independent association of physical activity or smoking.

Table 6.4. Prospective studies of physical activity and type 2 diabetes mellitus incidence.

Author	Population (no. of subjects)	Follow-up (years)	Age	Comparison	RR (ARR)	95% CI	Adjustment
Medalie et al. 1974[103]	Israel Ischemic Heart Disease Study (10059)	5	40+	Not stated	No association		RR not stated
Manson et al. 1991[104]	US Nurses Health Study (87253)	8	40–65	Weekly vigorous vs. not	0.83 (8.8/10 000 PY)	0.74–0.93	Age, BMI, family history, time period
Hu et al. 1999[105]	US Nurses Health Study (70102)	8	40–65	Q2 vs. Q1	0.77	0.66–0.90	Age, smoking, hypertension, family history, menopause, high cholesterol
				Q3 vs. Q1	0.75	0.65–0.88	
				Q4 vs. Q1	0.62	0.52–0.73	
				Q5 vs. Q1	0.54	0.45–0.64	
				Q5 vs. Q1	0.74	0.62–0.89	As above and BMI
Helmrich et al. 1991[106,125]	University of Pennyslvania male alumni (5990)	15	39–68	Moderate vs. none	0.90	0.65–1.26	Age
				Vigorous vs. none	0.69 (7.5/10 000 PY)	0.41–1/17	Age
				500 kcal/wk	0.94 (1.6/10 000 PY)	0.90–0.98	Age, BMI, hypertension, family history
Schranz et al. 1991[108]	Malta residents (259)	2	15+	Moderate/vigorous vs. low	0.49 (2.4/100 PY)	0.09–2.85	Similar with age adjustment
Kaye et al. 1991[109]	Iowa women (41 837)	2	55–69	Moderate vs. low	0.70	0.50–0.90	Age
				High vs. low	0.50	0.40–0.70	Age
Manson et al. 1992[110]	US physicians Health Study (men) (21 271)	5	40–84	Weekly vs. not weekly	0.64 (10.9/10 000 PY)	0.51–0.82	Age
				Weekly vs. not weekly	0.70	0.53–0.92	Age, BMI, hypertension
Gurwitz, et al. 1994[111]	East Boston Elderly EPESE (2797)	6	65+	Moderate vs. low	0.67		Age, sex, BMI, alcohol, BP, self-reported high blood sugar
				High vs. low	0.93		
Burchfiel et al. 1995[113]	Honolulu Heart Study (8006 Japanese-American men)	6	45–68	Q2 vs. Q1	0.86 (10.4/1000 PY)	0.64–1.14	Age
				Q3 vs. Q1	0.81 (12.9/1000 PY)	0.61–1.09	
				Q4 vs. Q1	0.72 (19.6/1000 PY)	0.54–0.98	
				Q5 vs. Q1	0.46 (38.2/1000 PY)	0.33–0.66	Age, BMI, skin folds, SBP, triglycerides, glucose, hematocrit, family history
				Q5 vs. Q1–4	0.49	0.34–0.72	

Table 6.4. contd.

Study	Population (n)	Years	Age	Comparison	RR	95% CI	Adjustments
Perry et al. 1995[116]	British Regional Heart Study, men (7577)	12.8	40–59	Moderate vs. inactive	0.40	0.20–0.70	Age, BMI, multiple factors – no change
Monterrosa et al. 1995[117]	San Antonio Heart Study, men (353), women (491)	8	25–64	Men	0.41	0.18–0.93	Age, BMI, SES, structural assimilation
				Women	1.43	0.85–2.41	
Eriksson and Lindgarde, 1996[76]	Malmö Feasibility Study, men (4637)	6	48	1 liter increase in vital capacity	0.51	0.37–0.69	BMI, FBG, 2 h insulin, delta insulin at 40 min
Hara, et al. 1996[114]	Japanese-Americans, Los Angeles (592)	6.3	40+	1 SD more activity	0.60		Age, sex, ns with BMI
	Japanese-Americans, Hawaii (552)		40+	1 SD more activity	0.75		Age, sex, BMI, ns without BMI
Lynch et al. 1996[107]	Finnish men (751)	4.2	42–60	5.5+ METs and 40+ min/wk	0.44 (11.6/1000 PY)	0.22–0.88	Age, BMI
Paffenbarger et al. 1997[118]	Harvard Alumni men (9124)	12	45–84	1000–2499 kcal/wk vs. <1000	0.72 (7.6/1000 PY)		Age, BMI, family history, hypertension, ETOH, chronic disease, sports in college
Haapanen et al. 1997[119]	NE Finnish men (891)	10	35–63	Moderate leisure activity vs. low	0.79		Age
				High leisure time vs. low	0.65 (2.8/1000 PY)		
	Women (973)		35–63	Moderate leisure activity vs. low	0.47 (4.1/1000 PY)		
				High leisure time vs. low	0.34 (5.1/1000 PY)		
Morin et al. 2000[120]	S. Colorado men and women (1,069)	10	20–74	Moderate and/or vigorous vs. low	0.72	0.49–1.08	Age, gender, ethnicity, BMI, skin folds, family hx diabetes
				High/vigorous vs. low	0.64	0.42–0.98	
Folsom et al. 2000[121]	Iowa women (34 257)	12	55–69	Any vs. none	0.69	0.63–0.77	Age, education, BMI, smoking, alcohol, estrogen use, diet, family history of diabetes
Hu, et al. 2001[122]	Health Professionals' Follow-up Study, men (37 918)	10	40–75	METs Q1	1.00		Age, smoking, alcohol, diet, family history of diabetes, vitamin E, increased TV watching, increased DM risk
				Q2	0.78	0.66–0.93	
				Q3	0.65	0.54–0.78	
				Q4	0.58	0.48–0.70	
				Q5	0.51	0.41–0.63	

RR = relative risk or rate ratio; ARR = absolute risk reduction (if not present, data were not present to calculate).

Within the clinical prevention trial of US male physicians, Manson and colleagues explored the role of activity measured at baseline in a cohort of over 21 000 men followed for five years[110]. There was a significant, graded reduction in risk with increasing amount of physical activity, and the overall age- and BMI-adjusted RR was 0.71 (CI 0.56–0.91; ARR = 10.9/10 000 person-years) for at least weekly physical activity versus less than weekly. The effect was greatest in men who were most overweight; however, no effect was seen in men with BMIs less than 23.

While most studies have been conducted in middle-aged cohorts, Gurwitz *et al.* studied 2797 people aged 65 years and older in the East Boston Established Populations for the Epidemiologic Study of the Elderly (EPESE) cohort with six-year follow-up[111]. The outcome was self-reported use of hypoglycemic medication, which will underestimate the frequency of actual glucose intolerance in this age group, whose average age was 75 years. Moderate activity was associated with a reduction in adjusted RR of hypoglycemic medication use of 0.67 compared to low activity, however no graded risk was seen. Among people reporting 'high' levels of activity (defined as working up a sweat at least once per week), the RR was 0.93 and not significantly different from 1.0. These are the only data suggesting that physical activity may continue to be protective in people over the age of 65 years.

The Honolulu Heart Study has studied a cohort of 8006 Japanese-American men since 1965. Burchfiel and co-workers explored the development of clinically diagnosed and treated diabetes[112,113]. Physical activity indices which estimated total activity throughout a 24-hour period were used. They found a graded reduction in risk with increased physical activity index, ranging from 0.86 (CI 0.64–1.14; ARR = 10.4/1000 person-years) for quartile 2 versus 1 (lowest activity index) to 0.46 (CI 0.33–0.66; ARR = 38.2/1000 person-years) for the highest quartile of activity, quartile 5 versus 1. Adjustment for obesity, fat patterning, blood pressure or family history of diabetes did not change the results. While there were problems in definition of the non-diabetic population at risk, since no glucose tolerance testing was conducted at baseline, multiple analyses with increasing likelihood of removing misclassification showed similar patterns. This study showed no suggestion of a threshold effect for the amount of activity and no important confounding with obesity.

Hara *et al.* also examined Japanese-Americans living in Hawaii and Los Angeles over 6.3 years[114]. The absolute incidence in these people was 17.2 per 1000 person years, slightly higher than adult Nauruans[115]. This means the incidence is one of the highest in the world. Results similar to those in the Honolulu Heart Study were found, though in the Hawaiian-Japanese, diabetes risk was only reduced (RR = 0.75, p = 0.033 for +1 SD of activity scale) when age, gender and BMI were included in models. In the Los Angeles cohort of Japanese-Americans, an age- and gender-adjusted RR of 0.60 was seen (p = 0.029), but in this cohort, adjustment for BMI removed the effect seen in the simpler models.

In a study of 7577 men in the British Regional Heart Study, Perry *et al.* followed subjects from general practices throughout the UK for 12.8 years[116]. Self-reported but clinically validated diabetes and mortality records were used as the outcome. They also saw a stepwise reduction in risk of diabetes for each category of activity from sedentary through to moderately vigorous. A non-significant reduction in risk was also present for the vigorous group, perhaps due to small numbers of subjects. Patterns were the same when adjustment for multiple factors was used.

In one of the few studies which has explored the effects of leisure time physical activity separately by gender, Monterrosa *et al.* explored a simple scale of activities in Mexican-American men and women in San Antonio, Texas[117]. Eight-year diabetes incidence was lower in men (OR = 0.41) (CI 0.18–0.93), but not in women (OR = 1.43) (CI 0.85–1.41). Exclusion of BMI from the models slightly increased the protective effect of physical activity among men (OR = 0.38), but 'dropped out of the model' for women, and no point estimate was reported, although the model including BMI was not significant either. This result seems likely to be due to variability from small numbers rather than a real gender difference.

While many studies have included only men or adjusted for gender without providing sex-specific estimates, the findings from the Nurses Health Study[105] and a study in northeastern Finland[118] of significant strong effects in women suggests that physical activity acts similarly in both genders.

Using a measure of vital capacity to index fitness rather than self-reported physical activity allowed Eriksson and Lingarde to explore diabetes incidence over six years in men in Malmö, Sweden[76]. They found an adjusted RR of 0.51 (CI 0.37–0.69) for an increase of one liter in vital capacity, which was moderately correlated with leisure time physical activity by self-report. This study, like that of Schranz[108], found no effect in people with IGT. The RCT results of the Finnish[69] and US prevention trials[72] among persons with IGT indicate that a lifestyle intervention that includes increases in activity can reduce diabetes incidence, but the interventions were not designed to isolate the independent effect of physical activity. Further subgroup analyses may be informative. In the DaQing study[55], the group randomized to exercise alone showed a reduction in incidence, suggesting that subjects with IGT will respond to increases in activity levels.

Physical activity and diabetes incidence were also studied in the Ischemic Heart Disease Risk Factor cohort of 751 men in Kuopio, Finland by Lynch and colleagues[107]. After an average of 4.2 years of follow-up, they found a signifi-cant reduction in diabetes risk for men who had participated in leisure time activity over the past year at moderate levels of intensity and duration (5.5 METS or greater for 40 minutes per week; OR = 0.44, CI 0.22–0.88;

ARR = 11.6/1000 person-years). These ORs were adjusted for age, baseline fasting glucose and BMI. This suggests that a threshold effect for diabetes incidence might exist. However, among higher risk men (those with a positive family history, BMI ≥ 26.8 and hypertension) the MET level for protection was lower than seen in all men, suggesting a different threshold level. Also, among all men, an age-adjusted effect was seen at lower intensities, which was reduced by adjustment for BMI. These results suggest several possibilities: (1) Lower levels of activity are more mediated by obesity than higher levels, as suggested by the authors; (2) The patterns of lower and higher levels of activity in Finnish men overlap and make detection of only lower level effects difficult, also implied by the authors; or (3) Relatively small numbers of cases (46 total) and a single measure of activity at baseline preclude identification of benefits for lower levels of activity. This study disagrees with observations on larger cohorts[113,116] which did not find a threshold effect, since graded risk reduction was seen for even occasional physical activity.

In contrast to a suggestion of a threshold effect, Paffenbarger and co-workers found less evidence of benefit from higher levels of activity in the long-term follow-up of male Harvard alumni[118]. The adjusted RR was 0.72 (p <0.05) for 1000–2499 Kcal/week of leisure time activity reported at baseline, 12 years prior to follow-up (ARR = 7.6/1000 person-years). Activity at higher levels (≥ 2500 Kcal/week) was not associated with reduced risk (RR = 0.97) and there was no dose–response gradient in multiply-adjusted models. While there were limited data on change in physical activity after baseline, these did not predict diabetes risk in either direction. Maintenance of a BMI < 26 over the 12-year time period did have a significantly lower RR of 0.39. Studies such as this, with limited data both at baseline and during follow-up, suggest that physical activity, which is difficult to measure, may have a stronger effect than previously estimated, since the inherent misclassification of imprecise measures, if random, will bias the estimates of relative risk toward the null.

Haapanen and colleagues conducted a follow-up of a community-based cohort of men and women in the Tampere area of northeastern Finland[119]. At baseline, people were questioned about clinically diagnosed diabetes (as well as CHD and hypertension) and leisure time physical activity, along with other risk factors. There were 1864 people eligible for diabetes incidence who were followed over 10 years, with morbidity surveys at five and 10 years. Mortality records were also traced. Review of self-reported diabetes and medical records at baseline suggested reasonable validity of these self-reports (Kappa = 0.71–0.79).

The age-adjusted RR for men was 0.65 (CI 0.35–1.19; ARR = 2.8/1000 person-years) for high total leisure time energy expenditure versus low, and was 0.79 (CI 0.45–1.40) for moderate activity. In women, similar trends were seen, but the gradient was stronger and statistically significant (high versus low RR = 0.34, (CI 0.17–0.68; ARR = 5.1/1000 person-years); moderate versus low

RR = 0.47 (CI 0.24–0.90; ARR = 4.1/1000 person-years). Intensity of activity (greater than or equal to one session per week of vigorous activity versus less than this amount) was significantly associated with reduced diabetes incidence in women (p = 0.043), and nearly so in men (p = 0.082).

A recent prospective study of physical activity is from the San Luis Valley Diabetes Study in Colorado[120] in Hispanics and non-Hispanic whites (NHWs). Non-diabetic persons (WHO criteria) at baseline (1984–1988) were followed for an average of 10 years. Among the 1280 eligible at baseline, 1069 had 1+ follow-up visits (73% had 2+ visits). Persons reporting high levels of vigorous activity (>3 times/week for a minimum of 20 minutes each time), or moderate levels (some vigorous activity but not at a high level) were compared to persons reporting no vigorous activity. Both high (OR = 0.46, CI 0.31–0.69) and moderate (OR = 0.54, CI 0.37–0.80) levels of vigorous activity were significantly protective in univariate models. The protective effect was slightly diminished by adjustment for age, gender, ethnicity, family history of diabetes, BMI and subscapular skin-fold, but remained statistically significant for high activity levels (OR = 0.64, CI 0.42–0.98). High activity levels were associated with a lower risk of type 2 diabetes in both Hispanics (higher risk of diabetes) and NHWs (lower risk of diabetes) at both high and low BMIs. High activity levels appeared somewhat more protective among persons with a family history of diabetes (interaction p = 0.08).

Results from the Iowa Women's Health Study have also shown protection from clinically diagnosed and self-reported diabetes after 12 years of follow-up[121]. The RR for diabetes was 0.69 (CI 0.63–0.77) among 34 257 women comparing any reported activity to no activity, adjusted for age, education, smoking, alcohol intake, estrogen use, diet variables and family history of diabetes.

The most recent prospective study analyzed health professional men (veterinarians, podiatrists, dentists, optometrists, etc.) aged 40–75 years and followed for 10 years[122]. Using MET hours per week as the summary of leisure activity, a gradient of reduced incidence was seen with increasing MET hours (Table 6.4). MET hours are metabolic equivalents – they are calculated by multiplying the metabolic cost of an activity by the number of hours activity is at that level. Interestingly, hours of TV-watching followed the opposite trend and were independent of self-reported activity. The RRs across categories of average hours of TV watching per week were: 1.00, 1.66, 1.64, 2.16 and 2.87 for 0–1 hours, 2–10, 11–20, 21–40, and 40+ respectively (p <0.001 for trend).

A small number of prospective studies have also looked at the relationship of physical activity to measures of glucose or insulin levels. Leonetti and colleagues noted that increased energy expenditure was associated with lower levels of 2 h glucose in Japanese-Americans in Seattle with IGT and among people with a positive family history after five years, but found nothing among people with normal glucose tolerance[123]. Rankinen *et al.*[124] showed that decreases in activity over 30 months were associated with increased fasting insulin levels, after adjustment for weight change and other important risk factors. The small number of people who increased their physical activity had lower levels of fasting insulin at follow-up.

The prospective observational evidence is consistent that higher levels of physical activity are associated with lower risk of type 2 diabetes. This protective effect appears to exist in people across the age span[111], and is likely to be similar in both men and women, since several studies (with the exception of one[117]) have found lower risk in women with higher activity. Larger studies find that there is usually a graded decrease in risk with increases in activity level from sedentary to even low levels of activity, though this is an area where additional data would be useful, since studies such as that by Lynch[107] suggest a possible threshold effect at fairly vigorous levels.

Methodological issues may be at play, since the first report of the Nurses Health Study found no graded risk using a simple scale of vigorous activity[104] but, with more detailed exposure data, a graded risk was seen[105]. The data are less complete concerning the types and intensities of physical activity, but the recent study by Hu *et al.*[105], with more power than most, suggests that brisk walking is vigorous enough to be associated with lower risk. Given the limited number of end-points in most prospective studies, it has not been possible to detect many interactions; that is, subgroups where the effects of activity are different.

In many studies of physical activity and diabetes, the adjustment for obesity measures presents a challenge, since activity also determines obesity, which is in the pathway from activity to diabetes risk. Epidemiological teaching suggests that such pathway variables should not be adjusted for, since this may overadjust or remove effects that actually exist. In some studies reviewed above, adjustment for obesity attenuated or removed the effects of activity, whereas in others, only small changes with adjustment occurred. Effects of activity that remain after adjustment for obesity suggest that either: (1) other effects exist (such as improved muscle blood flow and decreased insulin resistance independent of absolute obesity levels); or (2) that incomplete adjustment for obesity has occurred.

Some subgroups should be explored: two studies found no effect in people with IGT[76,123], and two found the greatest effect in the most obese people, with little effect in people near the normal weight range[110,125]. In a reanalysis of the Pennsylvania Alumni cohort, Helmrich *et al.*[125] found that increased physical activity was associated with decreased diabetes risk among high-risk men (BMI $\geq$ 25, hypertension and family history of diabetes) but no effect was seen among low-risk men. It is also possible that interactions with dietary intake of total or saturated fats, or family history could exist. In the case of dietary fats, cross-sectional analyses by Feskens *et al.*[126] and Marshall and co-workers[127] suggest this, as does the prospective analysis by Leonetti[123]. Family history has been explored in two studies, which noted similar effects in people with, and without, diabetes in relatives[104,105,108].

These findings have been surprisingly consistent. Interestingly, many of these studies are plagued by simple measures of activity, often collected only at baseline, with many intervening years of follow-up, a design which seems likely not to find consistent effects. In the dietary studies that follow, such consistency has not been found. In addition, only one of the studies in Table 6.4 explored changes in physical activity[118], which were not predictive. In addition, changes in weight, and other factors, were rarely measured. It is tempting to ask whether physical activity measures in observational studies are good surrogate measures for a complex of behaviors that mark overall lower risk. This is especially likely since the small number of clinical trials suggests that physical activity alone has limited effects on glucose levels in the absence of weight loss. The only RCT which suggests otherwise is the DaQing study[55], in which the physical activity intervention group had a lower incidence of diabetes. Thus, while the evidence from a single large clinical trial and most of the prospective studies supports a major role for physical activity, larger longer-term clinical trials are still needed to answer the question of whether increasing physical activity, independent of weight loss can prevent diabetes.

Diet composition

Composition of the diet has been explored as an etiological factor in the risk of type 2 diabetes for many years. Because of major recent changes in 'Western' diets (including increases in simple refined carbohydrates and in dietary fat from animal sources, with decreased complex carbohydrates and fiber intake), dietary constituents have received significant attention. An early hypothesis was that refined and simple sugars played a major role. This early debate has been summarized by Mann[128] who noted that a number of studies both supported and did not support this hypothesis. It is important to note that the majority of those early studies were methodologically weak, and few were prospective in design. West also provided a review of nutrition in the etiology and prevention of type 2 diabetes with published evidence from before 1975[129,130]. His primary conclusion was that total calories and obesity seem to be of primary importance, and he found little support for specific diet constituents, including dietary fat, simple carbohydrates and fibre[131].

Dietary fat intake has been explored in numerous studies, since it may play a role in development of obesity, alterations of insulin action or in diabetes incidence itself. Willett reviewed the evidence relating dietary fat to the development of obesity, and concluded that 'Diets high in fat do not appear to be the primary cause of the high prevalence of excess body fat in our society, and reductions in fat will not be a solution'[132]. Hannah and Howard came to a similar conclusion about glucose tolerance and the role of dietary fats[133], though Virtanen and Aro's review did suggest a role for high dietary fats based on their synthesis of the literature[134]. A recent review by Hu and colleagues updates this literature, and notes that the quality of dietary fat and carbohydrate, rather than simply quantity, may be the important variables[135].

Thus, there are conflicting opinions about the role of dietary fats in the etiology of type 2 diabetes. Based on a synthesis of animal and human studies, it appears likely that high saturated fat diets do play a role in increasing insulin resistance[136], although the type of fat and fatty acid composition of the diet play a major role[137]. The following section reviews the current evidence on dietary constituents in diabetes prevention.

RCTs

There have been no RCTs of specific dietary constituents on the incidence of diabetes in humans. Such trials would require the identification and follow-up of large numbers of high-risk subjects, with modification of carbohydrate, fat type or content, or protein with maintenance of energy balance, to be independent of weight change. Consequently, the only RCTs are those that have explored effects of dietary composition on defined changes in intermediate end-points such as insulin levels or action, glucose levels and lipids over short time periods (e.g.[138,139]). While providing physiological insight, such studies beg the question of the influence of long-term dietary intake in free-living populations. Thus, the primary evidence for dietary intake has come from prospective epidemiological studies of populations. This evidence is summarized in Table 6.5.

Prospective observational epidemiological studies

In the earliest reported prospective study of diet and incidence of diabetes, Medalie and colleagues showed no relationship with any dietary factor (total calories, carbohydrate, percentage of intake from saturated fat) and diabetes[103,140]. However, they did not report their methods or analysis in detail, and suggested that the short dietary assessment interview might be of limited validity.

In the only prospective dietary study reported among Pima Indians[141, 187] women aged 25–44 were followed from 1968 to an unspecified time prior to 1984; 87 developed diabetes. The only nutrient significantly predicting diabetes was higher total carbohydrate and starch intake. However, in each tertile of higher total energy and total fat intake there was a higher incidence (although this was not statistically significant). No multivariate analyses were performed. There was no relationship with tertiles of sugar intake. This small sample of young women may have lacked the power to identify major nutrients and represents only a limited exploration of nutrition in the population with the world's highest diabetes risk.

Table 6.5. Prospective studies of diet and type 2 diabetes.

Author, reference	Population	Follow-up (years)	Calories	Carbohydrates	Fat	Other
Medalie et al. 1974[107,140]	**Israeli Ischemic Heart Disease Study** 8688 men. Outcome: diabetes (including OGTT in some)	5	0*	0	0	0 protein
Bennett et al. 1984[141]	**Pima Indians** 187 women. Outcome: diabetes by OGTT	5	+ trend p = ns	+ total CHO + starch 0 sugar	0	
Snowdon and Phillips 1985[142]	**Seventh-day Adventists, California USA** 25 698 persons. Outcome: diabetes mortality	21	NA	NA	NA	+ non-vegetarian (increased meat)
Lundgren et al. 1989[143]	**Gothenburg, Sweden** 1154 women. Outcome: clinical diabetes or fasting glucose ≥7.0 mmol/L	12	0	0	0	0 protein; 0 potatoes, bread
Feskens et al. 1995[146]	**Seven Countries Study, Finnish and Dutch cohorts** 338 nondiabetic men, 1970–1990. Outcome: 2 h glucose	20	0	− total CHO − dietary fiber	+ total + saturated	− Vitamin C − vegetables, legumes
Feskens et al. 1991[147]	**Rotterdam, Netherlands, general practice** 175 normoglycemic persons. Outcome: OGTT, IGT + diabetes	4	0	+ total CHO (%) + pastries 0 fiber	0	− legumes
Feskens et al. 1991[148]	**Rotterdam, Netherlands, general practice** 175 normoglycemic persons. Outcome: OGTT, IGT + diabetes	4	0	+ total CHO (%)	0	− Fish
Stern 1991[5]	**San Antonio Heart Study, Texas, USA** 1093 Mexican-American and nonHispanic whites (NHW). Outcome: diabetes by OGTT, therapy	8	− Kcal/kg	0 total 0 starch 0 sucrose	0 total, saturated − poly-unsaturated − fat avoidance	
Marshall et al. 1994[149]	**San Luis Valley Diabetes Study, Colorado, USA** 134 Hispanic. NHW persons with IGT. Outcome: diabetes by OGTT, therapy	2	0	− total CHO (%) (p = 0.08)	+ total	

Table 6.5. contd.

Reference	Study	Follow-up		Carbohydrate	Fat	Other
Marshall et al. 1997[150]	**San Luis Valley Diabetes Study, Colorado, USA.** 1069 Hispanic, NHW normoglycemic persons. Outcome: fasting insulin	x̄ = 4.3	0	− starch − fiber	+ total + saturated	0 Ω-3 fatty acids
Leonetti et al. 1996[123]	**Seattle Washington, USA.** 124 Japanese-American nondiabetic men. Outcome: 2 h glucose	5	0	0	+ total + animal	
Hara et al. 1996[114]	**Los Angeles and Hawaii, USA.** 1144 Japanese-Americans. Outcome: diabetes by OGTT	6.3	0	0	0	
Colditz et al. 1992[154]	**Nurses Health Study, USA.** 84 360 white women. Outcome: self-reported diabetes	6	0	0 total 0 fiber 0 sucrose	0 animal − vegetable	− Potassium, calcium, magnesium
Salmerón et al. 1997[158]	**Nurses Health Study, USA.** 65 173 women. Outcome: self-reported diabetes	6	+	+ glycemic index − total, cereal fiber	0 animal − vegetable p = ns	− Magnesium
Salmerón et al. 1997[155]	**Health Professionals Follow-up Study, USA.** 42 759 men. Outcome: self-reported diabetes	6	0	+ glycemic index − total, cereal fiber	0 animal 0 vegetable	− Magnesium
Ford et al. 2000[162]	**NHANES I Epidemiologic Follow-up Study (NHEFS).** 9665 men and women in NHANES I. Outcome: diabetes by self report, hospital record, death certificate	10				− ≥5 fruit or vegetable servings/day
Ford 2001[238]	**NHANES I Epidemiologic Follow-up Study (NHEFS).** 9573 men and women in NHANES I. Outcome: diabetes by self report, hospital record, death certificate	10				− multivitamin use at baseline, adjusted for multiple factors
Meyer et al. 2000[159]	**Iowa Women's Health Study.** 35 988 women aged 55–69 years. Outcome: self-reported diabetes	6	adjusted	− whole grains − total dietary fiber − cereal fiber 0 glycemic index 0 refined grains		− magnesium 0 fruits/vegetables

Table 6.5. contd.

Meyer *et al.* 2001[161]	**Iowa Women's Health Study** 35 988 women aged 55–69 years. Outcome: self-reported diabetes	11	adjusted as above	– vegetable as above – poly-unsaturated fatty acids – trans-fatty acids
Salmerón *et al.* 2001[157]	**Nurses Health Study, USA** 84 204 women aged 38–63 in 1984. Outcome: self-reported diabetes	14		– poly-unsaturated fat + trans-fatty acids

*+ = positive association, – = negative association, 0 = no association

Seventh-day Adventists choose to eat primarily a lacto-ovo-vegetarian diet, although a range of red meat and poultry intake is seen. Snowden and Phillips investigated whether the intake of meat in this group increased the risk of diabetes[142]. They studied self-reported, cross-sectional prevalence and 21-year mortality using linked death certificates in 25 698 California Adventists.

Among males, there was a significant excess mortality from diabetes among red meat eaters (RR = 1.9) (1.2–3.1) adjusted for BMI, age, physical activity and other variables, but this was not seen in women (RR = 1.1) (CI 0.8–1.6). Meat consumption was also more common among persons with prevalent diabetes at baseline. Given the inaccuracies of death certificates, and only a single measure of diet 21 years prior to follow-up, it is surprising that these results, including a dose-response for increased meat consumption, were seen. It is likely that the dietary patterns were consistent and existed over long periods, so that a single measure gave a reasonable index of habits.

No other studies of diet have explored this issue of meat consumption (or conversely, the complex dietary differences between lacto-ovo-vegetarians and non-vegetarians) given the small numbers of such individuals in the larger cohorts studied by others. This study also provides no useful information about specific dietary constituents, since the diet questionnaire was relatively simple given the large number of subjects seen in 1960.

Lundgren completed a 12-year follow-up of 1242 Swedish women and explored baseline dietary differences in a nested case-control analysis[143]. No association was seen with total calories, dietary protein, carbohydrate or fat intake, though analyses were largely univariate in nature. Fiber was not investigated in detail, though there was no association with bread, fruit or potato consumption. In a companion paper reporting the role of obesity-related variables, he found that incidence of diabetes was strongly related to baseline BMI, sum of skin-folds and waist–hip ratio[144]. In addition, increases in BMI and skin-folds were also highly related to increases of serum glucose in normoglycemic women.

Consistent with the findings of Medalie[140], Feskens *et al.* reported no associations between dietary factors and clinical diabetes incidence in the 25-year follow-up of 841 middle-aged men in the Zutphen Study, which was the Netherlands portion of the Seven Countries Study[145]. This analysis used men enrolled from 1960 to 1985 with clinical diabetes as the end-point. In a later publication which used a portion of this same cohort, Feskens and colleagues analyzed 20-year follow-up data from the same Dutch cohort and added the Finnish cohorts of the Seven Countries Study[146]. In this later analysis, an OGTT was conducted at the 30-year follow-up visit, but diet data were used from the 1969–1970 visit, so only 20 years of follow-up were available. The authors now excluded people with clinical diabetes and used 2 h glucose among people not known previously to have diabetes as the primary end-point. This included 8% with newly diagnosed diabetes and 21% with IGT at follow-up.

Thorough multiple regression analysis revealed that prior intake of fat (especially saturated fat) was significantly associated with 2 h glucose, adjusted for BMI and age. There was a trend toward higher total and saturated fat intake (as percentage of energy) among people with newly diagnosed diabetes, but this was not statistically significant. They also noted an inverse association with 2 h glucose and vitamin C intake, also with increases in fish, potatoes, vegetables and legume intake between the surveys.

This report shows the differences that may result from different end-point definition within the same study. Significant associations with dietary fat were seen with 2 h glucose levels, but no association was seen using previously undiagnosed diabetes on the OGTT, which may have been due to smaller numbers of categorical end-points. This study has the advantage of very long-term follow-up, but suffers from limited numbers of dietary assessments and relatively small numbers of outcomes. It is also difficult to compare to the previously reported negative 25 year follow-up study using clinical diabetes as an end-point[145]. These two reports highlight the difficulties of these types of dietary studies. Here, the same dietary methods were used in all subjects, but the length of follow-up, proportion of the original cohort surviving, and the outcome all differed, as did the results between the reports.

Positive findings were also reported by Feskens and colleagues[147,148] in two publications from a general practice study of elderly people in Rotterdam, the Netherlands. Among people aged 64–87 years at baseline who were followed for four years with annual OGTTs, higher intake of carbohydrates and pastries and lower intake of legumes high in water-soluble fiber were associated with increased risk of glucose intolerance (IGT plus diabetes)[147]. In a parallel analysis, they identified a lower incidence of glucose intolerance with increased fish intake (OR = 0.47) (CI 0.23–0.93) adjusted for age, gender, past MI, BMI, energy intake/kg body weight and carbohydrate intake[148]. No relationship was seen with total or saturated fat intake. They noted that increased habitual fish intake would increase omega-3 fatty acids, which have been shown in animal studies to improve insulin resistance.

The Zutphen studies and these general practice studies used identical measures of dietary intake (the cross-check method). However, the length of follow-up and definition of outcomes differed substantially. Whether the use of OGTT defined glucose intolerance (including IGT)[146] compared with clinical diabetes[145] is primarily responsible for the different findings is not clear.

Stern explored dietary intake and behavior in the San Antonio Heart Study[5]. He found no relationship of any carbohydrate intake variable (total, starch, sucrose) after eight years of follow-up among 1093 Mexican-American and non-Hispanic whites, using a repeat OGTT or hypoglycemic therapy to define an incident case of diabetes. Total calories per kilogram of body weight showed an inverse association, such that people who remained non-diabetic reported higher calorie intake per unit of body weight.

Stern and colleagues noted that this seemingly counterintuitive finding could be due to under-reporting by obese people who were at higher risk, had lower physical activity or a more efficient metabolic state, such that people at risk actually ate fewer calories but were more likely to store them as fat. They found no significant associations with total or saturated fat intake as percentage of calories, although people who developed diabetes did report higher fat intake. People who remained free of diabetes were significantly more likely to report avoiding fat intake, using a fat avoidance scale developed locally. These results provide modest support for the role of dietary fat. However, they are limited by the lack of interim dietary measures and the use of a single test for diabetes at eight years.

In a two-year follow-up of 134 Hispanic and non-Hispanic white people with IGT, Marshall and colleagues explored dietary relationships with the development of diabetes diagnosed by OGTT[149]. An estimated increase of 40 g/day in total dietary fat was associated with an increase in diabetes (OR = 7.4) (1.3– 40.6), adjusted for energy intake, gender, age, BMI, waist–hip ratio, centrality index, and fasting and 1 h insulin fasting glucose at baseline. These are some of the strongest results supporting the role of dietary fat in a prospective study.

A recent analysis of longitudinal data from the San Luis Valley Diabetes Study was also reported by Marshall *et al.*[150.] There were 1069 non-diabetic subjects who were seen for a minimum of one and up to three visits over nine years (average 4.3 years). Complex longitudinal analyses were used which allowed multiple dietary intake data and fasting insulin levels to be examined allowing for both intra- and inter-individual variability over time. This technique, based on the Laird–Ware longitudinal models[151], improves power substantially with repeated continuous measures[152].

Marshall found that higher intake of total and saturated fat were strongly associated with higher fasting insulin levels, adjusted for BMI, waist circumference, physical activity, age, gender and ethnicity. Dietary fiber and starch intake were inversely associated with fasting insulin concentrations. No associations with fasting insulin concentrations were observed for monounsaturated fat, polyunsaturated fat, omega-3 fatty acids, sucrose, glucose and fructose intake. These results support animal studies and a limited number of human population studies that have suggested that increased saturated and total fat intake and decreased fiber and starch intake increase fasting insulin concentrations and may also increase insulin resistance.

Leonetti and colleagues studied 124 Japanese-American men in Seattle for five years[123]. They explored both nutrient content of the diet and reported energy expenditure. Among people with IGT, the percentage of calories from total dietary fat and animal fat were associated with the development of diabetes (higher fat) or reversion to normal glucose tolerance (lower fat). There was no overall effect of energy expenditure. A small effect was only seen in subgroups with a positive family history of diabetes or with IGT at baseline. Exploration of the interaction of diet and physical activity revealed that the percentage of calories from animal fat was also related to 2 h glucose levels after multiple adjustment, but only in those with less than the highest levels of energy expenditure. There was no effect of refined or complex carbohydrates. The relatively small numbers of subjects made it impossible to detect changes in categories of glucose tolerance (e.g. development of diabetes diagnosed by OGTT) with any power. The careful analysis of interactions which are biologically plausible (e.g. dietary fat effect strongest in sedentary people) provides a useful example for others to emulate in larger studies.

Hara and colleagues followed Japanese-Americans from the mid-1970s through to the 1980s for an average of 6.3 years in Los Angeles or Hawaii[114]. Subjects were ethnically pure Japanese emigrants from Hiroshima, Japan with an average age of 61 years. While the primary focus of the analysis was on physical activity (see above) and biochemical predictors, the authors note in the discussion that they found no associations between any dietary intake variable and the incidence of diabetes, although, in the abstract of the report, they suggest dietary fat intake is important. Detailed dietary intake data were available[153] so it is unclear whether or not this represents a thorough analysis of these data.

Several analyses of the large health professionals cohorts in the USA (Nurses Health Study[154-157], Health Professions Follow-up Study[158]) have explored dietary factors and risk of type 2 diabetes prospectively. Among 84 360 nurses followed for six years (1980–1986) for the development of clinically diagnosed diabetes (no OGTT was conducted) no excess risk was seen for high intakes of animal fat. Lower diabetes risk with higher intake of vegetable fat was seen[154].

In the second report from the Nurses Health Study, women who had not yet developed diabetes and who completed a more detailed diet questionnaire in 1986 were analyzed[155]. Follow-up every two years for a subsequent six years (1986–1992) occurred on the remaining 65 173 eligible women. Women with diabetes in the first analysis were excluded. Again, no relationship was seen for higher intake of animal or saturated fat, and the trend for an inverse association with vegetable fat seen in the first study was present, but was not significant. Foods with a high glycemic index, and low cereal fiber intake were found to independently increase diabetes risk. There was evidence of inter-action; that is, diets lowest in cereals and highest in glycemic index carried the highest risk (RR = 2.5). Foods with a high glycemic index increase insulin demand and hyperinsulinemia, which may lead to a high demand for endo-genous insulin production, stressing pancreatic reserve.

Similar findings were also observed among US male dentists, veterinarians, pharmacists, optometrists, osteopaths and podiatrists[158], although the trend for high glycemic foods was less clear until simultaneous adjustment for cereal fiber intake occurred. The primary effect in this analysis appeared to be restricted to men in the category with both the highest glycemic index and lowest cereal intakes, and little dose–response existed for men in groups with intermediate intake.

In a follow-up analysis of the Nurses Health Study, Liu *et al.* explored whole-grain intake on risk of type 2 diabetes in women[156]. In 10-year follow-up data, women who consumed wholegrain products (e.g. dark bread, wholegrain breakfast cereal, cooked oatmeal, popcorn) were 27% less likely to develop clinical diabetes (RR = 0.73, CI 0.63–0.89 adjusted for multiple factors) and 31% more likely to develop diabetes with a higher intake of refined grain products (RR = 1.31, CI 1.12–1.53). Analysis exploring potential interactions with BMI, saturated fat intake and other variables did not significantly alter these relationships.

Among nurses[154,155] and other health professionals[158], lower magnesium intake was also noted to increase risk of diabetes in a dose–response fashion, with the relative risk steadily dropping as intake increased to the highest quartile (nurses RR = 0.62, CI 0.50–0.78)[155]; male health professionals RR = 0.72, CI 0.54–0.96)[158]. Among nurses, lower intakes of calcium and potassium were also associated with increased diabetes risk[154], though this was not noted in the later analysis[155]. Similar findings for magnesium have also been reported from the Iowa Women's Health Study[159].

The most recent analysis of the Nurses Health Study cohort explored specific types of dietary fat on diabetes incidence[157]. Using the 14-year follow-up data on 84 204 women aged 34–59 years at baseline, Salmerón *et al.* again reported no effect of increased total dietary fat (RR = 0.98, CI 0.94–1.02 for a 5% increase in intake). Saturated and monounsaturated fatty acids were not found to be related, however, for every 5% increase in energy intake from polyunsaturated fatty acids, there was a reduction in diabetes risk (RR = 0.63, CI 0.53–0.76), and for a 2% increase in trans-fatty acids, there was excess risk (RR = 1.39, CI 1.15–1.67). An accompanying editorial notes that this novel hypothesis and finding are substantially limited by the methods used, and should be investigated in more detailed studies[160].

Meyer *et al.* have also conducted detailed dietary analyses on the Iowa Women's Health Study cohort[161]. After 11 years of follow-up with four interim diet assessments similar to those used in the Nurses Health Study, 1890 self-reported cases of diabetes developed among the 35 988 women aged 55–69 years at baseline. No relationship was seen with total dietary fat. Incidence was negatively associated with dietary polyunsaturated fatty acids, vegetable fat and trans-fatty acids, whereas trans-fatty acids were positively associated with diabetes risk in the Nurses Health Study[157]. With detailed adjustment for magnesium and cereal fiber intake, both significantly related to diabetes incidence in this cohort[159], as well as subsitution of other dietary fat components, the multiply-adjusted relative risks declined across quintiles of vegetable fat intake from 1.00, 0.90, 0.87, 0.84 and 0.82 (p = 0.02), although polyunsaturated fatty acids and trans-fatty acids no longer remained significant. Subsitution of polyunsaturated fatty acids for saturated fatty acids, and vegetable fat for animal fat, gave similar results. No effect modification by BMI, activity, alcohol or vitamin E intake was seen. Given the very high correlation with dietary fat intake components, some degree of attenuation between them is likely, making identification of specific fat subtypes difficult.

Ford and Mokdad reported on fruit and vegetable consumption in the 20-year follow-up of the NHANES-I Epidemiologic Follow-up Study (NHFES) cohort[162] using clinically reported diabetes, hospitalizations or death certificates as end-points. No OGTTs were conducted. Persons eating five or more servings of fruits and vegetables per day, adjusted for demographics, smoking, medications, activity, BMI and alcohol use, were 27% less likely to develop incident diabetes (HR = 0.73, CI 0.54–0.98; ARR $\cong$ 1.9/1000 person-years). This effect was primarily seen in women, and was attenuated when education was added to the model, but was not changed when percentage of calories from fat, total energy intake and use of vitamins were added. Given the details available about diet, incomplete adjustment for type of fat intake and levels of activity is likely, and no measures of glycemic load were available. Thus, it is not clear if fruit and vegetable intake is itself associated with lower incidence of diabetes, or whether it marks healthy behaviors in general. It appears consistent with results of Feskens[146].

The results of the several prospective studies presented in Table 6.5 present a somewhat inconsistent picture. This may be due in part to the different type and quality of nutrient intake data, which included 24-hour recalls, food frequencies of varying detail, and simple scales. Each of these allowed different levels of nutrient aggregation, some with more detailed nutrient databases underlying them than in other studies. Outcomes also varied, from use of 2 h glucose levels or insulin levels, to clinically diagnosed diabetes, to diabetes detected by OGTT, and including mortality. Each of these end-points may identify different portions of the phenotypic and etiological spectrum and may at least partially explain divergent results. In addition, the amount of interim data between baseline and follow-up varied, as did the analytic complexity, with earlier studies often being largely univariate, while later studies used time-to-event methods or longitudinal models. It is likely that each of these differences accounts for some of the between-study variability, and highlights the fact that there are very few studies with methods in common.

Findings for total energy intake varied, and dietary fiber had an inconsistent association with diabetes as an outcome, though higher intakes were associated with lower levels of glucose[146] or insulin[150]. The only prospective studies that identified a role for higher levels of dietary fat used 2 h glucose as an outcome[123,146], or fasting insulin[150], or OGTT diabetes among people with IGT[149]. The study by Stern[5] also found that persons 'avoiding fat' (on a scale no one else has replicated) had lower risk of developing clinical or OGTT diabetes.

The largest prospective studies of clinical diabetes among non-diabetics at baseline did not find a role for total dietary fat[154,155,157,158,161]. Consistently, these studies differed from those that were positive by not having any glucose tolerance testing either at baseline or at follow-up. It is unclear whether this could explain the reported differences. In addition, few of the studies explored composition interaction (e.g. dietary fat intake in persons with low versus high fiber intake) with the exception of the Health Professionals studies that reported glycemic index-fiber, and wholegrain–dietary fat interactions. Whether such analyses would clarify the picture remains unclear.

At present, the evidence still does not support a consistently replicated role for specific nutrients in diabetes incidence, though dietary fat subtypes and a role for cereal fiber and wholegrains is accumulating. A diet that combines limited energy intake for weight maintenance, low saturated fat content, high fruit and vegetable and wholegrain intake appears prudent for the reduction of cardiovascular disease, some cancers and diabetes. Use of such a diet in both the DPS[69] and the DPP[72] was one of the lifestyle changes that resulted in reduction of diabetes incidence.

Weight change and diabetes

Several types of studies have explored weight change and subsequent diabetes. These include RCTs aimed at weight loss or obesity prevention with diabetes as the outcome and observational studies that prospectively explore the influence of weight change[163,164]. They also include animal studies that allow unique observations not possible in humans.

Animal studies

Animal studies are mentioned briefly since two models of type 2 diabetes are relevant to the human condition and have allowed calorific restriction over much of the lifespan, which is difficult to achieve in humans. In the first model, using Israeli sand rats (*Psammomys obesus*), Walder and colleagues showed that restriction of food intake to 75% of *ad libitum* levels post-weaning led to complete restriction of the hyperglycemia that develops in this animal in laboratory settings[165]. Hyperinsulinemia was not completely prevented, however, and this led the authors to conclude that a genetic component may also exist to raise insulin levels.

The second model is the primate rhesus monkey (*Macaca mulatta*). Hansen and colleagues, in a series of elegant prospective studies, studied the development of obesity, hyperinsulinemia, beta-cell responsiveness and other parameters in male adult monkeys who are prone to the development of obesity and diabetes with characteristics similar to type 2 in humans[166,167]. They identified sequential stages of development of diabetes which began with obesity, followed by elevations in fasting insulin and decreases in insulin stimulated glucose disposal. Acute insulin secretion then rose to compensate, and later declined as hyperglycemia developed[168].

These studies were followed by a prevention trial in which eight male monkeys were fed three meals a day (13% fat, 17% protein, 70% carbohydrate as monkey chow) and calories were titrated to maintain stable young adult body weight[167]. Age-matched control monkeys (n = 19) were fed *ad libitum* (AL) on the same diet, and both groups were followed for five to nine years. Four (21%) of the AL fed monkeys developed diabetes by human OGTT criteria, and six (32%) had IGT, compared with no glucose intolerance among weight-stable monkeys. Fasting and glucose stimulated insulin levels were also significantly lower among weight-stable monkeys, and beta-cell responsiveness was maintained. Body fat remained at young adult levels as well. This prevention study in monkeys strongly suggests that obesity prevention can delay, if not completely prevent, type 2 diabetes. A 10-year follow-up of these monkeys showed that a significant and sustained long-term reduction in energy expenditure occurred as a result of the calorific restriction[169].

Human studies

Most of the over 600 human weight loss studies were recently critically reviewed using standardized criteria[29]. Relevant studies from this review have been included above as appropriate. Rather than review these studies for their weight loss aspects again here, the summary conclusions from the portion of the report relevant to diabetes prevention are shown in Table 6.6.

The authors felt that there was evidence from multiple well-conducted RCTs that weight loss produced by lifestyle modifications reduced blood glucose levels in overweight and obese people without type 2 diabetes. They did not conclude that weight loss prevented diabetes, however, since most of the studies were of relatively short duration, and were not large enough to directly test whether a categorical end-point such as diabetes was avoided. The other conclusions were based on fewer RCTs or on observational results alone. The use of weight loss medication has not been shown to be any better than weight loss through lifestyle modification for improving blood glucose levels in overweight or obese people, and may have unexpected side-effects of significant magnitude[163].

Based on observational studies, decreases in abdominal fat appear to improve glucose tolerance in overweight individuals with IGT, although this has not been shown to be independent of the total amount of weight loss. In addition, increased cardiorespiratory fitness improves glucose tolerance in overweight individuals, but there is no evidence that shows this relationship to be independent of weight loss, even though several studies have shown short-term improvements in hyperinsulinemia.

Table 6.6. Summary of findings on weight loss and diabetes from evidence-based review[29].

Observations	Quality of evidence*
Weight loss produced by lifestyle modifications reduces blood glucose levels in overweight and obese persons without type 2 diabetes (and reduces blood glucose levels and HbA$_{1c}$ in some patients with type 2 diabetes)	A
Weight loss produced by weight loss medications has not been shown to be any better than weight loss through lifestyle modification for improving blood glucose levels in overweight or obese persons with or without type 2 diabetes	B
Decreases in abdominal fat improve glucose tolerance in overweight individuals with impaired glucose tolerance, although this has not been shown to be independent of weight loss	C
Increased cardiorespiratory fitness improves glucose tolerance in overweight individuals, but no evidence has shown this relationship to be independent of weight loss	C

*Summarized in Table 6.1.

Thus, it appears that the benefits of weight loss in people without diabetes are reasonably well established, but are limited to small but significant reductions in glucose levels. Ultimately, the authors only recommended weight loss to lower elevated blood glucose levels in overweight and obese persons with type 2 diabetes, but not in people without diabetes. Since people at risk for diabetes are often dyslipidemic, the report also recommended weight loss for such people to lower LDL cholesterol and triglycerides, and raise HDL cholesterol. The authors left unanswered the questions of how to achieve long-term weight loss and, ultimately, whether this would prevent diabetes.

A recent publication from the British Regional Heart Study adds important observational evidence to weight change as a risk factor for diabetes[164]. The authors studied over 7700 men in 24 British towns with 12 years of follow-up. Substantial weight gain, defined as >10% of baseline weight, was associated with a 61% increase in type 2 diabetes risk (RR = 1.61; CI 1.01–2.56) compared to weight-stable people. A gradient of risk was also seen in multiply-adjusted models, such that people who lost >4% of baseline weight had a reduced risk (RR = 0.66), and people who gained 4–10% had a RR = 1.21, while people gaining >10% had an RR = 1.81 (P$_{trend}$ = 0.0009). Increased duration of obesity was also associated with increased risk of type 2 diabetes, though weight fluctuation had no influence.

These results are reasonably consistent with other prospective analyses of weight change and risk of type 2 diabetes. While several studies have shown that weight gain increases risk of type 2 diabetes[144,170-174], the beneficial effects of weight loss have not always been seen[174], and in some studies, weight loss has been associated with increased risk of diabetes[175,176]. This may perhaps result from failure to exclude people who were losing weight in the early stages of undiagnosed diabetes. In the British Regional Heart Study[164], exclusion of people developing diabetes within the first four years after baseline increased the risk of weight gain for diabetes in the subsequent eight years. Weight gain from age 20 to middle age has also been reported to increase the risk of the insulin resistance syndrome[177], though no data on weight loss were presented. An economic analysis of the benefits of modest weight reduction based largely on observational data suggests that 0.5–1.7 fewer years of life with diabetes would occur, accompanied by modest cost savings[178].

A recent publication from the Nurses Health Study combined several of the lifestyle factors reviewed in the prior sections of this chapter in an analysis of diabetes incidence over 16 years of follow-up[179]. Almost 85 000 nurses were followed from 1980 to 1996 who did not have diagnosed diabetes or heart disease at baseline. Clinically diagnosed diabetes was the outcome, and no OGTTs were conducted. A low risk group was defined as: (1) BMI <25; (2) no current smoking; (3) drinking half a unit or more of alcohol per day; (4) diet high in cereal fiber and polyunsaturated fat and low in trans-fat and glycemic load; and (5) at least half an hour of moderate to vigorous activity per day. Only 3.4% of the nurses were in this low risk group. Each of the low risk factors were significantly related to diabetes, as had been seen in several prior publications from the same study. Overweight or obesity was the most important predictor, but lack of activity, poor diet, smoking and non-drinking were independent risk factors. The relative risk of developing diabetes decreased as the number of protective factors increased. Women with three factors in the low risk group (diet, BMI and exercise as above) had a RR = 0.12 (CI 0.08–0.16) and a population attributable risk (PAR%) of 87%. This suggests that 87% of incident diabetes cases could be prevented if all women had these three factors present (other things being equal). The PAR% rose to 91% among women with all five factors present (RR = 0.09, CI 0.05–0.17). This analysis of a large observational cohort suggests that findings from RCTs like the DPS[69] and DPP[72] are likely to apply to a large group of women, at least, and that the average reductions in incidence seen in the RCTs could be even greater among persons adopting between three and five lifestyle changes. Substantial impact on diabetes incidence in the population was estimated from these analyses – that perhaps 85–90% of type 2 diabetes could be reduced if everyone were able to adopt these lifestyle changes. It seems likely that these results also apply to men, and to people in many ethnic and racial groups, given the consistency of the lifestyle results from the DPP[72].

Pharmacological studies

Pharmacological interventions to prevent diabetes or its complications early in the natural history have been published since the 1960s[180]. The rationale for drug intervention includes: (1) the drug may reverse one or more specific pathophysiological defects; (2) changes in lifestyle for otherwise healthy people are difficult to make and have not yet been shown to have long-term efficacy; (3) some people are unable to change their lifestyle due to disability or other disease; and (4) it may be easier to take a drug over longer periods than it is to make significant behavioral changes. While each of these issues has a certain amount of validity, it is also important to show, through well designed clinical trials, that pharmacological interventions are efficacious before they enter widespread use, especially if they are to be given to otherwise healthy, non-diseased persons as preventive agents[5].

Reviews of the use of such agents have been published[10,180-182]. Early trials were often aimed at subjects with 'chemical diabetes', considered to be 'early diabetes' by older criteria. Such studies often included a majority of people with what would now be considered IGT, and thus are reasonably relevant to a review of primary prevention. Agents available in the 1960s included first-generation sulfonylureas and biguanides. Similar to lifestyle studies, criteria for outcomes varied and were a mixture of glucose tolerance, fasting glucose and other end-points. Table 6.7 summarizes the RCTs that have been published.

Sulfonylureas

Belknap *et al.* investigated the impact of sulfonylurea on plasma lipids and glucose tolerance in 34 men from Seattle, Washington State, USA[183]. This was a double-blind crossover trial with random allocation of either 500 mg of tolbutamide twice daily or placebo taken for one year in random order. Subjects had a range of glucose intolerance from normal through to diabetic, though none were symptomatic. Baseline glucose levels suggest only three out of 34 subjects met current ADA criteria for diabetes. Nine men (21%) did not complete the two year trial (one year on each drug).

Very limited results were presented. No diabetes incidence was reported; however, it appeared that the active drug kept glucose levels from rising over baseline levels (+1 mg/dl, 0.056 mmol/L) whereas placebo levels increased more (+6 mg/dl, 0.33 mmol/L) leading to a significant difference at study end between active and control periods. The authors say that there were significant improvements in intravenous glucose tolerance, but present no results. No weight change occurred, and no improvements in triglycerides or total cholesterol were found. The small effects of tolbutamide seen in this crossover study with incomplete data presentation make it of limited use.

Another early trial of tolbutamide was conducted by Englehardt and Vecchio among oil company employees in Texas undergoing diabetes screening[184]. Forty-two people with abnormal glucose tolerance by Fajans and Conn criteria were enrolled in a randomized, blinded study of 500 mg of tolbutamide

Table 6.7. Pharmacological interventions (including mixed interventions) – randomized controlled trials (RCTs).

Author, Reference	Population	Intervention	Results	Comments
Sulfonylureas				
Belknap et al. 1967[183] 1-b	**Seattle, WA, USA** 34 men aged 33–75 ($\bar{x}$ = 57 years) with abnormal IV and OGTT; randomized cross-over design; follow-up 1 yr on each arm, 2 yrs total. Outcome: F glucose, IVGTT	**Tolbutamide** (N = 34) 500 mg bid **Placebo** (N = 34) cross-over design	**Tolbutamide:** diabetes incidence not reported; fasting glucose showed no increase on drug (+1 mg/dl); significantly different than placebo at end (p <0.01); no weight loss, no effect on lipids; IVGT said to improve, but data not shown. **Placebo:** fasting glucose increased +6 mg/dl; no weight change	Dropouts = 21%; order of randomization masked, double-blind. Very limited data presented; drug may have had effect by limiting increase in glucose levels. Drug stopped 12 hours before test
Engelhard and Vecchio, 1967[184] 1-a	**Humble Oil Co. employees, Houston, TX, USA** 42 persons aged 25–67 ($\bar{x}$ = 47) years with IGT by old criteria; follow-up 14 months. Outcome: OGTT	**Tolbutamide** (N = 20) 500 mg bid **Placebo** (N = 22)	**Tolbutamide:** Lower 1 h post-load glucose levels (−36.4 mg/dl, −2.0 mM/L); no differences in 2 h or 3 h levels at 14 months. No report of diabetes incidence. Essentially negative	23–25% drop-out at one year. No changes in weight, though placebo group was 8.2 lbs (3.7 kg) heavier at randomization. Allocation not masked; results were blinded. Considered patients to be asymptomatic diabetics, though most would be IGT by current criteria. Drug stopped for 12 hrs before test
Camerini-Davalos 1967[185] 1-c	**New York, NY, USA** 97 subjects with chemical diabetes aged 15–44 ($\bar{x}$ = 34 years); follow-up 10–24 months. Outcome: OGTT	**Tolbutamide** (N = 38) 500 mg bid **Placebo** (N = 59)	**Tolbutamide:** RR = 0.73 (0.45–1.18, p = 0.25 intent to treat. ARR = 14/100 PY)[1] for impaired OGTT at follow-up; no weight change; triglycerides increased (p <0.01). **Placebo:** similar improvement in glucose levels on OGTT	No randomization or allocation method noted, no blinding, variable follow-up duration across groups, no multivariate analysis. Drug stopped for 3 days before test
Feldman et al. 1967, 1973[187,188]	**Kaiser Permanente, Oakland, CA** 350 subjects aged 15–59 from screening, with chemical diabetes; follow-up 5 yrs. Outcome: diabetes incidence	**Tolbutamide** (N = 174) 500 mg bid **Phenformin** (N = 91) 100 mg/day **Placebo** (N = 85)	**Tolbutamide:** 0.6/100 PY diabetes at 5 years RR = 0.16 (0.02–1.54, p = 0.20, ARR = 2.9/100 PY)[1] vs placebo. **Phenformin:** 0/100 PY diabetes (p = 0.22) vs. placebo. **Placebo:** 3.5/100 PY diabetes	Most would have IGT by current criteria: double-blind; dropouts 22%. Greatest declines in 2 h glucose for tolbutamide, although placebo decreases were almost as great, and both returned to baseline by 42 months. Phenformin had no lowering of 2 h glucose levels. Drug stopped for 3 days prior to testing

Table 6.7. contd.

Keen et al. 1968[192] I-a	**Bedford, UK.** 248 persons with moderate hyperglycemia aged 20+; follow-up 5 yrs. Outcome: cardiovascular disease, diabetes	**Tolbutamide** 500 mg bid + No diet (N = 62); **Tolbutamide + diet** (N = 64); **Placebo + No diet** (N = 63); **Placebo + Diet** (N = 59)	No diet intake differences between groups at 6–9 months. **Tolbutamide + diet:** lowest CVD event rates of all groups, but not significant. **Tolbutamide (pooled):** frequency of definite CVD events said to be significantly lower than placebo (pooled), RR = 0.76 (0.50–1.15)[1], suggesting no difference in intention to treat analysis	**Diet:** restricted total carbohydrate to 120 g; restricted table sugar, sweets. Only ~50% took most drug each 6 months. No excess of arterial events on drug. No masking of allocation; no multivariate analysis. Double-blind. Drug stopped for 10 days before testing. Dropouts: 6% plus deaths
Keen et al. 1973[190] I-a	**Bedford, UK.** Follow-up 8.5 yrs	**Placebo** (N = 125) **Tolbutamide** (N = 123). As above; diet intervention ignored as ineffective.	**Tolbutamide:** RR = 1.12 (0.49–2.54) for diabetes incidence vs. placebo. No excess of vascular disease outcomes, and small nonsignificant advantage in selected subgroup analysis	Numbers differ from prior reports due to previous errors. No multivariate analysis
Keen et al. 1982[194] I-a	**Bedford, UK.** Follow-up 10 yrs	As above	No effect of tolbutamide (OR = 1.04, p = 0.9) or diet on incidence of diabetes in logistic analyses	
Paasikivi et al. 1970[186] I-b	**Karolinska Institute, Stockholm, Sweden.** 178 survivors from first MI, randomly allocated; follow-up x̄ = 2.9 yrs. Outcomes: total mortality, IVGTT, K_0	**Tolbutamide** (N = 95) 500 mg bid **Placebo** (N = 83)	**Tolbutamide:** Total mortality RR = 0.71 (0.36–1.39)[1], greatest difference at 18 months, less thereafter. No difference in glucose disappearance (K_0) on IVGTT among persons with normal or borderline K_0 at baseline compared with placebo; but significant improvement in K_0 among those in diabetic K_0 range only. No differences in fasting glucose levels compared with placebo. 0/95 developed diabetes vs. 3/83 on placebo (p = 0.20)	Randomization by even or odd date of birth; single-blind. Dropouts 1.8% up to 18 months, then 15.7% in placebo, 5.3% in tolbutamide
Tan et al. 1977[195] I-c	**Joslin Clinic, Boston, USA.** 120 men with chemical diabetes; follow-up 5 years. Outcome: normal glucose tolerance	**Chlorpropamide** (N = 18) 100 mg qd **Tolbutamide** (N = 28) 500 mg bid **Phenformin** (N = 23) 50 mg qd	No differences in F glucose, percent with normal OGTT, AUC insulin, triglycerides, or cholesterol at any year during 5-year follow-up, except in chlorpropamide group at 1 year, which was not sustained. No	Dropouts at 5 years ranged from 30–50%. No mention of randomization method or masking. No intention to treat

Table 6.7. contd.

Sartor et al. 1980[196] 1-b	**Malmöhus Study** 267 men with IGT 10-year follow-up 1962–65 entry; follow-up completed 1974–76 – average 10 yrs. Outcome: Diabetes, mortality	**Acetohexamide** (N = 14) 250 mg qd **Placebo** (N = 37) All groups received diet **Tolbutamide + diet** (N = 49) **Placebo + diet** (N = 48) **Diet alone** (N = 50) **No therapy** (N = 591)	differences in weight gain between groups Intention to treat: **Tolbutamide** = 10.2/100 diabetes incidence; **Placebo** = 12.5/100; **Diet alone** = 14.0/100; **No therapy** = 28.8/100. Tolbutamide vs. placebo: RR = 0.82 (0.27–2.50, ARR = 2.3/100 PY)[1]. RR = 0.73 (0.25–2.14, ARR = 3.8/100 PY)[1] vs. diet. Efficacy: TOLB = 0%	Vital status and clinical diabetes status verified for 100% at follow-up. 29 dropouts did not have OGTT at follow-up. Pre-WHO criteria for IGT, type 2. 79% of men had normal glucose tolerance, 18% IGT, 3% DM by WHO criteria[27]. Used consecutive randomization with known schedule. Double-blind until 1972, then unmasked. No therapy group was drawn retrospectively at study end – no criteria given for method
Knowler et al. 1997[197] 1-b	**Malmöhus Study** 149 men in 3 groups above; mortality follow-up 22 yrs	As above	Tolbutamide treated group vs. Placebo + Diet combined: RR = 0.66 (0.39–1.10) all causes of death RR = 0.42 (0.16–1.12) ischemic heart disease deaths among 49 men treated with tolbutamide and diet for up to 10 years	
Page et al. 1993[281] 1-b	**Oxford, UK** Pilot study for Fasting Hyperglycemia Study (see below); abnormal fasting glucose or CIGMA tests similar to IGT; follow-up 6 months. Outcome: CIGMA (glucose infusion)	**Glicazide** (N = 6) 40 mg bid **Placebo** (N = 8)	**Glicazide:** decreased fasting glucose and CIGMA glucose (p <0.01), without change in insulin sensitivity, but improved β-cell function (p <0.05). Glucose levels returned to normal 1 month after stopping drug. **Placebo:** no changes in glucose or insulin levels	Lifestyle results from this trial at two years are shown in Table 6.3[90]. Blinded, short duration of follow-up, small numbers
Karunakaran et al. 1997[56,199] I-a	**Fasting Hyperglycemia Study (FHS) II** – drug outcomes; UK and France 227 persons aged 30–65 (x̄ = 50 yrs); follow-up	**Glicazide**, 80 mg bid (N = 112) **Control** (N = 115) in factorial design with lifestyle[294].	**Glicazide:** fasting glucose, HbA$_{1c}$ significantly lower, 2 h glucose and AUCg both higher ; β-cell function improved slightly; no changes in insulin sensitivity, no change in percentage with diabetes. **Control:**	Selection based on fasting glucose meant that at baseline, 37% were normal, 37% had WHO IGT, and 26% had WHO NIDDM with IFG. Randomization allocation not masked

Table 6.7. contd.

Reference	Study	Groups	Results	Comments
	1 year. Outcome: OGTT			lower or no change in control group; weight loss in control group only; no changes in insulin sensitivity; no change in percentage with diabetes
Biguanides				
Papoz *et al.* 1978[202] I-a	**Hotel Dieu, Paris, France** 120 men aged 25–55 years (x̄ = 45) with borderline glucose tolerance; follow-up 2 years. Outcome: OGTT	**Glibenclamide** (N = 28) 2 mg bid **Biguanide** (N = 30) 0.85g bid **G + B** (N = 29) **Placebo** (N = 33)	**Biguanide:** no effect on glucose and insulin; significant weight loss. **Glibenclamide:** no effect on glucose and insulin; less weight loss than in other three groups	Most men would be IGT by current criteria. Double-blind. 28% dropouts, similar across groups. 14/120 subjects stopped drug for 1 month or less. No differences in weight loss (~4 kg) between placebo, G+B and B groups. 95% power to detect a 21 mg/dl drop in 2 h glucose level. Actual differences only 0–2 mg/dl. Drug not stopped for OGTT except at 2-year test, when stopped for 15 days before OGTT
Jarrett *et al.* 1979[204,205] I-a	**Whitehall, London, UK** 204 men with borderline glucose tolerance aged 40–64 years (x̄ = 57); follow-up 5 yrs. Outcome: diabetes incidence	**Diet** (N = 44) limit to 120 g/day carbohydrate **Phenformin** (N = 49) 50 mg/day **Diet + Phenformin** (N = 43) **Placebo** (N = 45)	**Diet:** 18.2/100 worsened to diabetes. **Phenformin:** 18.4/100. **Diet + Phenformin:** 9.3/100. **Placebo:** 13.3/100. Phenformin vs. no phenformin: RR = 0.90 (0.45–1.80)[1]	Most men would have IGT by current criteria. 23/204 men dropped out (11.3%). No relation of weight change to diabetes incidence. Diabetes required 2 or more positive tests. Drug arms were double blind. Randomization method not specified. Multiple logistic regression used to account for minor imbalances at entry
Kasperska *et al.* 1986[206] I-c	**Warsaw, Poland** 73 persons with borderline or chemical diabetes aged 23–74 (x̄ = 54); follow-up 5 yrs. Outcome: OGTT	**Diet** (N = 36) **Phenformin + Diet** (N = 37) 50 mg/day	**Phenformin + Diet:** RR = 0.89 (0.25–3.14)[1] for worsening OGTT among all subjects vs. diet. **Diet:** among those with borderline tolerance only, no differences. Small, nonsignificant changes in glucose and insulin levels at 5 years in persons with borderline glucose tolerance	Alternate allocation, no mention of blinding. Dropouts = 33%, equal in groups. At entry, ~60% had 'borderline' glucose tolerance by EASD criteria
Fontbonne *et al.* 1996[207–210] I-a	**BIGPRO 1, France** 457 subjects with high waist-hip ratio, aged	**Metformin** (N = 164) 850 mg bid **Placebo** (N = 160)	**Metformin:** −2.0 kg weight loss; less rise in F glucose and insulin; lower LDL cholesterol; tPA antigen, von	28–30% dropout at one year. 21.5% had abnormal OGTT at entry. Assuming all persons with diabetes

Table 6.7. contd.

	35–60; follow-up 1 yr. Outcome: OGTT	Both groups given diet and exercise	Willebrand factor: no change in two hour glucose or insulin. BP, triglycerides, HDL cholesterol. No diabetes developed. Fasting glucose improved only in those with IGT at baseline. **Placebo:** 5 persons developed diabetes. Increase in fasting glucose	were detected, absence of cases in Metformin group and 5 in placebo group gives exact p = 0.06[f]. Double-blind, randomization not said to be masked
Charles *et al.* 1999[210,211] 1-a	**BIGPRO 1.2, France** 168 men with high waist-hip ratio, mild hypertension, fasting glucose <7.8 mmol/L; follow-up 3 months. Outcome: fasting glucose, lipids	**Metformin** (N = 83) 850 bid **Placebo** (N = 83) No lifestyle changes	**Metformin:** −0.5 kg weight loss (ns), decreases in fasting glucose, insulin, LDL cholesterol, Apo B, tPA, as in BIGPRO 1. No change in BP or triglycerides. No diabetes developed in either group	Double-blind, randomization not said to be masked. Short follow-up. Dropouts only 3%
Li *et al.* 1999[212] 1-a	**Beijing, China** 90 subjects with IGT × 2 (2 years apart) in large corporation; aged 30–60 years ($\bar{x}$ = 50); follow-up 1 yr. Outcome: OGTT diabetes, IGT	**Metformin** (N = 42) 250 mg tid **Placebo** (N = 43)	**Metformin:** 7.1% incidence of DM, RR = 0.51 (0.14–1.91)[1], p = 0.50. Less IGT at follow-up than placebo. F glucose, AUC glucose and AUC insulin, albumin excretion all lower at 1 year in efficacy analysis. Slight weight loss (−1.4 BMI units). **Placebo:** 14.0% incidence of DM	Intention to treat analysis (85/90 subjects) shown. Efficacy analysis had RR = 0.19 (0.02–1.47). Double blind; allocation scheme not reported to be masked
DPP Research Group 2001[70-72] 1-a	**Diabetes Prevention Program (DPP)** 27 US centers, 3234 men and women; 45% nonCaucasian; aged $\bar{x}$ = 51 years, BMI = 34; follow-up 2.8 years. Outcome: diabetes by ADA criteria	**Metformin** (N = 1073) 850 mg twice/day **Placebo** (N = 1082) Tablets twice a day; annual meeting with written material on lifestyle	Metformin incidence rate = 7.8/100 PY vs. placebo = 11.0/100 PY; 31% reduction in incidence; ARR = 3.2/100 PY: less effect in BMI <30; age >60 years	72% took at least 80% of medication, 77% took placebo; NNT = 13.9 to prevent one case.

Thiazolidinediones

Nolan *et al.* 1994[216] 1-a	**San Diego, CA, USA** 18 nondiabetic obese persons, age $\bar{x}$ = 44.5 ys;	**Troglitazone** (N = 12) 200 mg, bid	**Troglitazone:** lower fasting and OGTT glucose and insulin levels, increased	Allocation was masked. Small numbers, short follow-up; no

Table 6.7. contd.

Study	Intervention (N)	Results	important side-effects noted
follow-up 3 months. Outcome: OGTT, clamp	Placebo (N = 6) Weight maintenence diet and physical activity	insulin sensitivity by clamp; 6/7 with IGT reverted to normal; lower SBP, DBP; no change in LDL-, HDL-cholesterol or triglycerides in either group. **Placebo:** no change in glucose or insulin levels, sensitivity or lipids. No data on reversion of IGT subjects	
Berkowitz et al. 1996[218] I-a	**Gestational Diabetes and IGT**, Los Angeles, CA. 42 post-GDM women aged x̄ = 33 yrs; follow-up 3 months. Outcome: OGTT, FSIGT	**Troglitazone** (N = 12) 200 mg qd **Troglitazone** (N = 13) 400 mg qd **Placebo** (N = 12)	**Troglitazone:** Dose-dependent increase in insulin sensitivity (Si) on IVGTT up to 88% in 400 mg group. Lower fasting insulin (−20%), no change in fasting or AUC glucose, lipids, BP, weight, % body fat. No development of diabetes. **Placebo:** No changes in Si, fasting insulin or glucose	Dropouts 12%, similar across groups. Double-blind; masking of allocation not mentioned
Antonucci et al. 1997[217] I-a	**Multicenter study of Troglitazone in IGT** 51 subjects aged 24–77 (x̄ = 47 years) with IGT; follow-up 3 months. Outcome: OGTT	**Troglitazone** (N = 25) 400 mg qd **Placebo** (N = 26)	**Troglitazone:** RR = 0.38 (0.15–1.00) to remain IGT vs. placebo; lower glucose and insulin AUC, triglyceride levels; no change in fasting glucose, insulin or C-peptide, LDL or HDL-C, BP, weight. HbA_{1c} in either group	80% of troglitazone subjects returned to normal OGTT vs. 48% of placebo group. Dropouts 20%, similar in each group. Said to be lower, but text disagrees with tables. Allocation was masked, double-blind
Cavaghan et al. 1997[221] I-a	**β-cell response to Troglitazone, Chicago, IL** 26 overweight subjects aged x̄ = 44 yrs with F glucose ≤ 140 mg/dl; follow-up 3 months. Outcome: OGTT, FSIGT, infusion	**Troglitazone** (N = 14) 400 mg qd **Placebo** (N = 7)	**Troglitazone:** glucose AUC decreased 10% (p = 0.03), fasting insulin lower, S_i and disposition index increased, insulin secretion adj for S_i increased 52%, improved β-cell entrainment to glucose. HbA_{1c} decreased; no change in fasting glucose. **Placebo:** no changes	Five dropouts (19%), similar between groups. Allocation masked, double-blind. Number of persons with IGT vs. diabetes not stated. Not a prevention trial, rather a mechanistic study with randomization
Buchanan et al. 2001[220]	**Troglitazone in the prevention of diabetes (TRIPOD)** Los Angeles, California 235 Latina women, hx of GDM; 30 month follow-up. Outcome: diabetes.	**Troglitazone** 400 mg/day (N = 114) **Placebo** (N = 121)	**Troglitazone:** 5.4/100 PY. **Placebo:** 12.3/100 PY. RR = 0.44. ARR = 6.9/100 PY. p = 0.001	Largest reduction in diabetes incidence seen in women with most improvement in insulin sensitivity in subset analysis. Effects appear to continue for up to 8 months off drug in preliminary results. Dropouts not reported

Table 6.7. contd.

Alpha-glucosidase inhibitors

Chiasson et al. 1996[222] I-a	**Acarbose Pilot, Montreal, Canada** 18 subjects with IGT; ($\bar{x}$ = 55 years); follow-up 4 months. Outcome: OGTT	**Acarbose** (N = 10) 100 mg tid **Placebo** (N = 8)	**Acarbose:** lower glucose and insulin (32%) AUC; no change in fasting glucose or insulin, BMI, lipids, BP. HbA_{1c}. **Placebo:** no changes in AUC, or fasting values, as above	Masking of allocation not noted. Short follow-up. Side-effects not mentioned
Chiasson et al. 1998[223] I-b	**STOP-NIDDM Trial** Canada, Europe 1429 men and women ($\bar{x}$ = 54.5 years). WHO IGT × 1; follow-up 3.3 years. Outcome: diabetes	**Acarbose** 100 mg tid or **Placebo**	**Acarbose:** HR = 0.75 (0.63–0.90; ARR = 9.1/100 PY) vs. placebo. Higher reversion to normal glucose tolerance (p <0.0001)	NNT = 11 persons with IGT to prevent one case; dropouts 23.9%, higher in acarbose (221) than placebo (130). Prepublication results

Other agents

Hansson et al. 1999[224] I-a	**Captopril Prevention Project (CAPPP)** 10985 subjects in Sweden, Finland, primary care; follow-up 6.1 years. Outcome: diabetes	**Captopril** (N = 5183 nondiabetic); 50 mg qd or bid **Conventional** (N = 5230 nondiabetic); β-blockers and/or diuretics	**Captopril:** RR = 0.86 (0.74–0.99) vs. **Conventional** treatment of hypertension. Efficacy analysis: RR = 0.79 (0.67–0.94)	Subgroup analysis of nondiabetic persons at baseline; more diabetes in captopril group at baseline; randomization by sealed envelope; dropouts 0.25%. Captopril group added thiazide diuretic in an unspecified percentage
Hansson et al. 1999[226] I-b	**Swedish Trial of Old People with Hypertension – 2 (STOP-2)** 6614 patients in primary care; 5-year follow-up. Outcome: diabetes by FPG × 2	Diuretic/beta-blocker strategy. ACE-inhibitors strategy. Calcium antagonist strategy	No difference in diabetes incidence by treatment group	Subgroup analysis
HOPE investigators 2000[225] I-b	**Heart Outcomes Prevention Evaluation Project (HOPE)** 267 centers in Canada, North and South America, and Europe	**Ramipril** (N = 2837 nondiabetic); 10 mg qd **Placebo** (N = 2883 nondiabetic) in 2 × 2 factorial with Vitamin E	**Ramipril:** RR = 0.66 (0.51–0.85) vs. placebo for incidence of new diabetes. No interaction with Vitamin E noted	Ramipril discontinued in 29%, placebo in 27%; 18% of placebo group used an ACE-inhibitor. Dropouts not stated. Side-effects primarily cough that differed from placebo

Table 6.7. contd.

Freeman *et al.* 2001[240] 1-b	9297 subjects aged 55 yrs and older (x̄ = 66); follow-up 5 years. Outcome: diabetes **West of Scotland Coronary Prevention Study (WOSCOPS)** Primary care practices; 5974 men. (x̄ = 55 years), nondiabetic, elevated cholesterol; 4.9-yr follow-up. Outcome: diabetes by modified ADA criteria	**Pravastatin** (40 mg/day) vs. Placebo	**Pravastatin:** multivariate HR = 0.7 (0.50–0.99) vs. placebo	Subgroup post-hoc analysis, requires confirmation. Absolute incidence rates not given by group; side-effects minimal. Approximately 30% withdrawals at 5 years in primary study

‡ Calculated from data available in the paper, not by the authors; FSIGT = frequently sampled intravenous glucose tolerance test; HR = hazard ratio; RR = relative risk or risk ratio; ARR = absolute risk reduction (if not present, data were not available to calculate).

twice a day compared with placebo. Subjects had a fasting blood glucose level <6.2 mmol/l (112 mg/dl) and 1 h >9.4 mmol/l (170 mg/dl) or 2 h >6.7 mmol/l (120 mg/dl), levels that would be considered mostly in the normal or IGT range by current criteria. After an average follow-up of 14 months, fasting glucose levels of approximately 91 mg/dl (5.05 mmol/L) on tolbutamide were significantly lower than the approximately 100 mg/dl (5.56 mmol/L) levels on placebo (p <0.05), but there were no significant differences in 1, 2 or 3 h levels. Analysis was confusing, with some results 'adjusted for baseline levels', and others averaged over various time periods. Only 15 subjects in each group were tested at 14 months (23–25% drop-out rate) and changes in diabetes status to normal were not reported. This study is difficult to interpret, but appears negative by current criteria, since there were only small differences in fasting glucose, and no differences in 2 h glucose levels.

At around the same time, Camerini-Davalos, in another study of the effect of sulfonylureas on diabetes outcomes[185], assigned 38 subjects with 'chemical diabetes' (normal fasting glucose, impaired oral tolerance, no symptoms, but criteria not stated – most would be current IGT) to 500 mg of tolbutamide twice daily and gave 59 subjects a placebo. Randomization or blinding were not specified. After variable follow-up of 10–24 months, the RR for continuing to have any degree of IGT was 0.73 (CI 0.45–1.18, ARR = 14/100 person-years; intention to treat, post-hoc analysis). The primary effect appeared to be a reduction in the sum of glucose levels among people who remained abnormal, without significant reduction in the percentage of people who remained glucose-intolerant. No weight change occurred between groups and triglyceride levels actually increased significantly on therapy. The numerous methodological problems with this study, and the use of early criteria and method of data presentation, make it difficult to interpret, though contemporary authors also considered it a negative result[186].

Feldman and colleagues took advantage of the multiphasic screening program at Kaiser-Permanente in northern California to identify subjects with glucose intolerance[187,188]. People with chemical diabetes by Fajans and Conn criteria[189] (most now classified as IGT) were randomly assigned to tolbutamide (n = 174, 500 mg twice daily), the biguanide phenformin (n = 91, 100 mg/day) or placebo (n = 85) in a double-blind design.

After five years of follow-up, the incidence of diabetes was 0.6% on tolbutamide, with a RR = 0.16 (CI 0.02–1.54; ARR ≅3/100 person-years, intention to treat, not accounting for losses, post-hoc analysis), there were no cases among those treated with phenformin (p = 0.22 versus placebo), and the rate in placebo treated subjects was 3.5%[188]. The 2 h glucose decline below entry levels was greatest in people taking tolbutamide, but was closely followed by those on placebo, and in both these groups glucose levels had returned to baseline levels after 42 months and were not different from each other. People taking phenformin had almost no change in 2 h glucose levels over the period.

Drop-outs averaged 22%[188] and no excess of cardiovascular mortality was seen.

The relatively low diabetes incidence, even among people on placebo, is probably a reflection of the criteria for the outcome of diabetes ('overt diabetes', probably requiring substantially elevated glucose levels), the relatively low blood glucose levels at entry, and the relatively young age of subjects. These results suggest that tolbutamide may lower the incidence of diabetes, though the lack of glucose lowering with phenformin suggests it is not likely to be effective, and it is no longer on the market due to adverse side-effects.

Keen and colleagues conducted a long-term randomized double-blind study of tolbutamide (500 mg twice daily) versus placebo (3 mg tolbutamide, twice daily), in a factorial design adding dietary restriction of carbohydrate up to a maximum of 120 g/day ('diet') or avoidance of simple sugars at the table ('no diet')[190]. The primary goal was to determine if cardiovascular disease endpoints were lessened (or increased) on tolbutamide, given the temporal relationship of the Bedford study with the University Group Diabetes Program (UGDP), which had reported increased CVD mortality in the tolbutamide group[191]. Subjects were seen twice a year for five years, then less frequently for the remaining five years.

In a series of reports spanning the study period[190,192-194], the authors noted that diet had no effect within six months and that only about 50% of subjects took most of the assigned medication[192]. Compliance and continuation of treatment were not mentioned in the later reports. By the 8.5-year follow-up, it was clear that there was no benefit from tolbutamide versus placebo on the incidence of diabetes[190] (RR = 1.12, CI 0.49–2.54), which was confirmed in the 10-year report using modern logistic analyses[194]. No excess of vascular events was seen in the tolbutamide group, in contrast to reports from the UGDP, but other adverse effects (e.g. hypoglycemia) were not reported. Thus, this reasonably conducted trial provides no evidence for the long-term efficacy of tolbutamide for diabetes prevention. Whether this is due to actual lack of efficacy or to limited drug exposure remains unclear.

Paasikivi[86] randomly assigned 178 survivors of a first myocardial infarction (MI) at the Karolinska Institute in Stockholm, Sweden to 500 mg of tolbutamide, twice daily (n = 95) or placebo (n = 83) using odd/even allocation on birth date. The trial was blinded only to the patient, and the primary outcome was changes in intravenous glucose tolerance (IVGT), making it hard to compare with current standards.

Total mortality was slightly but not significantly lower on active drug (RR = 0.71, CI 0.36-1.39) but there were minimal changes in glucose outcomes. There were no differences in fasting glucose between treated and control groups over several follow-up examinations. While none of the subjects had overt diabetes at entry, 23% (tolbutamide) or 29% (placebo) had 'diabetic' IVGT results, categorized as low levels of glucose disappearance (K0) based on prior studies. This prevalence of abnormal K_0 changed very little over the trial, which lasted up to five years, but was 2.9 years on average. None of the subjects remaining in the trial on tolbutamide developed overt diabetes, whereas three did so on placebo (p = 0.20, intention to treat, post-hoc analysis). Subjects with diabetic values for K_0 did have improvements in their values, but none of the subjects with borderline or normal K_0 showed changes. This trial, while interpreted as positive in subgroups by its author, was essentially negative by current intention-to-treat standards. There was a lower conversion to overt diabetes among treated subjects (0 versus. 3), but the trial was too small to detect a significant difference in this outcome or in total mortality at five years.

Investigators at the Joslin Clinic in Boston studied 120 men with chemical diabetes randomly allocated to placebo, chlorpropamide, tolbutamide, phenformin or acetohexamide for five years[195]. All subjects had normal fasting glucose (<100 mg/dl, 5.5 mmol/L) at entry, and most would have had normal glucose tolerance or IGT by current criteria.

Over the five-year follow-up, between 30–50% of men dropped out of the trial. No significant differences in the percentage with normal glucose tolerance were seen between the placebo group and all other groups at any time, and there were no changes sequentially within any group toward improved OGTT results. The only exception was a small improvement at one year in the chlorpropamide group, which was not sustained from years 2 to 5. In addition, there were no improvements in insulin area during the OGTT, and no changes in lipids. This study, while suffering from small numbers, rather high losses to follow-up and univariate analysis, was otherwise reasonably conducted, and found no improvements on any drug regimen.

Sartor and colleagues conducted a community screening in Malmöhus, Sweden from 1962 to 1965[196]. They conducted OGTTs on people who were glycosuric during screening, then sequentially randomized 267 men with IGT (by local criteria) to one of four groups: (1) diet alone, (2) diet plus 500 mg tolbutamide three times daily, (3) diet plus placebo or (4) no therapy. The first three groups underwent annual OGTT testing until the mid-1970s, and tolbutamide was unmasked in 1972, about two years before completion of follow-up.

While the primary analysis was conducted as an efficacy analysis ('per protocol'), i.e. comparing compliant and non-compliant subjects, it is possible to reconstruct an intention-to-treat result. This indicated no significant difference between tolbutamide (10.2% diabetes at 10 years), placebo (12.5%) and diet only (14.0%). Group 4 above, the 'no therapy' group was made up of an unspecified retrospective sample of 59 men originally randomized to no therapy in which the cumulative incidence of diabetes was 28.8%. Drop-outs were about 11.2% of total subjects.

Only limited conclusions are possible from this study, given its small size and efficacy analysis. Based on intention-to-treat analysis, there was no effect of tolbutamide therapy over 10 years, compared to placebo or diet alone, though the overall incidence was slightly lower (RR = 0.82, CI 0.27–2.50 versus placebo; RR = 0.73, CI 0.25–2.14 versus diet, post-hoc analyses). In the efficacy analysis, none of the subjects continuing to take tolbutamide developed diabetes at 10 years, an observation which has caused many to be hopeful of the potential benefit of the sulfonylureas [10].

A later follow-up of these subjects has been published[197]. Several useful clarifications appear here. First, it appears that the IGT criteria used in the 1960s included many normal subjects. On average, 79% of subjects in the groups randomized to tolbutamide, placebo or diet only had normal glucose tolerance by WHO criteria, and 18% had WHO IGT, while 3% had diabetes. Cumulative mortality rate ratios for the tolbutamide-treated men (compared to non-treated men) up until 1987 (~22 years) were 0.66 (CI 0.39–1.10) for all causes of death, and 0.42 (CI 0.16–1.12) for ischemic heart disease (IHD) deaths. Thus, it appears that the long-term IHD mortality in the tolbutamide group was lower than in men not taking it, for up to 10 years, rather than increased (as suggested by the UGDP results) among people with diabetes[191,198]. No additional insights concerning diabetes incidence were published.

A small pilot study was conducted in Oxford, the UK using the sulfonylurea glicazide (40 mg twice daily) versus placebo[44]. In the same pilot, a 'healthy living' group was included, and two-year follow-up of this portion of the study were reported[44] as noted above. Only the six-month follow-up of the drug group has been reported. Subjects with abnormal fasting glucose levels or glucose infusion tests with results said to be similar to WHO IGT were included. Six were given glicazide and eight were given placebo in blinded fashion.

At six months, fasting glucose and 1 h CIGMA glucose were decreased significantly without change in insulin sensitivity, but with improved beta-cell function. No significant changes were noted in the placebo group. One month after stopping the drug, people were retested, with reversion of fasting glucose to baseline levels. The authors concluded that drug therapy, to be effective, must be continued. This pilot led to the development of the Fasting Hyperglycemia Study summarized below, since larger numbers were needed with a longer follow-up period.

The Fasting Hyperglycemia Study (FHS) II was designed to identify high-risk subjects for prevention therapy using lifestyle and/or glicazide[56]. The basic design was described previously under combined lifestyle trials. In the pharmacological portion of the FHS, 227 subjects with IFG were randomly allocated to glicazide, 80 mg twice daily (n = 112) or control (n = 115), with 58 of the 115 controls given placebo tablets, and 57 given no tablets[199].

At one year of follow-up in the drug group, fasting glucose and HbA_{1c} were significantly lower. However, there was no change in the proportion of people with diabetes. Two-hour glucose and the area under the OGTT curve were both higher in the drug group at one year, though they were lower or showed no change in the control group. Beta-cell function improved slightly in the drug group, but there were no changes in insulin sensitivity in either group. Mild symptoms of hypoglycemia were twice as common among glicazide-treated subjects, though they were no different at one year. After six years, there were only 188 subjects available for analysis. Fewer subjects in the glicazide group (3.2%) developed overt diabetes (two fasting plasma glucose values >180 mg/dL or 10 mmol/L); than in the control group (10.8%) (p = 0.047; ARR = 7.6/100 person-years)[200]. However, there were no differences in the rate of development of WHO diabetes (FPG ≥140 mg/dL or 7.8 mmol/L or OGTT) and no differences in Homeostasis Model Assessment (HOMA) derived measures of resistance or secretion. The authors also conducted a two-month drug washout in a subsample, which found small increases in FPG (5.4 mg/dL, 0.3 mmol/L, p = 0.022), but no difference in two hour glucose, HbA_{1c}, or the proportion with diabetes between drug and control groups.

Clinical non-randomized studies

There is one non-randomized pharmacological intervention which provides limited additional insight into the utility of sulfonylureas. Ratzmann *et al.* assigned 27 subjects to the sulfonylurea glibeclamide and diet (n = 27, 2 mg/day) or diet alone (n = 18) in a non-randomized two-year study[201]. The diet included 30% dietary fat, and limited energy intake only slightly.

At 1 and 2 years, no weight loss occurred in either group. In the analysis, they stratified subjects by level of insulin response to an IVGTT. However, no real differences were seen across these groups. There was a small improvement in glucose tolerance in the low insulin responders, but no changes in fasting or 2 h glucose levels at two years. This study did not find a beneficial effect of sulfonylurea on insulin secretion or glucose tolerance, though the study groups were small. Without randomization or adjustment for baseline differences between groups, it appears that this study, like others conducted in the same period[187,195,202], provides limited evidence of benefit for sulfonylureas in prevention or improvement of glucose tolerance. One study which used chlorpropamide did not use controls[203] and is not included.

These studies using tolbutamide suffer from a number of methodological weaknesses. However, there are four studies which randomized reasonably large numbers of subjects, who were followed over several years and used intention-to-treat analysis, or reported data that could be calculated this way post-hoc. The study by Feldman *et al.*[187,188] had a substantially lower, though not significantly lower, RR of 0.16 (CI 0.02–1.54). The other widely quoted study by Sartor *et al.*[196] also had non-significant risk reductions when analyzed by intention to treat (RR = 0.82 (CI 0.27–2.50) vs. placebo, RR = 0.73 (CI 0.25–2.14) versus diet, post-hoc analyses). The Bedford study[194] was also of 10 years duration, and found no decrease in risk (OR = 1.04), which is consistent with the prior studies, given their wide confidence intervals. The six-year follow-up of the FHS-II[200] does not support an effect on diabetes incidence using current fasting criteria, and the effect on 'overt diabetes' (fasting glucose >180 mg/dL, 10 mmol/L) may simply be a treatment effect of the drug. The remaining studies were essentially negative or uninformative. Thus, the current evidence does not support a consistent role for tolbutamide derivatives in the prevention of type 2 diabetes.

Biguanides (including combinations)

Papoz and colleagues at the Hotel Dieu, Paris conducted a randomized, double-blind trial of a sulfonylurea (S) (glibenclamide, 2 mg twice daily), biguanide (B) (dimethylbiguanide, 0.85 g twice daily), alone and in combination (S+B) in a 2×2 factorial design with placebo[202]. Men aged 25–55 years ($\bar{x} = 45$ yrs) who had borderline glucose tolerance (most would have IGT by current criteria) were randomized from 1969 to 1971 and tested for glucose and insulin levels every six months for two years.

There were 28% drop-outs, with similar levels across treatment groups. At two years, there were no significant differences in glucose or insulin levels in any group, though B, S+B and placebo groups all lost about 4 kg of weight, more than the 2 kg in the S group. Worsening to diabetes was not reported. The trial could have detected as significant drop of 21 mg/dl (1.2 mmol/L) in 2 h glucose with 95% power, though actual differences were very small (0–2 mg/dl, 0-0.1 mmol/L) between groups. This study was well conducted, even by modern criteria, and indicates no benefit of either drug to lower glucose levels or enhance insulin secretion. In addition, the authors note that OGTT testing was conducted while on medication, except for the last test, which was done 15 days after stopping the drug. Even the interim results showed essentially no differences in glucose and insulin levels while on medication.

Jarrett and co-workers identified a group of Whitehall civil service workers with borderline glucose tolerance from a large (n = 20 000) survey[204]. Men aged 40–64 years were asked to participate in an RCT of dietary carbohydrate restriction and the biguanide phenformin (50 mg/day) for five years. Progression to diabetes was confirmed by OGTT or development of intercurrent symptoms and elevated glucose levels.

Overall, 27 of the 181 men (14.9%) completing the trial developed diabetes, with no significant differences between the treatment groups. Combining the phenformin groups across diet or no diet, the RR was 0.90 (CI 0.45–1.80) for the development of diabetes on drug. In logistic regression analyses adjusting for baseline imbalances at randomization, no effect of either diet or drug were seen. Only the level of fasting glucose predicted deterioration.

In a related report, no benefit (or harm) of phenformin on vascular or total mortality was noted[205] using either intention-to-treat or efficacy (per protocol) analysis. This study, like that of Papoz *et al.*[202], offers no evidence that phenformin will prevent diabetes for up to five years.

Phenformin (50 mg) plus diet was compared to diet alone in Polish subjects starting in 1976 and continuing for five years as reported by Kasperska *et al.*[206]. Seventy-three people aged 23–74 ($\bar{x}$ = 54 years) were alternately allocated to interventions. At baseline, approximately 60% had 'borderline' glucose intolerance by older EASD criteria, similar to current IGT levels. Only 67% completed the five year trial, and over all subjects there was no benefit of phenformin in preventing worsening of glucose intolerance (RR = 0.89, CI 0.25–3.14). Among those with 'IGT', small differences in glucose and insulin levels were noted, which were not significant. This study provides no support for the use of phenformin for prevention of diabetes. The high rate of lactic acidosis with phenformin led to its removal from the market.

French investigators conducted two studies using the second-generation biguanide metformin, to determine the impact of this agent on components of the insulin resistance syndrome. In the first study, **BIG**uanides and **P**revention of **R**isks of **O**besity, BIGPRO-1)[207,208] they selected 457 people with high waist–hip ratio (men ≥0.95, women ≥0.80) aged 35–60 ($\bar{x}$ = 49 years), randomly allocated them to 850 mg of metformin twice daily or placebo, and followed them every three months for one year. Both groups were given diet and physical activity instruction.

The metformin group showed small (−2 kg) but significant weight loss, less rise in fasting glucose, and marginally greater fall in fasting insulin, without changes in 2 h glucose or insulin. Lower LDL cholesterol, but no change in BP, triglycerides or HDL cholesterol were found. Of a number of hemostatic factors explored, the metformin group showed decreases in tissue plasminogen activator (tPA) antigen, and vonWillebrand factor[209], but no change in plasminogen activator inhibitor-1 (PAI-1) activity or antigen not accounted for by weight loss. Five in the placebo group developed diabetes, versus none in the metformin group (exact p = 0.06, post-hoc analysis). The results are difficult to interpret since there was a 28% and 30% drop-out rate in the two groups at one year. While subjects who dropped out were similar to those remaining in the trial, unexplained bias could have accounted for the results.

The investigators undertook a confirmatory study (BIGPRO-1.2) among 168 men who had slightly higher BP and triglyceride levels[210,211]. A similar randomization procedure and dose of metformin were used, though men were followed only for three months. Results were quite consistent with those of BIGPRO-1, in that fasting glucose, insulin, LDL cholesterol, ApoB (Apolipoprotein B) and tPA antigen declined, withouts change in BP or triglycerides. No diabetes occurred in either group and weight loss was only −0.5 kg.

In both studies, metformin produced more diarrhea, nausea and vomiting, but no hypoglycemic episodes[208]. The authors concluded that metformin would be an acceptable intervention in a type 2 diabetes prevention trial, but, with minimal changes in important cardiovascular risk factors, it would be less suitable for a CVD prevention study.

Li and colleagues evaluated the use of low-dose metformin (250 mg three times a day) compared to placebo to prevent the development of diabetes[212]. Subjects with IGT were identified during screening of a large workforce in Bejing, People's Republic of China, and 90 were randomly assigned to metformin or placebo.

After one year of follow-up, three people on metformin developed diabetes (7.1%), compared to six on placebo (14.0%) (RR = 0.51,CI 0.02–1.91, ARR = 6.9/100 person-years, post-hoc intention-to-treat analysis) There were also fewer people remaining with IGT and more reverting to normal glucose tolerance (p = 0.091). Using an efficacy analysis (including only the 70 persons who were compliant and continued in follow-up), the reduction in risk was naturally greater (RR = 0.19, CI 0.02–1.47), but it was not statistically significant unless the lower frequency of people with IGT were also included (p = 0.011).

This is one of the few pharmacological prevention studies using random-ization, a placebo and a double-blind design where the primary end-point was conversion to diabetes using modern criteria. While the results suggest that a 50% or greater reduction in diabetes incidence occurred, the duration of follow-up (one year) and the number of subjects were both limited. Glucose tolerance testing was conducted quarterly and conversion on a single test was considered diabetes, so the relatively high conversion rates may be due in part to frequent testing. Nonetheless, both placebo and intervention groups had an equal testing frequency, and intention-to-treat analyses were presented. The rate of drop out for gastrointestinal side-effects was 4.4% among people randomized to metformin versus 0% on placebo, and the non-compliance rate (which could have included people with mild side-effects) was also higher among metformin subjects (15.6% versus 11.1%).

The Diabetes Prevention Program (DPP) also included metformin (850 twice daily) or placebo with simple annual lifestyle advice, in a double-blind design[70]. The design and intensive lifestyle results were discussed earlier in this chapter. The primary end-point was clinical or OGTT diabetes, confirmed on at least two tests. Randomization procedures and drug assignments were carefully masked to investigators, and the metformin and placebo groups were extremely similar at baseline on all risk factors measured[71].

Metformin significantly reduced the incidence of diabetes by 31% compared to placebo (95% CI = 17–43%) (average annual incidence of 7.8/100 person-years versus 11.0/100 person-years in placebo; ARR = 3.2/100 person-years)[72]. Seventy-two percent of participants reported ≥80% adherence to the drug. In contrast to consistent results in subgroups for the DPP lifestyle intervention, metformin was less effective in persons with lower BMI, and in persons aged 60 years or greater. The lifestyle intervention was 39% more effective than metformin (p <0.001). Based on three-year lifetable cumulative estimates of diabetes development (28.9%, 21.7% and 14.4% in placebo, metformin and lifestyle groups respectively), the number needed to treat (NNT) was 6.9 to prevent one case using lifestyle, and was 13.9 for metformin. There were no differences in the rates of serious adverse events (hospitalizations, mortality) between groups, though mild gastrointestinal symptoms were significantly more common in the metformin group[72].

The DPP is the first large, carefully randomized study to show that metformin will delay or prevent diabetes in high-risk IGT subjects. The effect was smaller than that seen in the study in China by Li *et al.*[212] Interestingly, in the DPP, fasting plasma glucose levels were reduced similarly in the metformin and lifestyle groups, though two-hour glucose levels were reduced much more by lifestyle intervention, consistent with metformin's action on hepatic glucose production. It is not known whether the reduction in incidence is due to an acute metabolic effect of treatment of hyperglycemia, or a more fundamental change in glucose homeostasis. A washout study is underway to explore this question. The long-term duration of the metformin effect is also not known.

Other published studies have been excluded since they included only a small number of subjects[213] or were not randomized[214].

Thiazolidinediones

A new class of insulin-sensitizing agents has become available in the past few years, the thiazolidendiones[215]. These agents act by reducing insulin resistance at the cellular level, lowering plasma insulin and perhaps other components of the insulin resistance syndrome. The first generation agent, troglitazone, has been taken off the market and replaced with pioglitazone and rosiglitazone at time of writing.

The first study to explore this class of agents used the drug troglitazone in 18 non-diabetic obese (BMI >27) subjects, of whom 50% had IGT[216]. Nolan and colleagues randomly allocated 12 subjects to 200 mg twice daily troglitazone and six to placebo in a double-blind fashion. They were given a weight maintenance diet and activity instructions, and followed weekly for 12 weeks. At study end, subjects taking troglitazone had lower fasting and OGTT glucose and insulin levels, and higher insulin sensitivity by glucose clamp.

Six out of seven people with IGT on active drug had reverted to normal glucose tolerance, however. There were only two subjects with IGT on placebo, so no comparison was given. Side-effects were mild and well tolerated. The authors suggested that this drug might have a role in prevention of diabetes. Because the study was only 12 weeks in duration, longer studies will be required to understand the potential of this agent.

A second study of troglitazone was conducted in six sites[217] and included only people with IGT by WHO criteria, in contrast to the previous study.

Antonucci and colleagues randomized 51 subjects with IGT on a single OGTT to either 400 mg of troglitazone a day (n = 25) or placebo (n = 26). This is one of the few studies reviewed here to clearly note that allocation was masked to investigators since randomization was carried out by the drug company.

After 12 weeks of follow-up, 80% of people on troglitazone had reverted to normal glucose tolerance compared with 48% of placebo subjects (p = 0.016). The RR for remaining IGT was 0.38 (CI 0.15–1.00, unadjusted, ARR = 32/100 persons) for troglitazone subjects. Glucose and insulin areas under the OGTT curve were significantly improved. However, there were no changes in fasting glucose, insulin or C-peptide levels. Triglycerides decreased significantly on active drug, but there were no changes in other lipids, blood pressure, weight or HbA_{1c}. No one in this short study developed diabetes. Drop-out was approximately 20% in each group and there was no detail given of adverse events.

Change in insulin sensitivity using troglitazone was the primary outcome in a study of 42 women with prior gestational diabetes and current IGT carried by Berkowitz *et al.*[218]. Women were randomized to placebo, 200 mg or 400 mg of troglitazone and studied before treatment and after 12 weeks using the frequently sampled intravenous glucose tolerance test (FSIGT) with minimal model assessment to determine changes in insulin sensitivity (SI). There was a dose-dependent improvement in SI to a maximum of 88% in the 400 mg group. Interestingly, there were no significant changes in fasting or post-challenge glucose levels, in contrast to the study by Nolan *et al.*[216], but consistent with the results of Antonucci[217] for fasting glucose. Though not statistically significant, there were declines in AUC (area under the curve) glucose on the 400 mg dose among women with prior GDM, which is also consistent with people with IGT and no prior GDM[217].

Whether these results (improved SI with limited improvements in glucose tolerance) reflect underlying biological differences in women with prior GDM or simply variation between small studies with limited follow-up is unclear. It is possible that a history of GDM and current IGT reflects a greater degree of beta-cell compromise than is present in people with a single OGTT result of IGT. If so, then short-term treatment with the sensitizing agent troglitazone may have limited potential to improve glucose tolerance. Longer-term, larger studies among people with both types of history will be required to resolve this question. This study served as the pilot study for the larger TRIPOD study now underway.

The **TR**oglitazone **I**n the **P**revention **O**f **D**iabetes (TRIPOD) trial is a single-center, randomized, placebo-controlled, double-blinded five-year study to determine if troglitazone will prevent or delay the onset of type 2 diabetes in high-risk Latina women with a history of gestational diabetes (GDM)[219,220]. Two hundred and sixty-six women with confirmed GDM were randomized to placebo or 400 mg of troglitazone per day and 235 had at least one follow-up visit. The primary end-point was the development of OGTT diabetes (single 2 h glucose ≥200 mg/dl (11.1 mmol/L) or single fasting glucose ≥140 mg/dl (7.8 mmol/L). After a median of 30 months follow-up, the incidence rates in the placbo group were 12.3/100 person-years and were 5.4/100 person-years in the troglitazone group (RR = 0.44, ARR = 6.9/100 person-years, p = 0.001). Subgroup analysis showed that the majority of the effect was in women who improved their insulin sensitivity and reduced beta-cell workload. In the sub-group with a small fall in insulin area (n = 42), diabetes developed at 5.8% per year, whereas in the subgroup with a large fall in insulin area (n = 31), no cases of diabetes developed. In the group with no response to the drug, diabetes occurred at 9.8% per year. Troglitazone was discontinued in the study on removal from the market, and subjects are being tested an average of eight months after stopping the drug. In preliminary results on a subset of 27 subjects tested to date[220], only one subject has developed diabetes, although models using their baseline characteristics would predict that 37% would have decompensated if the drug were simply treating diabetes. Thus, it appears that reduction in beta-cell workload through improvements in insulin sensitivity reduce diabetes in these very high-risk women.

In a small study to explore further the usefulness of troglitazone, Cavaghan and co-workers randomly assigned 14 overweight people to troglitazone and seven to placebo[221]. This was not a primary prevention trial, since an undis-closed number of subjects had 2 h glucose levels > 200 mg/dl (11.1 mmol/L), but all persons had fasting glucose <140 mg/dl (7.8 mmol/L), so there was a mixture of people with IGT and diabetes. As in the other studies using troglit-azone, measures of insulin sensitivity improved, but the additional finding was that insulin secretion adjusted for insulin sensitivity also improved, and entrainment of beta-cell function (a marker of improved islet responsiveness to changes in glucose) was increased by 49%. The authors speculated that the mechanisms underlying the improved insulin secretion (using an insulin sensi-tizing agent) could be elimination of beta-cell glucotoxicity, improvements in peripheral insulin resistance or free fatty acid metabolism, or previously undocumented effects of the drug on the beta-cell itself.

Agents in this class which have acceptable adverse event profiles hold promise as preventive agents, since they improve insulin action and may also independently increase insulin secretion. The Diabetes Prevention Program (DPP), a 27-center RCT diabetes prevention program, originally chose troglit-azone as one of the agents to be tested (see below). After 585 people were randomized to troglitazone, a participant experienced hepatic failure and death, causing the investigators and NIH to stop its use in the trial. The subjects in the DPP who were randomly allocated to troglitazone were followed off-drug, but the results of this group have not been published. Troglitazone was withdrawn from the market. A trial of the second generation agent rosiglitazone is under-way (DREAM, see below).

Alpha-glucosidase inhibitors

Chiasson and colleagues in Montreal conducted a small pilot study (n = 18) of acarbose, an alpha-glucosidase inhibitor[215], in people with IGT[222]. Acarbose delays intestinal absorption of glucose and lowers peak glucose and insulin levels after eating. After four months, subjects on acarbose showed lower post-meal and 12 h glucose and insulin profiles, with no change among those on placebo. During an insulin suppression test, post-treatment steady-state glucose levels were significantly lower at the same level of insulin, suggesting improved insulin sensitivity. No changes in BMI, HDL cholesterol or triglycerides, fasting glucose or insulin, HbA_{1c} or BP were seen in either group. No comments were made concerning the side effects of acarbose, which is known to include increased flatulence and diarrhea[215]. Results in this short-term study suggest the utility of acarbose to improve glucose tolerance and insulin sensitivity, and led the authors to begin the STOP-NIDDM multicenter trial[223] in Canada and Europe.

The Study to Prevent NIDDM (STOP-NIDDM) was designed to test whether acarbose would delay or prevent type 2 diabetes among people with IGT by WHO criteria[223]. Results are not yet published but were available in preliminary form from the study investigators. A total of 1429 subjects were recruited with IGT and other eligibility criteria and were followed for an average of 3.3 years. Randomization was to acarbose (100 mg three times daily) or placebo. Mean age at baseline was 54.5 years, with a mean BMI of 30.9. The outcome was diabetes diagnosed annually on OGTT. After exclusions, there were 1368 persons in the intention-to-treat analysis, of whom 341 (23.9%) discontinued prematurely; 211 in the acarbose group and 130 in the placebo group. Acarbose treatment reduced overall risk of diabetes by 25% using proportional hazards (hazard ratio = 0.75, CI 0.63–0.90; ARR = 9.1/100 person-years over 3.3 years). It also resulted in a significant increase in conversion from IGT to normal glucose tolerance (p <0.0001). There was a higher drop-out rate in the active treatment group, a relatively high drop-out rate overall, and no additional details of analysis or subgroup effectiveness are available. However, STOP-NIDDM adds to the increasing list of pharmacological interventions that reduce the incidence of diabetes, at least over three years.

Angiotensin converting enzyme (ACE) inhibitors (ACE-I)

The Captopril Prevention Project (CAPPP)[224] compared this ACE-I against standard antihypertensive therapy with beta-blockers and diuretics. For most cardiovascular end-points there was no difference by treatment group at five years. However, diabetes incidence was reduced compared with standard antihypertensive treatment (RR = 0.86) (CI 0.74–0.99), and an efficacy analysis (including eligible subjects who took most of their assigned therapy) found a RR = 0.79 (CI 0.67–0.94) versus standard blood pressure medications.

Ramipril, one of the newer ACE-I, has also been studied in a cardiovascular prevention trial among high-risk subjects, including people both with diabetes and at risk for it. The Heart Outcomes Prevention Evaluation (HOPE) Study[225] found, in a subset analysis, that people at risk for type 2 diabetes who were randomized to ramipril had a lower incidence of diabetes than subjects on placebo (RR = 0.66) (CI 0.51–0.85, ARR = 1.8/100 person-years) over an average of five years of follow-up.

The STOP-2 study also used ACE-I[226]. Hypertensive persons aged 70–84 (with a baseline BP ≥180 mm systolic, 105 mm diastolic or both) were included; 5893 had no DM history at baseline. They were randomized to either a conventional diuretic and/or beta-blocker strategy, an ACE-I strategy (enalapril 10 mg/day or lisinopril 10 mg/day) or a calcium channel blocking agent strategy. No differences were seen in the incidence of diabetes by therapy strategy. However, about 40% of patients on ACE-I were also treated with hydrochlorothiazide to control BP, which may have increased diabetes risk and counteracted the ACE-I effects. In addition, the incidence of diabetes in the two groups not taking ACE-Is was very low (~1%/year), so clinically important risk reductions could have been missed.

Results from two of the three large RCTs indicate that ACE-I appear to decrease the incidence of diabetes, though the mechanism(s) for these findings is not clear. While diabetes incidence was a planned subset analysis in both CAPPP and HOPE, each includes only a portion of the randomized cohort at entry (without diabetes). Further analyses are required to remove the possibility that randomization imbalance or other subset effects are responsible for these findings. The DREAM study now underway (see below) is using ramipril in persons with IGT to confirm or refute these observations.

Other interventions

Chromium

Chromium (Cr) has been shown to play an important role in the regulation of glucose, insulin and lipid metabolism, as reviewed by Anderson[227] and Mertz[228]. Whether it plays an important role in primary prevention of diabetes is unclear at present, though observational data on chromium deficiency and clinical trial data on small numbers of non-diabetic subjects suggested it might hold promise[228]. Unfortunately, human studies to date have been small, and the term 'impaired glucose tolerance' has been used in a non-standardized way to include multiple glucose end-points. Thus, it is very difficult to know whether chromium would have preventive effects in large numbers of carefully defined high-risk subjects.

It is likely that the response to chromium depends on the chromium nutritional status of the subject, so that heterogeneous results may have occurred due to the inclusion of subjects in various nutritional states at entry. Methods for the evaluation of chromium status or diagnosis of chromium deficiency are not clinically established[227]. These facts present obstacles in defining risk groups or clinical responders. Observational studies have shown that lower chromium levels occur in people with type 2 diabetes compared with controls, and people with diabetes have been shown to have limited improvements in glucose tolerance and lipids (reviewed in Davies *et al.*[229]).

Davies and colleagues also showed that there are significant age-related declines in chromium levels in sweat, hair and serum using current analytical techniques[229] as well as lower levels in middle-aged males than in females. Notwithstanding these results, many of which come from less rigorously controlled studies, there are important negative clinical trials, which often were better designed (see Thomas and Gropper[230], Abraham *et al.*[231] and Uusitupa *et al.*[232] for review).

In a recent trial, Uusitupa and colleagues gave chromium-rich yeast supplementation (160 μg/day) or placebo to 26 subjects aged 65–74 years who had IGT on two OGTTs[232]. After six months, there were no significant improvements in glucose or insulin at fasting or during an OGTT. Insulin levels were non significantly lower at 1 and 2 h post-challenge, but this was associated with a small weight loss in this supplemented group. No changes in lipids were seen. Their review presents the counter-argument that chromium may not be effective in improving glucose tolerance, and calls into question how essential chromium is for human nutrition. Thus, chromium cannot be recommended as a preventive agent for type 2 diabetes on the basis of current evidence.

Antioxidants and other vitamins

Several studies have explored the role of antioxidants in diabetes and on related variables such as glucose levels, HbA_{1c} etc. In the prospective follow-up of the Finnish and Dutch cohorts of the Seven Countries Study, Feskens *et al.*[146] found that intake of vitamin C at baseline was inversely related to 2 h glucose level 20 years later, independent of dietary fat intake, BMI and energy expenditure. An inverse cross-sectional association sectionally was also seen in non-diabetics for vitamin C in Beaver Dam, Wisconsin[233] for levels of HbA_{1c}. No relationship was seen in this study for vitamins E or beta-carotene. Sargeant *et al.* also reported that plasma levels of vitamin C were associated with lower levels of HbA_{1c}[234] in a cross-sectional analysis in Norfolk, the UK. Persons with previously undiagnosed diabetes ($HbA_{1c} \geq 7\%$ and no medication) also had lower plasma levels of vitamin C. The OR for having undiagnosed diabetes for each 20 μmol/L increase in vitamin C level was 0.70 (CI 0.52–0.95).

After four years of prospective follow-up of 944 men in eastern Finland, Salonen *et al.*[235] found that low plasma vitamin E was independently associated with a 3.9-fold (CI 1.8–8.6) increase in diabetes incidence. Their results were consistent with a small crossover trial where vitamin E improved insulin action as measured by clamp[236]. A recently published multicenter study of vitamin E supplementation and cardiovascular incidence among high-risk subjects for cardiovascular disease and diabetes (HOPE[237]) did not mention any effects on diabetes incidence. Since the companion paper from this study specifically identified reduced diabetes incidence among people in the 2×2 factorial trial who were assigned angiotensin-converting enzyme inhibitors[225], this end-point was likely to have been examined.

In the only large RCT of antioxidants reported to date, Liu and co-workers gave 50 mg of beta-carotene every other day or placebo to over 22 000 US male physicians[238]. After a median of 12 years of follow-up, there was no difference in diabetes incidence rates (RR = 0.98, CI 0.85–1.12) adjusted for other risk factors. Thus, there is no evidence that supplementation with beta-carotene alters diabetes risk.

In the observational follow-up of the National Health and Nutrition Examination Survey – I Epidemiologic Follow-up survey[239], Ford found that persons who developed diabetes over approximately 20 years were significantly less likely to report use of multivitamins (21.4%) during the previous month at baseline than persons who did not develop diabetes (33.5%). After adjusting for demographics, BMI, smoking, activity, dietary variables and medications, the hazard ratio for the use of multivitamins was 0.76 (CI 0.63–0.93; ARR $\cong$1.6/1000 person-years). Persons reporting more sustained use had greater reductions, and persons starting vitamin intake after baseline had no reduction in risk. Whether this finding is due to the vitamin use itself, or to other aspects of lifestyle clustering in persons who use multivitamins, remains unclear.

Whether antioxidants have protective effects on diabetes incidence remains unanswered, though the limited RCT data do not support it. However, it is possible that longer-term studies of antioxidants may be required to understand their effects, since they may act at an earlier stage in disease[240] (requiring a cohort at lower risk at entry). They may also require intake of multiple antioxidants and other co-factors to be effective, as would occur in a diet higher in combinations of fruits and vegetables rather than single vitamin supplements[237].

Pravastatin

Freeman and colleagues recently reported a subgroup analysis of the West of Scotland Coronary Prevention Study (WOSCOPS)[241]. There were 5974 men aged 45–64 years ($\bar{x}$ = 55 years) without diabetes at baseline among the 6595 persons randomized to either pravastatin (40 mg/day) or placebo. Subjects at entry had normal fasting glucose levels, elevated LDL cholesterol and no history of diabetes, myocardial infarction or unstable angina or coronary revascularization at entry. Diabetes was defined by modified ADA criteria, requiring two fasting glucose levels ≥7.0 mmol/L (126 mg/dL) and an increment from baseline of ≥2.0 mmol/L (36 mg/dL) or treatment with diabetes medications. After 4.9 years of follow-up, men randomized to pravastatin had a 30% lower incidence of diabetes (p = 0.042) (multivariate hazard ratio = 0.7, 0.50–0.99). The authors noted that this could be due to effects on lowering of triglycerides and attendant changes in insulin resistance, or perhaps via anti-inflammatory mechanisms of the statins. Since this was a post-hoc analysis of WOSCOPS, confirmation in a second trial should be completed before fully accepting these results. They provide an important possibility that a widely prescribed drug class may have important effects on diabetes incidence.

Other factors

There have been reports of other potential risk factors for type 2 diabetes noted in observational studies which could hold some potential for preventive interventions. These include such metabolites as low potassium[154], low magnesium[154,159,242–245], and inadequate vitamin D intake[246]. RCTs are not available to determine the role supplementation might play in reducing diabetes incidence.

Observational results increasingly support the role of cigarette smoking as a reversible risk factor for diabetes. Manson and colleagues recently reported results from the Physicians Health Study[247], which found a dose-dependent increased risk for development of type 2 diabetes compared with never smokers. After adjustment for BMI, activity and alcohol consumption (but not dietary factors), the RR for smoking were 1.0 (CI 0.8–1.3) for 1–19.9 pack-years; 1.3 (CI 1.0–1.6) for 20–39.9 pack-years, and 1.6 (CI 1.3–2.1) for 40+ pack-years (p <0.001 for trend). The other Health Professional follow-up studies showed consistent elevations in diabetes risk[248,249], as did the Zutphen Study[145], a Japanese worker cohort[250] and the Osaka Health Survey[251]. Three other prospective studies found no associations[140,194,252]. Each of these negative studies had fewer cases of incident diabetes than seen in the positive studies. Smoking cessation for diabetes prevention has not been evaluated in randomized studies, though it now appears to be well established as a risk factor, based on observational studies[247].

Elective alcohol consumption has also been studied in several observational prospective studies as well, and moderate intake appears to reduce risk for diabetes, as it does for cardiovascular disease[253], though higher amounts may increase the risk. Moderate alcohol consumption has been shown to have dose-dependent protection for incident diabetes in the US Physician's Health Study[254], the Nurses Health Study[255], the Health Professional Follow-up

Study[249] and the British Regional Heart Study[116]. Higher risks for intake of 20 g/day or more have been seen in the Paris Prospective Study[256] and the Rancho Bernardo Study[257]. Recent results from the Atherosclerosis Risk in Communities (ARIC)[258] study showed reduced risk in women at all levels of consumption, but a higher risk of diabetes among men with the highest alcohol consumption (>21 drinks per week). Moderate levels of intake among men were consistent with reduced risk, but were not statistically significant. No RCTs have yet examined the use of moderate alcohol intake as a possible prevention for diabetes.

Bariatric surgery

Use of surgery to limit food intake and induce long-term weight loss is one of the most radical and costly approaches to induce weight loss and treat obesity[163]. The most common approaches include vertical banded gastroplasty or gastric bypass, which have been the subject of a National Institutes of Health consensus conference[259]. Since surgery is a way to induce weight loss, rather than a prevention therapy in its own right, it will not be evaluated further. There is reasonably convincing evidence that the significant weight loss induced by surgery can markedly reduce obesity, diabetes incidence[260], hypertension, hyperinsulinemia and hypertriglyceridemia[261].

PREVENTION OF OBESITY

Studies that aim to reduce obesity or prevent it from developing are relevant to the prevention of type 2 diabetes, since obesity is one of the major modifiable risk factors. Like diabetes, overweight and obesity have been the outcomes for a large number of clinical trials and observational studies exploring risk factors for their development and reduction. Comprehensive reviews of obesity prevention issues and approaches have been published[13,163,262-264] and it is not possible to review them here. The interventions studied have been similar to those for type 2 diabetes, and have focused on lifestyle modification as well the use of selected pharmacological agents that may reduce weight. No large RCTs have investigated the prevention of obesity (in contrast to obesity reduction) as it relates to type 2 diabetes.

Several community-based cardiovascular prevention studies have included obesity as one of several outcomes, often with limited success[265-267]. However, hypertension prevention trials with individual, rather community interventions, have often used weight loss and prevention of weight gain to decrease BP. While BP was the primary outcome, it is of interest to note that several of these studies achieved and maintained significant weight loss over 18 months to five years[268-270]. These studies, seldom cited in the diabetes or weight loss literature, offer hope that sustainable weight loss and weight gain prevention are possible using intensive interventions. Had these studies included measures of glucose tolerance, we would be much closer to an answer about the role of weight loss and obesity prevention on the incidence of diabetes.

TYPE 2 DIABETES PREVENTION STUDIES CURRENTLY UNDERWAY

There are several primary prevention trials currently underway or in the late planning stages which should add substantially to the knowledge base by 2002–2003. One lifestyle study and five pharmacological interventions are currently in progress and are summarized in Table 6.8.

Lifestyle trials

Community Diabetes Prevention Project (CDDP)

The CDDP was developed in Minneapolis, Minnesota, USA to determine if a low intensity community-based intervention could alter the natural history of insulin resistance, IGT and type 2 diabetes[67]. Subjects were identified using a simple screening interview, then randomized to a nutrition, physical activity and stress management intervention group or control, as described in Table 6.3. After two years, this low intensity intervention has reported no differences in diabetes incidence between intervention and control groups, however, four-year follow-up is currently being completed, with results to be reported in the near future. The other lifestyle studies underway differ from this community-based low intensity approach by including higher risk subjects and using more intensive interventions.

Pharmacological trials

Dutch Acarbose Trial (DAISI)

A three-year primary prevention study is underway in Hoorn, the Netherlands, also using acarbose among 150 subjects with IGT. After screening of potentially eligible subjects, those who have a mean of two fasting plasma glucose levels <7.8 mmol/l (140 mg/dl) and the mean of two 2 h post-load glucoses >8.6 – <11.1 mmol/l (>155.0 – <200 mg/dl) have been randomized to either 50 mg of acarbose three times a day or placebo. Subjects will have three-monthly fasting glucose levels, and an OGTT at 1.5 and three years for the primary endpoint of type 2 diabetes. A useful addition to this small trial is the performance of a hyperglycemic clamp at randomization and at three years to assess insulin resistance. Completion is expected in 2002.

Table 6.8. Primary prevention trials for type 2 diabetes mellitus underway as of 2002.

Study, author, reference	Population	Intervention	Randomization Start	Completion	Study end
		Lifestyle			
Community Diabetes Prevention Project (CDPP) Bergenstal et al. 1998[67]	Minneapolis, MN, USA 418 men and women Age x̄ = 46 yrs, BMI x̄ = 30. Outcome: Insulin resistance and diabetes	**Intervention:** low-intensity diet, exercise and stress management advice twice per year with monthly phone calls. **Control:** not stated. No difference in diabetes rates at 2 years.	1995	1996	2000–01
		Pharmacological			
DAISI – Dutch Acarbose Trial	Hoorn, Netherlands 150 men and women Age 45–70, IGT × 2. Outcome: diabetes	**Acarbose:** 50 mg tid or **placebo**	1998		2002
NANSY Melander et al. 1999[271]	Sweden, Norway 2224 subjects with impaired fasting glucose; five-year follow-up. Outcome: diabetes	**Glimepiride:** 1 mg qd or **placebo**	2000	2002	2007
Early Diabetes Intervention Trial (EDIT) Citroën et al. 2001[200]	United Kingdom, 9 centers, 631 men and women, aged x̄ = 52 years; fasting glucose 5.5 to 7.7 mmol/L; 3-year follow-up reported to date. Outcome: diabetes and insulin sensitivity, β-cell function	**Metformin** (500 tid) or placebo; **Acarbose** (50 tid) or placebo; 2 × 2 factorial design; preliminary report shows less adherence to acarbose or metformin than to placebo; suggests nonsignificant lowering of elevated plasma glucose levels at three years	1996	1998	2002
DREAM: Diabetes REduction Assessment with ramipril and rosiglitazone Medication	International, multicenter; 4000 subjects aged 30+ years with IGT; 3-year follow-up. Outcome: diabetes	**Ramipril** (10–15 mg/day) or placebo; **rosiglitazone** (8 mg/day) or placebo; 2 × 2 factorial design.	2000	2002	2005–6
Navigator: Nateglinide and Valsartan in Impaired Glucose Tolerance. Outcomes Research. Novartis-sponsored trial	600–800 centers in 40 countries; 7500 subjects with IGT: age 50+ with at least one CV disease or 55+ with at least one CV risk factor. Outcomes: diabetes (phase 1); CVD (phase 2)	**Nateglinide** (60 mg before meals), **Valsartan** (160mg daily), both, or placebo. 2 × 2 factorial design	2001	2003	2006–7

Early Diabetes Intervention Trial (EDIT)

EDIT is a six-year, prospective, randomized, placebo-controlled study in subjects with two consecutive fasting plasma glucose levels in the range 5.5–7.7 mmol/L (100–139 mg/dl). Nine UK clinical centers have recruited 631 subjects. The primary aim of the trial is to determine whether deterioration in glycemic tolerance towards diabetes can be delayed or prevented using the alpha-glucosidase inhibitor acarbose or the biguanide metformin, in a 2 × 2 factorial design. Three-year interim results have been presented in abstract form[200]. No significant effect has yet been seen on diabetes incidence, though both drug groups were said to have lower rates than the placebo group, but data were not presented for comparison. Small improvements in insulin sensitivity and beta-cell function, triglyceride levels and glucose levels were seen in both groups. Weight, HbA_{1c} and lipid profiles were not improved. The study will continue for three more years.

The NEPI ANtidiabetes StudY (NANSY)

The Network for Pharmacoepidemiology in Scandinavia is beginning a randomized-placebo controlled study of the sulfonylurea glimepiride (Amaryl) at a dose of 1 mg a day among persons with IGT[271]. Subjects will be men and women of European ancestry living in Sweden and Norway who are 40–70 years of age with an initial fasting blood glucose ≥5.6 mmol/l (100 mg/dl) and the mean of initial and subsequent tests ≥5.6 and <6.1 mmol/l (whole blood, <110 mg/dl) . All participants will receive initial advice about diet and physical activity, although no special lifestyle program is included. Randomization began in February 2000 and recruitment will last about two years. Participants will be followed for five years or until diabetes develops, when they will be placed on open label glimepiride. It is planned that 1112 participants per group (2224 total) will be enrolled, which will allow the detection of a 33% reduction in diabetes incidence. Results are expected in 2007.

Diabetes REduction Assessment with Ramipril and Rosiglitazone Medication (DREAM)

The DREAM trial is an international, multicenter, double-blind RCT aimed at recruiting at least 4000 participants with IGT. Participants will be randomly allocated to either ramipril and/or rosiglitazone using a 2 × 2 factorial design and followed for at least three years. Ramipril, an ACE-I, was suggested to reduce diabetes incidence in the Heart Outcomes Prevention Evaluation (HOPE) Study[225] in a subset analysis. DREAM will attempt to replicate these findings in a more homogeneous subset of subjects with IGT. The use of rosiglitazone, a second-generation thiazolidinedione insulin-sensitizing agent, is predicated on the positive preliminary results using troglitazone reviewed previously. Randomization began in 2000 and the trial will follow subjects for three years after randomization.

Nateglinide And Valsartan in Impaired Glucose Tolerance Outcomes Research (Navigator)

The Navigator Trial is industry-sponsored and will test the prevention of type 2 diabetes using two novel agents in a 2×2 factorial design with placebo. Nateglinide is an amino acid derivative that reduces post-prandial glycemia when taken immediately before meals[272]. Valsartan is an angiotensin-II receptor blocker, indicated for high blood pressure and heart failure[273]. The goal is to determine whether restoration of early phase insulin secretion and improvements in insulin sensitivity can arrest decline to type 2 diabetes and prevent cardiovascular disease. The study will be conducted in 600–800 centers in 30 countries, and will recruit 7500 subjects who have IGT and either a history of cardiovascular disease (if aged 50 or older) or one or more cardiovascular risk factors (if aged 55 or older). Diabetes incidence will be examined at three years (phase 1) and CVD prevention at five or six years (phase 2). Recruitment began in 2001 and the trial is expected to continue until 2006–2007.

PREVENTION STRATEGIES

Type 2 diabetes has multiple risk factors and, at the current state of knowledge, is regarded as a heterogeneous disorder. Given these facts, interventions can be targeted at the multiple risk factors, either in the entire population or in high-risk subjects, perhaps using both approaches. Tuomilehto and colleagues have succinctly summarized these approaches[6]. Given the widespread and increasing prevalence of obesity in the USA and other countries[274,275], a population-based strategy to reduce obesity is likely to lead to widespread benefits for diabetes and related disorders.

The evidence to date, however, does not suggest that obesity prevention or reduction is effective on a large scale. Community- and population-based approaches have been tried in limited numbers of studies with, at best, small impacts on obesity. This is an area that needs further work, especially given the strong environmental components working to reduce physical activity and increase energy intake in Western societies[276].

The studies of obesity prevention in children must be confirmed and expanded. Public policy must be addressed and changes made in order to increase activity, maintain weight for adults at near normal levels, and induce weight loss for overweight and obese people[277]. Such strategies echo the recommendations of Joslin over 80 years ago[1], mentioned at the beginning of this chapter.

A high-risk strategy involves identification of persons with levels of pre-diabetic risk factors that place them at high risk to develop diabetes in the near future[6]. This is the approach that was taken in all of the larger clinical trials recently completed. These studies have identified persons with IFG or post-challenge glucose levels characteristic of IGT, obesity, family history of diabetes, history of gestational diabetes, etc., for lifestyle or pharmacological intervention. These approaches have now been shown to work for lifestyle change, which has been replicated in three studies[55,69,72] and in very different populations. Results for metformin have been significant in only one large trial[72], and were consistent but non-significant in one smaller study[212]. Further details are required to more fully understand the recent acarbose results[223], but a second trial is underway (DAISI) and should soon provide information.

With efficacy of lifestyle changes established, it remains to be determined what the most efficient, cost-effective strategies are to identify and intervene in such high-risk subjects. In addition, longer-term follow-up is needed to determine the duration of the effects of lifestyle change, before beginning to understand the impacts on chronic complications and mortality. Pharmacological treatment approaches in high-risk subjects who are otherwise well must be carefully considered from a side-effect and cost standpoint, as well as for their efficacy. High-risk approaches must complement a wider public health approach aimed at general reduction of obesity and physical inactivity, since it is not possible to medically treat all subjects at the relatively late stages of diabetes development when IGT and declining beta-cell function are already evident[278,279].

A number of questions in the high-risk strategy remain unanswered. While it is now known that diabetes incidence can be reduced among persons with IFG or IGT, it is not clear whether there are additional subsets of high-risk subjects among those with IFG or IGT who can be identified. Such people might include those with low insulin response, or higher levels of obesity, who may respond to specific subinterventions as suggested by the TRIPOD study[220]. The evidence available suggests that weight loss is important if glucose levels are to be lowered. However, physical activity improves insulin action, even in the absence of weight loss. The effect of these different components of risk over the longer term remains largely unknown. Will it be useful to identify high-risk patterns of genes in individuals to target for intervention? The current epidemic of obesity and increasing diabetes rates has occurred over too short a time to implicate changes in the genetic structure of populations, but with evolving technology it might be cost-effective to identify genetically high risk subjects for intervention in the near future. Such issues remain unknown at present. Genetic screening of people currently involved in prevention trials may prove useful, once specific genes can be targeted. This may allow the identification of subjects who responded to the intervention due to their combination of genes and environmental changes.

SUMMARY

The available data now provide a firm answer that type 2 diabetes can be delayed or prevented in high-risk subjects. Trials currently underway should provide substantial evidence about the impact of specific pharmacologic interventions on diabetes prevention.

With the current level of information, it is reasonable to recommend a programme of moderate levels of physical activity, weight maintenance or modest weight loss (for overweight people), and a low-fat, calorie-moderated diet for the positive effects this will have on cardiovascular and other risks for large numbers of people. In addition, subjects at high risk should have specific risk factors for cardiovascular disease treated (e.g. lipids, blood pressure). The recent results from ACE-inhibitor trials suggest that such agents may also lower diabetes risk as an important benefit.

REFERENCES

1. Joslin EP (1921) The prevention of diabetes mellitus. *J.A.M.A* **76**: 79–84 American Medical Association.
2. Tuomilehto J (1988) Strategies for primary prevention of non-insulin dependent diabetes mellitus. *Adv. Exp. Med. Biol.* **246**: 403–411.
3. Zimmet PZ (1988) Primary prevention of diabetes mellitus. *Diabetes Care* **11**: 258–262.
4. King H, Dowd JE (1990) Primary prevention of type 2 (non-insulin-dependent) diabetes mellitus. *Diabetologia* **33**: 3–8.
5. Stern MP (1991) Kelly West Lecture. Primary prevention of type II diabetes mellitus. *Diabetes Care* **14**: 399–410.
6. Tuomilehto J, Knowler WC, Zimmet P (1992) Primary prevention of non-insulin-dependent diabetes mellitus. *Diabetes Metab. Rev.* **8**: 339–353.
7. WHO Study Group (1994) Prevention of diabetes mellitus. WHO Technical Report Series. 844, 1–100. Geneva World Health Organization.
8. Manson JE, Spelsberg A (1994) Primary prevention of non-insulin-dependent diabetes mellitus. *Am. J. Prev. Med.* **10**: 172–184.
9. Knowler WC, Narayan KM, Hanson RL, Nelson RG, Bennett PH, Tuomilehto J, Schersten B, Pettitt DJ (1995) Preventing non-insulin-dependent diabetes. *Diabetes* **44**: 483–488.
10. Melander A (1996) Review of previous impaired glucose tolerance intervention studies. *Diabet. Med.* **13**(Suppl 2): S20–2.
11. Bourn DM (1996) The potential for lifestyle change to influence the progression of impaired glucose tolerance to non-insulin-dependent diabetes mellitus. *Diabet. Med.* **13**: 938–945.
12. Dornhorst A, Merrin PK (1994) Primary, secondary and tertiary prevention of non-insulin- dependent diabetes. *Postgrad. Med. J.* **70**: 529–535.
13. Broussard BA, Sugarman JR, Bachman-Carter K, Booth K, Stephenson L, Strauss K, Gohdes D (1995) Toward comprehensive obesity prevention programs in Native American communities. *Obesity Research* **3 (Suppl 2)**: 289s–297s.
14. Daniel M, Gamble D (1995) Diabetes and Canada's aboriginal peoples: the need for primary prevention. *Int. J. of Nursing Studies* **32**: 243–259.

15. Mudaliar SR, Henry RR (1997) Strategies for preventing type II diabetes. What can be done to stem the epidemic? *Postgrad. Med.* **101**: 181–6, 189.
16. Goldberg RB (1998) Prevention of type 2 diabetes. *Med. Clin. North Am.* **82**: 805–821.
17. Songer TJ (1992) The economic costs of NIDDM. *Diabetes Metab. Rev.* **8**: 389–404.
18. Jonsson B (1998) The economic impact of diabetes. *Diabetes Care* **21**: C7–C10.
19. Javitt JC, Chiang Y-P (1995) Economic impact of diabetes. In: *Diabetes in America*, 2nd edn. National Diabetes Data Group, Ed. Bethesda, National Institutes of Health, pp. 601–611.
20. Brown JB, Nichols GA, Glauber HS, Bakst AW (1999) Type 2 diabetes: Incremental medical care costs during the first 8 years after diagnosis. *Diabetes Care* **22**: 1116–1124.
21. Selby JV, Ray GT, Zhang D, Colby CJ (1997) Excess costs of medical care for patients with diabetes in a managed care population. *Diabetes Care* **20**: 1396–1402.
22. Eastman RC, Javitt JC, Herman WH, Dasbach EJ, Harris MI (1996) Prevention strategies for non-insulin-dependent diabetes mellitus: an economic perspective. In *Diabetes Mellitus* (eds LeRoith D, Taylor SI, Olefsky JI) Philadelphia: Lippencott-Raven, pp. 621–630.
23. Segal L, Dalton AC, Richardson J (1998) Cost-effectiveness of the primary prevention of non-insulin dependent diabetes mellitus. *Health Promotion International* **13**: 197–209.
24. WHO Study Group (1985) *Diabetes Mellitus – Technical Report Series 727*. Geneva: World Health Organization.
25. WHO Expert Committee on Diabetes Mellitus (1980) *Second Report*. Geneva: World Health Organization.
26. Report of the Expert Committee on the Diagnosis and Classification of Diabetes Mellitus (1997) *Diabetes Care* **20**: 1183–1197.
27. Edelstein SL, Knowler WC, Bain RP, Andres R, Barrett-Connor EL, Dowse GK, Haffner SM, Pettitt DJ, Sorkin JD, Muller DC, Collins VR, Hamman RF (1997) Predictors of progression from impaired glucose tolerance to non-insulin-dependent diabetes mellitus: an analysis of six prospective studies. *Diabetes* **46**: 701–710.
28. US Preventive Services Task Force (1996) *Guide to clinical preventive services*. Alexandria, VA: International Medical Publishing.
29. Clinical guidelines on the identification, evaluation and treatment of overweight and obesity in adults. 1998. Bethesda, MD, NIH, NHLBI.
30. Harris MI (1995) Classification, diagnostic criteria, and screening for diabetes. In *Diabetes in America*, 2nd edn. National Diabetes Data Group, Ed. Bethesda, MD, NIH, NIDDK No. 95-1468, pp. 15–35.
31. Kobberling J, Tillil H (1990) Genetic and nutritional factors in the etiology and pathogenesis of diabetes mellitus. *World Rev. Nutr. Diet.* **63**: 102–115.
32. Bennett PH, Bogardus C, Tuomilehto J, Zimmet P (1992) Epidemiology and natural history of NIDDM: Non-obese and obese. In *International Textbook of Diabetes* (eds Alberti KGMM, DeFronzo RA , Keen H, Zimmet P) Chichester: John Wiley & Sons pp. 148–176.
33. Zimmet PZ (1992) Kelly West Lecture 1991. Challenges in diabetes epidemiology – from West to the rest. *Diabetes Care* **15**: 232–252.
34. O'Dea K (1992) Obesity and diabetes in 'the land of milk and honey'. *Diabetes Metab. Rev.* **8**: 373–388.
35. Knowler WC, Saad MF, Pettitt DJ, Nelson RG, Bennett PH (1993) Determinants of diabetes mellitus in the Pima Indians. *Diabetes Care* **16**: 216–227.

36. Hamman RF (1992) Genetic and environmental determinants of non-insulin-dependent diabetes mellitus (NIDDM). *Diabetes Metab. Rev.* **8**: 287–338.
37. Rewers M, Hamman RF (1995) Risk factors for non-insulin-dependent diabetes. In *Diabetes in America* – 1995 (ed. Harris MI) Washington, DC: US Government Printing Office.
38. Golay A, Felber JP (1994) Evolution from obesity to diabetes. *Diabete. Metab.* **20**: 3–14.
39. Haffner SM (1998) Epidemiology of type 2 diabetes: risk factors. *Diabetes Care* **21** (Suppl 3): C3–6.
40. King H, Zimmet P, Raper LR, Balkau B (1984) Risk factors for diabetes in three Pacific populations. *Am. J. Epidemiol.* **119**: 396–409.
41. Hazuda HP, Mitchell BD, Haffner SM, Stern MP (1991) Obesity in Mexican American subgroups: findings from the San Antonio Heart Study. *Am. J. Clin. Nutr.* **53**: 1529S–1534S.
42. Cederholm J (1985) Short-term treatment of glucose intolerance in middle-aged subjects by diet, exercise, and sulfonylurea. *Upsala J. Med. Sci.* **90**: 229–242.
43. Nilsson PM, Lindholm LH, Schersten BF (1992) Lifestyle changes improve insulin resistance in hyperinsulinaemic subjects: a one-year intervention study of hypertensives and normotensives in Dalby. *J. Hypertens.* **10**: 1071–1078.
44. Page RCL, Harnden KE, Cook JTE, Turner RC (1992) Can lifestyles of subjects with impaired glucose tolerance be changed? A feasibility study. *Diabetic Med.* **9**: 562–566.
45. Katzel LI, Bleecker ER, Colman EG, Rogus EM, Sorkin JD, Goldberg AP (1995) Effects of weight loss vs aerobic exercise training on risk factors for coronary disease in health, obese, middle-aged and older men: A randomized controlled trial. *J.A.M.A.* **274**: 1915–1921.
46. Singh RB, Singh NK, Rastogi SS, Mani UV, Niaz MA (1993) Effects of diet and lifestyle changes on atherosclerotic risk factors after 24 weeks on the Indian Diet Heart Study. *Am. J. Cardiol.* **71**: 1283–1288.
47. Coon PJ, Bleecker ER, Drinkwater DT, Meyers DA, Goldberg AP (1989) Effects of body composition and exercise capacity on glucose tolerance, insulin, and lipoprotein lipids in healthy older men: A cross-sectional and longitudinal intervention study. *Metabolism* **38**: 1201–1209.
48. Hellenius ML, Brismar KE, Berglund BH, de Faire UH (1995) Effects on glucose tolerance, insulin secretion, insulin-like growth factor 1 and its binding protein, IGFBP-1, in a randomized controlled diet and exercise study in healthy, middle-aged men. *J. Intern. Med.* **238**: 121–130.
49. Hellenius ML, de Faire U, Berglund B, Hamsten A, Krakau I (1993) Diet and exercise are equally effective in reducing risk for cardiovascular disease. Results of a randomized controlled study in men with slightly to moderately raised cardiovascular risk factors. *Atherosclerosis* **103**: 81–91.
50. Colman E, Katzel LI, Rogus E, Coon P, Muller D, Goldberg AP (1995) Weight loss reduces abdominal fat and improves insulin action in middle-aged and older men with impaired glucose tolerance. *Metabolism* **44**: 1502–1508.
51. Holme I (1993) The Oslo Diet and Exercise Study (ODES): design and objectives. *Control. Clin. Trials* **14**: 229–243.
52. Anderssen SA, Hjermann I, Urdal P, Torjesen PA, Holme I (1996) Improved carbohydrate metabolism after physical training and dietary intervention in individuals with the "atherothrombogenic syndrome'. Oslo Diet and Exercise Study (ODES). A randomized trial. *J. Intern. Med.* **240**: 203–209.
53. Anderssen SA, Holme I, Urdal P, Hjermann I (1998) Associations between central obesity and indexes of hemostatic, carbohydrate and lipid metabolism. Results of a

one-year intervention from the Oslo Diet and Exercise Study. *Scand. J. Med. Sci. Sports* **8**: 109–115.

54. Torjesen PA, Birkeland KI, Anderssen SA, Hjermann I, Holme I, Urdal P (1997) Lifestyle changes may reverse development of the insulin resistance syndrome. The Oslo Diet and Exercise Study: A randomized trial. *Diabetes Care* **20**: 26–31.

55. Pan XR, Li GW, Hu YH, Wang JX, Yang WY, An ZX, Hu ZX, Lin J, Xiao JZ, Cao HB, Liu PA, Jiang XG, Jiang YY, Wang JP, Zheng H, Zhang H, Bennett PH, Howard BV (1997) Effects of diet and exercise in preventing NIDDM in people with impaired glucose tolerance. The Da Qing IGT and *Diabetes Study. Diabetes Care* **20**: 537–544.

56. Hammersley MS, Meyer LC, Morris RJ, Manley SE, Turner RC, Holman RR (1997) The Fasting Hyperglycaemia Study: I. Subject identification and recruitment for a non-insulin-dependent diabetes prevention trial. *Metabolism* **46**: 44–49.

57. Eriksson KF, Lindgarde F (1991) Prevention of type 2 (non-insulin-dependent) diabetes mellitus by diet and physical exercise. The six-year Malmö feasibility study. *Diabetologia* **34**: 891–898.

58. Bourn DM, Mann JI, McSkimming BJ, Waldron MA, Wishart JD (1994) Impaired glucose tolerance and NIDDM: Does a lifestyle intervention program have an effect? *Diabetes Care* **17**: 1311–1319.

59. Wing RR, Venditti E, Jakicic JM, Polley BA, Lang W (1998) Lifestyle intervention in overweight individuals with a family history of diabetes. *Diabetes Care* **21**: 350–359.

60. Narayan KM, Hoskin M, Kozak D, Kriska AM, Hanson RL, Pettitt DJ, Nagi DK, Bennett PH, Knowler WC (1998) Randomized clinical trial of lifestyle interventions in Pima Indians: a pilot study. *Diabet. Med.* **15**: 66–72.

61. Kumanyika SK, Obarzancek E, Stevens VJ, Hebert PR, Whelton PK (1991) Weight-loss experience of black and white participants in NHLBI-sponsored clinical trials. *Am. J. Clin. Nutr.* **53**: 163S–168S.

62. Weinstock RS, Dai H, Wadden TA (1998) Diet and exercise in the treatment of obesity: effects of 3 interventions on insulin resistance. *Arch. Intern. Med.* **158**: 2477–2483.

63. Simkin-Silverman LR, Wing RR, Boraz MA, Meilahn EN, Kuller LH (1998) Maintenance of cardiovascular risk factor changes among middle-aged women in a lifestyle intervention trial. *Womens Health* **4**: 255–271.

64. Kuller LH, Simkin-Silverman LR, Wing RR, Meilahn EN, Ives DG (2001) Women's Healthy Lifestyle Project: A randomized clinical trial: results at 54 months. *Circulation* **103**: 32–37.

65. Bergenstal R, Monk A, List S, Upham P, List S (1997) The Community Diabetes Prevention Project (CDPP): Identification of the natural history of the insulin resistance syndrome (IRS) and whether progression to type II diabetes can be altered (Abstract). Diabetes.

66. Monk A, Upham P, Bergenstal R (1997) Community Diabetes Prevention Project (CDPP): Baseline characteristics. Diabetes Educ.

67. Bergenstal R, Monk A, Upham P, Nelson JB, List S (1998) The Community Diabetes Prevention Project (CDPP): Identification of the natural history of the insulin resistance syndrome (IRS) and whether progression to Type 2 diabetes can be altered – year 2 data (Abstract). *Diabetes* **47**:

68. Eriksson J, Lindstrom J, Valle T, Aunola S, Hamalainen H, Ilanne-Parikka P, Keinanen-Kiukaanniemi S, Laakso M, Lauhkonen M, Lehto P, Lehtonen A, Louheranta A, Mannelin M, Martikkala V, Rastas M, Sundvall J, Turpeinen A,

Viljanen T, Uusitupa M, Tuomilehto J (on behalf of the Finnish Diabetes Prevention Study Group) (1999) Prevention of Type II diabetes in subjects with impaired glucose tolerance: the Diabetes Prevention Study (DPS) in Finland – Study design and one-year interim report on the feasibility of the lifestyle intervention programme. *Diabetologia* **42**: 793–801.

69. Tuomilehto J, Lindstrom J, Eriksson JG, Valle TT, Hamalainen H, Ilanne-Parikka P, Keinanen-Kiukaanniemi S, Laakso M, Louheranta A, Rastas M, Salminen V, Uusitupa M (2001) Prevention of type 2 diabetes mellitus by changes in lifestyle among subjects with impaired glucose tolerance. *N. Engl. J. Med.* **344**: 1343–1350.

70. Diabetes Prevention Program Research Group (1999) The Diabetes Prevention Program: Design and methods for a clinical trial in the prevention of type 2 diabetes mellitus. *Diabetes Care* **22**: 623–634.

71. The Diabetes Prevention Program Research Group (2000) The Diabetes Prevention Program: Baseline characteristics of the randomized cohort. *Diabetes Care* **23**: 1619–1629.

72. The Diabetes Prevention Program Research Group (in press) Lifestyle modification and metformin reduce the incidence of Type 2 diabetes mellitus. See www.niddk.nih.gov/welcome/releases/8_8_01.htm.

73. O'Dea K (1984) Marked improvement in carbohydrate and lipid metabolism in diabetic Australian Aborigines after temporary reversion to traditional lifestyle. *Diabetes* **33**: 596–603.

74. Ravussin E, Valencia ME, Esparza J, Bennett PH, Schulz LO (1994) Effects of a traditional lifestyle on obesity in Pima Indians. *Diabetes Care* **17**: 1067–1074.

75. Eriksson K-F, Lindgarde F (1991) Prevention of type 2 (non-insulin-dependent) diabetes mellitus by diet and physical exercise. *Diabetologia* **34**: 891–898.

76. Eriksson KF, Lindgarde F (1996) Poor physical fitness and impaired early insulin response but late hyperinsulinaemia, as predictors of NIDDM in middle-aged Swedish men. *Diabetologia* **39**: 573–579.

77. Eriksson KF, Lindgarde F (1998) No excess 12-year mortality in men with impaired glucose tolerance who participated in the Malmö Preventive Trial with diet and exercise. *Diabetologia* **41**: 1010–1016.

78. Viswanathan M, Snehalatha C, Viswanathan V, Vidyavathi P, Indu J, Ramachandran A (1997) Reduction in body weight helps to delay the onset of diabetes even in non-obese with strong family history of the disease. *Diab. Res. Clin. Pract.* **35**: 107–112.

79. Ramachandran A, Snehalatha C, Shobana R, Vidyavathi P, Vijay V (1999) Influence of lifestyle factors in development of diabetes in Indians – scope for primary prevention. J. Assoc. Phys. India **47**: 764–766.

80. Saltin B, Lindgarde F, Houston M, Horlin R, Nygaard E, Gad P (1979) Physical training and glucose intolerance in middle-aged men with chemical diabetes. Diabetes **28 (Suppl 1)**: 30–32.

81. Ramaiya KL, Swai ABM, Alberti KGMM, McLarty D (1992) Lifestyle changes decrease rates of glucose intolerance and cardiovascular (CVD) risk factors: a six-year intervention study in a high risk Hindu Indian sub-community (Abstract). *Diabetologia* **35**: A60.

82. Simmons D, Fleming C, Voyle J, Fou F, Feo S, Gatland B (1998) A pilot urban church-based programme to reduce risk factors for diabetes among Western Samoans in New Zealand. *Diabet. Med.* **15**: 136–142.

83. McKenzie SB, O'Connell J, Smith LA, Ottinger WE (1998) A primary intervention program (pilot study) for Mexican American children at risk for type 2 diabetes. *Diabetes Educ.* **24**: 180–187.

84. Trevino RP, Pugh JA, Hernandez AE, Menchaca VD, Ramirez RR, Mendoza, M (1998) Bienestar: a diabetes risk-factor prevention program. *J. Sch. Health* **68**: 62–67.

85. Holcomb JD, Lira J, Kingery PM, Smith DW, Lane D, Goodway J (1998) Evaluation of Jump Into Action: a program to reduce the risk of non-insulin dependent diabetes mellitus in school children on the Texas–Mexico border. *J. Sch. Health* **68**: 282–288.

86. Luepker RV, Perry CL, McKinlay SM, Nader PR, Parcel GS, Stone EJ, Webber LS, Elder JP, Feldman HA, Johnson CC, et al.: (1996) Outcomes of a field trial to improve children's dietary patterns and physical activity. The Child and Adolescent Trial for Cardiovascular Health. CATCH collaborative group. *J.A.M.A.* **275**: 768–776.

87. Harrell JS, Gansky SA, McMurray RG, Bangdiwala SI, Frauman AC, Bradley CB (1998) School-based interventions improve heart health in children with multiple cardiovascular disease risk factors. *Pediatrics* **102**: 371–380.

88. Gortmaker SL, Peterson K, Wiecha J, Sobol AM, Dixit S, Fox MK, Laird N (1999) Reducing obesity via a school-based interdisciplinary intervention among youth: Planet Health. *Arch. Pediatr. Adolesc. Med.* **153**: 409–418.

89. Robinson TN (1999) Reducing children's television viewing to prevent obesity. *J.A.M.A.* **282**: 1561–1567.

90. Resnicow K, Robinson TN (1997) School-based cardiovascular disease prevention studies: review and synthesis. *Ann. Epidemiol.* **7**: 514–531.

91. Kriska AM, Blair SN, Pereira MA (1994) The potential role of physical activity in the prevention of non-insulin-dependent diabetes mellitus: the epidemiological evidence. *Exerc. Sport Sci. Rev.* **22**: 121–143.

92. Mayer EJ, Alderman BW, Regensteiner JG, Marshall JA, Haskell WL, Baxter J, Hamman RF (1991) Physical-activity-assessment measures compared in a biethnic rural population: the San Luis Valley Diabetes Study. *Am. J. Clin. Nutr.* **53**: 812–820.

93. Kriska AM, Bennett PH (1992) An epidemiological perspective of the relationship between physical activity and NIDDM: from activity assessment to intervention. *Diabetes Metab.* Rev. **8**: 355–372.

94. Pate RR, Pratt M, Blair SN, Haskell WL, Macera CA, Bouchard C, Buchner D, Ettinger W, Heath GW, King AC, Kriska A, Leon AS, Marcus BH, Morris J, Paffenbarger RS, Patrick K, Pollock ML, Rippe JM, Sallis J, Wilmore JH (1995) Physical activity and public health: A recommendation from the Centers for Disease Control and Prevention and the American College of Sports Medicine. *J.A.M.A.* **273**: 402–407.

95. Spelsberg A, Manson JE (1995) Physical activity in the treatment and prevention of diabetes. *Comp. Therapy* **21**: 559–562.

96. Blair SN, Kohl HW, Gordon NF, Paffenbarger RS Jr. (1992) How much physical activity is good for health? *Annu. Rev. Public Health* **13**: 99–126.

97. Clark DO (1997) Physical activity efficacy and effectiveness among older adults and minorities. *Diabetes Care* **20**: 1176–1182.

98. Blair SN, Horton E, Leon AS, Lee IM, Drinkwater BL, Dishman RK, Mackey M, Kienholz ML (1996) Physical activity, nutrition, and chronic disease. *Med. Sc. Sports Exercise* **28**: 335–349.

99. NIH Consensus Development Panel on Physical Activity and Cardiovascular Health (1995) Physical activity and cardiovascular health. *NIH Consens.Statement* **13**: 1–33.

100. Zurlo F, Ferraro RT, Fontvieille AM, Rising R, Bogardus C, Ravussin E (1992) Spontaneous physical activity and obesity: cross-sectional and longitudinal studies in Pima Indians. *Am. J. Physiol.* **263**: E296–E300.

101. Selby JV, Newman B, King MC, Friedman GD (1987) Environmental and behavioral determinants of fasting plasma glucose in women. A matched co-twin analysis. *Am. J. Epidemiol.* **125**: 979–988.

102. Kujala UM, Kaprio J, Sarna S, Koskenvuo M (1998) Relationship of leisure-time physical activity and mortality. *J.A.M.A.* **279**: 440–444.

103. Medalie JH, Papier CM, Herman JB, Goldbourt U, Tamir S, Neufeld HN, Riss E (1974) Diabetes mellitus among 10000 adult men: I. Five-year incidence and associated variables. *Isr. J. Med. Sci.* **10**: 681–697.

104. Manson JE, Rimm EB, Stampfer MJ, Colditz GA, Willett WC, Krolewski AS, Rosner B, Hennekens CH, Speizer FE (1991) Physical activity and incidence of non-insulin-dependent diabetes mellitus in women. *Lancet* **338**: 774–778.

105. Hu FB, Sigal RJ, Rich-Edwards J, Colditz GA, Solomon CG, Willett WC, Speizer FE, Manson JE (1999) Walking compared with vigorous physical activity and risk of type 2 diabetes in women. *J.A.M.A* **282**: 1433–1439.

106. Helmrich SP, Ragland DR, Leung RW, Paffenbarger RS Jr. (1991) Physical activity and reduced occurrence of non-insulin-dependent diabetes mellitus. *N. Engl. J. Med.* **325**: 147–152.

107. Lynch J, Helmrich SP, Lakka TA, Kaplan GA, Cohen RD, Salonen R, Salonen JT (1996) Moderately intense physical activities and high levels of cardio-respiratory fitness reduce the risk of non-insulin-dependent diabetes mellitus in middle-aged men. *Arch. Int. Med.* **156**: 1307–1314.

108. Schranz A, Tuomilehto J, Marti B, Jarrett RJ, Grabauskas V, Vassallo A (1991) Low physical activity and worsening of glucose tolerance: results from a two-year follow-up of a population sample in Malta. *Diabetes Res. Clin. Pract.* **11**: 127–136.

109. Kaye SA, Folsom AR, Sprafka JM, Prineas RJ, Wallace RB (1991) Increased incidence of diabetes mellitus in relation to abdominal adiposity in older women. *J. Clin. Epidemiol.* **44**: 329–334.

110. Manson JE, Nathan DM, Krolewski AS, Stampfer MJ, Willett WC, Hennekens CH (1992) A prospective study of exercise and incidence of diabetes among US male physicians. *J.A.M.A.* **268**: 63–67.

111. Gurwitz JH, Field TS, Glynn RJ, Manson JE, Avorn J, Taylor JO, Hennekens CH (1994) Risk factors for non-insulin-dependent diabetes mellitus requiring treatment in the elderly. *J. Am. Geriatr. Soc.* **42**: 1235–1240.

112. Burchfiel CM, Curb JD, Rodriguez BL, Yano K, Hwang LJ, Fong KO, Marcus EB (1995) Incidence and predictors of diabetes in Japanese–American men. The Honolulu Heart Program. *Ann. Epidemiol.* **5**: 33–43.

113. Burchfiel CM, Sharp DS, Curb JD, Rodriguez BL, Hwang LJ, Marcus EB, Yano K (1995) Physical activity and incidence of diabetes: the Honolulu Heart Program. *Am. J. Epidemiol.* **141**: 360–368.

114. Hara H, Egusa G, Yamakido M (1996) Incidence of non-insulin-dependent diabetes mellitus and its risk factors in Japanese–Americans living in Hawaii and Los Angeles. *Diabet. Med.* **13**: S133–42.

115. Balkau B, King H, Zimmet P, Raper LR (1985) Factors associated with the development of diabetes in the micronesian population of Nauru. *Am. J. Epidemiol.* **122**: 594–605.

116. Perry IJ, Wannamethee SG, Walker MK, Thomson AG, Whincup PH, Shaper AG (1995) Prospective study of risk factors for development of non-insulin-dependent diabetes in middle aged British men. *BMJ* **310**: 560–564.

117. Monterrosa AE, Haffner SM, Stern MP, Hazuda HP (1995) Sex difference in lifestyle factors predictive of diabetes in Mexican–Americans. *Diabetes Care* 1995
118. Paffenbarger RS Jr., Lee IM, Kampert JB (1997) Physical activity in the prevention of non-insulin-dependent diabetes mellitus. *World Rev. Nutr. Diet.* 82: 210–218.
119. Haapanen N, Miilunpalo S, Vuori I, Oja P, Pasanen M (1997) Association of leisure time physical activity with the risk of coronary heart disease, hypertension and diabetes in middle-aged men and women. *Int. J. Epidemiol.* 26: 739–747.
120. Morin CL, Hamman RF, Shetterly SM, Marshall JA (2000) Does physical activity lower diabetes risk similarly in high versus low risk groups? (Abstract). *Diabetes* 49: 2000.
121. Folsom AR, Kushi LH, Hong CP (2000) Physical activity and incidence of diabetes mellitus in postmenopausal women. *Amer. J. Public Health* 90: 134–138.
122. Hu FB, Leitzmann MF, Stampfer MJ, Colditz GA, Willett WC, Rimm EB (2001_ Physical activity and television watching in relation to risk for type 2 diabetes mellitus in men. *Arch. Int. Med.* 161: 1542–1548.
123. Leonetti DL, Tsunehara CH, Wahl PW, Fujimoto WY (1996) Baseline dietary intake and physical activity of Japanese–american men in relation to glucose tolerance at 5-year follow-up. *Am. J. Hum. Biol* 8: 55–67.
124. Rankinen T, Suomela-Markkanen T, Vaisanen S, Helminen A, Penttila I, Berg A, Bouchard C, Rauramaa R (1997) Relationship between changes in physical activity and plasma insulin during a 2.5-year follow-up study. *Metabolism* 46: 1418–1423.
125. Helmrich SP, Ragland DR, Paffenbarger RS Jr. (1994) Prevention of non-insulin-dependent diabetes mellitus with physical activity. *Med. Sci. Sports Exer.* 26: 824–830.
126. Feskens EJ, Loeber JG, Kromhout D (1994) Diet and physical activity as determinants of hyperinsulinemia: the Zutphen Elderly Study. *Am. J. Epidemiol.* 140: 350–360.
127. Marshall JA, Hamman RF (1993) Dietary lipids and glucose tolerance: The San Luis Valley Diabetes Study. *Ann. NY Acad. Sci.* 683: 46–56.
128. Mann JI, Houston A (1983) The aetiology of non-insulin-dependent diabetes mellitus. In *Diabetes in Epidemiological Perspective.* (eds Mann JI, Pyorala K, Teuscher A) Edinburgh: Churchill Livingstone, pp. 122–164.
129. West KM (1975) Prevention and therapy of diabetes mellitus. *Nutr. Rev.* 33: 193–198.
130. West KM (1978) Epidemiology of Diabetes and its Vascular Lesions. New York: Elsevier Biomedical Press.
131. West KM (1976) Diet and diabetes. *Postgrad. Med.* 60: 209–216.
132. Willett WC (1998) Is dietary fat a major determinant of body fat? *Am. J. Clin. Nutr.* 67: 556S–562S.
133. Hannah JS, Howard BV (1994) Dietary fats, insulin resistance, and diabetes. *J. Cardiovasc. Risk.* 1: 31–37.
134. Virtanen SM, Aro A (1994) Dietary factors in the aetiology of diabetes. *Ann. Med.* 26: 469–478.
135. Hu FB, van Dam RM, Liu S (2001) Diet and risk of Type II diabetes: the role of types of fat and carbohydrate. *Diabetologia* 44: 805–817.
136. Storlien LH, Baur LA, Kriketos AD, Pan DA, Cooney GJ, Jenkins AB, Calvert GD, Campbell LV (1996) Dietary fats and insulin action. *Diabetologia* 39: 621–631.

137. Storlien LH, Kriketos AD, Jenkins AB, Baur LA, Pan DA, Tapsell LC, Calvert GD (1997) Does dietary fat influence insulin action? *Ann. NY Acad. Sci.* **827**: 287–301.
138. Sarkkinen E, Schwab U, Niskanen L, Hannuksela M, Savolainen M, Kervinen K, Kesaniemi A, Uusitupa MI (1996) The effects of monounsaturated-fat enriched diet and polyunsaturated-fat enriched diet on lipid and glucose metabolism in subjects with impaired glucose tolerance. *Eur. J. Clin. Nutr.* **50**: 592–598.
139. Howard BV, Abbott WG, Swinburn BA (1991) Evaluation of metabolic effects of substitution of complex carbohydrates for saturated fat in individuals with obesity and NIDDM. *Diab. Care* **14**: 786–795.
140. Medalie JH, Papier CM, Goldbourt U, Herman JB (1975) Major factors in the development of diabetes mellitus in 10000 men. *Arch. Intern. Med.* **135**: 811–817.
141. Bennett PH, Knowler WC, Baird HR, Butler WJ, Pettitt DJ, Reid JM (1984) Diet and development of diabetes mellitus: An epidemiological perspective. In *Diet, Diabetes, and Atherosclerosis* (ed Pozza B) New York: Raven Press, pp. 109–119.
142. Snowdon DA, Phillips RL (1985) Does a vegetarian diet reduce the occurrence of diabetes? *Am. J. Public Health* **75**: 507–512.
143. Lundgren H, Bengtsson C, Blohme G, Isaksson B, Lapidus L, Lenner RA, Saaek A, Winther E (1989) Dietary habits and incidence of non-insulin-dependent diabetes mellitus in a population study of women in Gothenburg, Sweden. *Am. J. Clin. Nutr.* **49**: 708–712.
144. Lundgren H, Bengtsson C, Blohme G, Lapidus L, Sjostrom L (1989) Adiposity and adipose tissue distribution in relation to incidence of diabetes in women: results from a prospective population study in Gothenburg, Sweden. *Int. J. Obes.* **13**: 413–423.
145. Feskens EJ, Kromhout D (1989) Cardiovascular risk factors and the 25-year incidence of diabetes mellitus in middle-aged men. The Zutphen Study. *Am. J. Epidemiol.* **130**: 1101–1108.
146. Feskens EJ, Virtanen SM, Rasanen L, Tuomilehto J, Stengard J, Pekkanen J, Nissinen A, Kromhout D (1995) Dietary factors determining diabetes and impaired glucose tolerance. A 20-year follow-up of the Finnish and Dutch cohorts of the Seven Countries Study. *Diab. Care* **18**: 1104–1112.
147. Feskens EJ, Bowles CH, Kromhout D (1991) Carbohydrate intake and body mass index in relation to the risk of glucose intolerance in an elderly population. *Am. J. Clin. Nutr.* **54**: 136–140.
148. Feskens EJM, Bowles CH, Kromhout D (1991) Inverse association between fish intake and risk of glucose intolerance in normoglycemic elderly men and women. *Diab. Care* **14**(11): 935–941.
149. Marshall JA, Hoag S, Shetterly SM, Hamman RF (1994) Dietary fat predicts conversion from impaired glucose tolerance to NIDDM: The San Luis Valley Diabetes Study. *Diab. Care* **17**: 50–56.
150. Marshall JA, Bessesen DH, Hamman RF (1997) High saturated fat and low starch and fibre are associated with hyperinsulinaemia in a non-diabetic population – the San Luis Valley Diabetes Study. *Diabetologia* **40**: 430–438.
151. Laird NM, Ware JH (1982) Random-effects models for longitudinal data. *Biometrics* **38**: 963–974.
152. Marshall JA, Scarbro SL, Shetterly SM, Jones RH (1998) Improving power with repeated measures: diet and serum lipids. *Amer. J. Clin. Nutr.* **67**: 934–939.
153. Kawate R, Yamakido M, Nishimoto Y, Bennett PH, Hamman RF, Knowler WC (1979) Diabetes mellitus and its vascular complications in Japanese migrants and on the island of Hawaii. *Diab. Care* **2**: 161–170.

154. Colditz GA, Manson JE, Stampfer MJ, Rosner B, Willett WC, Speizer FE (1992) Diet and risk of clinical diabetes in women. *Am. J. Clin. Nutr.* **55**: 1018–1023.
155. Salmeron J, Manson JE, Stampfer MJ, Colditz GA, Wing AL, Willett WC (1997) Dietary fiber, glycemic load, and risk of non-insulin-dependent diabetes mellitus in women. *J.A.M.A.* **277**: 472–477.
156. Liu S, Manson JE, Stampfer MJ, Hu FB, Giovannucci E, Colditz GA, Hennekens CH, Willett WC (2000) A prospective study of whole-grain intake and risk of type 2 diabetes mellitus in US women. *Amer. J. Public Health* **90**: 1409–1415.
157. Salmeron J, Hu FB, Manson JE, Stampfer MJ, Colditz GA, Rimm EB, Willett WC (2001) Dietary fat intake and risk of type 2 diabetes in women. *Am. J. Clin. Nutr.* **73**: 1019–1026.
158. Salmeron J, Ascherio A, Rimm EB, Colditz GA, Spiegelman D, Jenkins, DJ, Stampfer MJ, Wing AL, Willett WC (1997) Dietary fiber, glycemic load, and risk of NIDDM in men. *Diab. Care* **20**: 545–550.
159. Meyer KA, Kushi LH, Jacobs DR Jr., Slavin J, Sellers TA, Folsom AR (2000) Carbohydrates, dietary fiber, and incidence of type 2 diabetes in older women. *Am. J. Clin. Nutr.* **71**: 921–930.
160. Clandinin MT, Wilke MS (2001) Do trans-fatty acids increase the incidence of type 2 diabetes? *Am. J. Clin. Nutr.* **73**: 1001–1002.
161. Meyer KA, Kushi LH, Jacobs DR Jr., Folsom AR (2001) Dietary fat and incidence of type 2 diabetes in older Iowa women. *Diab. Care* **24**: 1528–1535.
162. Ford ES, Mokdad AH (2001) Fruit and vegetable consumption and diabetes mellitus incidence among US adults. *Prev. Med.* **32**: 33–39.
163. Maggio CA, Pi-Sunyer FX (1997) The prevention and treatment of obesity. Application to type 2 diabetes. *Diab. Care* **20**: 1744–1766.
164. Wannamethee SG, Shaper AG (1999) Weight change and duration of overweight and obesity in the incidence of type 2 diabetes. *Diab. Care* **22**: 1266–1272.
165. Walder K, Dascaliuc CR, Lewandowski PA, Sanigorski AJ, Zimmet P, Collier GR (1997) The effect of dietary energy restriction on body weight gain and the development of non-insulin-dependent diabetes mellitus (NIDDM) in Psammomys obesus. *Obes. Res.* **5**: 193–200.
166. Hansen BC, Bodkin NL (1990) Beta-cell hyper-responsiveness: earliest event in development of diabetes in monkeys. *Am. J. Physiol* **259**: R612–R617.
167. Hansen BC, Bodkin NL (1993) Primary prevention of diabetes mellitus by prevention of obesity in monkeys. *Diabetes* **42**: 1809–1814.
168. Bodkin NL, Ortmeyer HK, Hansen BC (1994) Longitudinal study of the insulin resistance trajectory preceding non-insulin-dependent diabetes mellitus in Rhesus monkeys (Abstract). *Diabetes* 43.
169. DeLany JP, Hansen BC, Bodkin NL, Hannah J, Bray GA (1999) Long-term calorie restriction reduces energy expenditure in aging monkeys. *J. Gerontol. A. Biol. Sci. Med. Sci.* **54**: B5–11.
170. Holbrook TL, Barrett-Connor E, Wingard DL (1989) The association of lifetime weight and weight control patterns with diabetes among men and women in an adult community. *Int. J. Obes.* **13**: 723–729.
171. Chan JM, Rimm EB, Colditz GA, Stampfer MJ, Willett WC (1994) Obesity, fat distribution, and weight gain as risk factors for clinical diabetes in men. *Diab. Care* **17**: 961–969.
172. Hanson RL, Narayan KMV, McCance DR, Pettitt DJ, Jacobsson LTH, Bennett PH, Knowler WC (1995) Rate of weight gain, weight fluctuation, and incidence of NIDDM. *Diabetes* **44**: 261–266.

173. Colditz GA, Willett WC, Rotnitzky A, Manson JE (1995) Weight gain as a risk factor for clinical diabetes mellitus in women. *Ann. Intern. Med* **122**: 481–486.

174. Ford ES, Williamson DF, Liu SM (1997) Weight change and diabetes incidence – findings from a national cohort of US adults. *Am. J. Epidemiol.* **146**: 214–222.

175. Noppa H (1980) Body weight change in relation to incidence of ischemic heart disease and change in risk factors for ischemic heart disease. *Am. J. Epidemiol.* **111**: 693–704.

176. Higgins M, D'Agostino R, Kannel W, Cobb J, Pinsky J (1993) Benefits and adverse effects of weight loss. Observations from the Framingham Study. *Ann. Intern. Med* **119**: 758–763.

177. Everson SA, Goldberg DE, Helmrich SP, Lakka TA, Lynch JW, Kaplan GA, Salonen JT (1998) Weight gain and the risk of developing insulin resistance syndrome. *Diab. Care* **21**: 1637–1643.

178. Oster G, Thompson D, Edelsberg J, Bird AP, Colditz GA (1999) Lifetime health and economic benefits of weight loss among obese persons. *Am. J. Public Health* **89**: 1536–1542.

179. Hu FB, Manson JE, Stampfer M, Colditz G, Liu S, Solomon CG, Willett WC (2001) Diet, lifestyle, and the risk of type 2 diabetes mellitus in women. *N.E.J.M.* **345**: 790–797.

180. Fuller JH (1983) Clinical trials in diabetes mellitus. In *Diabetes in Epidemiological Perspective* (eds Mann JI, Pyorala K, Teuscher A) Edinburgh: Churchill Livingstone, pp. 265–285.

181. Melander A, Bitzen PO, Sartor G, Schersten B, Wahlin-Boll E (1990) Will sulfonylurea treatment of impaired glucose tolerance delay development and complications of NIDDM? *Diab. Care* **13** (Suppl 3): 53–58.

182. Charles MA, Eschwege E (1999) Prevention of type 2 diabetes: role of metformin. Drugs

183. Belknap BH, Bagdade JD, Amaral JAP, Bierman EL (1967) Plasma lipids and mild glucose tolerance. A double-blind study of the effect of tolbutamide and placebo in mild adult diabetic outpatients. *Excerpta Med. Int. Congr. Ser.* **149**: 171–176.

184. Engelhardt HT, Vecchio TJ (1965) The long-term effect of tolbutamide on glucose tolerance in adults, asymptomatic, latent diabetes. *Metabolism* **14**: 885–890.

185. Camerini-Davalos RA (1967) Treatment of 'chemical' diabetes. Excerpta *Med. Int. Congr. Ser.* **149**: 228–242.

186. Paasikivi J (1970) Long-term tolbutamide treatment after myocardial infarction. *Acta Med. Scand.* (Suppl. 507:

187. Feldman R, Fitterer D (1967) The prophylactic use of oral hypoglycemic drugs in asymptomatic diabetes. *Excerpta Med. Int. Congr. Ser.* **149**: 243.

188. Feldman R, Crawford D, Elashoff R, Glass A (1973) Progress report on the prophylatic use of oral hypoglycemic drugs in asymptomatic diabetes: neurovascular studies. *Adv. Metab. Dis.* 2(Suppl. 2): 557–567.

189. Fajans SS, Conn JW (1954) An approach to the prediction of diabetes mellitus by modification of the glucose tolerance test with cortisone. *Diabetes* **3**: 296.

190. Keen H, Jarrett RJ, Fuller JH (1973) Tolbutamide and arterial disease in borderline diabetics. *Excerpta Med. Int. Congr. Ser.* **312**: 588–602.

191. University Group Diabetes Program (1976): A study of the effects of hypoglycemic agents on vascular complications in patients with adult-onset diabetes. *Diabetes* **25**: 1129–1153.

192. Keen H, Jarrett RJ, Chlouverakis C, Boyns DR (1968) The effect of treatment of moderate hyperglycemia on the incidence of arterial disease. *Postgrad. Med .J.* **44**: 960–965.

193. Keen H, Jarrett RJ, Ward JD, Fuller JH (1973) Borderline diabetics and their response to Tolbutamide. *Adv. Metab. Dis.* **2**(Suppl. 2): 521–531.
194. Keen H, Jarrett RJ, McCartney P (1982) The ten-year follow-up of the Bedford Survey (1962–1972): Glucose tolerance and diabetes. *Diabetologia* **2**: 73–78.
195. Tan MH, Graham CA, Bradley RF, Gleason RE, Soeldner JS (1977) The effects of long-term therapy with oral hypoglycemic agents on the oral glucose tolerance test dynamics in male chemical diabetics. *Diabetes* **26**: 561–570.
196. Sartor G, Schersten B, Carlstrom S, Melander A, Norden A, Persson G (1980) Ten-year follow-up of subjects with impaired glucose tolerance. Prevention of diabetes by tolbutamide and diet regulation. *Diabetes* **29**: 41–49.
197. Knowler WC, Sartor G, Melander A, Schersten B (1997) Glucose tolerance and mortality, including a substudy of tolbutamide treatment. *Diabetologia* **40**: 680–686.
198. University Group Diabetes Program (1970) A study of the effects of hypoglycemic agents on vascular complications in patient with adult-onset diabetes. II. Mortality results. *Diabetes* **19**: 789–830.
199. Karunakaran S, Hammersley MS, Morris RJ, Turner RC, Holman RR (1997) The Fasting Hyperglycaemia Study: III. Randomized controlled trial of sulfonylurea therapy in subjects with increased but not diabetic fasting plasma glucose. *Metabolism* **46**: 56–60.
200. Holman RR, North BV, Tunbridge FKE: Possible prevention of type 2 diabetes with acarbose or metformin (Abstract). *Diabetes* **49**: (Suppl. 1): A111; 200.
201. Ratzmann KP, Witt S, Schulz B (1983) The effect of long-term glibenclamide treatment on glucose tolerance, insulin secretion and serum lipids in subjects with impaired glucose tolerance. *Diab. Metab.* **9**: 87–93.
202. Papoz L, Job D, Eschwege E, Aboulker JP, Cubeau J, Pequignot G, Rathery M, Rosselin G (1978) Effect of oral hypoglycemic drugs on glucose tolerance and insulin secretion in borderline diabetic patients. *Diabetologia* 15: 373–380.
203. Stowers JM (1973) Treatment of chemical diabetes with chlorpropamide and the associated mortality. *Adv. Metab. Dis.* **2**(Suppl. 2): 549–555.
204. Jarrett RJ, Keen H, Fuller JH, McCartney M (1979) Worsening to diabetes in men with impaired glucose intolerance ('borderline diabetes'). *Diabetologia* **16**: 25–30.
205. Jarrett RJ, Keen H, Fuller JH, McCartney M (1977) Treatment of borderline diabetes: controlled trial using carbohydrate restriction and phenformin. *Brit. Med. J.* **2**: 861–865.
206. Kasperska-Czyzykowa T, Jaskolska K, Galecki A, Trzcaski M, Woy-Wojciechowski J (1986) Effect of biguanide derivatives (phenformin) on carbohydrate tolerance in 'borderline' and asymptomatic ('chemical') diabetes. Results of a five-year prospective study. *Acta Med. Pol.* **27**: 141–152.
207. Fontbonne A, Andre P, Eschwege E (1991) BIGPRO (biguanides and the prevention of the risk of obesity): study design. A randomized trial of metformin versus placebo in the correction of the metabolic abnormalities associated with insulin resistance. *Diab. Metab.* **17**: 249–254.
208. Fontbonne A, Charles MA, Juhanvague I, Bard JM, Andre P, Isnard F, Cohen JM, Grandmottet P, Vague P, Safar ME, Eschwege E (1996) The effect of metformin on the metabolic abnormalities associated with upper-body fat distribution. *Diab. Care* **19**: 920–926.
209. Charles MA, Morange P, Eschwege E, Andre P, Vague P, Juhan-Vague I (1998) Effect of weight change and metformin on fibrinolysis and the von Willebrand

factor in obese nondiabetic subjects: the BIGPRO1 Study. Biguanides and the Prevention of the Risk of Obesity. *Diab. Care* **21**: 1967–1972.

210. Charles MA, Eschwege E and the BIGPRO Study Group (1999) Metformin and the treatment of the insulin resistance syndrome. The BIGPRO studies. In *Proceedings of the 7th European Symposium on Metabolism* (eds Crepaldi G, Tiengo A, DelPrato S) Padova, Italy. Amsterdam: Elsevier pp. 237–242.

211. Charles MA, Eschwege E, Grandmottet P, Isnard F, Cohen JM, Bensoussan JL, Berche H, Chapiro O, Andre P, Vague P, Juhan-Vague I, Bard J-M, Safar M (2000) Treatment with metformin of non-diabetic men with hypertension and hypertriglyceridaemia and central fat distribution. The BIGPRO 1.2 Trial. *Diab. Metab.* 16

212. Li CL, Pan CY, Lu JM, Zhu Y, Wang JH, Deng XX, Xia FC, Wang HZ, Wang HY (1999) Effect of metformin on patients with impaired glucose tolerance. *Diab. Med.* **16**: 477–481.

213. Giugliano D, De Rosa N, Di Maro G, Marfella R, Acampora R, Buoninconti R, D'Onofrio F (1993) Metformin improves glucose, lipid metabolism, and reduces blood pressure in hypertensive, obese women. *Diab. Care* **16**: 1387–1390.

214. Landin K, Tengborn L, Smith U (1991) Treating insulin resistance in hypertension with metformin reduces both blood pressure and metabolic risk factors. *J. Intern. Med.* **229**: 181–187.

215. Bressler R, Johnson DG (1997) Pharmacological regulation of blood glucose levels in non- insulin-dependent diabetes mellitus. *Arch. Intern. Med.* **157**: 836–848.

216. Nolan JJ, Ludvik B, Beerdsen P, Joyce M, Olefsky J (1994) Improvement in glucose tolerance and insulin resistance in obese subjects treated with troglitazone. *N.E.J.M.* **331**: 1188–1193.

217. Antonucci T, Whitcomb R, Norris RM, McLain R, Lockwood D (1997) Impaired glucose tolerance is normalized by treatment with the thiazolidinedione troglitazone. *Diab. Care* **20**: 188–193.

218. Berkowitz K, Peters R, Kjos SL, Goico J, Marroquin A, Dunn ME, Xiang, A, Azen S, Buchanan TA (1996) Effect of troglitazone on insulin sensitivity and pancreatic beta-cell function in women at high risk for NIDDM. *Diabetes* **45**: 1572–1579.

219. Azen SP, Peters RK, Berkowitz K, Kjos S , Xiang A, Buchanan TA (1998) TRIPOD (TRoglitazone In the Prevention Of Diabetes): a randomized, placebo-controlled trial of troglitazone in women with prior gestational diabetes mellitus. *Control. Clin. Trials.* **19**: 217–231.

220. Buchanan TA, Xiang A, Peters RK, Kjos SL, Marroquin A, Goico J, Ochoa C, Tan S, Azen SP (2001) Protection from type 2 diabetes persists in the TRIPOD cohort eight months after stopping troglitazone (Abstract). *Diabetes* **50 (Suppl 2)**: A81.

221. Cavaghan MK, Ehrmann DA, Byrne MM, Polonsky KS (1997) Treatment with the oral antidiabetic agent troglitazone improves beta cell responses to glucose in subjects with impaired glucose tolerance. *J. Clin. Invest.* **100**: 530–537.

222. Chiasson JL, Josse RG, Leiter LA, Mihic M, Nathan DM, Palmason C, Cohen RM, Wolever TMS (1996) The effect of acarbose on insulin sensitivity in subjects with impaired glucose tolerance. *Diab. Care* **19**: 1190–1193.

223. Chiasson JL, Gomis R, Hanefeld M, Josse RG, Karasik A, Laakso M (1998) The STOP-NIDDM Trial: an international study on the efficacy of an alpha-glucosidase inhibitor to prevent type 2 diabetes in a population with impaired glucose tolerance: rationale, design, and preliminary screening data. Study to Prevent Non-Insulin-Dependent Diabetes Mellitus. *Diab. Care* **21**: 1720–1725.

224. Hansson L, Lindholm LH, Niskanen L, Lanke J, Hedner T, Niklason A, Luomanmaki K, Dahlof B, deFaire U, Morlin C, Karlberg BE, Wester PO, Bjorck J-E, (for the Captopril Prevention Project (CAPPP) study group) (1999) Effect of angiotensin-converting-enzyme inhibition compared with conventional therapy on cardiovascular morbidity and mortality in hypertension: the Captopril Prevention Project (CAPPP) randomized trial. *Lancet* **353**: 611–616.

225. The Heart Outcomes Prevention Evaluation Study Investigators (2000) Effects of an angiotensin-converting-enzyme inhibitor, ramipril, on cardiovascular events in high-risk patients. *N. Engl. J. Med.* **342**: 145–153.

226. Hansson L, Lindholm LH, Ekbom T, Dahlof B, Lanke J, Schersten B, Wester PO, Hedner T, de Faire U (1999) Randomised trial of old and new antihypertensive drugs in elderly patients: cardiovascular mortality and morbidity in the Swedish Trial in Old Patients with Hypertension-2 study. *Lancet* **354**: 1751–1756.

227. Anderson RA (1997) Nutritional factors influencing the glucose/insulin system: chromium. *J. Am. Coll. Nutr.* **16**: 404–410.

228. Mertz W (1993) Chromium in human nutrition: a review. *J. Nutr.* **123**: 626–633.

229. Davies S, McLaren Howard J, Hunnisett A, Howard M (1997) Age-related decreases in chromium levels in 51 665 hair, sweat, and serum samples from 40 872 patients – implications for the prevention of cardiovascular disease and type II diabetes mellitus. *Metabolism* **46**: 469–473.

230. Thomas VL, Gropper SS (1996) Effect of chromium nicotinic acid supplementation on selected cardiovascular disease risk factors. *Biol. Trace Elem. Res.* **55**: 297–305.

231. Abraham AS, Brooks BA, Eylath U (1992) The effects of chromium supplementation on serum glucose and lipids in patients with and without non-insulin-dependent diabetes. *Metabolism* **41**: 768–771.

232. Uusitupa MI, Mykkanen L, Siitonen O, Laakso M, Sarlund H, Kolehmainen P, Rasanen T, Kumpulainen J, Pyorala K (1992) Chromium supplementation in impaired glucose tolerance of elderly: effects on blood glucose, plasma insulin, C-peptide and lipid levels. *Br. J. Nutr.* **68**: 209–216.

233. Shoff SM, Mares-Perlman JA, Cruickshanks KJ, Klein R, Klein BE, Ritter LL (1993) Glycosylated hemoglobin concentrations and vitamin E, vitamin C, and beta-carotene intake in diabetic and nondiabetic older adults. *Am. J. Clin. Nutr.* **58**: 412–416.

234. Sargeant LA, Wareham NJ, Bingham S, Day NE, Luben RN, Oakes S, Welch A, Khaw KT (2000) Vitamin C and hyperglycemia in the European Prospective Investigation into Cancer–Norfolk (EPIC-Norfolk) study: a population-based study. *Diab. Care* **23**: 726–732.

235. Salonen JT, Nyyssonen K, Tuomainen TP, Maenpaa PH, Korpela H, Kaplan GA, Lynch J, Helmrich SP, Salonen R (1995) Increased risk of non-insulin-dependent diabetes mellitus at low plasma vitamin E concentrations: a four-year follow-up study in men. *BMJ.* **311**: 1124–1127.

236. Paolisso G, D'Amore A, Giugliano D, Ceriello A, Varricchio M, D'Onofrio F (1993) Pharmacologic doses of vitamin E improve insulin action in healthy subjects and non-insulin-dependent diabetic patients. *Am. J. Clin. Nutr.* **57**: 650–656.

237. Yusuf S, Dagenais G, Pogue J, Bosch J, Sleight P (2000) Vitamin E supplementation and cardiovascular events in high-risk patients. The Heart Outcomes Prevention Evaluation (HOPE) Study Investigators. *N. Engl. J. Med* **342**: 154–160.

238. Liu S, Ajani U, Chae C, Hennekens C, Buring JE, Manson JE (1999) Long-term ß-carotene supplementation and risk of type 2 diabetes mellitus. *J.A.M.A* **282**: 1073–1075.
239. Ford ES (2001) Vitamin supplement use and diabetes mellitus incidence among adults in the United States. Amer. J. Epidemiol. 153: 892-897, 2001
240. Steinberg D (1995): Clinical trials of antioxidants in atherosclerosis: are we doing the right thing? *Lancet* **346**: 36–38.
241. Freeman DJ, Norrie J, Sattar N, Neely RD, Cobbe SM, Ford I, Isles C, Lorimer AR, Macfarlane PW, McKillop JH, Packard CJ, Shepherd J, Gaw A (2001) Pravastatin and the development of diabetes mellitus: evidence for a protective treatment effect in the west of Scotland Coronary Prevention Study. *Circulation* **103**: 357–362.
242. Lind L, Lithell H, Hvarfner A, Ljunghall S (1990) Indices of mineral metabolism in subjects with an impaired glucose tolerance. *Exp. Clin. Endocrinol*. **96**: 109–112.
243. Manolio TA, Savage PJ, Burke GL, Hilner JE, Liu K, Orchard TJ, Sidney S, Oberman A (1991) Correlates of fasting insulin levels in young adults: the CARDIA study. *J. Clin. Epidemiol* **44**: 571–578.
244. Ma J, Folsom AR, Melnick SL, Eckfeldt JH, Sharrett AR, Nabulsi AA, Hutchinson RG, Metcalf PA (1995) Associations of serum and dietary magnesium with cardiovascular disease, hypertension, diabetes, insulin, and carotid arterial wall thickness: the ARIC study. Atherosclerosis Risk in Communities Study. *J. Clin. Epidemiol*. **48**: 927–940.
245. de Valk HW (1999) Magnesium in diabetes mellitus. *Neth. J. Med*. **54**: 139–146.
246. Boucher BJ (1998) Inadequate vitamin D status: does it contribute to the disorders comprising syndrome 'X'? *Br. J. Nutr*. **79**: 315–327.
247. Manson JE, Ajani UA, Liu S, Nathan DM, Hennekens CH (2000) A prospective study of cigarette smoking and the incidence of diabetes mellitus among US male physicians. *Am. J. Med*. **109**: 538–542.
248. Rimm EB, Manson JE, Stampfer MJ, Colditz GA, Willett WC, Rosner B, Hennekens CH, Speizer FE (1993) Cigarette smoking and the risk of diabetes in women. *Am. J. Public Health* **83**: 211–214.
249. Rimm EB, Chan J, Stampfer MJ, Colditz GA, Willett WC (1995) Prospective study of cigarette smoking, alcohol use, and the risk of diabetes in men. *BMJ* **310**: 555–559.
250. Kawakami N, Takatsuka N, Shimizu H, Ishibashi H (1997) Effects of smoking on the incidence of non-insulin-dependent diabetes mellitus – replication and extension in a Japanese cohort of male employees. *Am. J. Epidemiol*. **145**: 103–109.
251. Uchimoto S, Tsumura K, Hayashi T, Suematsu C, Endo G, Fujii S, Okada K (1999) Impact of cigarette smoking on the incidence of type 2 diabetes mellitus in middle-aged Japanese men: the Osaka Health Survey. *Diabet. Med* **16**: 951–955.
252. Wilson PW, Anderson KM, Kannel WB (1986) Epidemiology of diabetes mellitus in the elderly. The Framingham Study. *Am. J. Med*. **80**: 3–9.
253. Colsher PL, Wallace RB (1989) Is modest alcohol consumption better than none at all? An epidemiologic assessment. *Annu. Rev. Public Health* **10**: 203–219.
254. Ajani UA, Hennekens CH, Spelsberg A, Manson JE (2000) Alcohol consumption and risk of type 2 diabetes mellitus among US male physicians. *Arch. Intern. Med* **160**: 1025–1030.
255. Stampfer MJ, Colditz GA, Willett WC, Manson JE, Arky RA, Hennekens CH, Speizer FE (1988) A prospective study of moderate alcohol drinking and risk of diabetes in women. *Am. J. Epidemiol*. **128**: 549–558.

256. Balkau B, Eschwege E, Ducimetiere P, Richard JL, Warnet JM (1991) The high risk of death by alcohol related diseases in subjects diagnosed as diabetic and impaired glucose tolerance: the Paris Prospective Study after 15 years of follow-up. *J. Clin. Epidemiol.* **44**: 465–474.

257. Holbrook TL, Barrett-Connor E, Wingard DL (1990) A prospective population-based study of alcohol use and non-insulin-dependent diabetes mellitus. *Am. J. Epidemiol.* **132**: 902–909.

258. Kao WH, Puddey IB, Boland LL, Watson RL, Brancati FL (2001) Alcohol consumption and the risk of type 2 diabetes mellitus: Atherosclerosis Risk In Communities Study. *Am. J. Epidemiol.* **154**: 748–757.

259. Gastrointestinal surgery for severe obesity: NIH Consensus Development Conference Statement 1991 March 25-27. *Am. J. Clin. Nutr.* **55**: 615S–619S. 1992

260. Long SD, O'Brien K, MacDonald KG, Leggett-Frazier N, Swanson MS, Pories WJ, Caro JF (1994) Weight loss in severely obese subjects prevents the progression of impaired glucose tolerance to type II diabetes: A longitudinal intervention study. *Diab. Care* **17**: 372–375.

261. Sjostrom CD, Lissner L, Wedel H, Sjostrom L (1999) Reduction in incidence of diabetes, hypertension and lipid disturbances after intentional weight loss induced by bariatric surgery: the SOS Intervention Study. *Obes. Res.* **7**: 477–484.

262. Stern MP (1995) The case for randomized clinical trials on the treatment of obesity. *Obes. Res.* **3**(Suppl. 2): 299s–306s.

263. Williamson DF (1996) Dietary intake and physical activity as 'predictors' of weight gain in observational, prospective studies of adults. *Nutr. Rev.* **54**: S101–S109.

264. Williamson DF (1999) The prevention of obesity. *N. Engl. J. Med* **341**: 1140–1141.

265. Taylor CB, Fortmann SP, Flora J, Kayman S, Barrett DC, Jatulis D, Farquhar JW (1991) Effect of long-term community health education on body mass index. The Stanford Five-City Project. *Am. J. Epidemiol.* **134**: 235–249.

266. Jeffery RW (1995) Community programs for obesity prevention: the Minnesota Heart Health Program. *Obes. Res.* **3 (Suppl 2)**: 283s–288s.

267. Cambien F, Richard JL, Ducimetiere P, Warnet JM, Kahn J (1981) The Paris Cardiovascular Risk Factor Prevention Trial. Effects of two years of intervention in a population of young men. *J. Epidemiol. Community Health* **35**: 91-97.

268. Stevens VJ, Corrigan SA, Obarzanek E, Bernauer E, Cook NR, Hebert P, Mattfeldt-Beman M, Oberman A, Sugars C, Dalcin AT (1993) Weight loss intervention in phase 1 of the Trials of Hypertension Prevention. The TOHP Collaborative Research Group. *Arch. Intern. Med.* **153**: 849–858.

269. Cutler JA (1991) Randomized clinical trials of weight reduction in nonhypertensive persons. *Ann. Epidemiol.* **1**: 363–370.

270. Elmer PJ, Grimm R Jr., Laing B, Grandits G, Svendsen K, Van Heel N, Betz E, Raines J, Link M, Stamler J (1995) Lifestyle intervention: results of the Treatment of Mild Hypertension Study (TOMHS). *Prev. Med.* **24**: 378–388.

271. Melander A, Vaaler S, Lindblad U, Lindberg G (1999) The Nepi Antidiabetes Study (NANSY). Prevention of type 2 diabetes. Malmö, Sweden, NEPI Institute.

272. Nateglinide for type 2 diabetes. *Medical Letter on Drugs & Therapeutics* **43**: 29–30. 2001

273. Thurmann PA (2000) Valsartan: a novel angiotensin type 1 receptor antagonist. *Expert Opin. Pharmacother.* **1**: 337–350.

274. Mokdad AH, Serdula MK, Dietz WH, Bowman BA, Marks JS, Koplan JP (1999) The spread of the obesity epidemic in the United States. *J.A.M.A* **282**: 1519–1522.

275. Mokdad AH, Bowman BA, Ford ES, Vinicor F, Marks JS, Koplan JP (2001_ The continuing epidemics of obesity and diabetes in the United States. *J.A.M.A.* **286**: 1195–1200.
276. Hill JO, Peters JC (1998) Environmental contributions to the obesity epidemic. *Science* **280**: 1371–1374.
277. Koplan JP, Dietz WH (1999) Caloric imbalance and public health policy . *J.A.M.A* **282**: 1579–1581.
278. Vinicor F (1998) The public health burden of diabetes and the reality of limits. *Diab. Care* **21**: C15–C18.
279. Glasgow RE, Wagner EH, Kaplan RM, Vinicor F, Smith L, Norman J (1999) If diabetes is a public health problem, why not treat it as one? A population-based approach to chronic illness. *Ann. Behav. Med.* **21**: 159–170.
280. Dyson PA, Hammersley MS, Morris RJ, Holman RR, Turner RC (1997) The Fasting Hyperglycaemia Study: II. Randomized controlled trial of reinforced healthy-living advice in subjects with increased but not diabetic fasting plasma glucose. *Metabolism* **46**: 50–55.
281. Page RCL, Harnden KE, Walravens NK, Onslow C, Sutton P, Levy JC, Hockaday DT, Turner RC (1993) 'Healthy living' and sulphonylurea therapy have different effects on glucose tolerance and risk factors for vascular disease in subjects with impaired glucose tolerance. *Q. J. Med.* **86**: 145–154.

7

Missed and Newly Recovered Potential for the Prevention of Type 2 Diabetes: A Commentary

JAAKKO TUOMILEHTO
University of Helsinki, 00300 Helsinki, Finland

MISSED OPPORTUNITY

It is difficult to understand, and for the medical community to explain, why primary prevention of type 2 diabetes did not receive more attention before the 1990s. In fact, Dr E. Joslin was encouraging the primary prevention of type 2 diabetes in the early 1900s[1]. The literature between 1922 and 1979 hardly mentions this matter. Yet, during this period multiple applications of primary prevention of cardiovascular diseases (CVD) and cancer were successfully developed[2–8], although these diseases emerged much later than diabetes. Why did primary prevention of type 2 diabetes not begin in the early 1900s as Dr Joslin had argued? Reviewing the papers related to diabetes published in medical journals over the last decades illustrates the reasons for this; other matters around diabetes were receiving more attention. The massive review work done in Chapter 6 by Professor Hamman gives useful insights into this dilemma. On the other hand, the scope of diabetes research in general provides further understanding for this unfortunate and unbalanced development in medical history.

LACK OF KNOWLEDGE AT THE POPULATION LEVEL

The reason was not that the medical community did not know about the growing problem of diabetes, since Dr Joslin, in the early 1920s, had been

The Evidence Base for Diabetes Care. Edited by R. Williams, W. Herman, A.-L. Kinmonth and N. J. Wareham.
© 2002 John Wiley & Sons, Ltd

alerted to its growing prevalence. The first population-based survey of diabetes in the community was carried out in Oxford, MA, USA and published in 1947[9] by Dr L Krall, who later became the head of the Joslin Diabetes Clinic. Also at that time the first proper epidemiological studies of CVD and cancer were initiated. Nevertheless, epidemiological research into diabetes developed much more slowly than research into CVD and cancer until the 1980s.

One reason for this disproportionate development in epidemiological research between these chronic diseases might be the improvement in mortality statistics. Since acute CVD events and many types of cancer are often fatal, and their contribution to morbidity could be identified by history or autopsy, they were attractive targets for epidemiologic research. Type 2 diabetes, however, is seldom the immediate cause of death, and its contribution to an individual's death may be difficult to define. Thus, other methods than mortality studies are required to reveal the epidemiology of type 2 diabetes and to estimate its public health impact[10]. Since epidemiology should be regarded as the science of public health, it is not hard to conclude that the lack of comprehensive epidemiological data on diabetes has limited public health applications related to diabetes, such as primary prevention. Still, at the start of the twenty-first century, no country worldwide has outlined a strategy for prevention of type 2 diabetes. Yet the disease has been known and described for a very long time.

THE TREATMENT OF DIABETES

Soon after Dr Joslin wrote his strong recommendations stressing the import- • ance of the primary prevention of diabetes, insulin was discovered. Diabetic patients could be treated and their fate could be changed, particularly in type 1 diabetic patients. What about type 2 diabetes? Until the late 1950s, insulin was the only drug therapy available for type 2 diabetic patients. The good results of insulin therapy are certainly among the best in the history of medicine, dramatically decreasing mortality from acute complications of diabetes. There was a lengthy period in the diabetes field dealing with insulin therapy when hopes were raised that the 'cure for diabetes' had been found.

The development and introduction of oral antidiabetic drugs raised similar hopes. Why should people worry about diabetes or talk about its prevention when 'easy' treatment was available? This is seen in the paper from C. Best's group in 1940 (the next paper after Joslin's 1921 paper with the words 'prevention of diabetes' in the title) suggesting that early insulin therapy could also be a solution for the prevention of diabetes[11]. More than 40 years later US investigators tested this hypothesis in the Diabetes Prevention Trial – 1 and concluded that this 'preventive treatment' was inefficient (Skyler J, personal communication (2001), ADA Scientific Sessions, Philadelphia, PA, USA).

Meanwhile, in the 1970s a number of small trials attempted to determine whether diabetes could be prevented in people with milder elevation of blood glucose. These studies in many ways do not meet the current criteria of controlled clinical trials and may thus be considered uninformative. From the public health perspective they are, however, very informative. These first attempts at primary prevention of type 2 diabetes used mainly pharmacological interventions rather than trying to reduce the disease burden by interventions lowering the risk factors for the disease, a strategy that was used in preventive studies against CVD and cancer. Also, target populations were not selected because they had risk factors for diabetes, but for their glucose level alone. Up to now it has been argued that different diseases require specific treatments and preventative actions. However, when dealing with multifactorial chronic diseases it is not possible to use such a single-target approach but instead is necessary to intervene with multiple methods, since these diseases are developed due to multiple exposures. Good recent examples of failures to prevent CVD and cancer are antioxidant vitamin supplementation trials[12], while epidemiological evidence convincingly shows that foods rich in such elements are associated with reduced mortality and morbidity[13].

DIFFICULTIES IN DIAGNOSING DIABETES AND IN DEFINING HYPERGLYCEMIA

Diabetes is defined as hyperglycaemia exceeding a certain level of blood glucose. Only after the beta-cell function has been reduced significantly, (usually by approximately 50%), do people get the typical symptoms of diabetes. Scientists who started to carry out more extensive epidemiological research, particularly Dr K. West, realised in the 1970s that there were no unequivocal criteria used to diagnose diabetes[14]. This led to the development of the first standard diagnostic criteria for diabetes by the US National Diabetes Data Group in 1979[15] and by the WHO Expert Committee in 1980[16], which were slightly refined in 1985[17]. Small adjustments were made to these previous recommendations by the ADA Expert Committee in 1997[18] and the WHO Consultation Group in 1999[19], but the main previous principles were retained.

Two main factors that formed the basis of the diagnostic criteria for type 2 diabetes in all these recommendations were: (1) glucose levels and (2) the prevalence of retinopathy. No other outcome, particularly macrovascular disease, was used to define the level of hyperglycaemia that would require medical attention. This is in a strong contrast to practices with high blood pressure and dyslipidemia[20–23] where the recommended cut-points are defined according to the probability of the most important and severe outcomes such as myocardial infarction or stroke. The argument that these outcomes are due to multiple risk factors, not just hyperglycaemia, is illogical, since these diseases cause the majority of deaths among diabetic patients.

This 'glucocentric' attitude has probably prevented a more comprehensive look at the public health aspects of type 2 diabetes. Today, in developed countries the vast majority (>70%) of health care resources for diabetic patients with type 2 diabetes are used for the treatment of macrovascular complications. The only cost-effective way to cut these costs, which make up over 10% of total health budgets, would be to prevent or postpone the rise in blood glucose levels for as long as possible. In the past, with lower prevalence of obesity and more physical activity, it was possible to treat glucose levels even in people with a high predisposition to type 2 diabetes.

ECOLOGICAL FALLACY OR ECOLOGICAL REALITY?

Ecological fallacy is usually defined as a problem occurring when a correlation between the exposure variable (e.g. obesity) and the outcome (e.g. diabetes) is studied in several populations, and conclusions are drawn from differences in outcomes between populations. 'Ecological fallacy' means that some other unmeasured genetic or environmental factor between populations is responsible for the differences observed. In the past it was difficult in most populations to find an association between type 2 diabetes and obesity or physical inactivity since these risk factors were not particularly common in young and middle-aged populations. Thus, a 'reverse ecological fallacy' was contemplated, arguing that in many populations diabetic people are not necessarily obese and physically inactive. While this observation was indeed true, the point was missed: to investigate the effect of environmental risk factors on disease development in a population, there must be a sufficient range of variation in the exposure variable. The lack of prospective studies with proper environmental exposure assessments was one of the main problems faced when trying to provide consistent and sufficiently clear evidence of the importance of these factors in the development of type 2 diabetes.

Even today, it is obvious that in many Asian populations obesity cannot be the only and the most important risk factor since most diabetic patients are not obese[24]. Yet, in these populations the avoidance of obesity has been and is likely to be the primary factor in preventing diabetes or postponing the onset of clinical disease. In this way, it is possible to prevent the onset of diabetic complications long enough for them to no longer be an issue during most of active life.

GENETIC FACTORS

It has been known for decades, even for centuries, that diabetes has a strong familial component[25,26]. It is therefore obvious that children of parents with type 2 diabetes are at a higher risk of the disease. In the past, however, predictions based on family history had been troubled by the facts that: (1)

only about half of the offspring of diabetic subjects inherit the same susceptibility genes; (2) the 'penetrance' of the genes is not complete, and is largely determined by environmental factors: people were lean and physically active and thus avoided diabetes even though they may have carried the genes for diabetes; (3) survival was much lower due to the prevalence of many diseases and other events such as wars, etc. and thus they did not reach the age needed to show clinical signs of the disease; (4) the diagnosis of diabetes was done post-mortem in asymptomatic patients and the diagnosis of symptomatic diabetes might also have been missed in the past. Therefore, due to the high probability of false-negative family history, it has not been a very sensitive indicator of the risk of diabetes. Nevertheless, when we look at the importance of family history from the prevention perspective, positive evidence for a family history of type 2 diabetes in first-degree relatives is always an indication for at least 50% to have inherited the genetic predisposition to diabetes.

Since type 2 diabetes may only develop in people who have a genetic predisposition to it, the presence of environmental risk factors such as obesity and physical inactivity in non-predisposed subjects has sometimes created misleading inferences and arguments that these factors may not be causal risk factors for diabetes. Only during the last few decades has the importance of gene–environmental interaction been understood properly. On the other hand, it is likely that the prevention and control of obesity and physical inactivity will result in other health benefits even in people who are not predisposed to diabetes, and will thus be useful from a public health point of view. To what extent genetic information is needed or useful to prevent type 2 diabetes is not known, but none of the current attempts have used genetics. Whether the recent successful trials in diabetes prevention have really prevented the disease or have simply postponed its clinical onset needs to be seen. One may argue that once the susceptibility genes are unequivocally known, with good genetic information the identification of genetically predisposed individuals will become possible and real primary prevention can be targeted to such people from very early on. On the other hand, positive family history will reveal such information anyway without information about specific genetic markers. Thus, in principle, we could now initiate this kind of targeted primary prevention, if such a strategy is considered appropriate

AT WHAT AGE ARE PREVENTIVE MEASURES NEEDED?

It has been well established that the development of a fetus in an abnormal intrauterine environment implies structural and functional adaptations with long-lasting consequences for the metabolism of the offspring in later life. A phenotype has been proposed in which inadequate fetal nutrition alters the development of glucose and insulin metabolism in adulthood[27]. Disproportionate size at birth is a fairly recently discovered risk factor for type 2 diabetes. The proposed biological mechanisms involve both pancreatic beta-cell dysfunction and insulin resistance, and therefore the effect is plausible, given the multiple observational studies and animal experiments that agree with this theory.

UK studies have originally shown that babies born with the lowest birth weights, i.e. <2.5 kg, were almost seven times more likely to have some degree of impairment in their glucose tolerance compared with heavier babies[28]. Similar findings have now been made globally in a variety of populations and ethic groups[29-31]. In keeping with the phenotype hypothesis are findings from twin studies; twins with type 2 diabetes had a lower birth weight[32] than the twins without type 2 diabetes. Monozygotic twins share the same genetic make-up, suggesting that the mechanism of the link between low birth weight and subsequent type 2 diabetes is environmental. This should not be interpreted as there being no role for genetics in the development of type 2 diabetes, but it certainly shows that the link between low birth weight and type 2 diabetes can occur independently of genetic influence.

The importance of exposure before birth on the lifetime occurrence of chronic diseases has recently been shown in many populations and for many diseases[32]. In the past, when infectious diseases were more common, it was evident that fetal and childhood health affected health in adult life. Now current observations also stress the importance of fetal life as a crucial period for the natural history of type 2 diabetes. The thrifty phenotype hypothesis suggests that the fetal nutritional environment has a programming effect on various physiological functions, including glucose and lipid metabolism and blood pressure[32]. It is the mismatch between a relatively poor intrauterine environment and a nutritionally rich environment in later life that increases the risk of diabetes and other diseases. Adaptation to lack of nutrition in utero may limit the extent of dietary change to which a generation can be exposed without adverse effects. Such individuals are more susceptible to type 2 diabetes if they catch up in weight and body mass index (BMI) during childhood, as shown by a recent Finnish study[31]. Since children born small and thin have proportionally less muscle mass, catch-up growth would mean a disproportionate increase in weight and fat mass in relation to lean body mass during early childhood. Therefore, prevention of obesity during childhood seems particularly important among children with low birth-weights.

THE PREVENTATIVE EFFECT OF LIFESTYLE CHANGES

THE FINNISH DIABETES PREVENTION STUDY (DPS)

The DPS was carried out between 1992–2000 in five clinics in different parts of Finland, aimed at preventing type 2 diabetes with lifestyle modification alone[33,34]. A total of 522 individuals at high risk of developing diabetes were recruited into the study, mainly by opportunistic screening for impaired glucose tolerance (IGT) in middle-aged (aged 40–64), overweight (BMI >25 kg/m^2) subjects. The presence of IGT was confirmed in two successive 75 g oral glucose tolerance tests; the mean of the two values had to be within the IGT range. From previous research it was estimated that the cumulative diabetes incidence in such a high-risk group would be approximately 35% in six years. The study subjects were randomly allocated either into the control group or the intensive intervention group. The subjects in the intervention group had frequent consultation visits with a nutritionist and received individual advice to reduce their weight and fat intake and increase their fibre intake. They were asked to increase everyday activity and were offered supervised, circuit-type exercise sessions aiming at increasing muscle mass, in addition to aerobic exercise. The control group subjects were also given general advice about healthy lifestyles during their annual visits to the study clinic. An oral glucose tolerance test was done annually and if diabetic values were found, a confirmatory OGTT was performed.

During the first year of the study, body weight decreased on average by 4.2 kg in the intervention group and by 0.8 kg in the control group subjects (p = 0.0001). Weight reduction was mostly maintained during the second year. Also, indicators of central adiposity and fasting glucose and insulin, 2 h post-challenge glucose and insulin, and HbA$_{1c}$ reduced significantly more in the intervention group than in the control group at both one- and two-year follow-up examinations. At these examinations, intervention group subjects reported significantly more beneficial changes in their dietary and exercise habits, based on diaries they had kept.

A total of 86 cases of diabetes were diagnosed among the 522 subjects randomised into the DPS trial with median follow-up duration of three years. Of these, 27 occurred in the intervention group and 59 in the control group. The cumulative incidence in the intervention group was 58% lower than in the control group (Figure 1).

The difference between the groups was statistically significant after only two years: 6% in the intervention group and 14% in the control group. After four years, the cumulative incidences were 11% and 23% respectively. The absolute risk of diabetes was 32/1000 person-years in the intervention group and 78/1000 person-years in the control group. In men, the incidence of diabetes was reduced by 63% in the intervention group compared with the control group, and in women by 54%.

According to these results, 22 people with IGT will need to be treated for one year or five people for five years with lifestyle intervention to prevent one case of diabetes. The public health implications of these results are far-reaching. The primary prevention of type 2 diabetes is possible by non-pharmacological intervention that can be implemented in the primary health

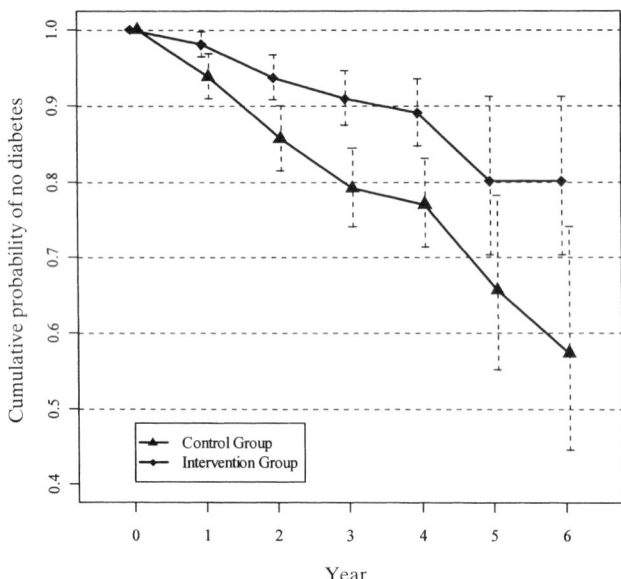

Figure 7.1. Development of diabetes in subjects with IGT at baseline during the lifestyle intervention trial by the randomisation group[34].

care setting. It is necessary for such an intervention to become a part of routine preventative care in order to reduce the burden of type 2 diabetes, which is reaching epidemic proportions in many countries. At the same time, it is also necessary to develop national programmes for the primary prevention of type 2 diabetes that include not only those at high risk but also the general population.

The US Diabetes Prevention Program (DPP) recently reported that the reduction in risk of diabetes in people with IGT was (58%) through reinforced lifestyle intervention as that in the Finnish study[35]. Thus, we now know that type 2 diabetes is preventable in high-risk subjects, and we also know the magnitude of the effect, at least from the perspective of a few years.

THE FUTURE

The primary prevention of type 2 diabetes should receive more attention than it has received in the past, even though the WHO Study Group recommended in 1994[36] that national diabetes prevention programmes should be set up. However, no country has yet initiated a prevention programme for type 2 diabetes. Why? The plethora of observational data demonstrate that lifestyle factors such as physical inactivity and obesity are increasing worldwide and that these trends have been accompanied by a steep increase in type 2 diabetes. These unfavourable lifestyle changes are no longer an issue only among adults but also among children and adolescents. As a consequence, the age at onset of type 2 diabetes has lowered, not only in ethnic groups but in many societies in both developed and developing countries. The main question now is, how should the available information be applied in public health practice?

The data from intervention studies obtained thus far in various settings have provided unequivocal evidence that the risk of type 2 diabetes in high-risk individuals can be reversed. It has worked in different societies, in different ethnic groups and age groups, and in both men and women. Thus, the evidence is now clearly sufficient to initiate intensive community-wide, even global action to prevent type 2 diabetes. The identification of high-risk subjects for type 2 diabetes is relatively easy; no biochemical or other costly tests are required, and most high-risk subjects are already regular customers of primary health care services. What is needed is a systematic approach to target lifestyle intervention at these individuals. This is not an easy task, but we know for instance from cardiovascular prevention programmes that such interventions are possible and efficient[37]. When these activities were initiated in the early 1970s, there was considerable debate over whether the prevention of cardiovascular disease was possible and whether lifestyle changes are possible. This debate is now history. From now on, such a debate will not be needed with regard to the prevention of type 2 diabetes. However, this step has been delayed by some 80 years and is long overdue.

REFERENCES

1. Joslin E (1921) The prevention of diabetes mellitus. *JAMA* **76**: 79–84.
2. Doll R (1967) *Prevention of Cancer. Pointers from Epidemiology*. Whitefriars Press: London.
3. Hakama M, Pukkala E (1977) Selective screening for cervical cancer. Experience of the Finnish mass screening system. *Br. J. Prev. Soc. Med.* **31**: 238–44.
4. Stamler J (1967) *Lectures on Preventive Cardiology*. Grune & Stratton: New York and London.
5. Anonymous (1970) Report of inter-society commission for heart disease resources: primary prevention of the atherosclerotic disease. *Circulation* **42**(Suppl.).
6. Farquhar JW (1978) The community-based model of lifestyle intervention trials. *Lancet* **i**: 1192–5.
7. Anonymous (1976) Prevention of coronary heart disease. Report of a joint working party of the Royal College of Physicians of London and the British Cardiac Society. J. Royal Coll. Physicians10.
8. Puska P, Tuomilehto J, Salonen J, Nissinen A, Virtamo J, Björkqvist S, Koskela K, Neittaanmäki L, Takalo T, Kottke T, Mäki J, Sipilä P, Varvikko P (1981) The North Karelia Project: community control of cardiovascular diseases. Evaluation of

a comprehensive community programme for control of cardiovascular diseases in North Karelia, Finland, 1972–1977. WHO/EURO Monograph: Copenhagen.

9. Wilkerson HLC, Krall LP (1947) Diabetes in a New England town: a study of 3516 persons in Oxford, Mass. *JAMA* **135**: 209–16.

10. Fuller J, Elford J, Goldblatt P, Adelstein AM (1983) Diabetes mortality: new light on an underestimated public health problem. *Diabetologia* **24**: 336–7.

11. Haist RE, Campbell J. Best CH (1940) The prevention of diabetes. *New Engl. J. Med.* **223**: 607–15.

12. The ATBC Cancer Prevention Study Group (1994) The effect of vitamin E and beta carotene on the incidence of lung cancer and other cancers in male smokers. *New Eng.l J. Med.* **330**: 1029–35.

13. National Research Council (1982) *Diet, Nutrition and Cancer*. National Academy Press: Washington D.C.

14. West K (1978) *Epidemiology of Diabetes and its Vascular Lesions*. New York: Elsevier.

15. National Diabetes Data Group (1979) Classification and diagnosis of diabetes mellitus and other categories of glucose intolerance. *Diabetes* **28**:1039–57.

16. WHO Expert Committee (1980) Diabetes Mellitus, Second Report. Technical Report Series No. 640. WHO: Geneva.

17. WHO Study Group (1985) Diabetes Mellitus. Technical Report Series No. 727. WHO: Geneva.

18. Expert Committee on the Diagnosis and Classification of Diabetes Mellitus (1997) Report of the Expert Committee on the Diagnosis and Classification of Diabetes Mellitus. *Diab. Care* **20**:1183–97.

19. WHO consultation (1999) Definition, Diagnosis and Classification of Diabetes Mellitus and its Complications. Report of a WHO Consultation. Part 1: Diagnosis and Classification of Diaebtes Mellitus. WHO/NCD/99.2. WHO: Geneva..

20. Expert Panel on Detection, Evaluation and Treatment of High Blood Cholesterol in Adults (2001) Executive Summary of the Third Report of the National Cholesterol Education Program (NCEP) Expert Panel on Detection, Evaluation, and Treatment of High Blood Cholesterol in Adults (Adult Treatment). *JAMA* **285**: 2486–94.

21. Guidelines Subcommittee (1999) World Health Organization – International Society of Hypertension Guidelines for the Management of Hypertension. *J. Hypertens.* **17**: 151–83.

22. Ramsay LE, Williams B, Johnston GD, MacGregor GA, Poston L, Poulter NR, Russell G (1999) Guidelines for management of hypertension: Report of the third working party of the British Hypertension Society. *J. Human Hypertens.* **13**: 569–92.

23. WHO Expert Committee. Community prevention and control of cardiovascular diseases. Technical Report Series No. 732. WHO: Geneva.

24. Qiao Q, Nakagami T, Tuomilehto J, Borch-Johnsen K, Balkau B, Iwamoto Y, Tajima N (for the DECODA Study Group on behalf of the International Diabetes Epidemiology Group) (2000) Comparison of the fasting and the 2-h glucose criteria for diabetes in different Asian cohorts. *Diabetologia* **43**: 1470–75.

25. Neel JV (1962) Diabetes mellitus: a 'thrifty' genotype rendered detrimental by progress? *Am. J. Human Genet.* **14**: 353–62.

26. Pyke D (1997) Preamble: the history of diabetes. In (eds Alberti KGMM, Zimmet P, DeFronzo RA) *International Textbook of Diabetes Mellitus*, 2nd edition. John Wiley & Sons: Chichester.

27. Hales C, Barker D (1992) Type 2 (non-insulin-dependent) diabetes mellitus: the thrifty phenotype hypothesis. *Diabetologia* **35**:595–601.

28. Hales C, Barker D, Clark P, Cox L, Fall C, Osmond C, Winter PD (1991) Fetal and infant growth and impaired glucose tolerance at age 64. *BMJ* **303**: 1019–22.

29. Lithell H, McKeigue P, Berglund L, Mohsen R, Lithell U, Leon D (1996) Relation of size at birth to non-insulin dependent diabetes and insulin concentrations in men aged 50–60 years. *BMJ* **312**: 406–10.

30. Rich-Edwards J, Colditz G, Stampfer M, Willett W, Gillman M, Hennekens C, Speizer F, Manson J (1999) Birthweight and the risk for type 2 diabetes mellitus in adult women. *Ann. Intern. Med.* **130**: 278–84.

31. Forsén T, Eriksson J, Tuomilehto J, Reunanen A, Osmond C, Barker D (2000) The fetal and childhood growth of persons who develop type 2 diabetes. *Ann. Intern. Med.* **133**: 176–82.

32. Barker D (1998) *Mothers, Babies, and Health in Later Life*. 2nd ed. Edinburgh: Churchill Livingstone.

33. Eriksson J, Lindström J, Valle T, Aunola S, Hämäläinen H, Ilanne-Parikka P, Keinänen-Kiukaanniemi S, Laakso M, Lauhkonen M, Lehto P, Lehtonen A, Louleranta A, Mannelin M, Martikkala V, Rastas M, Sundvall J, Turpeinen A, Viljanen T, Uusitupa M, Tuomilehto J on behalf of the Finnish Diabetes Prevention Study Group (1991) Prevention of type II diabetes in subjects with impaired glucose tolerance: the Diabetes Prevention Study (DPS) in Finland–Study design and one-year interim report on the feasibility of the lifestyle intervention programme. *Diabetologia* **42**: 793–801.

34. Tuomilehto J, Lindström J, Eriksson J, Valle T, Hämäläinen H, Ilanne-Parikka P, Keinanen-Kiukaanniemi S, Laakso M, Louheranta A, Rastas M, Salminen V, Aunola S, Cepaitis Z, Moltchanov V, Hakumaki M, Mannelin M, Martikkala V, Sundvall J, Uusitupa M, the Finnish Diabetes Prevention Study Group (2001) Prevention of type 2 diabetes mellitus by changes in lifestyle among subjects with impaired glucose tolerance. *N. Engl. J. Med.* **344**: 1343–1350.

35. The Diabetes Prevention Program Research Group (1999) The Diabetes Prevention Program. Design and methods for a clinical trial in the prevention of type 2 diabetes. *Diab. Care* **22**(4): 623–634.

36. WHO Study Group (1994) Primary Prevention of Diabetes Mellitus. Technical Report Series No. 844. WHO: Geneva.

37. Puska P, Tuomilehto J, Nissinen A, Vartiainen E (1995) The North Karelia Project. 20-year results and experiences. National Public Health Institute: Helsinki.

Part III

EARLY DETECTION, SCREENING AND CASE FINDING IN TYPE 2 DIABETES

8

The Evidence to Screen for Type 2 Diabetes Mellitus

MICHAEL M. ENGELGAU
K. M. VENKAT NARAYAN

Division of Diabetes Translation Mailstop K-10, Atlanta GA 30341-3724, USA

INTRODUCTION

In 1995, an estimated 135 million people worldwide had diabetes. By the year 2025 this figure is expected to be 300 million[1]. A complex disease that frequently has devastating consequences, diabetes is also an economic scourge around the world[2,3]. The epidemic level of diabetes has clearly established it as a major public health problem.

What role should screening for undiagnosed type 2 diabetes play in combating the worldwide diabetes epidemic? Because type 2 diabetes accounts for 90–95% of all diabetes cases, it represents the majority of the public health burden and is the form of the disease considered in this chapter[4–6]. At present, even though improved levels of care can clearly help delay the development of complications and prevent disability[7], the benefits of early detection of type 2 diabetes through screening are not clearly established[8–10]. Despite scant evidence for diabetes screening, several health organizations have already decided to recommend it[11–14]. Why might screening be recommended? First, the fact that undiagnosed diabetes is common and widespread has been demonstrated repeatedly; population-based surveys have found one-third to one-half of the total cases to be undiagnosed[1,15–21]. Second, numerous studies[22–28] have found diabetic complications to be common at clinical diagnosis. Existing recommendations, primarily based on expert opinion, perhaps, in part, reflect the clinical experience and frustration among health care providers at seeing newly diagnosed persons with established complications. Finally, even without data to support their arguments, some have contended that treatment of early disease improves health outcomes and saves resources[29].

The Evidence Base for Diabetes Care. Edited by R. Williams, W. Herman, A.-L. Kinmonth and N. J. Wareham.
© 2002 John Wiley & Sons, Ltd

Although detecting type 2 diabetes early might intuitively be expected to yield health benefits, the decision to screen should be based on the best available quantitative evidence[30]. Perhaps screening for diabetes and earlier exposure to treatment may potentially reduce the incidence of complications, require fewer resources, and improve quality of life. However, screening pitfalls such as biases in evaluation, side-effects of treatment, and other adverse consequences need consideration. The purpose of this chapter is to examine the evidence for type 2 diabetes screening.

HISTORICAL PERSPECTIVE

Some of the first organized diabetes screening activities were conducted in the USA among insurance applicants during the early 1900s[31]. Later, large scale diabetes screening was conducted among inductees into the armed services during World Wars I and II. The advent of automated glucose measurement techniques in the latter half of the twentieth century led to even more widespread screening activity in many communities, in workplaces, and at health fairs. Still, despite broad implementation, at that time, little was known or understood about what these efforts accomplished.

Although initial qualitative assessments of diabetes screening tests in the USA during the 1950s found high false positive and false negative rates and overall poor performance[31], it was not until the 1970s that evaluating diabetes screening efforts were considered[32]. In both that decade and in the 1980s, problems were noted with mass indiscriminate screening, and the value of such initiatives was questioned[33–38]. Two of the major issues raised were the criteria for a positive screening test and the need for standardized diagnostic criteria for diabetes. Diagnostic criteria were more firmly established in the early and mid-1980s[39,40]. In the late 1980s and early 1990s, following the widespread implementation of diagnostic criteria as well as reports from population-based studies that nearly half of all diabetes cases were undiagnosed, some organizations began to recommend screening.

PRINCIPLES OF TYPE 2 DIABETES SCREENING

There is a major distinction between screening and diagnostic testing for type 2 diabetes. Screening involves attempts to detect asymptomatic disease and screening tests differentiate those at high risk from those at low risk using a variety of methods (risk assessment questionnaires, capillary blood assessments, laboratory-based assessments, all with various thresholds or cut-points) that are typically rapid, simple and safe[10,41–43]. By contrast, when individuals exhibits symptoms or sign of disease, diagnostic tests are performed and such tests do not represent screening. Diagnostic tests using standard criteria[14] are required after screening tests to establish a diagnosis. Finally, once a diagnosis has been made from screening, treatment must provide additional benefit over starting treatment following routine clinical diagnosis.

From a public health perspective, is screening for type 2 diabetes appropriate? A good way to answer this question is to consider responses to seven queries[10,41-52]: (1) Does diabetes represent an important health problem imposing a significant burden from losses in quality and quantity of life? (2) Does it have a natural history that is understood? (3) Is there a preclinical (asymptomatic) state during which the disease can be diagnosed? (4) Are treatments available following early detection that yield benefits superior to those obtained by delayed treatment? (5) Are there tests that can detect the preclinical state that are reliable and have acceptable risks? (6) Are the costs of case finding and treatment reasonable and balanced in relationship to health expenditures as a whole, and are there resources available to treat detected cases? (7) Will screening be a continuing systematic process incorporated into routine health care, not a single effort? We will critically review the available evidence for each of these issues; because questions 4 and 5 are critical to this evaluation, we will devote most of this chapter to these two issues.

ISSUE 1: DOES DIABETES REPRESENT AN IMPORTANT HEALTH PROBLEM THAT IMPOSES A SIGNIFICANT BURDEN FROM LOSSES IN QUANTITY AND QUALITY OF LIFE?

The global burden of diabetes is large and increasing. The worldwide prevalence of diabetes was estimated to be 4.0% in 1995 and is expected to increase to 5.4% over the next 30 years[1]. The three countries with the largest burden, India, China and the USA, are currently estimated to have 19.4 million, 16.0 million and 13.9 million affected persons, respectively.

Diabetes is a complex disease that damages nearly every organ in the body. It is a major cause of visual impairment and blindness[53-56], end-stage renal disease (ESRD)[57,58], and lower-extremity amputations[59-62]. It is also a significant cause of cardiovascular disease (CVD), stroke, peripheral vascular disease, congenital malformations, perinatal mortality, disability and premature mortality[59,63-66]. Currently diabetes is the seventh leading cause of death overall in the USA, but ranks even higher among some US minority populations[67].

Diabetes consumes an extraordinary amount of resources and places a heavy economic burden on societies. The annual cost in the USA alone is estimated to be US$98.2 billion and persons with diabetes account for approximately 15% of all national health care expenditures[2,3]. Diabetic populations tend to consume health care resources at a rate of two to three times that of non-diabetic populations[2]. Indirect costs from losses in productivity, although poorly characterized, are significant in both developed and developing countries.

ISSUE 2: DOES TYPE 2 DIABETES HAVE A NATURAL HISTORY THAT IS UNDERSTOOD?

A chronic degenerative condition, diabetes progresses through several identifiable states. Biological onset is followed by a period during which the disease remains undiagnosed[4,15,17-20,68]. After a person develops typical diabetes symptoms or following incidental tests, a diagnostic test (or tests) is performed. Diabetic microvascular complications (retinopathy, nephropathy and neuropathy) and macrovascular disease (cardiovascular, cerebrovascular and peripheral vascular disease) develop in most patients and can result in major disability and, ultimately, death. Major risk factors for microvascular complications include poor glycaemic control and hypertension; for macrovascular disease they include hypertension, smoking, dyslipidemia and possibly poor glycaemic control.

Understanding the natural history of diabetes within and across populations requires standard diagnostic criteria. Events of the past two decades illustrate how diagnostic criteria have improved. In 1979–1980, the National Diabetes Data Group (NDDG) in the USA and the World Health Organization (WHO), in parallel, reviewed the available scientific knowledge and developed and widely disseminated recommendations for diagnosing diabetes[39,40]. In 1995–1997, the International Expert Committee on the Diagnosis and Classification of Diabetes Mellitus revised these recommendations[14]; currently a WHO committee is completing a similar review[12]. Following careful review of data from three population-based studies, the Expert Committee recommended new diagnostic criteria (Table 8.1). When typical diabetes symptoms (polyuria, polydipsia or unexplained weight loss) are present, a casual (i.e. any time during the day without regard to the last meal) plasma glucose of 11.1 mmol/L ($\geq$200 mg/dl) confirms the diagnosis. Alternatively, the diagnosis can be made with fasting glucose or oral glucose tolerance test measures (OGTT). The Expert Committee lowered the previous fasting diagnostic criterion of a plasma glucose of 7.7 mmol/l ($\geq$140 mg/dl) to 7.0 mmol/l ($\geq$126 mg/dl)[14]. Although it retained the two-hour (2)-h OGTT value of 11.0 mmol/l ($\geq$200 mg/dl), it eliminated routine use of this test. The Expert Committee recom-

Table 8.1. Criteria for the diagnosis* of diabetes mellitus[14]

1.	Symptoms of diabetes** and a casual*** plasma glucose $\geq$200 mg/dl (11.1 mmol/l)
2.	Fasting plasma glucose $\geq$126 mg/dl (7.0 mmol/l)
3.	Two-hour plasma glucose on an oral glucose tolerance test $\geq$200 mg/dl

*   Note: Need only meet one criterion. Test must be repeated and remain positive on a separate day except when symptoms of unequivocal hyperglycaemia with acute metabolic decompensation are present.
**   Polyuria, polydipsia and unexplained weight loss.
*** Any time during the day without regard to the time since the last meal.

mended that persons with only one positive diagnostic test have a repeat test on a different day to confirm the diagnosis.

Thus, the natural history of diabetes has been described in several populations, and diagnostic criteria are well established. While variations exist in diabetes risk factor profiles, the magnitude of risk associated with each factor, and the progression rates across different populations, the diabetes-related clinical states are common to all.

ISSUE 3: DOES DIABETES HAVE A RECOGNIZABLE AND DIAGNOSABLE PRECLINICAL STATE?

Using the same diagnostic criteria as for symptomatic cases[14], diabetes can be detected in the preclinical state (Figure 8.1). Population-based prevalence studies designed to identify all cases (diagnosed and undiagnosed) test many asymptomatic persons and commonly detect undiagnosed cases[4,15,17-20,68].

Establishing the duration of the preclinical state is a difficult task.[69] Attempts using currently available data have required major assumptions. One study estimated the duration of preclincial diabetes at 9–12 years before clinical diagnosis when assuming that the prevalence of retinopathy is linear with the duration of diabetes and that the prevalence is zero in non-diabetic persons[26]. Another study used a non-linear regression model and estimated the preclinical duration at between 7 and 8 years[70]. Thus, depending on the investigators' assumptions and the populations studied, the preclincal phase may vary widely but may last for several years.

Complications are by no means uncommon at this stage. Among people with either undiagnosed or newly diagnosed type 2 diabetes detected during population studies or in clinical trials, 2–39% have retinopathy[22-26], 8–18%

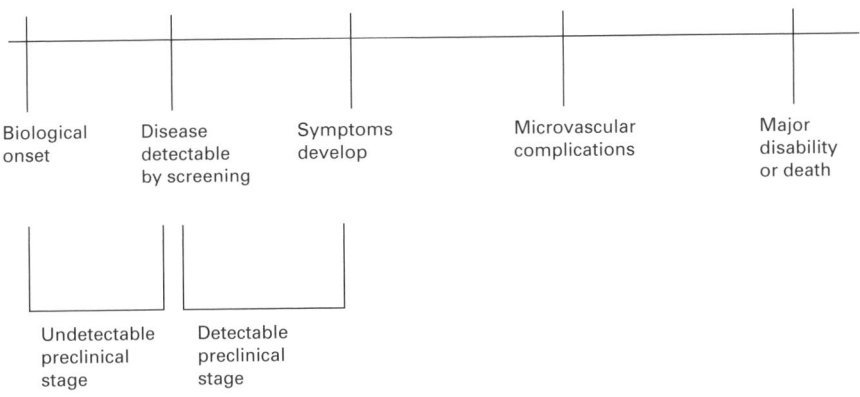

Figure 8.1. Clinical stages in the natural history of type 2 diabetes mellitus relevant to screening.

have nephropathy[27,71,72], 5–13% have neuropathy[4,22,73], and 8% have cardio-vascular disease[71]. Futhermore, the prevalence of cardiovascular and peripheral vascular disease as well as premature death among those with undiagnosed diabetes is similar to that found among those with diagnosed diabetes[28,74,75].

ISSUE 4: DOES TREATMENT FOLLOWING EARLY DETECTION OF TYPE 2 DIABETES YIELD BENEFITS SUPERIOR TO THOSE OBTAINED WHEN TREATMENT IS DELAYED?

This issue is of major importance to the evidence base for screening. In this section we discuss methods to assess benefits and then review studies that help determine the potential benefits from screening, improved glycaemic control that might occur following early detection, and diabetic complication detection and treatment. Finally, we examine the potential risks of early treatment.

Assessing Benefit

Four measures can be used to assess the benefits of screening and early treatment[44,76-78]: (1) the relative reduction in morbidity or mortality rates; (2) the absolute reduction in morbidity and mortality rates; (3) the number of patients needed to treat to prevent one adverse event (in a given time period); and (4) the total cohort mortality rate (all causes of mortality, not just diabetes-related). Absolute differences are preferred because they measure the actual units of benefit whereas relative risks do not. For example, a relative risk reduction of 50% could mean going from 1% to 0.5% or from 20% or 10%. However, the absolute risk reductions of 0.5% and 10% yield markedly different benefit units. The number needed to treat (NNT) for a given duration to prevent one adverse event is the inverse of the absolute risk reduction (i.e. the inverse of the difference in the absolute risk between screened and unscreened groups). For example, if the absolute risk reduction is from 20% to 10%, the number needed to treat is 100/10 or 10; and from 1% to 0.5% yields 100/0.5 or 200. The total mortality rate accounts for competing mortality risks from chronic diseases (e.g. cardiovascular diseases and cancer) and other causes (e.g. infectious diseases, injury, etc.) and can be used to determine additional life years and quality-adjusted life years (QALYs). QALYs take into account whether years are lived with disabilities such as blindness, amputation and ESRD[76,79].

Finally, when assessing the net benefit of screening, there are four types of potential bias that may lead to spurious conclusions: selection, lead time, length time and overdiagnosis bias (Table 8.2)[42,45]. Selection bias occurs if screen-detected persons are more likely than the general population to have good health outcomes. For example, if those who participate in screening programmes are more likely to follow health recommendations than those

Table 8.2. Types of bias and their effect on screening evaluations.

Type	Effect
Selection	Having healthy participants leads to better outcomes in screen-detected persons
Lead time	Earlier diagnosis results in screen-detected persons living longer with disease than persons diagnosed through standard procedures
Length time	Persons detected through screening have a slower natural progression of disease and a better prognosis than those detected through standard procedures
Overdiagnosis	Enthusiasm for screening leads to erroneous diagnosis among persons who do not have true disease

diagnosed through standard procedures, they may prevent or delay diabetic complications for reasons other than early detection.

Lead time is the period between screen-detection of disease and diagnosis through standard procedures. If early treatment of screen-detected diabetes during the lead time is ineffective, compared to persons diagnosed through standard procedures, those detected through screening would appear to have a longer interval before diabetes complications develop because of their earlier diagnosis. However, closer examination would demonstrate that early detection did not alter the natural history of disease. Length time bias occurs if people with screen-detected disease have a slower natural progression of disease than those diagnosed through standard practice which results in lower morbidity and mortality. The chance that diabetes is detected through screening depends on the duration of the preclinical disease state[42]. Thus, a person who has a short preclinical state has little chance for detection before becoming symptomatic. On the other hand, those with long preclinical states are more likely to be detected in a screening programme. Thus, screening would tend to detect disease with a slower progression. Finally, overdiagnosis bias can occur when vigorous screening efforts result in diagnoses being made among those who do not have true disease.

Although conditions or behaviours that accelerate diabetic complications (such as hypertension, hyperlipidemia or smoking) might also be detected at diabetes diagnosis[51], these conditions can be detected without diabetes screening and their presence does not specifically warrant screening for type 2 diabetes[8]. Furthermore, screening, identifying and treating these other conditions in the population directly may be more efficient[8]. Thus, examination of studies that might support diabetes screening should primarily consider the benefit gained from improved glycaemic control alone.

Randomized controlled trials (RCTs) would be the best means to evaluate the benefits and risks of early diabetes treatment and are superior to case-control designs or observational studies because they measure the effect of the screening procedure alone and not other health behaviours that make an individual submit to screening[80]. In an RCT, a control group (not screened) receiving currently available routine care after clinical diagnosis (usually at onset of symptomatic hyperglycaemia) could be compared with an intervention group diagnosed earlier (before symptomatic hyperglycaemia) following active screening.

RCTs of diabetes screening have not been conducted to date and may be difficult to conduct in the future because of ethnical concerns and costs. Random assignment to the control group (no screening) might be seen as unethical because several organizations have already recommended it. Second, because the benefits may be small and accrue over many years, the large numbers of participants and long-term follow-up would require substantial resources. These issues may be part of the reason that diabetes screening has not been on research agendas[81,82].

Other forms of evidence of the effectiveness of screening may be derived from observational data either by comparison of outcomes before and after commencement of screening or by comparison of similar geographically defined communities that adopt different screening policies. Future observational studies may characterize some of the benefits because screening recommendations are at various levels of implementation and may create screened and not-screened groups for comparisons. In addition, better health care system data and health services research techniques may facilitate such comparisons. These types of studies have not been conducted to date, but could provide evidence of an intermediate level between RCTs and disease models.

Potential Benefits of Screening

Scant empirical data exist about the benefits of screening *per se*. However, two small observational studies from the 1960s should be noted. The first, conducted in the former German Democratic Republic (East Germany), was a follow-up study of 250 diabetic patients detected by glycosuria screening who were compared with matched patients (by age, sex and weight) diagnosed through standard clinical practice[65]. No difference between the groups was noted in mortality, survival times and vascular complications at 10 and 20 years. A second study conducted in Italy compared 105 patients with diabetes detected through screening to 104 matched patients (age, sex, weight, family history, therapy and smoking) diagnosed through standard clinical practice[83]. After six years of follow-up the average glycaemia was significantly less in the screen-detected group, although there was no difference between the groups with regard to development of retinopathy, cataracts, neuropathy, lipid levels, CVD or peripheral vascular disease (PVD). These older studies, while interesting, are of limited value. Neither was a RCT and the understanding of the benefits of glycaemic control and the clinical practice patterns during this era were very different from our current understanding and practices.

Potential Benefits from Glycaemic Control

In the face of such limited empirical data on the benefits of screening, we examine less direct evidence of the benefit of glucose control for preventing microvascular and macrovascular complications by reviewing observational studies, RCTs of glycaemic control, and disease models (Table 8.3). We do have good evidence that persons with new clinically diagnosed diabetes typically have glucose levels that warrant treatment. For example, in the United Kingdom Prospective Diabetes Study (UKPDS), the average HbA_{1c} among persons with newly diagnosed type 2 diabetes at recruitment was 9.0%[71]. Therefore, it is relevant to this review to examine benefits (i.e. microvascular, macrovascular and mortality outcomes), and the risks (i.e. hypoglycaemia, weight gain, quality of life) associated with improved glycaemic control in type 2 diabetes. Here the data are much stronger and suggest a favourable benefit–risk ratio. However, it must be borne in mind that these benefits may not translate to persons diagnosed through screening.

Observational studies of glycaemia and diabetic complications

The Wisconsin (USA) Epidemiologic Study of Diabetic Retinopathy (WESDR) is an ongoing observational study examining the relationship between glycaemia exposure and diabetic complications[84]. Glycosylated haemoglobin at baseline has been found to be a significant predictor of the 10-year incidence

Table 8.3. Studies examining the benefit of glucose control in type 2 diabetes mellitus for preventing microvascular and macrovascular diabetic complications.

Study Type	Microvascular	Macrovascular
Observational		
Wisconsin Epidemiological Study of Diabetic Retinopathy[84]	+	+
Pima Indians[85]	+	+/–
Meta-analysis		
Coutinho *et al.*[86]	NA*	+
Randomized-controlled trials		
University Group Diabetes Study[87]	NA	–
Kumomoto Study[88]	+	–
Veterans Affair Cooperative Study[90]	–	NA
United Kingdom Propective Diabetes Study[91–93]	+	–
Disease models		
Vijan *et al.*[94]	+	NA
CDC Diabetes Cost-Effectiveness Study Group [76]	+	–

NA* – Not a goal of study, or not addressed
+ = benefit
– = benefit not shown

of diabetic retinopathy, macular oedema proliferative retinopathy, stroke and survival. The longitudinal study of diabetes and its complications in the Pima Indians of North America found that the five-year cumulative incidence of retinopathy was about 3 to 10 times higher (20% versus approximately 2–6%) in persons with fasting and 2 h glucose concentrations and haemoglobin A1 levels in the tenth decile than it was in persons with values in the ninth decile (10th versus 9th deciles: fasting, 10.2 and 6.8 mmol/l; 2 h, 18.1 and 11.5 mmol/l; HbA_{1c}, 9.1% and 7.4%).[85] A similar pattern was observed for nephropathy.

A recent meta-regression analysis examined the relationship between glucose concentrations and cardiovascular risk in persons without diagnosed diabetes but including persons with undiagnosed diabetes[86]. The 20 published prospective studies reviewed for this analysis included 95 783 persons who had suffered 3707 cardiovascular events (coronary artery disease, stroke, mortality) over 12.4 years (1 193 231 person-yr). Using a reference value for fasting glucose of 4.2 mmol/l, a fasting glucose of 6.1 mmol/l (the lower limit of impaired fasting glucose[14]) was found to carry a relative risk for cardiovascular events of 1.33 (95% CI 1.06–1.67). In addition, a 2 h glucose following a glucose challenge of 7.8 mmol/l (the lower limit of impaired glucose tolerance[14]) was determined to carry a relative risk for cardiovascular events of 1.58 (95% CI 1.19–2.10). Studies reported events by several glucose intervals, the highest of which included glucose values in the diabetic range (both fasting and 2 h values) that carried significantly higher relative risks for cardiovascular events. A limitation of this analysis was that the risk of cardiovascular events could not be adjusted directly for other cardiovascular risk factors, although such an adjustment was reported in 14 of the 20 studies. Of these 14, five showed a significant effect of glucose even after adjusting for one or more of the following: age, blood pressure, body mass index, weight, lipid concentrations or smoking habits.

Randomized Controlled Trials of Glycaemia and Diabetes Complications

The effect of glycaemic control on type 2 diabetes complications has been studied directly in four RCTs. In the first, the University Group Diabetes Study[87] conducted in a US diabetic population, no benefit from glycaemic control was found for the major outcomes of interest: cardiovascular outcomes and mortality (cardiovascular and total). The second, the Kumomoto Study[88] was conducted in Japanese subjects with diagnosed diabetes and found that intensive glycaemic control yielded a 30%–60% reduction in development and progression of microvascular complications – reductions similar to those found in the Diabetes Control and Complications Trial (DCCT) among persons with type 1 diabetes[89]. The Veterans Affairs (VA) Cooperative Study on Glycaemic Control and Complications in Type 2 Diabetes found no difference in cardiovascular events after two years of intensive glycaemic control[90].

The fourth RCT, the recently completed United Kingdom Prospective Diabetes Study (UKPDS), also studied directly the relationship between improved glycaemic control and complications[91-93]. In this large study (n = 5102) of persons with newly diagnosed type 2 diabetes (not identified through screening) who were followed for an average of 10 years, the intensive treatment group using oral hypoglycaemic agents and insulin achieved an average HbA_{1c} of 7.0%; the conventional therapy group averaged 7.9%. Overall, the intensive group had a 25% lower rate of aggregate microvascular endpoints and there was a 16% statistically non-significant decrease (p = 0.52) in the risk of non-fatal and fatal cardiovascular endpoints.

Modelling Studies of Glycaemia and Diabetic Complications

Recently, two computer-based disease models relevant to screening have been published. These types of disease models incorporate empirical data from several sources and make several assumptions. Thus, the assumptions and the results require cautious interpretation. However, they potentially can lend valuable insight to various issues and therefore are included in this review.

The first, a Markov model, examined the potential benefits of control for newly diagnosed, complication-free members of a health maintenance organization[94]. The model was constructed using the disease states (retinopathy, nephropathy and neuropathy) and rates for early development of microvascular disease from the DCCT and values from the literature for the end-stage outcomes. Mortality estimates were based on US vital statistics data and were not adjusted for level of glycaemic control. The lifetime benefits were determined for a hypothetical intervention that reduced HbA_{1c} from 9% to 7%. For a person diagnosed with diabetes aged 45 years, a reduction in HbA_{1c} from 9% to 7% was estimated to decrease lifetime risk of blindness by 2.3 percentage points (from 2.6% to 0.3%) and to lengthen life by 1.3 years. Benefits depended strongly on age and the baseline level of glycaemic control, however. For example, an improvement in HbA_{1c} from 9% to 7% in 65-year-old persons with newly diagnosed diabetes reduced blindness only 0.5 percentage points (from 0.5% to <0.1%). On the other hand, if 65-year-old persons improved their HbA_{1c} from 11% to 9%, their lifetime risk of blindness decreased 1.4 percentage points (1.9% to 0.5%). ESRD was found to have a similar pattern. The model assumed that following implementation of the intervention, glycaemic control remained constant until death, an assumption not consistent with the UKPDS, where glycaemic control worsened with duration despite continued intervention. Also, the model's incidence rates of retinopathy were lower than in the UPKDS and WESDR, possibly reflecting the lack of worsening glycaemic control over time.

The second published disease model directly examined the effect of improved glycaemic control in screen-detected diabetes[76]. A Monte Carlo simulation model estimated the lifetime benefits and costs associated with early detection and treatment of one-time opportunistic (clinic-based) screening for type 2 diabetes and compared them with the benefits and costs for persons diagnosed by current clinical practice (results are summarized in Table 8.4). Data for the model were obtained from clinical trials, epidemiological studies and population surveys. In brief, a hypothetical cohort of 10 000 persons from the general US population aged $\geq$25 years who had newly diagnosed diabetes were followed from onset of disease (assumed to be 10.5 years before clinical diagnosis, and 5.5 years before screening diagnosis) until death. The lifetime incidence of ESRD, blindness and lower extremity amputation were reduced in the screened group by 26%, 35% and 22%, respectively, and years lived free of these three major complications increased (0.08 years, 0.27 years and 0.15 years, respectively). The absolute lifetime risk reduction was greatest for blindness, where the number needed to treat was just 31 (i.e. to prevent one case of blindness). The benefits of early detection and treatment were found to accrue more from postponement of complications and the resulting improvement in the quality of life than from additional years of life gained.

This study did not include any potential benefit from early initiation of glycaemic control on the incidence of cardiovascular disease, as strong evidence was lacking[92]. It also did not include any possible benefits from the opportunity to influence macrovascular risk factors other than hyperglycaemia, e.g. hypertension, because of a paucity of empirical data. The model was found to be moderately sensitive to assumptions about the performance of the screening test (sensitivity and specificity), and the length of the pre-clinical diagnosis interval (a shorter interval was less cost-effective), the prevalence of undiagnosed diabetes (higher prevalence was more cost-effective) and the intensity of glycaemic control therapy. It should be pointed out that if intensive glycaemic control became the standard of care for type 2 diabetes, screening would become less cost-effective because average glycaemic concentrations would probably drop low enough to bring lifetime incidence of complications to a point where little room exists for further improvement through early diagnosis and treatment. Thus, benefits are directly related to current and future treatment patterns and the levels of glycaemic control they achieve; improvement will tend to yield less screening benefit while a decline would tend to yield greater benefits.

Potential Benefit from the Detection and Treatment of Diabetic Complications

Early diagnosis following screening may also provide an opportunity to prevent morbidity from major microvascular complications. Such complications are common at diagnosis; but timely laser therapy for retinopathy may prevent or delay visual loss[95-97], instituting angiotensin-converting-enzyme inhibitor

Table 8.4. Effectiveness of screening for type 2 diabetes from lifetime simulation model*.

	Lifetime cumulative incidence			Life-years gained	QALYs gained	Cost (US$)	
	ESRD	Blindness	LEA			Per life-year gained	Per QALY gained
Total population age ≥25							
Without screening	3.5%	9.1%	4.6%				
With screening	2.6%	5.9%	3.6%				
Absolute risk reduction	0.9%	3.2%	1.0%				
Number needed to treat	111	31	100	0.02	0.08	236 449	56 649
Total population age 25–34							
Without screening	19.2%	32.4%	19.0%				
With screening	15.9%	25.9%	16.0%				
Absolute risk reduction	3.3%	6.5%	3.0%				
Number needed to treat	30	15	33	0.12	0.35	35 768	13 376
Total population age ≥65							
Without screening	0.3%	1.7%	1.0%				
With screening	0.2%	1.1%	0.7%				
Absolute risk reduction	0.1%	0.5%	0.3%				
Number needed to treat	1000	200	333	0.00	0.01	NA	575 241

*See reference 76. ESRD, end-stage renal disease; LEA, lower extremity amputation; QALY, quality adjusted life-year; NA, not applicable because denominator is zero. Number needed to treat is over the lifetime.

therapy may prevent or delay nephropathy[98,99] and initiating comprehensive foot care may prevent lower extremity amputations[100,101].

Potential Risks of Early Treatment

To make a good policy decision about screening, any potential treatment benefits should be examined against possible adverse effects of screening or subsequent diagnostic tests. At present such negative effects are poorly understood, but should consider physical, psychological and social harm[44,47].

In terms of physical effects, one might consider the possibility that hyperinsulinaemia, which has been tied to atherosclerosis in prospective epidemiologic studies among non-diabetic populations[102-104], might result from intensified glycaemic control achieved through increased insulin doses. However, the UKPDS, the University Group Diabetes Study and the Kumomoto Study provide some supportive evidence that the risk of cardiovascular events did not increase and actually may have tended to be reduced with improved glycaemic control.

The risks associated with drugs or insulin therapy in screen-detected populations are not known[105]. However, in all the RCTs reviewed here hypoglycaemia occurred more frequently in the intensive treatment groups than among the conventional treatment groups. The UKPDS noted hypoglycaemic episodes in both groups, but the rate was higher in the intensive group (1.0–1.8% annual rate in oral- and insulin-treated intensive groups versus 0.7% in the conventional group; $p < 0.001$)[92].

Improved glycaemic control in persons with diagnosed diabetes may result in weight gain. Over the six years of the Kumamota Study there was a a slight increase in body mass index in both treatment groups that was not statistically significant[88]. However, in the UKPDS, there was a significantly greater increase in weight in the intensive treatment group compared to the conventional treatment group (2.9 kg, $p < 0.001$)[92].

Very little is known about how well asymptomatic persons who have been diagnosed following screening will comply with advice about diet and exercise, and little is known about the long-term safety and effectiveness of pharmacological therapy in this population. Improved glycaemic control may require more intensive self-care and substantial lifestyle change, which may affect quality of life (QOL). How QOL would be affected by instituting treatment in screen-diagnosed persons is unknown. Among subjects in the UKPDS (with diagnosed diabetes) there was neither improvement or decline in QOL assessments of mood, cognitive function, symptoms or general health between the two treatment groups[106]. However, QOL was affected by the occurrence of hypoglycaemia[106].

If patients largely ignore advice about diet and exercise and if pharmacological therapy is associated with substantial side-effects, any benefits of early detection thorough screening may be diminished. Finally, if a large percentage of those detected through screening are elderly, the benefits may be limited because of a shortened life expectancy [76,94] and the risk of morbidity associated with work-up and treatment may outweigh the relatively modest benefits[49,107].

In terms of psychological and social effects, patients may become overly frightened about where their 'disease' will lead them. In addition, after being told they have diabetes, they may have difficulty obtaining health insurance or employment even though they are apparently healthy.

Conclusions

In summary, observational studies, RCTs and one disease model provide evidence for a potential benefit from treating glycaemic levels found in newly diagnosed persons, and one disease model suggests that screening and early treatment decreases microvascular complications resulting from glycaemic control. The effects on macrovascular disease are less clear. Most of these studies however, were limited to populations with well-established diagnosed diabetes. Screening may prevent some disability from microvascular complications that are present at clinical diagnosis. On the other hand, the potential harm from early treatment is poorly understood. All things considered from both observational and clinical trial data and models, on balance, there appears to be modest evidence, at best, for benefit from early improved glycaemic control in type 2 diabetes.

ISSUE 5: ARE THERE TESTS THAT CAN DETECT PRECLINICAL DIABETES THAT ARE RELIABLE AND HAVE ACCEPTABLE RISKS?

This issue has been extensively studied, and a vast literature exists. Here we review the characteristics of screening tests, discuss the methodological issues for evaluating screening tests, examine the performance of both questionnaire and biochemical screening tests and, finally, discuss risks that can be associated with applying screening tests.

Screening Test Characteristics

Ideally, a diabetes screening test should be both sensitive (have a high probability of being positive when the person truly has diabetes) and specific (have a high probability of being negative when the persons does not have diabetes), but generally a trade-off must be made between sensitivity and specificity. When considering a test or evaluating studies, one will frequently examine the positive predictive value (PPV) (the probability of having diabetes when the screening test result is positive) as well[10,108-110]. The determinants of the PPV are the sensitivity and specificity of the screening test and the prevalence of disease in the population. When sensitivity and specificity are constant, the higher the prevalence of a disease, the higher the PPV of the screening test. Because an increase in PPV translates into more cases detected for each diagnostic test, it has significant implications for resource use. Information about the type of population (e.g. volunteers, community-based, clinic-based) and the distribution of risk factors (age, race or ethnicity, family history, obesity, physical activity) can be used to target groups with a higher prevalence of diabetes and thereby enhance the efficiency of the test.

Screening tests should also be reliable. Consistent results should be obtained when the test is performed more than once on the same person under the same conditions[108]. Uniform procedures and methods, standardized techniques, properly functioning equipment and quality control are necessary to ensure reliability.

Methodological Issues for Screening Test Evaluation Studies

When evaluating studies of the performance of type 2 diabetes screening tests, four issues must be considered: characteristics of the study population, referral policies for positive tests, the validity of the diagnostic test, and the selection of cut-points. The population's characteristics are important because they affect sensitivity and specificity. For example, both of these values will be higher in populations that include persons with severe hyperglycaemia, as is the case when persons with diagnosed diabetes are included, because it is easier to distinguish between those with frank diabetes and those without disease than between those with asymptomatic undiagnosed diabetes and those without disease. Thus, studies including persons with diagnosed diabetes should be interpreted cautiously. Second, referral policies are important because if participants with positive screening tests are preferentially referred to receive verification by the gold standard test, work-up bias may occur that substantially distorts sensitivity and specificity[111]. The third issue, the validity of the diagnostic test, is important because some studies have not performed definitive testing with a diagnostic gold standard.

Finally, the issue of cut-points is important, particularly in relation to sensitivity and specificity[10,108]. For example, selection of a high blood glucose cut-point for a positive test results in a low sensitivity and high specificity, and selection of a low cut-point results in a high sensitivity and low specificity. The choice of a cut-point may be influenced by policy, priorities and costs. Ideally, receiver operating characteristic (ROC) curve analyses, which can evaluate performance over the entire range of cut-points, should be used to compare tests[109,112-116]. Unfortunately, few studies have performed such analyses. Although not ideal, choosing a common specificity for each test allows for rough comparison of the sensitivity and, similarly, a common sensitivity allows comparisons of specificity.

Types of screening tests and their performance

The two major types of screen tests for type 2 diabetes are questionnaires and biochemical tests.

Questionnaires

With questionnaires, self-reported demographic, behavioural and medical information are used to assign a person to a high or low risk group. Community-based diabetes prevention programmes may use questionnaires to assess diabetes symptoms and risk factors and refer those at risk for a medical evaluation[117]. Questionnaires are popular and usually less expensive than biochemical tests, but when used alone they have generally performed poorly.

In 1989 the American Diabetes Association (ADA) published a questionnaire in which participants were asked about various diabetes risk factors (family history, obesity, at-risk race/ethnicity [American Indian, Hispanic, black], history of impaired glucose tolerance, hypertension or hyperlipidemia, and history of gestational diabetes or delivery of a >4 kg baby). The expected results were that persons with one or more risk factors would be more likely than those with none to have abnormal capillary glucose values. However, actual findings showed virtually no difference: 8% of those with no risk factors and 9% of those with one or more had elevated capillary glucose measurements[118]. Sensitivity of this discriminant (i.e. having one or more risk factors) was 69% and specificity was 34%. Significant increases in the odds of an elevated capillary measurement were found if a history of impaired glucose tolerance was reported or if there were three or more diabetes risk factors.

In 1993 the ADA disseminated a second questionnaire, called 'Take the Test. Know the Score', which was designed to increase public awareness as well assess risk[119]. Points were given for positive responses, and scores of ≤5 and >5 points were termed low risk and high risk, respectively. Subsequent use among both US[120] and UK[121] populations found the test performed rather poorly. For example, in the UK, when a score of >5 was used to predict persons with random capillary glucose measurements of >6.5 mmol/l, the sensitivity was 46% and the specificity was 59%. In addition, participants commonly reported symptoms of diabetes regardless of the capillary glucose measurement. Overall, approximately one-third of participants reported frequent urination, extreme fatigue and blurred vision, and nearly 20% reported excessive thirst.

A third risk assessment questionnaire was developed in the USA, in this instance with data from the US National Health and Nutritional Examination Survey II[122]. A test of the questionnaire in the population from which it was developed found a sensitivity of 79% and specificity of 65% for detection of undiagnosed diabetes using WHO criteria[40]. By ROC curve comparisons, it performed better than the ADA's 'Take the Test. Know the Score'. High risk groups were identified through only five risk factors for diabetes (older age, obesity, sedentary lifestyle, family history of diabetes and delivering a baby of more than 4 kg); participants were considered at high risk if they have one or more factors. The questionnaire did not depend on prior medical evaluations or care to ensure its applicability to all populations, including the medically underserved[123]. The ADA has incorporated an adaptation of this instrument in its current diabetes screening position statement as a risk test for use in community-based diabetes screening programmes[117]. Subsequently, this adapted risk test was used in a community screening program in Onondaga County, New York, where it had an overall sensitivity of 80% but a specificity of only 35% and a very low yield (PVP <10%)[123].

Finally, a questionnaire developed in the Netherland's Hoorn Study population incorporates symptoms (thirst, pain or shortness of breath during walking), demographic and clinical characteristics (age, sex, obesity, family history of diabetes, hypertension) and preferences (e.g. reluctance to use a bicycle for transportation)[124]. This questionnaire was subsequently evaluated in a separate sub-group of the Hoorn Study population and found to have a sensitivity of 56% and specificity of 72% and a performance better than the ADA questionnaires (as judged by ROC analyses).

In summary, in light of the rather poor performance of risk assessment questionnaires as a stand-alone test, they might best be limited to education and awareness efforts[125–127].

Biochemical tests

Measurements of glucose and highly correlated metabolites (e.g. HbA_{1c} and fructosamine) have been used extensively for diabetes screening. Urine glucose[38,128-134] or venous and capillary blood glucose[38,128-130,135-156] is measured under various conditions – fasting, at random, postprandial, or after glucose loading – to represent different metabolic states. For some tests, however, the immediate metabolic state is of relatively little importance; these include the glycosylated hemoglobin (total, A1 fraction, and the A1c fraction)[129,130,135,136,140,142,152,154,156-167] fructosamine,[140,143,158,163,167,168] and anhydroglucitol[135,169-171]. Characteristic of several biochemical screening tests are found in Table 8.5.

Use of trace glycosuria as a positive test tends to have low sensitivity and high specificity. Performance is usually better with random, postprandial or glucose-loaded measurements than with fasting measurements, perhaps in part because the renal threshold for glucose should be reached more often in the non-fasting state.

Studies of fasting venous blood screening tests often have used measurements collected as part of diagnostic testing and the 2 h glucose concentration serves as the gold standard test. In populations where persons with previously

Table 8.5. Sensitivity and specificity of various biochemical tests and combinations of tests for detecting undiagnosed type 2 diabetes.

Test	Metabolic state	Cut-point	Sensitivity (%)	Specificity (%)	Reference
Urine glucose*					
	Fasting	≥trace	16	98	130
	Fasting	≥trace	35	100	38
	Random	≥trace	18	99	128
	Random	≥trace	64	99	129
	1 h pp	≥trace	43	98	131,134
	2 h OGTT¶	≥trace	48	96	38
	2 4 h pp§	≥trace	39	98	38
Venous glucose†					
	Fasting	≥5.8	85	84	152
	Fasting	≥6.1	65	93	137
	Fasting	≥6.1	80	96	138
	Fasting	≥6.1	95	90	129
	Fasting	≥6.1	66	96	150
	Fasting	≥6.5	74	93	135
	Fasting	≥6.7	44	98	38
	Fasting	≥6.7	32	97	143
	Fasting	≥6.9	48	97	158
	Fasting	≥7.0	56	98	148
	Fasting	≥7.0	40	99	149
	Fasting	≥7.0	59	96	151
	Fasting	≥7.8	52	99	136
	1 h OGTT	≥11.1	87–93	89–90	138
	2 h OGTT	≥11.1	90–93	100	138
	2 4 h pp	≥7.2	50	99	38
Capillary glucose†					
	Fasting	≥5.5	90	94	130
	Fasting	≥6.7	65	94	153
	Fasting	≥6.7	90	90	154
	Random	age-, pp time-specific	50s-60s	90	172
	Random	≥7.2	80	80	154
	Random	≥8.0	69	95	128
	2 h OGTT	≥11.1	69	98	139
	2 h OGTT	≥8.6	90	93	130
	2 h OGTT	≥9.7	98	98	155
Glycosylated haemoglobin‡					
	–	≥5.6	35	100	158
	–	≥5.6	83	84	209
	–	≥5.8	92	89	129
	–	≥6.0	60	91	136
	–	≥6.03	85	91	159
	–	≥6.1	78	79	152
	–	>6.3	48	100	157
	–	≥8.0	87	87	154

Table 8.5. contd.

	–	≥8.1	37	96	160
	–	≥8.3	48	100	157
	–	≥8.3	43	96	164
	–	>8.42	27	88	161
	–	≥8.5	15	100	163
	–	≥8.6	67	97	167
Fructosamine†	–	≥1.18	19	99	143
	–	≥1.78	19	97	163
	–	≥1.92	74	95	168
	–	≥2.50	67	96	167
	–	≥2.90	23	98	158
Combination tests					
	Fasting glucose and HbA$_{1c}$	≥7.8mmol/l ≥6.0%	40	99	136
	Fasting glucose and HbA$_{1c}$	≥5.6 mmol/l ≥5.5%	83	83	152
	Fasting glucose and fructosamine	≥5.4 mmol/l ≥235μmol/l	82	83	152
	Fasting glucose and HbA$_{1c}$	≥6.1 mmol/l ≥6.1%	69	96	156

*Cut-point expressed as qualitative dipstick determination.
†Cut-point expressed as mmol/l.
‡Cut-point expressed as percentage of haemoglobin A$_{1c}$.
§Postprandial.
¶Oral glucose tolerance test.

diagnosed diabetes have been excluded or the population has not been enriched with high risk persons[38,136,137,148,149], sensitivity has ranged from 40% to 65% at a specificity of >90%. Other studies have reported higher sensitivity (up to 95%)[129,135,138,150-152], but some included persons with diagnosed diabetes or populations with an increased proportion of persons with abnormal glucose tolerance. Studies of fasting capillary glucose tests have had ranges in performance similar to that for fasting venous tests.

In some cases, random and postprandial venous and capillary glucose tests perform better than fasting tests. This happens because, compared to persons without diabetes, persons with undiagnosed diabetes are more likely to have postprandial hyperglycaemia than fasting hyperglycaemia.[172] Higher cut-points are needed to account for the postprandial state (and age in some cases) to obtain optimal performance from random and postprandial tests[172,173].

Glycosylated haemoglobin measurement, which is becoming more widely available[174], has a moderate to low sensitivity and moderate to high specificity at the cut-points generally reported. Sensitivity of 15% to 67% has been reported at a specificity of >90% (Table 8.5). Higher sensitivity at high specificity has been reported, but these were in populations that included persons with diagnosed diabetes or a high level of glucose intolerance[129,159].

Among problems with glycosylated haemoglobin measurements are the lack of widely used laboratory standard reference materials and variation in the reference method. In addition, HbA_{1c} (the most commonly used glycosylated haemoglobin measurement) may be fundamentally unsuited for diabetes screening. As evidence, a study in a small number of persons with normoglycaemia (no diabetes) failed to find a relationship between fasting venous glucose and HbA_{1c} values.[175] Others have found that only 2–30% of non-diabetic variance in glycosylated haemoglobin can be explained by fasting or postload blood glucose, while the remainder is presumably related to other factors independent of glycaemia, such as the rate of glycation and differences in red cell survival[176,177].

Among other biochemical screening tests that have been evaluated, both anhydroglucitol, a polyol sugar alcohol found in reduced serum concentrations in persons with diabetes[135], and serum fructosamine, a measure of glycosylated total serum proteins[140,143,158,163,167,168], are independent of fasting status, but neither has performed better than other available tests.

Combinations of biochemical tests have also been evaluated[136,152,156]. Using multiple tests in series (with second and subsequent screening tests performed only when the preceding test is positive) can enhance the yields from certain screening test strategies because it can increase the prevalence of disease in the screened population that ultimately receives diagnostic testing. For example, a second screening test performed only in the population of persons who had positive initial screening tests yields a 'double positive' population that will have a higher prevalence of disease than if either test were administered alone. Screening programmes can use a less expensive test first followed by the more complicated or expensive test (e.g. questionnaire followed by capillary glucose measurement). Strategies that use multiple screening tests will not detect more undiagnosed cases (i.e. will not improve sensitivity) but will potentially allow for more efficient use of resources.

Screening Test Risks

There are several risks associated with screening tests. Exposure to additional diabetes and other comorbidity tests may convey harmful risks[8,178] and may increase worry and reduce health-related quality of life. In addition, persons without diabetes who have positive screening tests (false positives) are subject to the costs (out-of-pocket expenses and missed work time) of unnecessary evaluations as well as hazards they present. Furthermore, the inconvenience of screening and such adverse effects such as 'labelling' of false positive persons must be considered[105]. On the other hand, persons with diabetes who have negative screening tests (false negatives) will not receive appropriate diagnostic testing and will be falsely reassured that they are disease free. Finally, among persons who do not have diabetes and have negative screening tests (true negatives), accurate interpretation and communication of their diabetes risk status may be challenging.

Although community level screening interventions may sometimes seem to be more effective than those in clinical practice[105,179], it may be difficult to ensure proper referral for screen positive persons and appropriate repeated testing in those who are screen negative[180]. Furthermore, screening outside of clinical settings may mean that abnormal tests are never discussed with the primary health care provider, that compliance with recommendations is low, and that a positive long-term impact on health is unlikely[178].

The issue of informed consent must also be considered; failure to obtain truly informed consent for screening may be unethical[46]. Before conducting screening, health care providers and public health workers need to be aware of the risks and benefits of complex information so they can fully inform their patients. Rarely is there sufficient time for providers to provide this information, and patients may have trouble assimilating the important parts.

Conclusions

Review of various screening methods for detecting undiagnosed type 2 diabetes shows that questionnaires tend to work poorly, while biochemical tests are a better alternative. Because test performance typically depends on the populations being evaluated and the cut-point reported, interpretation can be difficult and comparisons to other studies challenging. Finally, the risks associated with screening tests remain poorly understood.

POINT 6: ARE THE COSTS OF CASE FINDING AND TREATMENT BALANCED IN RELATIONSHIP TO HEALTH EXPENDITURES AS A WHOLE, AND ARE RESOURCES AVAILABLE TO TREAT DETECTED CASES?

Diabetes screening programmes include screening tests in populations, diagnostic tests in those with positive screening tests, and the initiation of lifelong care for those confirmed to have diabetes. Thus, determining the costs of programmes and the additional burden on the health care system requires a knowledge of the prevalence of undiagnosed diabetes, the method of case finding and the operation of the health care delivery system. As each of these three factors may vary widely by setting, making general statements about the costs and burden of screening is fraught with difficulty. One safe generalization is that for early detection to provide benefit, there needs to be ongoing access to diabetes care[8,51]. For countries with publicly funded national health care and universal access to services where most patients see a physician often, screening yields may be vanishingly low and not worth the effort[181]. Within the USA, in contrast, where there may be up to 40 million persons (nearly 18% of the population) with either no medical care coverage at all or inadequate medical coverage[182], yields may be greater than in other countries.

In the screening simulation model discussed earlier in this chapter, an opportunistic screening programme for the general US population aged 25 years and older, the cost per case identified was US$1200, which included a fasting plasma glucose screening test, an oral glucose tolerance test in those with a positive screening test, and physician time for test interpretation[76]. Diabetes was diagnosed approximately 5.5 years earlier with a screening programme and the estimated average annual cost for treatment of newly diagnosed persons was US$1007. The lifetime cost of diabetes treatment (routine care and treatment of complications) was US$3400 higher with screening (US$49 600 versus US$46 200). In addition, with screening, the benefit in additional life-years was less than the gain in QALYs; the cost per life-year gained (US$236 400) was four times the cost per QALY obtained (US$56 600) (Table 8.4). Compared to older persons, younger persons had greater benefits and more favourable cost-effectiveness. In addition, African-Americans had greater benefits and a more favorable cost-effectiveness ratio than the general population, primarily because of higher complication rates in this population. We note from reviews of guidelines and previous cost-effectiveness studies of interventions for diseases and conditions other than diabetes that interventions whose cost-effectiveness is between $20 000 and $100 000 per QALY are often provided, but availability may be somewhat limited[183].

From an economic, clinical and public health perspective, the issue of how diabetes screening complements efforts to control other diseases should be considered as well. The diagnosis of type 2 diabetes can be combined with detection efforts for other conditions (e.g. smoking, hypertension, hyperlipidemia)[8,51] and the optimal mix of screening tests that produce the most benefits could then be determined[51,79,81].

For a health care system to implement diabetes screening, either obtaining new resources or redirecting current resources away from other activities is required. Because health care budgets are finite, redirection is more common, and thus there is an 'opportunity' cost in taking on a new activity (i.e. other activities may have to be reduced or eliminated altogether)[79]. Health care policy leaders in each country will need to inventory their current situation and priorities and then assess where diabetes screening fits. Cost-effectiveness studies can help, but the absolute cost (for the entire population) of the effort must be considered, and the decision may be very different for developed counties as compared to developing countries.

In summary, the global impact of a screening programme on the health care system is likely to be substantial, but may vary greatly from country to country. Generally, there is scant information about the expected impact on health care systems.

POINT 7: WILL SCREENING BE A CONTINUING PROCESS, NOT A SINGLE EFFORT?

Screening programmes inevitably miss some cases (sensitivity is less than 100%; many people do not present themselves for screening) and new onset cases continue to replenish the pool of undiagnosed cases. Thus, to fully address the undiagnosed burden, screening programmes must be ongoing. To accomplish this, there must be a commitment to developing and sustaining screening capacity, which should include programme support, coordination and evaluation. If made part of routine preventive care, screening could be conducted in the clinic setting at designated intervals. However, the optimal interval between screenings is not clear and a few studies have examined the appropriate frequency of screening. In one UK study that conducted a repeat diabetes screening at 30 months using self-testing of postprandial glycosuria in 3200 persons registered at a general clinic, the repeat screening response rate was slightly lower than the initial (73% versus 79%, p <0.0001), but the yields were not significantly different (0.44% versus 0.72%, p = 0.2)[184]. The optimal interval would be one where the cost-effectiveness was equal for each screening.

THE YIELD OF DIABETES SCREENING PROGRAMMES

Direct evaluation of screening programme effectiveness has been limited to their ability to detect undiagnosed cases. Three approaches to diabetes screening programmes have been used, population-based, selective and opportunistic; results from all these types are presented in Table 8.6[178,185-187]. Classification for this chapter is based on the information within each report and what was deemed the dominant mode of the screening effort.

Population-based approaches screen every person. Health planning efforts and epidemiological studies designed to assess the magnitude of diabetes prevalence may use this method. Costly and potentially inefficient, this method is not widely favoured except in very high-prevalence populations. Selective screening, often conducted outside the health care system, targets sub-groups of the population with a high prevalence of risk factors for diabetes[117,188,189].

Table 8.6. Population-based, selective, and opportunistic screening program strategies and yields.

Type	Setting	Target population	Total tests	Screening test used	Total number positive screening tests	Total number new cases detected	Yield* (%)	Reference
Population								
	Community awareness campaign	Volunteers	NR	Self-referral after ad campaign	41	7	17	194
	Community sample for diabetes study	Volunteers responding to invitation	320	Risk score	21	4	19	210
	Community education and outreach	Volunteers	320	Risk score	18	3	17	210
			3031	CG	72	52	72	198
	Community screening	Volunteers	2016	CG	148	6	4	120
	Community health fair	Volunteers	3212	VG	120	25	21	211
	Community outreach	Volunteers	253 190	VG	9682	5370	55	212
	Community diabetes detection drive	Volunteers	559	VG, CG, urine	164	42	26	213
	Community diabetes promotion	Volunteers	23 228	CG	860	64	7	214
	Community outreach	Volunteers	396	Risk score	264	28	11	126
Selective	Hospital waiting room	Volunteers	548	CG	NR	5	–	196

Table 8.6. contd.

Dental clinic (distributed 35 000 urine kits)	All patients	119	VG	24	6	25	34
Pharmacy (preference to high risk: >40yr obese, FH, large baby)	Volunteers	3409	urine	164	2	13	197
Community Outreach (Mailed 7 426 risk questionnaires to households)	Volunteers (>60 yrs)	349	Risk score	181	11	6	125
Community physician's patients	20% sample of patients >40 yrs	1767	BG	48	19	40	181
Clinic population (mailed urine glucose kits)	Volunteers 45–70 yrs	2984	urine	73	17	23	35
Clinic population (mailed urine glucose kits)	Volunteers 45–70 yrs	3231	urine	52	10	19	188

Table 8.6. contd.

Clinic population (mailed urine glucose kit)	Volunteers 45–70 yrs	13 795	urine	343	99	29	134
Motor vehicle department licence renewal	Volunteers >70 yrs	410	CG	11	NR	–	199
Industry workers	Volunteers 18–74 yrs	4048	CG	267	13	5	215
Clinic registries	Volunteers 50–69 yrs	367	CG	28	5	18	195
Opportunistic							
Clinic population	Volunteers	3268	CG, urine	234	66	28	128
Health insurance beneficiaries	Volunteers >25 yrs	8818	VG	176	30	17	178

NR – not reported, CG – capillary glucose, VG – venous glucose, risk score – use of questionnaire or risk classification scheme, FH – family history.
*Positive Predictive Value (PPV)

Opportunistic screening tests all or a sub-group of persons during routine encounters with the health care system, such as primary care visits or periodic health evaluations[185-187, 190-193]. Both selective screening and opportunistic screening can significantly reduce the resources needed to reach at-high-risk groups, conduct screening tests and perform follow-up, but some important groups may be missed[187]. Opportunistic screening may often have poor coverage and have a tendency to be misdirected – some persons getting too many tests too often, others getting too few.

Most screening programmes report using either population, selective or a combined population/selective strategy (Table 8.6). Some of the selective programmes, for example, have begun with population-based health promotion and diabetes awareness programmes targeting entire communities, then screened volunteers with diabetes risk factors. Testing strategies used have included questionnaires as well as fasting, random, postprandial and glucose-loaded biochemical measurements. Some programmes have conducted public awareness campaigns which have resulted in increased patient requests for screening when making clinic visits[194], while others have advocated increasing professional alertness as an efficient approach[180]. The yields reported, which are highly variable and dependent on the screening test cut-point, have ranged from 5–72% (Table 8.6).

Selective screening has also occurred in such widely varied settings as doctors' offices and medical clinics[195], clinic and hospital waiting rooms[196], dental clinics[34], community pharmacies[197], shopping centres[198], community centres[198], drivers' licence registration centres[199], work sites and community churches[200]. Groups with an expected rate higher than the general population have been targeted using factors such as age and risk factors (e.g. family history of diabetes, obesity)[107,199]. Yields for selective screening have ranged from 5–40%.

Although data on the effectiveness of screening (from simulation models) are available only for opportunistic methods[76], few reports have used such methods. Strategies have included the sponsorship by health insurance companies of multichannel chemistry screening through widespread phlebotomy centres[178] and use of patient clinic registries[128].

CURRENT SCREENING POLICIES AND RECOMMENDATIONS AND PRACTICES

Several health agencies, task forces and professional organizations have provided recommendations for type 2 diabetes screening (Table 8.7)[11–14,105, 117,201–203]. Some of the recommendations were published several years ago, but none has been revised since the reporting of the results of the UKPDS[92] or the cost-effectiveness simulation model[76]. The most recent ADA recommendations were included in the report of the Expert Committee on the Diagnosis and Classification of Diabetes Mellitus[14]. The preliminary report by the WHO on diagnosis and classification did not address screening[12].

Because definitive studies on the benefits of screening are not available, all the recommendations relied on expert opinion and consensus. None encourages population-based screening, but some suggest using a selective or opportunistic approach in populations with diabetes risk factors. The WHO, the British Diabetic Association and the ADA statements all provide screening strategies and recommend repeat screening intervals. None of the strategies or recommended intervals have been formally evaluated.

The United States Preventive Services Task Force (USPSTF), in its current recommendations, which were published in 1996 and endorsed by the American Medical Association[204], cite insufficient evidence to recommend for or against routine screening[105]. Major limitations cited by the USPSTF are (1) lack of a practical screening test that is sufficiently sensitive and specific, and (2) insufficient evidence that detection during the preclinical phase will improve long-term outcomes. Noting that evidence of benefit from early detection was not available, however, the USPSTF suggests that clinicians may decide to screen high-risk individuals on other grounds (e.g. a screening test in high-prevalence populations has a better yield) and for the potential benefit, albeit unproven, that early treatment may provide. The report suggests that if the UKPDS trial demonstrates important clinical benefits from more intensive interventions in patients with minimally symptomatic diabetes, a sub-group study from the UKPDS that has not been performed, it would provide stronger support for screening in asymptomatic adults.

The current ADA recommendations, which were published in 1998, state that early detection and thus early treatment may well reduce the burden of type 2 diabetes and its complications and, accordingly, screening may be appropriate in certain circumstances. The recommendations suggest that screening be considered at any age if risk factors for diabetes are present (i.e. family history, obesity, belonging to high-risk minority group, abnormal glucose tolerance [IGT or IFG], hypertension, hyperlipidemia, previous gestational diabetes or history of delivery of a large baby [>4 kg]). In addition, the ADA recommends to consider screening all persons ≥45 years old regardless of risk factor status and repeating screening at three-year intervals. Its rationale for these latter recommendations is that there is a steep rise in the incidence of diabetes after age 45, there is a negligible likelihood of developing any significant complications of diabetes within three years of a negative test, and that the risk factors included in their recommendations are firmly established.

In the light of these recommendations, just how common is screening for type 2 diabetes? Scant information describing the level of screening activities is available and is limited to experience in the USA. A 1989 population-based survey found approximately 40% of persons who did not have diabetes reported being checked for the disorder during the previous year by a doctor

Table 8.7. Screening recommendations for type 2 diabetes by health agencies, professional organizations and associations, and health task forces*

Agency, Organization, Task Force	Strategy	Specimen	Type of collection	Positive test (mmol/l)	Repeat interval	Year published	Reference
WHO	Selective, target risk factors	Urine Blood	Not stated Plasma Fasting Random	≥6.5 ≥7.0 to 8.0	Not stated	1994	11
BDA	target risk factors	Selective, Urine Blood	2 h postprandial Plasma Fasting 2 h 75 OGTT	≥trace ≥6.7 ≥8.0	5 yr	1993	13
USPSTF	Selective, target risk factors	Blood	Plasma Fasting	Not stated	Clinical discretion	1996	105
CTFPHE	Selective, target risk factors	Urine Blood	Not stated Fasting, random	Not stated Not stated	Not stated	1979	202
ADA	Selective, using risk assessment questionnaire	Blood	Plasma Fasting (≥8 hrs) Random (<8 hrs) 2-hour post 75 oral glucose load Capillary (whole blood) Fasting (≥8 hrs) Random (<8 hrs)	≥7.0 ≥8.9 ≥11.1 ≥6.1 ≥7.8	3 yr	1998	14 117
ACP	Selective, target risk factors	Blood	Plasma Fasting	Not stated	Not stated	1991	201
AAFP	All children, adolescents, and adults	None	Counsel to engage in regular physical activity	–	Not stated	1998	203

*World Health Organization (WHO), British Diabetic Association (BDA), United States Preventive Services Task Force (USPSTF), Canadian Task Force on Periodic Health Examination (CTFPHE), American Diabetes Association (ADA), American College of Physicians (ACP), American Academy of Family Physicians (AAFP).

or other health professional[189], but this report did not describe the location or and circumstances of the screening tests. In 1998, a population-based survey in Montana found that 39% of persons without diabetes had been screened during the previous year[205]. With several organization and agencies recommending it, screening is, no doubt, taking place in several countries but it seems unlikely that it is systematically applied. It is more probable that it is left up to patients, health care providers, and various public health and health promotion workers. In addition there is certainly a good deal of 'accidental' diabetes screening in the health care setting, as the widespread use of multi-channel chemistry tests means that glucose values are frequently available when laboratory tests are conducted for other reasons.

SUMMARY

For this review, we have considered the evidence for each of seven issues to determine whether diabetes screening is appropriate clincal and public health activity. We have clearly shown that diabetes is an important public health problem, has a well characterized natural history, and that it can be diagnosed in the preclinical (asymptomatic) state. However, currently there appears to be little or no direct evidence to support diabetes screening. The effect of early treatment on long-term health outcomes and the risks associated with it are unclear. In addition, while several screening tests and some screening strategies have been evaluated, there is no clear evidence that broad implementation of these strategies will be effective and sustainable.

Definitive studies on the effectiveness of screening will probably not be forthcoming. RCTs would be the best means to assess effectiveness, but several barriers prevent these studies from being conducted. Future observational studies may characterize some of the benefits because screening recommendations are at various levels of implementation and may create screened and not-screened groups for comparisons. In addition, better health care system data and health services research techniques may facitate such comparisons.

Statistical models have already helped to answer some of the key questions and may continue to do so. This approach is attractive because of their relatively low cost (compared to a clinical trial), their ability to incorporate data from many clinical and epidemiological studies, to perform economic evaluations, and the capability of modifying treatment algorithms relatively easily. Current models need to be refined with new clinical and epidemiologic information such as the UKPDS results[91]. In addition, future models need to include: better information on the natural history of the preclinical phase, comprehensive cardiovascular disease modules and the influence of glucose and cardiovascular risk factor reduction[67], comprehensive quality of life information (physical, psychological and social consequences), and refined economic evaluations using common outcome measures (cost per additional life year or QALY gained)[10,79,206-208]. These studies should consider all costs associated with a comprehensive screening programme, including, at a minimum, the direct costs of screening, diagnostic testing and care for persons with type 2 diabetes detected through screening. However, it must be borne in mind that these models require multiple assumptions which must be considered when interpreting the results. Finally, various mixes of several disease screening interventions should be considered in economic studies to allows for selection of the optimal combination of interventions within the financial and resource limitations of the health care system[79].

CONCLUSIONS

The effectiveness of diabetes screening has not been directly demonstrated. Indirect examination of the potential benefits of screening using data from RCTs of treatment of diagnosed diabetes, observational studies and disease models lend some support to the idea that early improvement in glycaemic control may help reduce the lifetime occurrence of microvascular disease. There is little convincing evidence that there will be macrovascular disease reductions. The physical, psychological and social effects of screening and early diagnosis and treatment remain unclear. Thus, on balance, there is only modest evidence, at best, supporting screening for type 2 diabetes. (Level of evidence II-3; Strength of Recommendation B.)

REFERENCES

1. King H, Aubert RE, Herman WH (1998) Global burden of diabetes, 1995–2025: prevalence, numerical estimates, and projections. *Diab. Care* **21**: 1414–31.
2. Rubin RJ, Altman WM, Mendelson DN (1994) Health care expenses for people with diabetes mellitus, 1992. *J. Clin. Endocrinol. Metab.* **78**: 809A–809F.
3. American Diabetes Association (1998) Economic consequences of diabetes mellitus in the US in 1997. *Diab. Care* **21**: 296–309.
4. Harris MI (1993) Undiagnosed NIDDM: clinical and public health issues. *Diab. Care* **16**: 642–52.
5. Alberti KGMM, DeFronzo RA, Zimmet P (Eds) (1995) *International Textbook of Diabetes Mellitus*. New York: John Wiley & Sons.
6. Centers for Disease Control and Prevention (1997) National Diabetes Fact Sheet, 1997. Atlanta, GA. Division of Diabetes Translation, Centers for Disease Control and Prevention, Department of Health and Human Services.
7. Clark CM (1998) How should we respond to the worldwide diabetes epidemic? *Diab. Care* **21**: 475–6.
8. Knowler WC (1994) Screening for NIDDM. Opportunities for detection, treatment, and prevention. *Diab. Care* **17**: 445–50.

9. Harris MI, Modan M (1994) Screening for NIDDM. Why is there no national program? *Diab. Care* **17**: 440–44.
10. Engelgau MM, Aubert RE, Thompson TJ, Herman WH (1995) Screening for NIDDM in nonpregnant adults. A review of principles, screening tests, and recommendations. *Diab. Care* **18**: 1606–18.
11. World Health Organization Study Group on Prevention of Diabetes Mellitus (1994) Prevention of Diabetes Mellitus. Technical Report Series No. 844. Geneva: World Health Organization.
12. Alberti KG, Zimmet P (1998) Definition, diagnosis and classification of diabetes mellitus and its complications. Part 1: diagnosis and classification of diabetes mellitus. Provisional report of a WHO consultation. *Diabet. Med.* **15**: 539–53.
13. Patterson KR (1993) Population screening for diabetes mellitus. *Diabet. Med.* **10**: 77–81.
14. The Expert Committee on the Diagnosis and Classification of Diabetes Mellitus (1997) Report of the expert committee on the diagnosis and classification of diabetes mellitus. *Diab. Care* **20**: 1183–97.
15. Harris MI, Flegal KM, Cowie CC, Eberhardt MS, Goldstein DE, Little RR, Wiedmeyer HM, Byrd-Holt DD (1998) Prevalence of diabetes, impaired fasting glucose, and impaired glucose tolerance in US adults. The Third National Health and Nutrition Examination Survey, 1988–1994. *Diab. Care* **21**: 518–24.
16. Oliveira JE, Milech A, Franco LJ (1996) The prevalence of diabetes in Rio de Janeiro, Brazil. The Cooperative Group for the Study of Diabetes Prevalence in Rio De Janeiro. *Diab. Care* **19**: 663–6.
17. Harris MI, Hadden WC, Knowler WC, Bennett PH (1987) Prevalence of diabetes and impaired glucose tolerance and plasma glucose levels in the US population aged 20–74. *Diabetes* **36**: 523–34.
18. King H, Rewers M (1993) Global estimates for prevalence of diabetes mellitus and impaired glucose tolerance in adults. *Diab. Care* **16**: 157–77.
19. Harris MI (1990) Noninsulin-dependent diabetes mellitus in black and white Americans. *Diabetes Metab. Rev.* **6**: 71–90.
20. McLarty DG, Pollitt C, Swai ABM (1990) Diabetes in Africa. *Diabet. Med.* **7**: 670–84.
21. Flegal KM, Ezzati TM, Harris MI, Haynes SG, Juarez RZ, Knowler WC, Perez-Stable EJ. Stern MP (1991) Prevalence of diabetes in Mexican Americans, Cubans, and Puerto Ricans from the Hispanic Health and Nutritional Examination Survey, 1982–1984. *Diab. Care* **14**: 628–38.
22. Wang WQ, Ip TP, Lam KS (1998) Changing prevalence of retinopathy in newly diagnosed non-insulin dependent diabetes mellitus patients in Hong Kong. *Diabetes Res. Clin. Pract.* **39**: 185–91.
23. Harris MI, Klein R, Cowie CC, Rowland M, Byrd-Holt DD (1998) Is the risk of diabetic retinopathy greater in non-Hispanic blacks and Mexican Americans than in non-Hispanic whites with type 2 diabetes? A US population study. *Diab. Care* **21**: 1230–5.
24. Rajala U, Laakso M, Qiao Q, Keinanen-Kiukaanniemi S (1998) Prevalence of retinopathy in people with diabetes, impaired glucose tolerance, and normal glucose tolerance. *Diab. Care* **21**: 1664–9.
25. Kohner EM, Aldington SJ, Stratton IM, Manley SE, Holman RR. Matthews DR, Turner R (1998) United Kingdom Prospective Diabetes Study. Diabetic retinopathy at diagnosis of non-insulin-dependent diabetes mellitus and associated risk factors. *Arch. Ophthalmol.* **116**: 297–303.

26. Harris MI, Klein R, Welborn TA, Knuiman MW (1992) Onset of NIDDM occurs at least 4–7 years before clinical diagnosis. *Diab. Care* **15**: 815–9.
27. Ballard DJ, Humphrey LL, Melton LJ, Frohnert PP, Chu PC, O'Fallon WM, Palumbo PJ (1988) Epidemiology of persistent proteinuria in type II diabetes mellitus. Population-based study in Rochester, Minnesota. *Diabetes* **37**: 405–12.
28. Harris MI (1989) Impaired glucose tolerance in the US population. *Diab. Care* **12**: 464–74.
29. Pauker SG (1993) Deciding about screening. *Ann. Intern. Med.* **118**: 901–2.
30. Engelgau MM, Narayan KMV, Herman WH (2000) Screening for type 2 diabetes mellitus. *Diab. Care* **20**: 1563–80.
31. Davidson JK (Ed.) (1991) *Clinical Diabetes Mellitus. A Problem Oriented Approach, 2nd edn.* New York: Thieme Medical Publishers.
32. Galen RS, Gambino SR (1975) *Beyond Normality: The Predictive value of Efficiency of Medical Diagnosis.* New York: John Wiley & Sons.
33. Genuth SM, Houser HB, Carter JR, Merkatz IR, Price JW, Schumacher OP, Wieland RG (1978) Observations on the value of mass indiscriminate screening for diabetes mellitus based on a five-year follow-up. *Diabetes* **27**: 377–83.
34. Kupfer IJ (1970) Diabetes screening in an outpatient oral surgery clinic. *NY State Dent. J.* **36**: 31–2.
35. Hawthorne VM, Cowie CC (1984) Some thoughts on early detection and intervention in diabetes mellitus. *J. Chron. Dis.* **37**: 667–9
36. Bennett PH, Knowler WC (1984) Early detection and intervention in diabetes mellitus: is it effective? *J. Chron. Dis.* **17**: 653–66.
37. West K (1979) Community screening programs for diabetes? *Diab. Care* **2**: 381–4.
38. West KM, Kalbfleisch JM (1971) Sensitivity and specificity of five screening tests for diabetes in ten countries. *Diabetes* **20**: 289–96
39. World Health Organization Expert Committee on Diabetes Mellitus (1980) Second Report on Diabetes Mellitus. Technical Report Series No. 646, pp. 8–14. Geneva: World Health Organization.
40. National Diabetes Data Group (1979) Classification and diagnosis of diabetes mellitus and other categories of glucose intolerance. *Diabetes* **28**: 1039–57.
41. Calman K (1994) Developing screening in the NHS. *J. Med. Screen.* **1**: 101–5.
42. Morrison AS (1992) *Screening in Chronic Disease, 2nd edn.* New York: Oxford University Press.
43. Wilson JMG, Jungner G (1968) *Principles and Practice of Screening for Disease.* Geneva: World Health Organization.
44. Marshall KG (1996) Prevention. How much harm? How much benefit? 1. Influence of reporting methods on perception of benefits. *Can. Med. Assoc. J.* **154**: 1493–9.
45. Gordis L (1994) The scope of screening. *J. Med. Screen.* **1**: 98–100.
46. Marshall KG (1996) Prevention. How much harm? How much benefit? 4. The ethics of informed consent for preventive screening programs. *Can. Med. Assoc. J.* **155**: 377–83.
47. Marshall KG (1996) Prevention. How much harm? How much benefit? 3. Physical, psychological and social harm. *Can. Med. Assoc. J.* **155**: 169–76.
48. Marshall KG (1996) Prevention. How much harm? How much benefit? 2. Ten potential pitfalls in determining the clinical significance of benefits. *Can. Med. Assoc. J.* **154**: 1837–43.
49. Trilling JS (1990) Screening for non-insulin-dependent diabetes mellitus in the elderly. *Clin. Geriatr. Med.* **6**: 839–48.
50. Browder AA (1994) Screening for diabetes. *Prev. Med.* **3**: 220–4.

51. de Courten M, Zimmet P (1997) Screening for non-insulin-dependent diabetes mellitus: where to draw the line? *Diabet. Med.* **14**: 95–8.
52. Cadman D, Chambers L, Feldman W, Sackett D (1984) Assessing the effectiveness of community screening programs. *JAMA* **251**: 1580–5.
53. National Society to Prevent Blindness (1980) *Vision Problems in the US.* New York: National Society to Prevent Blindness.
54. Klein R, Klein BEK (1985) Vision disorders in diabetes. In (eds Harris MI, Hamman RF) *Diabetes in America.* Bethesda, MD: National Institute of Health.
55. Palmer PF (1977) Diabetic retinopathy. *Diabetes* **26**: 703–9.
56. Klein R, Klein BEK, Moss SE (1984) Visual impairment in diabetes. *Ophthalmology* **91**: 1–9.
57. Eggers PW (1988) Effect of transplantation on Medicare end-stage renal disease program. *N. Engl. J. Med.* **318**: 223–229.
58. Rettig BS, Teutsch SM (1984) The incidence of end-stage renal disease in type I and type II diabetes mellitus. *Diabet. Nephropathy* **3**: 26–7.
59. Centers for Disease Control (1993) *Diabetes Surveillance, 1993.* Atlanta, GA: US Department of Health and Human Services, Public Health Service.
60. Most RS, Sinnock P (1983) The epidemiology of lower extremity amputation in diabeticindividuals. *Diab. Care* **6**: 87–91.
61. Humphrey LL, Palumbo PJ, Butters MA, Hallett JW, Chu CP, O'Fallon M, Ballard DJ (1994) The contribution of non-insulin-dependent diabetes to lower-extremity amputation in the community. *Arch. Intern. Med.* **154**: 885–92.
62. Moss SE, Klein R, Klein BEK (1992) The prevalence and incidence of lower extremity amputation in a diabetic population. *Arch. Intern. Med.* **52**: 610–16.
63. Wetterhall SF, Olson DR, DeStefano F, Stevenson JM, Ford ES, German RR, Will JC, Newman JM, Sepe SJ, Vinicor F (1992) Trends in diabetes and diabetic complications. *Diab. Care* **15**: 960–7.
64. Carter Center of Emory University (1985) Closing the gap: The problem of diabetes mellitus in the United States. *Diab. Care* **8**: 391–406.
65. Panzram G (1987) Mortality and survival in type 2 (non-insulin-dependent) diabetes mellitus. *Diabetologia* **30**: 123–31.
66. Kleinman JC, Donahue RP, Harris MI, Finucane FF, Madans JH, Brock DB (1988) Mortality among diabetics in a national sample. *Am. J. Epidemiol.* **128**: 389–401.
67. Geiss LS, Engelgau M, Frazier E, Tierney E (1997) Diabetes Surveillance, 1997. Atlanta, GA: Centers for Disease Control and Prevention, US Department of Health and Human Services.
68. Papazoglou N, Manes C, Chatzimitrofanous P, Papadeli E, Tzounas K, Scaragas G, Kontogiannis I, Alexiades D (1995) Epidemiology of diabetes mellitus in the elderly in northern Greece: a population study. *Diabet. Med.* **12**: 397–400.
69. Brookmeyer R, Day NE, Moss S (1986) Case-control studies for estimation of the natural history of preclinical disease from screening data. *Stat. Med.* **5**: 127–38.
70. Thompson TJ, Engelgau MM, Hegazy M,. Ali MA, Sous ES, Badran A, Herman WH (1996) The onset of NIDDM and its relationship to clinical diagnosis in Egyptian adults. *Diabet. Med.* **13**: 337–40.
71. Turner R, Cull C, Holman R (1996) United Kingdom Prospective Diabetes Study 17: a 9-year update of a randomized, controlled trial on the effect of improved metabolic control on complications in non-insulin-dependent diabetes mellitus. *Ann. Intern. Med.* **124**: 136–45.
72. Klein R, Klein BEK, Moss SE (1993) Prevalence of microalbuminuria in older-onset diabetes. *Diab. Care* **16**: 1325–30.

73. Eastman RC (1996) Neuropathy in diabetes. In *Diabetes in America,*. 2nd edn. National Diabetes Data Group. Bethesda, MD: National Institute of Health, National Institute of Diabetes and Digestive and Kidney Diseases (NIH publication 95-1468).
74. Wingard DL, Barrett-Connor E (1996)Heart disease in diabetes. In *Diabetes in America,*. 2nd edn. National Diabetes Data Group, Bethesda, MD: National Institute of Health, National Institute of Diabetes and Digestive and Kidney Diseases (NIH publication 95-1468).
75. Eastman RC, Cowie CC, Harris MI (1997) Undiagnosed diabetes or impaired glucose tolerance and cardiovascular risk. *Diab. Care* **20**: 127–8.
76. CDC Diabetes Cost-Effectiveness Study Group (1998) The cost-effectiveness of screening for type 2 diabetes. *JAMA* **280**: 1757–63.
77. Gold MR, Siegel JE, Russell LB, Weinstein MC (1996) *Cost-Effectiveness in Health and Medicine.* New York: Oxford University Press.
78. Rembold CM (1998) Number needed to screen: development of a statistic for disease screening. *BMJ* **317**: 307–12.
79. Donaldson C (1994) Using ecomonics to assess the place of screening. *J. Med. Screen.* **1**: 124–9.
80. Sasco AJ (1991) Validity of case-control studies and randomized controlled trials of screening *Internat. Epidemiol.* **20**: 1143–4.
81. Davies M, Day J (1996) The Cochrane Collaborative Diabetes Review Group. *Diabet. Med.* **13**: 390–1.
82. Airey CM, Williams DRR (1995) Cochrane Collaboration Review Group: Diabetes. *Diabet. Med.* **12**: 375–6.
83. Manservigi D, Samori G, Graziani R, Bottoni L (1982) Impaired glucose tolerance and clinical diabetes: a 6-year follow-up of screened versus non-screened subjects. *Diabetologia* **23**: 185.
84. Klein R (1995) Hyperglycemia and microvascular and macrovascular disease in diabetes. *Diab. Care* **18**: 258–68.
85. Liu QZ, Knowler WC, Nelson RG, Saad MF, Charles MA, Liebow IM, Bennett PH, Pettitt DJ (1992) Insulin treatment, endogenous insulin concentration, and ECG abnormalities in diabetic Pima Indians. Cross-sectional and prospective analyses. *Diabetes* **41**: 1141–50.
86. Coutinho M, Gerstein HC, Wang Y, Yusef S (1999) The relationship between glucose and incident cardiovascular events. A metaregression analysis of published data from 20 studies of 95783 individuals followed for 12.4 years. *Diab. Care* **22**: 233–40.
87. University Group Diabetes Program (1970) A study of the effects of hypoglycemic agents on vascular complications in patients with adult-onset diabetes. *Diabetes* **19**: 747–830.
88. Ohkubo Y, Kishikawa H, Araki E, Miyata T, Isami S, Motoyoshi S, Kojima Y, Furuyoshi N, Shichiri M (1995) Intensive insulin therapy present in the original progression of diabetic microvascular complications in Japanese patients with non-insulin-dependent diabetes mellitus: a randomized prospective six-year study. *Diabetes Res. Clin. Pract.* **28**: 103–117.
89. The Diabetes Control and Complications Trial Research Group (1993) The effect of intensive treatment of diabetes on the development and progression of long-term complications in insulin-dependent diabetes mellitus. *N. Engl. J. Med.* **329**: 977–86.
90. Abraira C, Colwell J, Nuttall F, Sawin CT, Henderson W, Comstock JP, Emanuele NV, Levin SR, Pacold I, Lee HS (1997) Cardiovascular events and correlates in the Veterans Affairs Diabetes Feasibility Trial. Veterans Affairs Cooperative Study on

Glycemic Control and Complications in Type II Diabetes. *Arch. Intern. Med.* **157**: 181–8.

91. UKPDS Group (1998) Tight blood pressure control and risk of macrovascular and microvascular complications in type 2 diabetes: UKPDS 38. *BMJ* **317**: 703–13.

92. UKPDS Group (1998) Intensive blood-glucose control with sulphonylureas or insulin compared with conventional treatment and risk of complications in patients with type 2 diabetes (UKPDS 33). *Lancet* **352**: 837–53.

93. UKPDS Group (1998) Effect of intensive blood-glucose control with metformin on complications in overweight patients with type 2 diabetes (UKPDS 34). *Lancet* **352**: 854–65.

94. Vijan S, Hofer TP, Hayward RA (1997) Estimating benefits of glycemic control in microvascular complication in type 2 diabetes. *Ann. Intern. Med.* **127**: 788–95.

95. Ferris FL (1993) How effective are treatments for diabetic retinopathy? *JAMA* **269**: 1290–1.

96. Diabetic Retinopathy Study Group (1981) Photocoagulation treatment of proliferative diabetic retinopathy: Clinical application of diabetic retinopathy study (DRS) findings. *Ophthalmology* **88**: 583–600.

97. ETDRS Research Group (1985) Photocoagulation for diabetic macular edema. *Arch. Ophthalmol.* **103**: 1796–1806.

98. Lewis EJ, Hunsicker LG, Bain RP, Rohde RD (1993) The effect of angiotensin-converting- enzyme inhibition on diabetic nephropathy. *N. Engl. J. Med.* **329**: 1456–62.

99. Kasiske BL, Kalil RSN, Ma JZ, Liao M, Keane WF (1993) Effect of antihypertensive therapy on the kidney in patients with diabetes: A meta-regression analysis. *Ann. Intern. Med.* **118**: 129–38.

100. Reiber GE, Pecoraro RE, Koepsell TD (1992) Risk factors for amputation in patients with diabetes mellitus. A case-control study. *Ann. Intern. Med.* **117**: 97–105.

101. Bild DE, Selby JV, Sinnock P, Browner WS, Braveman P, Showstack JA (1989) Lower-extremity amputation in people with diabetes. Epidemiology and prevention. *Diab. Care* **12**: 24–31.

102. Welborn TA, Wearne K (1979) Coronary heart disease incidence and cardiovascular mortality in Busselton with reference to glucose and insulin concentrations. *Diab. Care* **2**: 154–60.

103. Pyorala K, Savolainen E, Kaukola S, Haapakoski J (1985) Plasma insulin as a coronary heart disease risk factor: relationship to other risk factors and predictive value during 9.5-year follow-up of the Helsinki Policeman Study Population. *Acta. Med. Scand.* **701**: 38–52.

104. Fontbonne A, Charles MA, Thibult N, Richard JL, Claude JR, Warnet JM, Rossellin GE, Eschwege E (1991) Hyperinsulinemia as a predictor of coronary heart disease mortality in a healthy population: the Paris Prospective Study, 15-year follow-up. *Diabetologia* **34**: 356–61.

105. US Preventive Services Task Force (1996). *Guide to Clinical Preventive Services,*. 2nd edn. Alexandria, VA: International Medical Publishing.

106. UKPDS Group (1999) Quality of life in type 2 diabetic patients is affected by complications but not by intensive policies to improve blood glucose or blood pressure control (UKPDS 37). *Diab. Care* **22**: 1125–36.

107. Bulpitt CJ, Benos AS, Nicholl CG, Fletcher AE (1990) Should medical screening of the elderly population be promoted? *Gerontology* **36**: 230–45.

108. Mausner JS, Kramer S (1985) *Epidemiology – An Introductory Text.* Philadelphia: W.B. Saunders.

109. Fletcher RH, Fletcher SW, Wagner EH (1988) *Clinical Epidemiology: The Essentials.* Baltimore: Williams and Wilkins.
110. Hennekens CH, Buring JE (1987) *Epidemiology in Medicine.* (Ed. Mayrent SL) Boston: Little Brown.
111. Reid MC, Lachs MS, Feinstein AR (1995) Use of methodological standards in diagnostic test research: getting better but still not good. *JAMA* **274**: 645–51.
112. Centor RM, Schwartz JS (1985) An evaluation of methods for estimating the area under the receiver operating characteristic (ROC) curve. *Med. Decis. Making* **5**: 149–58.
113. Hanley JA, McNeil BJ (1983) A method of comparing the areas under receiver operating characteristic curves derived from the same cases. *Radiology* **148**: 839–43.
114. Bamber D (1975) The area above the ordinal dominancy graph and the area below the receiver operating characteristic graph. *J. Math. Psychol.* **12**: 387–415.
115. Beck JR, Shultz EK (1986) The use of relative operating characteristic (ROC) curves in test performance evaluation. *Arch. Pathol. Lab. Med.* **110**: 13–20.
116. Centor RM (1985) A visicalc program for estimating the area under a receiver operating characteristic (ROC) curve. *Med. Decis. Making* **5**: 139–48.
117. American Diabetes Association (1999) Screening for type 2 diabetes. *Diab. Care* **21**: S20–S23.
118. Duncan WE, Linville N, Clement S (1993) Assessing risk factors when screening for diabetes mellitus. *Diab. Care* **16**: 1403–4.
119. American Diabetes Association (1993) American diabetes alert. *Diab. Forecast* **46**: 54.
120. Newman WP, Nelson R, Scheer K (1994) Community screening for diabetes. Low detection rate in a low-risk population. *Diab. Care* **17**: 363–5.
121. Burden ML, Burden AC (1994) The American Diabetes Association screening questionnaire for diabetes. Is it worthwhile in the UK? *Diab. Care* **17**: 97.
122. Herman WH, Smith PJ, Thompson TJ, Engelgau MM, Aubert RE (1995) Take the test: know the score. A new questionnaire to identify persons at increased risk for undiagnosed diabetes mellitus. *Diab. Care* **18**: 382–7.
123. Herman WH, Smith PJ, Thompson TJ, Engelgau MM, Aubert RE (1998) Response to Knudson *et al. Diab. Care* **21**: 1030–1.
124. Ruige JB, de Neeling JN, Kostense PJ, Bouter LM, Heine RJ (1997) Performance of an NIDDM screening questionnaire based on symptoms and risk factors. *Diab. Care* **20**: 491–6.
125. McGregor MS, Pinkham C, Ahroni JH, Herter CD, Doctor JD (1995) The American Diabetes Association risk test for diabetes. *Diab. Care* **18**: 585–6.
126. Knudson PE, Turner KJ, Sedore A, Weinstock RS (1998) Utility of the American Diabetes Association risk test in a community screening program. *Diab. Care* **21**: 1029–31.
127. McGregor MS, Pinkham C, Ahroni JH, Kerter CD, Doctor JD (1995) The American Diabetes Association risk test for diabetes. Is it a useful screening tool? *Diab. Care* **18**: 585–6.
128. Andersson DK, Lundblad E, Svardsudd K (1993) A model of early diagnosis in type 2 diabetes mellitus in primary health care. *Diabetic Med.* **10**: 167–73.
129. Hanson RL, Nelson RG, McCance DR, Beart JA, Charles MA, Pettitt DJ, Knowler WC (1993) Comparison of screening tests for non-insulin-dependent diabetes mellitus. *Arch. Intern. Med.* **153**: 2133–40.
130. Forrest RD, Jackson CA, Yudkin JS (1987) The glycohaemoglobin assay as a screening test for diabetes mellitus: The Islington Diabetes Survey. *Diabet. Med.* **4**: 254–9.

131. Davies M, Alban-Davies H, Cook C, Day J (1991) Self testing for diabetes mellitus. *BMJ* **303**: 696–8.

132. Anokute CC (1990) Epidemiologic studies of diabetes mellitus in Saudi Arabia. Part I–screening of 3158 males in King Saud University. *J. R. Soc. Health* **110**: 201–3.

133. Orzeck EA, Mooney JH, Owen JA (1971) Diabetes detection with a comparison of screening methods. *Diabetes* **20**: 109–16.

134. Davies MJ, Williams DRR, Metcalfe J, Day JL (1993) Community screening for non- insulin-dependent diabetes mellitus: self-testing for post-prandial glycosuria. *Q. J. Med.* **86**: 677–84.

135. Robertson DA, Albeti KGMM, Cowse GK, Zimmet P, Toumilehto J, Gareeboo H (1992) Is serum anhydroglucitol an alternative to the oral glucose tolerance test for diabetes screening? *Diabet. Med.* **10**: 56–60.

136. Simon D, Coignet MC, Thibilt N, Senan C, Eschwege E (1985) Comparison of glycosylated hemoglobin and fasting plasma glucose with two-hour post-load plasma glucose in the detection of diabetes mellitus. *Am. J. Epidemiol.* **122**: 589–93.

137. Modan M, Harris MI (1994) Fasting plasma glucose in screening for NIDDM in the US and Israel. *Diab. Care* **17**: 436–439.

138. Haffner SM, Rosenthal M, Hazuda HP, Stern MP, Franco LJ (1984) Evaluation of three potential screening tests for diabetes in a biethenic population. *Diab. Care* **7**: 347–53.

139. Forrest RD, Jackson CA, Judkin JS (1988) The abbreviated glucose tolerance test in screening for diabetes: the Islington Diabetes Study. *Diabetic Med.* **5**: 557–61.

140. Tsuji I, Nakamoto K, Hasegawa T, Hisashige A, Inawashiro H, Fukao A, Hisamichi S (1991) Receiver operating characteristic analysis on fasting plasma glucose, HbA$_{1c}$, and fructosamine on diabetes screening. *Diab. Care* **14**: 1075–7.

141. Blunt BA, Barrett-Conner E, Windgard D (1991) Evaluation of fasting plasma glucose as a screening test for NIDDM in older adults. Rancho Bernardo Study. *Diab. Care* **14**: 989–93.

142. Modan M, Halkin H, Karasik A, Lusky A (1984) Effectiveness of glycosylated hemoglobin, fasting plasma glucose, and a single post load plasma glucose level in population screening for glucose tolerance. *Am. J. Epidemiol.* **119**: 431–44.

143. Swai AB, Harrison K, Chuwa LM, Makene W, McLarty D, Alberti KG (1988) Screening for diabetes: Does measurement of serum fructosamine help? *Diabet. Med.* **5**: 648–52.

144. Bourn D, Mann J (1992) Screening for noninsulin dependent diabetes mellitus and impaired glucose tolerance in a Dunedin general practice – is it worth it? *N. Z. Med. J.* **105**: 208–10.

145. Abernathy MH, Andre C, Beaven DW, Taylor, HW, Welsh G (1977) A random blood sugar diabetes detection survey. *N. Z. Med.* **86**: 123–6.

146. Sigurdsson G, Gorrskalksson G, Thorsteinsson T, Davidsson D, Olafsson O, Samuelsson S, Sigfusson N (1981) Community screening for glucose intolerance in middle-aged Icelandic men. *Acta. Med. Scand.* **210**: 21–6.

147. Moses RG, Colagiuri S, Shannon AG (1985) Effectiveness of mass screening for diabetes mellitus using random capillary blood glucose measurements. *Med. J. Aust.* **143**: 544–6.

148. Lee CH, Fook-Chong S (1997) Evaluation of fasting plasma glucose as a screening test for diabetes mellitus in Singaporean adults. *Diabet. Med.* **14**: 119–22.

149. Chang CJ, Wu JS, Lu FH, Lee HL, Yang YC, Wen MJ (1998) Fasting plasma glucose in screening for diabetes in the Taiwanese population. *Diab. Care* **21**: 1856–60.
150. Nitiyanant W, Ploybutr S, Sriussadaporn S, Yamwong P, Vannasaeng S (1998) Evaluation of the new fasting plasma glucose cutpoint of 7.0 mmol/l in detection of diabetes mellitus in the Thai population. *Diabetes Res. Clin. Prac.* **41**: 171–6.
151. Wiener K (1997) Fasting plasma glucose as a screening test for diabetes mellitus. *Diabet. Med.* **14**: 711–2
152. Ko GT, Chan JC, Yeung VT, Chow CC, Tsang LW, Li JK, So WY, Wai HP, Cockram CS (1998) Combined use of a fasting plasma glucose concentration and HbA$_{1c}$ or fructosamine predicts the likelihood of having diabetes in high-risk subjects. *Diab. Care* **21**: 1221–5.
153. Bortheiry A, Malerbi DA, Franco LJ (1994) The ROC curve in the evaluation of fasting capillary blood glucose as a screening test for diabetes and IGT. *Diab. Care* **17**: 1269–72.
154. Ferrell RE, Hanis CL, Aguilar L, Tulloch B, Garcia C, Schull WJ (1984) Glycosylated hemoglobin determination from capillary blood samples. Utility in an epidemiologic survey of diabetes. *Am. J. Epidemiol.* **119**: 159–66.
155. Forrest RD, Jackson CA, Yudkin JS (1987) Screening for diabetes mellitus in general practice using a reflectance meter system. The Islington Diabetes Survey. *Diabetes Res.* **6**: 119–22.
156. Ko GTC, Chan JCN, Cockram CS (1998) Supplement to the use of a paired value of fasting plasma glucose and glycated hemoglobin in predicting the likelihood of having diabetes. *Diab. Care* **21**: 2032–3.
157. Santiago JV, Davis JE, Fisher F (1978) Hemoglobin A$_{1c}$ levels in a diabetes detection program. *J. Clin. Endocrinol. Metab.* **47**: 578–80.
158. Sekikawa A, Tominaga M, Takahashi K, Watanabe H, Miyazawa K, Sasaki H (1990) Is examination of fructosamine levels valuable as a diagnostic test for diabetes mellitus? *Diabetes Res. Clin. Pract.* **8**: 187–92.
159. Little RR, England JD, Wiedmeyer HM, McKenzie EM, Pettitt DJ, Knowler WC, Goldstein DE (1988) Relationship of glycosylated hemoglobin to oral glucose tolerance: Implications in diabetes screening. *Diabetes* **37**: 60–64.
160. Orchard TJ, Daneman D, Becher D, Kuller LH, LaPorte RE, Drash AL, Wagener D (1982) Glycosylated hemoglobin: a screening test for diabetes mellitus? *Prev. Med.* **11**: 595–601.
161. Motala AA, Omar MAK (1992) The values of glycosylated haemoglobin as a substitute for the oral glucose tolerance test in the detection of impaired glucose tolerance (IGT). *Diabetes Res. Clin. Prac.* **17**: 199–207.
162. Verrillo A, Teresa AD, Golia R, Nunziata V (1983) The relationship between glycosylated haemoglobin levels and various degrees of glucose intolerance. *Diabetologia* **24**: 391–3.
163. Guillausseau PJ, Charles MA, Paloaggi F, Timsit J, Chanson P, Peynet J, Godard V, Eschwege E, Rousselet F, Lubetzki J (1990) Comparison of HbA1 and fructosamine in diagnosis of glucose-tolerance abnormalities. *Diab. Care* **13**: 898–900.
164. Kesson CM, Young RE, Talwar D, Whitelaw JW, Robb DA (1982) Glycosylated hemoglobin in the diagnosis of non-insulin-dependent diabetes mellitus. *Diab. Care* **5**: 395–8.
165. Goldstein DE, Little RR, England JD, Wiedmeyer HM, McKenzie E (1989) Glycated hemoglobin: Is it a useful screening test for diabetes mellitus? In *Frontiers of Diabetes Research: Current Trends in Non-insulin-dependent Diabetes Mellitus* (eds Alberti KGMM, Mazze R) New York: Elsevier Science.

166. Lester E, Frazer AD, Shepard CA, Woodroffe FJ (1985) Glycosylated haemoglobin as an alternative to the glucose tolerance test for the diagnosis of diabetes mellitus. *Ann. Clin. Biochem.* **22**: 74–8.

167. Salemans THB, van Dieijen-Vissser MP, Brombacher PJ (1987) The value of HbA1 and fructosamine in predicting impaired glucose tolerance – an alternative to OGTT to detect diabetes mellitus or gestational diabetes. *Ann. Clin. Biochem.* **24**: 447–452.

168. Croxson SCM, Absalom S, Burden AC (1991) Fructosamine in diabetes screening of the elderly. *Ann. Clin. Biochem.* **28**: 279–82.

169. Frattali AL, Wolf BA (1994) 1.5-anhydroglucitol: A novel serum marker for screening and monitoring diabetes mellitus? *Clin. Chem.* **40**: 1991–3.

170. Tanabe T, Umegae Y, Koyashiki Y, Kato Y, Fukahori K, Tajima S, Yabuuchi M (1994) Fully antomated flow-injection system for quantifying 1.5-anhydro-d-glucitol in serum. *Clin. Chem.* **40**: 2006–12.

171. Fukumura Y, Tajima S, Oshitani S, Ushijima Y, Kobasyashi I, Hara F, Yamamoto S, Yabuuchi M (1994) Fully enzymatic method for detemining 1.5-anhydro-d-glucitol in serum. *Clin. Chem.* **40**: 2013–16.

172. Engelgau MM, Thompson TJ, Smith PJ, Herman WH, Aubert RE, Gunter EW, Wetterhall SF, Sous ES, Ali MA (1995) Screening for diabetes mellitus in adults: The utility of random capillary blood glucose measurements. *Diab. Care* **18**: 463–6.

173. Blunt BA, Barrett-Connor E, Wingard DL (1991) Evaluation of fasting plasma glucose as a screening test for NIDDM in older adults. Rancho Bernardo Study. *Diab. Care* **14**: 989–93.

174. Goldstein DE, Little RR, Wiedmeyer HM, England JD, Rohlfing CL, Wilke AL (1994) Is glycohemoglobin testing useful in diabetes mellitus? Lessons from the Diabetes Control and Complications Trial. *Clin. Chem.* **40**: 1837–40.

175. Kilpatrick ES, Maylor PW, Keevil BG (1998) Biological variation of glycated hemoglobin. Implications for diabetes screening and monitoring. *Diab. Care* **21**: 261–4.

176. Yudkin JS, Forrest RD, Jackson CA, Ryle AJ, Davie S, Gould BJ (1990) Unexplained variability of glycated hemoglobin in nondiabetic subjects not related to glycemia. *Diabetologia* **33**: 208–15.

177. Modan M, Meytes D, Roseman P, Yosef SB, Sehayek E, Yosef NB (1988) Significance of high HbA1 levels in normal glucose tolerance. *Diab. Care* **11**: 422–28.

178. Mold JW, Aspy CB, Lawler FH (1998) Outcomes of an insurance company-sponsored multichannel chemistry screening initiative. *J. Fam. Pract.* **47**: 110–7.

179. Frame PS, Berg AO, Woolf S (1997) US Preventive Services Task Force: highlights of the 1996 report. *Amer. Fam. Physician* **55**: 567–76, 581–2.

180. Home PD (1994) Diagnosing the undiagnosed with diabetes. *BMJ* **308**: 611–2.

181. Worrall G 1994) Screening the population for diabetes. *BMJ* **308**: 1639.

182. Davidoff F, Reinecke RD (1999) The 28th Amendment. *Ann. Inter. Med.* **130**: 692–4.

183. Laupacis A, Feeny D, Detsky AS, Tugwell PX (1992) How attractive does a new technology have to be to warrant adoption and utilization? Tentative guidelines for using clinical and economic evaluations. *Can. Med. Assoc. J.* **146**: 473–81.

184. Davies M, Day J (1994) Screening for non-insulin-dependent diabetes mellitus (NIDDM): how often should it be done? *J. Med. Screen.* **1**: 78–81.

185. Worrall G (1992) Screening for diabetes – an alternative view. *Br. J. Gen. Pract.* **42**: 304.

186. Santrach PJ, Burritt MF (1995) Point-of care testing. *Mayo. Clin. Proc.* **70**: 493–4.
187. Law M (1995) 'Opportunistic' screening. *J. Med. Screen.* **1**: 208.
188. Davies M, Day J (1994) Screening for non-insulin-dependent diabetes mellitus (NIDDM): how often should it be performed? *J. Med. Screen.* **1**: 18–81.
189. Cowie CC, Harris MI, Eberhardt MS (1994) Frequency and determinants of screening for diabetes in the US *Diab. Care* **17**: 1158–63.
190. Luckmann R, Melville SK (1995) Periodic health evaluation of adults: a survey of family physicians. *J. Fam. Prac.* **40**: 547–54.
191. Herbert CP (1995) Clinical health promotion and family physicians: a Canadian perspective. *Patient Educ. Couns.* **25**: 277–82.
192. Stange KC, Flocke SA, Goodwin MA (1998) Opportunistic preventive services delivery. Are time limitations and patient satisfaction barriers? *J. Fam. Prac.* **46**: 419–24.
193. Dickey LL, Kamerow DB (1996) Primary care physicians' use of office resources in the provision of preventive care. *Arch. Fam. Med.* **5**: 399–404.
194. Singh BM, Prescott JJ, Guy R, Walford S, Murphy M (1994) Effect of advertising on awareness of symptoms of diabetes among the general public: the British Diabetic Association Study. *BMJ* **308**: 632–6.
195. Bourn D, Mann J (1992) Screening for noninsulin-dependent diabetes mellitus and impaired glucose tolerance in a Dunedin general practice – is it worth it? *N.Z. Med. J.* **105**: 207–10.
196. Clement S, Duncan W, Coffey L, Dean K, Kinum N (1989) Screening for diabetes mellitus. *Ann. Intern. Med.* **110**: 572–3.
197. Solomon AC, Hoag SG, Kloesel WA (1977) A community pharmacist-sponsored diabetes detection program. *J. Am. Pharm. Assoc.* **17**: 161–3.
198. Bernard JA (1971) Diabetic screening program held in El Paso, November 19-21, 1970. *Southwestern Medicine* **2**: 33–34.
199. Ross BC (1985) Diabetes screening for over 70 motor drivers. *N.Z. Med. J.* **98**: 1093.
200. Engelgau MM, Narayan KM, Geiss LS, Thompson TJ, Beckles GL, Lopez L, Hartwell T, Visscher W, Liburd L (1998) A project to reduce the burden of diabetes in the African-American community: Project DIRECT. *J. Nat. Med. Assoc.* **90**: 605–13.
201. Hayward RSA, Steinberg EP, Ford DE, Roizen MF, Roach KW (1991) Preventive Care. Guidelines: 1991. *Ann. Intern. Med.* **114**: 758–83.
202. Canadian Task Force on Periodic Health Examination (1979) Periodic health examination. *Can. Med. Assoc. J.* **121**: 1193–1254.
203. www.aafp.org/policy/camp/app-d.html
204. Houston TP, Elster AB, Davis RM, Deitchman SD (1998) The U.S. Preventive Services Task Force Guide to Clinical Preventive Services, second edition. AMA Council on Scientific Affairs. *Am. J. Prev. Med.* **14**: 374–6.
205. Harwell TS, Smile JG, McDowall JM, Helgerson SD, Gohdes D (2000) Diabetes screening practice among individuals age 45 years and older. *Diab. Care* **23**: 125–6.
206. Amiel SA (1997) Screening for curly two disease: a transatlantic perspective. *Diabet. Med.* **14**: 635–6.
207. Quickel KE (1996) Diabetes in a managed care system. *Ann. Intern. Med.* **124**: 160–3.
208. Cairns JA, Shackley P (1994) Assessing value for money in medical screening. *J. Med. Screen.* **1**: 39–44.
209. Rohlfing CL, Little RR, Wiedmeyer HM, England JD, Madsen R, Harris MI, Flegal KM, Eberhardt MS, Goldstein DE (2000) Use of Ghb (HbA_{1c}) in screening for undiagnosed diabetes in the US population. *Diab. Care* **23**: 187–91.

210. Azzopardi J, Fenech FF, Junoussov Z, Mazovetsky A, Olchanski V (1995) A computerized health screening and follow-up system in diabetes mellitus. *Diabet. Med.* **12**: 271–6.
211. Abernethy MH, Andre C, Beaven DW, Taylor HW, Welsh G (1977) A random blood sugar diabetes detection survey. *N.Z. Med. J.* **86**: 123–6.
212. Kent GT, Leonards JR (1968) Analysis of tests for diabetes in 250000 persons screened for diabetes using finger blood after a carbohydrate load. *Diabetes* **17**: 274–80.
213. Orzech EA, Mooney JH, Owen JA (1971) Diabetes detection with a comparison of screening methods. *Diabetes* **20**: 109–16.
214. Moses RG, Colagiuri S, Shannon AG (1985) Effectiveness of mass screening for diabetes mellitus using random capillary blood glucose measurements. *Med. J. Aust.* **143**: 544–6.
215. Rand CG, Jackson RJD, Mackie CC (1974) A method for the epidemiologic study of early diabetes. *Can. Med. Assoc. J.* **111**: 1312–14.

9

Understanding and Avoiding the Adverse Psychological Effects of Screening: A Commentary

THERESA M. MARTEAU

King's College, London SE1 9RT, UK

Screening for disease has the potential to do harm as well as good. Given a clinically effective screening programme, the harm and benefits depend critically upon how people respond to the information they are given about their risks. How anxious are those with a positive result made? How likely are those with a positive result to follow advice to reduce their risks or treat their disease? Do those who receive a negative result understand that they still have a chance, albeit small, of developing the disease?

This commentary considers the emotional and behavioural consequences of screening, and describes the characteristics of screening programmes that avoid or produce least harm, and those that realise most benefits. The commentary draws upon examples from a range of screening programmes, including screening for diabetes, aimed at detecting disease or risk of disease in adults. This allows conclusions to be based upon a larger literature than would be possible if it were restricted to screening for diabetes only. The validity of this approach is suggested by the fact that the emotional and behavioural responses to risk information are broadly similar across screening for different diseases[1]. Thus the research findings on cardiovascular screening programmes are likely to be relevant in predicting individuals' responses to diabetes screening.

The Evidence Base for Diabetes Care. Edited by R. Williams, W. Herman, A.-L. Kinmonth and N. J. Wareham.
© 2002 John Wiley & Sons, Ltd

AVOIDING THE PSYCHOLOGICAL HARMS OF SCREENING

Screening for risk of various diseases has formed a significant part of health care in many countries for over 50 years[2]. The psychological impact of screening was largely unquestioned until the publication of a paper by Haynes and colleagues[3] describing increased rates of absenteeism following the detection of hypertension in a group of steelworkers. Since this time there have been numerous studies assessing the emotional and behavioural effects of screening. The two main harms that have been documented in those undergoing screening are psychological distress and false reassurance.

DISTRESS

The first systematic evaluation of the psychological impact of being invited for screening provides no evidence that being invited to participate in a screening programme raises anxieties or concerns about illness[4]. Nor is there any good evidence to suggest that participating in a screening programme and receiving a negative result causes distress[1]. There is, however, good evidence to show that receipt of a positive test result on screening is associated with raised levels of anxiety in the short term. In most studies this distress is found to be short-lived. For example, Johnson and Tercyak[5] described the psychological impact of identifying children and adults who were at risk for developing insulin-dependent diabetes by screening for islet cell antibodies (ICA). Identification of ICA-positive individuals resulted initially in clinically significant levels of anxiety for adults, children, parents and spouses. This, however, had dissipated by four months. But in about a quarter of studies, anxiety continues to be raised even when further investigations fail to find a problem. For example, 18 months after a false positive result on mammography screening for breast cancer, 29% of women reported anxiety about breast cancer compared with 13% of women who received a negative result[6].

Among those found to be at increased risk or with a confirmed diagnosis of diabetes, an element of concern is appropriate and may motivate individuals to reduce their risks or to reduce the burden of the disease. Johnston and Tercyak[5], for example, found that anxiety following disclosure of test results was positively associated with change in diet or increased activity, such that higher levels of anxiety were associated with greater changes in behaviour which would reduce the risk of developing diabetes. In those with diabetes, one study suggests the beneficial effects of raising anxiety about diabetic complications[7]. Patients who received an educational intervention comprising slides depicting infected diabetic feet and amputated limbs had lower amputation rates two years after the intervention than the group randomised to receive written information only on care of their feet. Too much anxiety can inhibit acting to reduce a threat[8], and in some cases can result in over-compliance which can damage health[9]. Similarly, depression significantly reduces the chances of individuals complying with health advice or medical treatment[10]. Raised anxiety, fear or concern are rarely sufficient to motivate behaviour change. Motivation to change behaviour requires individuals to perceive benefits to changing their behaviour as well as perceive that such change is possible. Motivation to change behaviour is more likely to occur if individuals are helped to form action plans specifying when, where and how the intended behaviour will occur[11,12]. Change is also more likely following participation in intervention programmes with evidence of effectiveness[13].

PREDICTING DISTRESS

Responses to any event are in part a reflection of individuals and in part a reflection of the situation in which they find themselves. Two of the characteristics of individuals that predict their responses are their emotional resources and prior awareness of risk. Emotional resources include general mood, coping skills and social support. The importance of these resources is illustrated in studies of individuals undergoing predictive genetic testing. Amongst those with a known family history of a genetic disorder, emotional responses to predictive testing are predicted more by pretest mood than by the results of testing[14]. In a study of the impact of screening on first-degree relatives screened for type 2 diabetes, Farmer and colleagues[15] found that while there was no main effect of screening upon anxiety, anxiety was raised following screening among those who had undergone previous treatment for anxiety or depression.

Those who are aware of an increased risk of a disease before screening experience less anxiety upon receipt of a positive test result than do those with no previous knowledge[16,17]. In keeping with this, screening of non-diabetic siblings of patients with NIDDM resulted in minimal changes in levels of anxiety[18]. By contrast, receipt of a false positive result following screening pregnant women with no previous awareness of their risk of gestational diabetes left them with a lowered perception of their health[19].

AVOIDING ANXIETY

Experimental studies from screening for conditions other than diabetes suggest how some of the very high levels of anxiety from screening may be avoided or reduced. Providing detailed information about their meaning when giving test results has been shown in several studies to avoid high levels of anxiety[1]. Reflecting this evidence, the General Medical Council in the UK has recently produced guidelines on the information needed for informed choice, including informed choice to undergo screening[20]. These state that, in order to ensure that screening is not contrary to the individual's interests, it is necessary to explain five points:

- the purpose of screening;
- the likelihood of positive and negative findings, along with the possibility of false positive and negative findings;
- the uncertainties and risks attached to the screening process;
- any significant medical, social or financial implications of screening;
- follow-up plans including the availability of counselling and support services.

Given evidence that some groups of individuals are more vulnerable to distress than others following participation in screening programmes, identifying these groups and providing them with more information and support both before the test is taken and when the results are given may be an efficient use of resources in screening programmes. Two vulnerable groups that have already been identified are those with positive test results who are anxious or depressed at the time of screening or who have a history of emotional problems, and those with a positive test result who were unaware prior to screening of having an increased risk for the screened condition. The latter group are most common in population-based screening programmes.

FALSE REASSURANCE

False negative results are inevitable in any screening programme, given that sensitivity will be less than 100%. There is growing recognition of the possible harm that could result from this. Such harm includes delay in seeking treatment if symptoms occur, poor psychological adjustment to the disease, and litigation. In contrast with the large amount of research carried out on the psychological consequences of positive results in screening, there has been little systematic research on the consequences of false negative results. In a recent systematic review[21], 6660 abstracts were screened and 420 potentially relevant papers identified. Only one paper presented evidence on the psychological consequences of false negative results in antenatal screening, and only two provided evidence on the economic consequences. There is some evidence that false negative results may have a large legal impact based on reports in the UK and the USA. In addition, the authors of the review suggested that there is a consensus in the literature that false negatives may have an adverse effect on public confidence in screening, although empirical evidence on this is lacking.

FACTORS CONTRIBUTING TO FALSE REASSURANCE

One of the main sources of false reassurance is the failure of those providing screening to give appropriate information on the performance of the test to those participating in their programmes. For example, a content analysis of mammography leaflets in Australia found that only 26% mentioned sensitivity and none mentioned specificity of the test[22]. One reason why leaflets may not contain such information is the belief that this may deter people from attending for screening. Such a position reflects a public health view of the purpose of screening being to reduce the prevalence of disease in the population. Such a position is no longer considered ethical if the public health aim is achieved at the cost of patients being able to exercise an informed decision about whether or not to participate in a screening programme[23]. Even where information is provided in writing, this may not be explained or reinforced by those presenting a screening test. One reason for this is that health professionals themselves can lack knowledge of test sensitivity and specificity[24].

Even if individuals are informed of the meaning of a negative test result, a number of psychological processes may prevent this information from being retained. First, individuals may not understand the information given. Second, they may understand but then forget it. Third, they may understand the information but perceive the residual risk of a negative result as so low as to be equivalent to no risk. There is a well-recognised tendency for probabilities to be perceived categorically, with low-probability events being seen as being equivalent to no risk. A final process that may undermine retention of information about a small residual risk is the tendency for people to recall information that underplays risk, sometimes referred to as threat minimisation[25].

AVOIDING FALSE REASSURANCE

A first step towards reducing false reassurance from screening is to correct misconceptions about the purpose of screening and the accuracy of screening tests in the general public, in those undergoing screening as well as health professionals[21]. Brief training of health professionals can increase their knowledge of screening as well as the quality and quantity of information they provide when offering screening[26]. However, such training may be difficult to implement in practice. Only 27% of those invited to participate in Smith *et al.*'s trial, aimed at improving communication of screening tests in antenatal care, completed the training, and those with the poorest skills were least likely to complete the trial. While the GMC guidelines state that the meaning of negative tests results should be explained, they provide no guidance on the most effective way of explaining them. The results of two experimental studies show that the proportion of those receiving negative results who understand the residual risk inherent in such a result can be increased significantly by the use of a simple sentence or the use of a numerical probability expressing the meaning of the result[27,28].

CONCLUDING COMMENT

Avoiding harm from screening is important not only from an ethical perspective but also from a clinical one. Screening programmes that result in high levels of distress among those with a positive result, or high rates of false reassurance for those with negative results will reduce the chances of individuals acting appropriately to reduce the risk of disease. The design and implementation of any screening trial or programme needs to incorporate this evidence. Different ways of providing information and support need to be evaluated, and perhaps tailored to address the different emotional and informational needs of participants. In addition, screening programmes such as those envisaged for diabetes need to consider not only how to deliver screening in order to avoid harm, but how to deliver screening in order to motivate individuals to reduce their risk of the disease. This is a great research and clinical challenge for the next decade. Linking the presentation of risk information to programmes facilitating behaviour change provides a great research and clinical challenge for the next decade.

ACKNOWLEDGEMENT

The author is funded by The Wellcome Trust.

REFERENCES

1. Shaw C, Abrams K, Marteau TM (1991) Psychological impact of predicting individuals' risk of illness: a systematic review. *Social Science & Medicine* **49**: 1571–1598.
2. Holland WW, Stewart S (1990) *Screening in Health Care. Benefit or Bane?* London: Nuffield Provincial Hospitals Trust.
3. Haynes RB, Sackett DL, Taylor DW, Gibson ES, Johnson AL (1978) Increased absenteeism from work after detection and labeling of hypertensive patients. *New England Journal of Medicine* **299**: 741–744.
4. Wardle J, Taylor T, Sutton S, Atkin W (1999) Does publicity about cancer screening raise fear of cancer? Randomised trial of the psychological effect of information about cancer screening. *British Medical Journal* **319**: 1037–1038.
5. Johnson SB, Tercyak KP (1995) Psychological impact of islet cell antibody screening for IDDM on children, adults, and their family members. *Diabetes Care* **118**: 1370–1372.
6. Gram IT, Lund E, Slenker SE (1990) Quality of life following a false positive mammogram. *British Journal of Cancer* **62**: 1018–1022.
7. Malone JM, Snyder M, Anderson G, Bernhard VM, Holloway Jr. GA, Bunt TJ (1989) prevention of amputation by diabetic education. *American Journal of Surgery* **158**: 520–524.
8. Kash K, Holland J, Halper M, Miller D (1992) Psychological distress and surveillance behaviors of women with a family history of breast cancer. *Journal of the National Cancer Institute* **84**: 24–30.

9. Lifshitz F, Moses N (1989) Growth failure. A complication of dietary treatment of hypercholesterolemia. *American Journal of Child Development* **143**: 505–507.
10. DiMatteo MR, Lepper HS, Croghan TW (2000) Depression is a risk factor for non-compliance with medical treatment. *Archives of Internal Medicine* **160**: 2101–2107.
11. Leventhal H (1970) Findings and theory in the study of fear communications. *Advances in Experimental Social Psychology* **5**: 119–186.
12. Sheeran P (2002) Intention–behaviour relations: A conceptual and empirical review. In Hewstone M, Stroebe W (eds) *European Review of Social Psychology*, Volume 12. Chichester: John Wiley & Sons, pp. 1–36.
13. Jepson R (2000) *The effectiveness of interventions to change health-related behaviours: a review of reviews*. Glasgow: MRC Social and Public Health Sciences Unit, Occasional Paper No. 3.
14. Broadstock M, Michie S, Marteau TM (2000) The psychological consequences of predictive genetic testing: a systematic review. *European Journal of Human Genetics* **8**: 731–738.
15. Farmer AJ, Doll H, Levy JC, Salkovskis PM (submitted to *Diabetic Medicine*) The impact of screening for type 2 diabetes in siblings of patients with established diabetes.
16. Bekker H, Modell M, Dennis G, Silver A, Mathew C, Bobrow M, Marteau TM (1993) Uptake of cystic fibrosis carrier testing in primary care: Supply push or demand pull? *British Medical Journal* **306**: 1584–1586.
17. Marteau TM, Kidd J, Cook R, Johnston M, Michie S, Shaw RW, Slack J (1988) Screening for Down's syndrome. *British Medical Journal* **297**: 1469
18. Farmer AJ, Levy JC, Turner RC (1999) Knowledge of risk of developing diabetes mellitus among siblings of type 2 diabetic patients. *Diabetic Medicine* **16**: 233–7.
19. Kerbel D, Glazier R, Holzapfel S, Yeung M, Lofsky S (1997) Adverse effects of screening for gestational diabetes: A prospective cohort study in Toronto, Canada. *Journal of Medical Screening* **4**: 128–132.
20. General Medical Council (1999) *Seeking patients' consent: the ethical considerations*. London: GMC.
21. Petticrew MP, Sowden AJ, Lister-Sharp D, Wright K (2000) False-negative results in screening programmes: systematic review of impact and implications. *Health Technology Assessment* **4**(5).
22. Slayter EK, Ward, JE (1998) How risks of breast cancer and benefits of screening are communicated to women: analysis of 58 pamphlets. *British Medical Journal* **317**: 263–264.
23. Raffle AE (2000) Honesty about new screening programmes is best policy. *British Medical Journal* **320**: 872.
24. Smith D, Shaw RW, Marteau T (1994) Lack of knowledge in health professionals: A barrier to providing information to patients. *Quality in Health Care* **3**: 75-78.
25. Axworthy D, Brock DJH, Bobrow M, Marteau TM (1996). Psychological impact of population-based carrier testing for cystic fibrosis: three-year follow-up. *Lancet* **347**: 1443–1446.
26. Smith DK, Shaw RW, Slack J, Marteau TM (1995) Training obstetricians and midwives to present screening tests: evaluation of two brief interventions. *Prenatal Diagnosis* **15**: 317–324.
27. Marteau TM, Saidi G, Goodburn S, Lawton J, Michie S, Bobrow M (2000) Numbers or words? A randomised controlled trial of presenting screen negative results to pregnant women. *Prenatal Diagnosis* **20**: 714–718.
28. Marteau TM, Senior V, Sasieni P (2001) Women's understanding of a 'normal smear test result': experimental questionnaire based study. *British Medical Journal* **322**: 526–528.

Part IV

GESTATIONAL DIABETES

10

Gestational Diabetes Mellitus

DAVID R. McCANCE

Regional Centre for Endocrinology and Diabetes,
Royal Victoria Hospital, Belfast, UK

There are few other areas of diabetes research which have aroused such confusion and controversy as the concept and diagnosis of gestational diabetes mellitus (GDM). The fundamental difficulty lies in the apparent absence of a threshold separating subjects into low and high risk groups for adverse pregnancy outcome. Any statistical definition will therefore be arbitrary and possibly divorced from clinical relevance. Unfortunately debate has been hindered by a lack of focus on the relevant end-points and entrenched geographical differences in diagnostic practice. Respected international bodies[1-5], four international workshops[6-9] and a number of position statements[10-14] have attempted to clarify the situation and offer a uniformity of approach, but after two decades this is still lacking on a global and even national perspective. Several authors have questioned whether diabetes during pregnancy is a disease, or simply a risk factor for disease[15], or whether glucose intolerance antedated the pregnancy[16] or indeed, whether it is worth diagnosing?[17,18]. A number of provocative reviews have recently challenged established dogma and thinking[19-21].

The concept of gestational diabetes was of course popularised before considerations of evidence-based medicine[22] and it is both appropriate and timely to subject current diagnostic practice in pregnancy to the same scrutiny which has taken place in the nonpregnant context. This chapter seeks to address the key issues in the form of three questions, although it will quickly be realized that the evidence base is limited. Congenital malformations are thought to be a reflection of hyperglycaemia during organogenesis (and hence hyperglycaemia antedating pregnancy) and are dealt with in Chapter 11.

The Evidence Base for Diabetes Care. Edited by R. Williams, W. Herman, A.-L. Kinmonth and N. J. Wareham.
© 2002 John Wiley & Sons, Ltd

IS HYPERGLYCAEMIA IN PREGNANCY ASSOCIATED WITH ADVERSE OUTCOMES FOR THE FOETUS AND MOTHER?

BIOLOGICAL HYPOTHESES

The concept of fuel-mediated teratogenesis was enunciated by Pedersen over 20 years ago[23]. The hypothesis envisaged that excess foetal growth associated with diabetic pregnancy was the consequence of foetal hyperinsulinism secondary to excess maternal glucose and other fuels. Subsequent experimental and clinical data would generally support this concept[24–29]. Pregnancies complicated by pre-existing diabetes indicate that stimulation of pancreatic beta-cells can occur as early as 11–15 weeks gestation[30], but the major impact seems to be from 28–32 weeks onward, most likely because the foetal capacity to store triglycerides in adipose tissue matures at that time[31]. Lipids and amino-acids[29,32] are elevated in pregnancies complicated by maternal diabetes and have been correlated with the risk of macrosomia[33,34]. Amino acids (e.g. arginine and leucine) are known to stimulate insulin secretion from human foetal islets[35]. These factors, however, cannot be measured routinely, and unless they mirror plasma glucose, their relation to foetal morbidity remains unclear. Equally, little is known of the factors which control the transfer of nutrients across the placenta[36] or of the influence of substances such as growth factors and leptin which are elaborated by the placenta during diabetic pregnancy. It seems likely, however, that the greatest level of complexity rests with the foetus, where growth and regulation manifestly are influenced by a combination of factors including parity, foetal sex, maternal height and birth weight, prepregnancy weight, weight gain in pregnancy and socioeconomic status[37–42]. Familial and ethnic variation in birth weight are well recognised, and thus, whether the estimated foetal weight in any individual pregnancy is appropriate for the level of glycaemia (or other fuels) remains conjectural. Moreover, only a subgroup of infants will be at risk for excessive growth in the presence of a diabetic maternal environment. The relevance of the intrauterine environment has been further highlighted by Barker and colleagues who have invoked a critical role for malnutrition *in utero* as an explanation for the epidemiological associations which they have demonstrated between low birth-weight and cardiovascular disease in adult life[43]. Perhaps the Barker and Pederson–Freinkel hypotheses should be viewed as one and the same, each proposing a fuel-related programming which exists at the extremities of foetal nutrition[44]. It seems likely, however, that both genetic and environmental factors are operative[44,45] as was recently illustrated by Hattersley *et al.*[46] who showed that mutations in the glucokinase gene of the foetus resulted in reduced birth-weight. These authors have also demonstrated that maternal hyperglycaemia during pregnancy and obesity postdelivery may alter the penetrance of HNF_{1a} genetic mutations (which are known to result in young-onset diabetes), again highlighting the enduring impact of the intrauterine glycaemic milieu[47].

Although the association of maternal glucose with maternal/foetal outcome is undoubtedly complex, and delineation of genetic mutations in the future may allow a more precise classification of pathophysiological mechanisms, hyperglycaemia remains the common denominator which seems to be critical in its influence, and from a practical perspective is the variable most easily measured. Thus, as in nonpregnant subjects, blood glucose measurement should remain the basis for diagnosis (Tables 10.1–10.3).

EVIDENCE IN RELATION TO SHORT-TERM OUTCOMES

Maternal morbidity

Maternal morbidity associated with diabetic pregnancy is well described[48] but few studies have attempted to use this as an outcome variable for diagnosis. Evidence of a relation is largely uncontrolled and often retrospective. In one study, prediabetic women had a higher rate of toxaemia (when they may have had glucose intolerance during pregnancy) compared with the general population (14.2% versus 7.0%)[49]. Another (uncontrolled) study reported higher rates of pre-eclampsia and chronic hypertension than would be expected in unaffected populations[50]. Operative delivery was more common in untreated women than in women treated with insulin and diet, though the reasons for this were not discussed[26]. Maternal morbidity with present-day practice is exceptionally rare.

Perinatal mortality

Early studies suggested a two- to four-fold increase in perinatal mortality[48,50–52] but this is very unlikely with modern obstetric techniques. O'Sullivan reported an increased incidence of perinatal mortality of 6.4% among 187 pregnancies in women with untreated gestational diabetes mellitus compared with 1.5% among 259 randomly selected normal pregnancies[52]. A study involving over 800 Pima Indian women who underwent a 75g oral glucose tolerance test (OGTT) in the third trimester but who received no treatment showed that in those with impaired glucose tolerance (IGT) (by WHO criteria), the perinatal morbidity was 4.4% compared with 0.5% in subjects with normal glucose tolerance. Similarly, Oats and Beischer[53], using a 50g 3 h OGTT, identified 2.5% of the population with a perinatal mortality twice that of the background population. In high-risk populations, with a high background prevalence of diabetes combined with limited access to medical and perinatal care, perinatal mortality was reduced after screening and treatment of gestational diabetes[54]. Retrospective studies suggest lower still-birth rates after the introduction of screening and treating gestational diabetes in low-risk populations[52], but demonstrating a benefit in prospective studies is more difficult. In

Table 10.1. Oral glucose tolerance test criteria during pregnancy.

Author	Sampling times				Load	Comment
	Fasting	1 h	2h	3h		
*O'Sullivan[82]	5.0 (90)	9.2 (165)	8.1 (145)	7.0 (125)	100g	2 or more met or exceeded
Gillmer[67]	+	+	+	+	50g	> 42 area units above baseline
Merkatz[141]	5.8 (105)	10.3 (185)	7.7 (140)	6.9 (125)	75g	2 values met or exceeded
Mestman[84]	6.1 (110)	11.1 (200)	8.3 (150)	7.2 (130)	100g	2 values met or exceeded
†NDDG[1]	5.8 (105)	10.6 (190)	9.2 (165)	8.1 (145)	100g	2 or more must be met/exceeded
Carpenter[73]	5.3 (95)	10.0 (180)	8.7 (155)	7.8 (140)	100g	2 values met or exceeded
WHO[1-3] (IGT,G-IGT)	<7.8 (140)		7.8–11.1 (140-199)			Both must be met
WHO[1-3] (DM,GDM)	≥7.8		≥200		75g	Either fasting or 2h value met or exceeded
Oats & Beischer[83]		9.0 (162)	7.0 (126)		50g	Both values met or exceeded

IGT (impaired glucose tolerance); G-IGT (gestational impaired glucose tolerance), DM (diabetes mellitus); GDM (gestational diabetes mellitus).

*Measured on whole blood using Somogyi-Nelson method. Figures are rounded to nearest 5 mg/dl. The remaining criteria are based on plasma using glucose oxidase/hexokinase methodology.

†Corrects for change from whole blood to plasma or serum glucose and for the use of glucose oxidase or hexokinase methodology. In nonpregnant state a 75 g glucose load is used. IGT is defined as fasting <140, 1 h ≥200, 2 h 140–199 (all three must be met). Diabetes: Fasting ≥140, 1 h ≥200, 2 h ≥200 (Either fasting or 1 h and 2 h values must be met).

Table 10.2a. Diagnostic scheme for gestational diabetes mellitus as defined by the Fourth International Workshop Conference on Gestational Diabetes Mellitus in 1998[9].

Plasma glucose	100 g OGTT diagnostic test			
Venous plasma glucose	Carpenter and Coustan		4th GDM Workshop	
	mmol/l	mg/dl	mmol/l	mg/dl
Fasting	5.3	95	5.3	95
1-hour	10.0	180	10.0	180
2-hour	8.6	155	8.6	155
3-hour	7.8	140		

The cut-off values for the diagnosis of GDM with a 100 g oral glucose load proposed by the 4th GDM Workshop and ADA are those of Carpenter and Coustan. The 4th GDM workshop also proposed that the 1 h and 2 h cut-off values be used for diagnosis of GDM after a 75 g oral glucose load (see text). Using a 75 g load, two or more of the venous plasma concentrations must be met or exceeded for a positive diagnosis. These cut-off values are of necessity arbitrary.

Table 10.2b. 1997 ADA/1998 WHO criteria for the diagnosis of diabetes mellitus.[5]

Normoglycaemia	IFG and IGT/G-IGT	Diabetes mellitus
FPG <6.1 mmol/l (110)	FPG ≥6.1 mmol/l(110) but <7.0 mmol/l (125) (IFG)	FPG ≥7.0 mmol/l (126)
2 h PG <7.8 mmol/l (140)	2 h PG ≥7.8 mmol/l (140) but <11.1 mmol/l (200) (IGT)	2 h PG ≥11.1 mmol/l (200)
		Symptoms of diabetes and casual plasma glucose ≥11.1 mmol/l (200)

Plasma glucose values mmol/l (mg/dl); FPG (fasting plasma glucose), 2 h PG (2 h postload plasma glucose); Impaired fasting glucose (IFG), Impaired glucose tolerance (IGT). New recommendations include reduction in FPG cutpoint from 7.8 to 7.0 mmol/l and creation of new IFG category. A diagnosis of diabetes must be confirmed on a subsequent day by any one of the three methods included in the chart. Fasting is defined as no caloric intake for at least 8 h. The term gestational diabetes is retained but now encompasses the groups formerly classified as gestational impaired glucose intolerance (G-IGT) and gestational diabetes mellitus (GDM).

Western populations which have a low prevalence of diabetes, good access to medical care and low perinatal mortality and morbidity rates, there are ethical constraints in mounting randomised trials with sufficient power to test whether treating gestational diabetes may reduce perinatal morbidity. More recent studies have almost universally found no increase in perinatal mortality among pregnancies identified by diagnostic criteria[55–59].

Surrogate markers of maternal–foetal outcome

Among the Pima Indians, Pettitt *et al.*[60] showed that the rate of complications (perinatal mortality, macrosomia, toxaemia, caesarian section) and the sub-

Table 10.3. European Guidelines for interpretation of the 75 g OGTT during pregnancy.

	Venous plasma glucose on the 75 g OGTT	
	Fasting	2 h
Diabetes	>7 mmol/l	>11 mmol/l
Gestational IGT	5.5–7.0 mmol/l	9–11 mmol/l
Normal	<5.5	<9

The Report of the British Pregnancy and Neonatal Care Group[197] defined three categories of fasting glucose: >8 mmol/l (diabetes), 6-8 mmol/l IGT and <6 mmol/l (normal) after a 75 g OGTT. Following the reduction in the fasting glucose diagnostic cut-point from 7.8 to 7.0 mmol/l, it would seem appropriate to lower the fasting glucose to 5.5 mmol/l, a value also adopted by the Scottish Intercollegiate Guidelines Network[198]. Since the fasting plasma glucose level falls and the 2 h value rises in normal, nondiabetic pregnancy, using such criteria 15% of women would be diagnosed as having gestational diabetes. The British Group thus adopted the recommendation of the Diabetic Pregnancy Study Group of the European Association for the Study of Diabetes (EASD) that the 95th centile of 2 h plasma glucose be used as the cut-off point for diagnosis (9.0 mmol/l).

sequent incidence of diabetes in the mother was continuous through the range of 2 h glucose concentrations studied. Among 249 women who had a 100 g OGTT at 28 weeks gestation and a negative test based on NDDG criteria, Tallarigo *et al.*[61] found that women with 2 h glucose values in the 'impaired' range (6.7–9.1 mmol/l) compared with those below 5.5 mmol/l had a significant increase in foetal macrosomia (27.5% versus 9.9%) and pre-eclampsia and/or Caesarian section (40.0% versus 19.9%). The results of Tallarigo *et al.* implied that the group of women at risk could be as large as 16% and not the 3–4% of subjects usually indicated by NDDG criteria. Other studies[62–64] also suggest that increasing carbohydrate intolerance among patients not meeting the current criteria for the diagnosis of GDM leads to unfavourable perinatal outcomes. Patients with an abnormal glucose challenge test but a normal OGTT are at increased risk of foetal macrosomia[64], as are those with one abnormal OGTT value rather than the two required by the NDDG criteria[63]. A positive relationship between gestational diabetes and foetal macrosomia has been demonstrated in several studies[65,66]. Langer reported a progressive increase in the risk of foetal macrosomia (birth weight >90th centile for age) with no obvious threshold in association with increasing mean maternal glycaemia in a large cohort of women with treated GDM. Gilmer derived criteria for GDM on the basis of risk for neonatal hypoglycaemia, and reported an increased likelihood of this outcome if the area under an 100g OGTT was >42 mmol/units[67]. Among low risk populations, some reports however have failed to find an association between GDM and foetal outcome[57,58].

An important study is that of Sacks *et al.*[68] which examined 3505 pregnant women who had a fasting glucose <5.8 mmol/l and 2 h <11.1 mmol/l during a 75 g OGTT performed at 24–28 weeks gestation. No clinically meaningful glucose threshold values relative to birth weight or macrosomia were found (Table 10.4) and these relationships were linear over only portions of the

Table 10.4. Venous plasma glucose results in relation to gestational age in 3505 unselected subjects undergoing a 75 g OGTT (Sacks *et al.*[68]). Reproduced by permission of Mosby Inc.

	Gestational age				
	0–23 weeks	24–28 weeks	29–36 weeks	≥37 weeks	*Significance
No	494	2094	857	55	
Fasting (mmol/l)	4.6 ± 0.5	4.6 ± 0.5	4.7 ± 0.5	4.5 ± 0.4	p = 0.1
(mg/dl)	83.5 ± 9.4	83.6 ± 8.9	84.0 ± 9.8	81.3 ± 8.1	
1 hour (mmol/l)	7.0 ± 1.9	7.1 ± 1.8	7.6 ± 1.9	7.5 ± 1.7	p = 0.0001
(mg/dl)	126.5 ± 34.2	128.4 ± 32.9	136.0 ± 34.2	134.8 ± 31.1	
2 hour (mmol/l)	5.9 ± 1.4	6.1 ± 1.4	6.2 ± 1.4	6.3 ± 1.5	p = 0.0008
(mg/dl)	107.1 ± 25.6	108.4 ± 24.8	111.1 ± 25.9	114.3 ± 26.5	

One-hour and two-hour values are significantly greater for 29 weeks to 36 weeks than for 24–28 weeks. Glucose values are expressed as mean ±SD.
*One-way analysis of variance. Sacks *et al.*[68].

ranges of glucose values. For those linear portions, the strongest positive association between birth weight and glucose values was for fasting plasma glucose (slope 0.29, p = 0.001).

Perhaps the most important evidence to date for the continuous relationship between glycaemia and maternal/foetal outcome comes from the Toronto Tri-Hospital Gestational Diabetes Project[69–72] in which 4274 women were screened and 3836 proceeded to a diagnostic 100 g OGTT. A major advantage of this prospective cohort study was the blinding of care-givers to the results of the 1 h glucose challenge test and 3 h OGTT unless the latter met NDDG criteria for gestational diabetes. Many women did meet the more inclusive criteria of Carpenter and Coustan[73] (Tables 10.1 and 10.2). Significant positive relationships were found between increasing carbohydrate intolerance (fasting, 1 h, 2 h, 3 h) and a number adverse outcomes including Caesarian section, preeclampsia, macrosomia, the need for phototherapy, and the length of maternal and neonatal hospital stay. In multivariate analysis, maternal hyperglycaemia was an independent risk factor for foetal macrosomia, as were maternal BMI and a history of a previous macrosomic infant. Of note was the fact that there was no apparent threshold for these outcomes (Table 10.5). Only a minority of infants, in any maternal glucose (quartile) category, had any perinatal morbidity.

The authors also examined the impact of foetal macrosomia on the risk of caesarean delivery by dividing the blinded cohort into three mutually

Table 10.5. Relationships of OGTT (mmol/l) by quartiles to adverse maternal–foetal outcomes among 3637 subjects without overt GDM. Toronto Tri-Hospital Gestational Diabetes Project (Sermer *et al.*[70]). Reproduced by permission of Mosby Inc.

	Pre-eclampsia		Macrosomia (>4000 g)		Caesarean section	
	%	P	%	P	%	p
OGTT (mmol/l)						
Fasting		NS		<0.001		NS
<4.1	5.1		9.7		20.6	
4.1–4.2	3.7		14.4		18.4	
4.3–4.5	5.9		14.1		22.5	
>4.5	5.9		20.5		22.9	
1 h level		0.004		<0.001		0.005
<6.4	3.5		12.1		18.5	
6.4–7.5	4.5		13.3		20.3	
7.6–8.7	6.7		14.1		21.7	
>8.7	5.9		17.5		23.8	
2 h level		0.0001		<0.001		0.003
<5.6	3.3		10.3		19.2	
5.6–6.4	4.7		14.4		18.7	
6.5–7.3	6.5		16.4		22.8	
>7.3	6.4		16.3		23.8	

exclusive groups: 1 h glucose <7.8 mmol/l, 1 h glucose ≥7.8 mmol/l but without GDM, and GDM diagnosed by Carpenter–Coustan criteria (but not NDDG). Within each of these groups, increasing Caesarean delivery occurred primarily with an increase in the prevalence of birth weights >4000g (19.1% versus 27.1%; 22.9% versus 30.0%; 23.2% versus 45.5%, respectively), implying foetal macrosomia *per se* accounted for most of the increase in Caesarean deliveries with increasing maternal glycaemia. The group with the highest glucose concentrations (positive both by Carpenter–Coustan and NDDG criteria), who were treated to reduce their glucose concentrations, had the lowest proportion of infants with macrosomia but the highest rate of caesarean section delivery.

Maternal risk factors

The relevance of age, body mass index (BMI), family history of diabetes and ethnicity to diabetic hyperglycemia and pregnancy outcome is well recognised[20,74–80] and many reports have failed to control for these factors. Some consider that the adverse outcome of hyperglycaemia during pregnancy is explicable by maternal risk factors while others believe that even minor degrees of hyperglycaemia present an independent risk for adverse pregnancy outcome[61,63]. The situation is further complicated by the fact that some clinical risk factors used to screen subjects (e.g obesity and family history of type 2 diabetes) also confer an increased risk of glucose intolerance in the non pregnant state, independent of knowledge of OGTT results during pregnancy[16]. Among the early studies, O'Sullivan found an excess perinatal mortality in women who were obese or at least 25 years old[52]. A number of studies have shown a direct relationship between the 2 h glucose response and foetal birth weight[62,77,79,81], controlled for maternal risk factors. The two large prospective studies from California[68] and Toronto[69–72] described above also provide important information in this respect. In the study of Sacks *et al.*[68], maternal race, parity, prepregnancy body mass index, weight gain, gestational age at testing, fasting and 2 h glucose were significantly associated with macrosomia using multiple logistic regression analysis. A positive association was found between maternal glucose values and birth weight centile. Using a multivariate analysis, the Toronto study also showed that increasing carbohydrate intolerance remained an independent predictor for various unfavourable foetal outcomes, but the strength of the associations was diminished: only the 3 h glucose (odds ratio 1.10; 95% CI 1.03–1.19) was an independent predictor of Caesarean section, only fasting glucose remained significant for macrosomia (birth weight >4000g: odds ratio 2.00, 95% CI 1.45–2.54) and no glucose variable predicted pre-eclampsia. When the models were re-run with only BMI and glucose variables to determine residual 'reversible risk', the association with operative delivery and the 3 h glucose value remained modest, but the fasting value had a moderately strong relationship to the risk of macrosomia (odds ratio 2.00;

95% CI 1.61–2.58). Compared with normoglycaemic control subjects, the untreated borderline GDM group had increased rates of macrosomia (28.7 versus 13.7%, p <0.001) and Caesarean delivery (29.6 versus 20.2%, p = 0.03). An increased risk of caesarian delivery among treated patients compared with normoglycaemic control subjects persisted after adjustment for multiple maternal risk factors, suggesting that recognition of GDM may lead to a lower threshold for surgical delivery.

The evidence would therefore suggest the glycaemic risk appears to be continuous for both maternal and foetal outcome, and results in a genuine increase in perinatal morbidity. The large majority of infants, however, incur no excess risk of morbidity with mild hyperglycaemia (e.g. Carpenter–Coustan) and the effect of glycaemia is weakened by controlling for other risk factors. Fasting hyperglycaemia may be one of the best predictors of macrosomia. It would appear that the diagnosis of GDM itself shifts obstetric practice style toward Caesarean delivery, as was clearly demonstrated in the Toronto study. (Level of evidence II–2; Strength of Recommendation B.)

EVIDENCE IN RELATION TO LONG-TERM OUTCOMES

MATERNAL DIABETES

It is difficult to compare studies because of the differing diagnostic criteria used in pregnant and nonpregnant states, differing background prevalence rates of diabetes in the populations studied, and the variable time periods elapsed since pregnancy. Data from various studies suggest that there is a 17–63% risk of gestational diabetes within five to 16 years after the index pregnancy[82–90.] The risk of diabetes depends predominantly on ethnicity and is also particularly high in women who have marked hyperglycaemia during[82–90,] or soon after pregnancy[87–90], women who are obese[88,89,91], and women whose gestational diabetes was diagnosed before 24 weeks gestation[86,90,92,93]. Other contributing factors are weight during pregnancy and subsequent weight gain, age, parity and family history[85,94]. In high-risk populations, such as Hispanic American women, about 50% of women with gestational diabetes develop diabetes within six years, which rises to 80% among those with impaired glucose tolerance (by WHO criteria) after birth[90,95]. In white Europeans the rate of progression to diabetes is slower – 20–40% within 20 years[87].

MATERNAL VASCULOPATHY

An acceleration of established microvascular disease is well recognised in diabetic pregnancy. Of interest are the findings of a recent study which demonstrated endothelial dysfunction in mothers with a previous history of gestational diabetes mellitus, compared with those who had normal glucose tolerance during pregnancy[96].

FOETAL OUTCOME

Foetal outcome is integral to any assessment of the value of detection and treatment. Several studies have reported an increased risk for both obesity and diabetes in offspring following diabetes in pregnancy[97–102]. Two of the most remarkable long-term studies have been among the Pima Indians[100] and the North Western Programme in Chicago[102]. It should be noted, however, that both these populations have very high rates of both obesity and type 2 diabetes, and the latter population was not only heterogenous in genotype but included subjects with both pregestational and gestational diabetes. In Pima Indians, children of a diabetic mother are at a greater risk of diabetes and childhood obesity than older siblings born before their mother became diabetic, emphasising the importance of the hyperglycaemic intrauterine environment. Both the Pima Indian and the North Western studies have demonstrated that offspring of diabetic mothers are at increased risk for both glucose intolerance and obesity. Among Pima Indians, the prevalence of diabetes at 10–39 years of age was over 40% and influenced by age, sex, birth weight, birthdate, maternal diabetes and breast-feeding. In the Chicago study, one-third of offspring of diabetic mothers had impaired glucose tolerance or type 2 diabetes by 17 years of age. In both studies, no correlation was seen between macrosomia or birth weight and the later development of obesity. In the Chicago study, after covariate adjustment for both sex and maternal weight, an association was found between BMI at 14–17 years and amniotic fluid insulin concentration, indicating an association between premature islet activation and the later development and maintenance of obesity.

Maternal carbohydrate metabolism may also influence future human foetal insulin secretion and function, as suggested by the studies on black and white American adolescents. Those born to diabetic mothers had greater insulin resistance and were more likely to be glucose-intolerant during puberty. There is relatively little data on other cardiovascular risk factors although higher blood pressures have been reported[101]. Several studies have suggested that the impact of intrapartum maternal metabolism on subsequent neurobehavioural development of the offspring is small[101,103], but this requires confirmation.

Among Pima Indians, there was a direct relation between these outcomes and increasing maternal glycaemic response to a 75 g OGTT[60]. In the Chicago study, Metzger *et al.*[88] showed that among 113 women diagnosed as having gestational diabetes by NDDG criteria, fasting plasma glucose during pregnancy was related to the development of an abnormal OGTT within the first year postpartum.

In summary, controlled but nonrandomised trials indicate that glucose intolerance detected in pregnancy is predictive of later maternal type 2 diabetes. However, the critical threshold of hyperglycaemia is not known, and this may simply reflect the predictive power of IGT for subsequent diabetes mellitus in the nonpregnant state. Increased maternal morbidity with lesser degrees of glycaemia is much less certain. In light of the fact that the onset of type 2 diabetes in women can be delayed by weight control and exercise, particularly among obese women with a family history of diabetes[104], it is recommended that that any women with GDM or impaired fasting glucose should have a 75 g OGTT after pregnancy. Recent studies of lifestyle and pharmacological agents strengthen the case for identification of these women during pregnancy[105,106]. (Maternal diabetes: Level of evidence II-2; Strength of recommendation A; Fetal outcome: Level of evidence II-2; Strength of recommendation B.)

HOW CAN HYPERGLYCAEMIA IN PREGNANCY BE DETECTED?

DEFINITION

The adverse outcome of pregnancy in type 1 diabetes mellitus has been recognised for over a century[107] although in early studies measurements were limited to glycosuria[108].

The exact origin of the term *gestational diabetes* is difficult to ascertain, but almost certainly grew from a realisation of the relationship between fetal survival, birth weight and hyperglycaemia in pregnancy[109,111]. The original concept of gestational diabetes required it to be a temporary state with a return to normal after delivery[112], and was the definition used by Jorgen Pedersen in his pioneering book, *the Pregnant Diabetic and her Newborn*[23]. The present-day situation is more confused. Two slightly different definitions espoused by differing international bodies and reflecting different diagnostic practices have evolved. The American Diabetes Association[2,10-14] and associated groups define the term as 'carbohydrate intolerance of varying severity with onset or first recognition during pregnancy'. This definition (which has remained unchanged in subsequent international workshops[7-9]) applies 'irrespective of whether or not insulin is used for treatment, or the condition persists after pregnancy'. By contrast, the World Health Organisation (WHO)[2-5] defines diabetes mellitus as 'a state of chronic hyperglycaemia' on the basis of guidelines used for nonpregnant adults, and includes an additional category of impaired glucose tolerance (G-IGT). This latter definition is applicable only to women in whom these criteria are first detected during pregnancy.

The meaning of the term 'gestational diabetes' therefore differs depending on which set of diagnostic criteria are used. Both definitions require the fulfilment of criteria after an oral glucose tolerance test, but the NDDG defines

only two categories – normal glucose tolerance and gestational diabetes –
while the WHO criteria include categories of normality, impaired glucose
tolerance and diabetes.

DIAGNOSIS

Tables 10.1–10.3 summarise some of the oral glucose tolerance test (OGTT)
criteria for diabetes in pregnancy. The diagnosis of symptomatic type 1 diabetes
is usually obvious, being readily confirmed by glycosuria and prompt blood
testing. There is international agreement that a random glucose ≥ 11.1 mmol/l
(200 mg/dl) suggests the diabetic state and warrants further investigation[2–5]. In
the recently revised WHO Diagnostic Criteria[5], the fasting threshold has been
reduced from 7.8 mmol/l to 7mmol/l[5] (Table 10.2). The basic problem in
pregnancy relates to those subjects found on screening with few, if any, related
symptoms or signs.

In North America the O'Sullivan and Mahan Criteria[82,113], endorsed by the
National Data Group (NDDG)[2], are widely used. These were derived from an
unselected group of 752 pregnant women recruited on registration in a Boston
hospital over a four-month period in the 1950s. On the basis of a 100 g OGTT
with sampling fasting, and at one, two and three hours, upper threshold values
were created by adding one, two or three standard deviations (SDS) above the
mean result for each time point. For each set of threshold values, the OGTT
was positive if blood glucose results for two or more time stages exceeded the
corresponding threshold. These criteria were then applied to a second group
of 1013 women to determine which set had the best sensitivity and specificity
for subsequent diabetes in the nonpregnant state (as defined by United States
Public Health Criteria, USPH) over periods ranging up to eight years. The
best set of threshold values were the mean plus two standard deviations for
each of the OGTT values which were rounded off for simplification and
adjusted to modern glucose measurement procedures. There has been criticism of the attempt to convert the O'Sullivan criteria to current methods of
measurement[21,114]. The NDDG criteria were derived by extrapolation of the
O'Sullivan data, correcting for the change from venous blood to plasma or
sera, and appear to lie outside the 95% confidence intervals (CIs)of three of
the four points chosen. Carpenter and Coustan have proposed alternative
figures to the O'Sullivan criteria, correcting not only for the change from
venous whole blood to plasma but also for the use of glucose oxidase or hexokinase methodology which yields values approximately 0.27 mmol/l (5 mg/dl)
lower than the Somogi–Nelson criteria[73] (Table 10.2). In several studies, these
revised criteria identified more patients with GDM whose infants had peri-
ntatal morbidity[69,115]. The Fourth International Workshop on GDM[9] and a
recent ADA consensus statement[14] recommended the Carpenter–Coustan
modification for diagnosis (Table 10.2).

In the late 1970s and early 1980s several authoritative bodies including the United States Diabetes Data Group and the WHO Expert Committee on Diabetes Mellitus[2–4] reviewed the available evidence and made recommendations about diagnostic standards (Table 10.2). There was agreement on the use of a 75 g OGTT, diagnostic cut-off levels and the creation of a new category of impaired glucose tolerance. The groups differed, however, on the application of glycaemic criteria to glucose intolerance in pregnancy: the WHO proposing the criteria for diabetes in nonpregnant adults should also be applied to pregnant adults with the proviso that the 'management of IGT during pregnancy should be the same as for diabetes'[4] (Table 2). By contrast, the NDDG recommended retention of the procedures and criteria based on those originally proposed by O'Sullivan and Mahan[73,82]. It was perceived by the WHO that this distinction between diabetes and IGT in pregnancy would allow further elucidation of conflicting reports[19,25,61,74] of the 'effects of minor degrees of glucose intolerance upon maternal and child health'[4].

Few studies have compared the two criteria, but there is some evidence to suggest that 'gestational diabetes', as defined by WHO criteria, will identify a greater number of pregnancies with maternal or perinatal complications associated with high plasma glucose[68,116,117]. It was the realisation that 10% of a diverse European population had 2 h values >8 mmol/l (140 mg/dl) that motivated the Diabetes in Pregnancy Study Group of the European Association for the Study of Diabetes (DPSG-EASD)[118] to increase the upper limit of the 2 h glucose from 8 to 9 mmol/l (162mg/dl) (Table 10.3). The WHO criteria are most widely used outside North America. Other European criteria have largely been based on various measures of outcome. Oats and Beischer[53] reported a 50 g 3 h OGTT which identified 2.5% of the population whose risk of perinatal mortality was approximately twice the background rate.

The Fourth International Workshop/Conference on Gestational Diabetes Mellitus[9] alluded to the international differences in diagnostic practice and by way of compromise suggested that the same numerical values for the fasting, 1 h and 2 h time points be used in both the 75 g OGTT and the Carpenter–Coustan 100 g test. The former cut-points were justified on the basis that they represented the mean plus 1.5 SDs of the OGTT in a study by Sacks *et al.*[68] (Table 10.2), but with the 2 h value being raised to 8.6 mol/l to provide consistency with the 100 g OGTT and the DPSG-EASD.

PROBLEMS THAT SHOULD BE ENCOUNTERED

Physiological considerations

The diabetogenic effect of pregnancy has long been recognised[106] but the exact mechanism remains incompletely understood[119–123]. Various lines of observation including an increase in both fasting and postprandial insulin levels with advancing pregnancy, a blunted response to the intravenous injection of exogenous insulin, the development of abnormal glucose tolerance late in gestation, the need for increasing doses of insulin during pregnancy and resolution of the process after delivery point to pregnancy as inducing a state of insulin resistance. It is generally accepted that fasting glucose values are lower during pregnancy than in non pregnant individuals[123,124] but are held within a restricted range. The glucose response to a mixed meal or pure glucose challenge is both delayed and increased[125,126]. Fasting glucose levels fall in the first trimester[25,124]. With advancing normal pregnancy, both fasting and postprandial blood glucose levels rise a little although still within the normal non-pregnant normal range. Sacks *et al.* found that fasting plasma glucose did not vary significantly with gestational age but there was a significant increase in post-challenge values in subjects tested after 28 weeks compared with those tested earlier (Table 4)[68]. The practical implication of these observations for diagnosis is that any perceived abnormality of glucose tolerance must be related to a nonpregnant, trimester-specific reference range. Centile values for each trimester have been established for the 100g OGTT[83,127] and more recently using a 75g load[68,118,128] and some have criticised the O'Sullivan criteria in this regard[20]. Similar trimester-specific data for glycated haemoglobin are also available[129,130].

The oral glucose tolerance test

Timing of the OGTT during pregnancy

The increased diabetogenic stress with advancing pregnancy is the rationale for customary diagnostic testing in the third trimester, but the possible benefit of earlier identification of women at risk for adverse maternal-fetal outcome cannot be excluded. There is some evidence that fetal macrosomia is associated with transient abnormalities in maternal glucose metabolism in the second trimester[129]. Conceivably, treatment may only be effective if instituted at an early stage.

Reproducibility

Methodological concern over the poor reproducibility of the OGTT applies both to the pregnant and nonpregnant individual. Reproducibility is of the order of 50–70% in nonpregnant subjects[131], but with few exceptions[132,133], has seldom been examined in pregnancy and was not considered in the derivation of the O'Sullivan criteria[82]. Patients and controls in various studies frequently differ in the presence or absence of a glucose challenge during an earlier screening procedure. Moreover, the whole category of IGT introduced by the WHO may be heterogenous[134].

Glucose load

The actual amount of glucose ingested (50 g, 75 g or 100 g) varies from centre to centre. A 100 g load is most commonly used in the USA. British Commonwealth countries have tended to use a 50 g load mainly because it causes less vomiting. Most European centres have adopted the 75 g OGTT interpreted by WHO criteria. It has been shown, however, that 75 g of glucose gives OGTT values that are virtually identical to those obtained with 100 g glucose[135]. The shorter duration (2 h) may decrease the opportunity to meet the 3 h O'Sullivan criteria.

Haemodilution in pregnancy alters the relation between plasma and whole-blood concentrations. Plasma contains more glucose than whole blood since after haemolysis there is less glucose inside the red cell; venous blood contains less glucose than arterial blood and capillary glucose approximates more to the arterial level. Fortunately venous plasma (measured in hospital) and capillary whole blood (measured by an impregnated test strip) are virtually equivalent[136]. These differences may have some importance in pregnancy.

Ethnic variation

International comparisons of the prevalence of diabetes during pregnancy are made difficult by the use of different methods and cut-off points for diagnosis. The general picture, however, seems to mirror geographical differences in the prevalence of type 1 and type 2 diabetes, being lowest in northernmost parts of Western civilised countries and highest in subtropical and tropical developing countries[137,138]. The contribution of undiagnosed diabetes preceding pregnancy will also vary with location. Gestational diabetes mellitus complicates approximately 4% (ranging from 1.4–12.3% depending on the population studied) of all pregnancies in the USA[139], and between 4.3–15% in Australia, depending on country of birth[140]. Using WHO criteria, diabetes during pregnancy was 40 times more prevalent in Pima Indians than in the South Boston population (60% white, 40% nonwhite) studied by O'Sullivan and 10 times more prevalent than in the Cleveland population (61% white, 39% nonwhite) studied by Merkatz *et al.*[141]. The Diabetes and Pregnancy Study Group of the European Association for the Study of Diabetes performed a multicentre study on glucose tolerance in normal pregnancy and showed that at least 10% of normal pregnant women had a 2 h test value of more than 8 mmol/l after a 75 g OGTT and thus were labelled as having IGT[118]. Adoption of population-specific criteria on a statistical basis will yield greatly differing prevalence rates. A universal framework of reference has a strong epidemiological appeal.

Pregnant/Nonpregnant definitions

The most recent GDM workshop[9] acknowledged that glucose intolerance may often antedate pregnancy. Harris[16] pointed to the similar rates of GDM/G-

IGT in pregnant and nonpregnant individuals together with their association with risk factors for type 2 diabetes, and suggested that the condition may represent the discovery of pre-existing glucose intolerance. Normal women destined to have gestational diabetes exhibit decreased insulin-stimulated glucose disposal before conception[142]. This has implications both for diagnosis and the concept and significance of minor degrees of hyperglycaemia.

Postpartum studies of glucose tolerance should be considered an integral part of the diagnostic process, but suffer from changing diagnostic practice and criteria for 'normality'. The 'diabetes' predicted by O'Sullivan criteria was defined by US Public Health Criteria and many, if not most, of these 'diabetics' would have had IGT by NDDG/WHO criteria. This disparity makes it difficult to compare estimates of the subsequent development of glucose intolerance. NDDG/WHO criteria state that women should be formally retested after pregnancy using a 75 g OGTT and reclassified according to their new nonpregnant results. Unfortunately for the NDDG criteria, this means that different tests will be used in the same person before and after pregnancy.

Defining relevant end-points

An inherent weakness and major criticism of the O'Sullivan criteria is their validation by prediction of subsequent maternal diabetes, not fetal outcome[82]. In the context of diabetic pregnancy, there are immediate and long-term outcomes for both mother and baby. Pregnancy outcome has undoubtedly been affected by improved obstetric practice and neonatal care to the extent that, for perinatal mortality, it may not be possible to further reduce existing rates. None of the surrogate markers of diabetic control are specific for diabetes and many are influenced by the practice of individual obstetricians, maternal obesity, age and parity[143]. Several studies have now examined more distant outcomes, but lack of universally agreed diagnostic criteria both during and after pregnancy make comparisons difficult and almost certainly have contributed to the disparate results obtained. There is also the additional supervision which inevitably attends any possible diagnosis of abnormality[51,81]. Treatment, whether intentional or incidental, has made the question more difficult to answer (100 g OGTT Level of evidence II-2; Strength of recommendation B; 75 g OGTT Level of evidence III; Strength of recommendation C).

DOES TREATMENT OF HYPERGLYCAEMIA IN PREGNANCY REDUCE ADVERSE OUTCOMES?

DIETARY INTERVENTION

Few studies have examined the effects of primary dietary therapy on fetal growth and neonatal outcomes in women identified as having gestational diabetes. The Cochrane database[144] reviewed four such trials, mostly small, some unpublished and of variable quality, involving 612 women. If dietary therapy did not achieve set targets, insulin was frequently added to the dietary regimen. The trial conducted by Li *et al.* 1987[145] randomised by alternate allocation. Trial design was complex, involving 216 women with an abnormal 100 g OGTT and results were based on those subsequently designated as having normal glucose tolerance (n = 111, 51%) and IGT (n = 98, 45%), by a 75 g OGTT. No information was given regarding the arm of the trial for the seven women requiring insulin, and 10% of the sample were excluded. The perinatal outcome was comparable in the control and treatment groups. In a randomised study involving 300 Canadian women with gestational diabetes, Garner and colleagues[146] found no difference in a variety of outcomes between treatment and control groups, but all women and physicians knew of the diagnosis and statistically the sample size was not large enough to allow any conclusions to be drawn[147]. In a meta-analysis of these four studies, no differences were detected between primary dietary therapy and no primary dietary therapy for birth weights greater than 4000g (OR 0.798, 95% CI 0.45–1.35) or Caesarean deliveries (OR 0.97, 95% CI 0.65–1.44), and it was concluded that there was insufficient evidence to evaluate the use of primary dietary therapy for women who show impaired glucose metabolism during pregnancy. Not included in the Cochrane data base were the recent results of Jovanovic *et al.*[148] who reported the effect of treatment of 83 women with a positive glucose challenge test but a negative 100 g OGTT. The 35 women who were randomised to dietary counselling and home glucose monitoring had a lower prevalence of macrosomia than did controls. Maternal complications did not differ between the groups (Level of evidence 1; Strength of recommendation B).

PHYSICAL ACTIVITY

Studies seeking to explore a beneficial role for physical activity are limited in number and not infrequently are combined with diet or insulin. Surrogate endpoints, such as avoidance of the need for insulin therapy, may be reported rather than clinical end-points. Bung *et al.*[149] randomised 41 patients with gestational diabetes requiring insulin to an exercise programme. Seventeen of the 21 patients completed the programme while maintaining normoglycaemia and obviating insulin therapy. Maternal and neonatal complications did not differ between the study and control groups. Jovanovic *et al.*[150] applied arm ergometer training to a population of women with GDM and compared their glycaemia to women receiving only dietary instruction. The two groups' glycaemic levels started to diverge by the fourth week of the programme, and by the sixth week, the women in the exercise group had normalised their HbA$_{1c}$, fasting plasma glucose and their response to a glucose challenge test compared with no change in glucose levels in those women treated with diet alone. Most studies suggest that exercise is safe[151] in women with gestational diabetes mellitus and does not cause fetal distress, low infant birth weight or uterine contractions (Level of evidence II-1; Strength of recommendation B).

INSULIN THERAPY

The major randomised trials to date that have utilised insulin therapy in pregnancy are shown in Table 10.6. The first, and probably the most extensive, study was published in 1966 by O'Sullivan *et al.* in Boston, where pioneering investigations into glucose tolerance in pregnancy had been undertaken[152]. During two time periods, 1954–1960 and 1962–1970, mothers with GDM (using their previously established criteria) were prospectively randomised to routine prenatal care or diet and insulin management. In addition, they randomly selected a further group of mothers known to have normal glucose tolerance who also received routine prenatal care. Insulin treatment consisted of 10 units NPH (isophane) insulin each morning from about 32 weeks gestation, with some increase judged by tests for glycosuria and occasional laboratory blood sugar measurements. Compared with the untreated gestational diabetic mothers, the number of babies over 9 lbs (4.0 kg) born to insulin treated mothers was significantly reduced and was no different from the number of big babies born to untreated normoglycaemic mothers. A significant reduction in perinatal mortality, as a result of treatment with insulin and diet, was only seen when data from the two different study periods were combined, and included only those mothers who were ≥25 years old and had entered the study before the thirty-second week of pregnancy[153].

Two other studies by Coustan and colleagues[27,154] confirmed these findings, particularly in the reduction of macrosomia. In the larger study in New Haven, Connecticut[153], a retrospective assessment of outcome of 115 diet and insulin treated and 184 nondiet or insulin treated mothers whose hyperglycaemia had been established by modified O'Sullivan and Mahan criteria[113] was compared with that of 146 untreated normoglycaemic mothers (Table 10.6). Insulin treatment commenced at a higher dose, 20 units NPH (isophane) and 10 units soluble (regular) each morning. In a careful analysis allowing for some potential bias in selection, they found a significantly reduced incidence of Caesarean sections, birth trauma and babies in more than the 90th centile for birth weight standard. A similar initial dose of insulin was used in a smaller randomised study in Alabama, and also resulted in a significant reduction in birth weights[155], but there were no differences in operative delivery, shoulder dystocia or neonatal metabolic complications. In a large population-based study, Langer compared conventional therapy with more intensive monitoring and found a significant improvement in the rates of macrosomia, Caesarean

Table 10.6. Trials of insulin therapy for gestational diabetes mellitus.

Author	Design	n	Outcome macrosomia	LGA	CS	Birth trauma
O'Sullivan (1966)[152]	RCT	305 (insulin) 306 (no Rx) 324 (control)	4.3%† 13.1% 3.7%			
Coustan and Imarah[154] (1984)	Retrospective	115(insulin) 184 (diet) 146 (untreated)	7%† 18.5% 17.8%		16.3%* 30.4% 28.5%	4.8%* 13.4% 20.4%
Thompson (1990)[155]	RCT	34 (diet + insulin) 34 (diet)	5.9%* 26.5%			
Langer (1994)[156]	Prospective cohort	1145 (intensive) 1316 (conventional)	7% 14%	13% 20%		
Persson (1995)[157]	RCT	97 (diet + insulin) 105 (diet)		4% 6%		
Buchanan (1997)[161]	RCT <75th Cent >75th Cent ≥75th Cent	171 (std diet) 29 (diet) 30 (insulin)	3444 ± 38g 3878 ± 72g↑ 3647 ± 67g§	14% 45%↑ 13%§	14% 14% 43%	

$*p = 0.05$. $†p < 0.01$. LGA = large for gestational age; CS = Caesarian section. In the study of Buchanan *et al.*, abdominal circumference (AC) (centile) was measured by ultrasound between 29 and 33 weeks gestation. ($↑p < 0.01$ versus <AC75th centile; $§p < 0.04$ versus diet-treated group in randomised trial).

section, shoulder dystocia and neonatal metabolic complications in the intensive compared with conventional therapy[156].

By contrast, in a prospective study of 202 pregnant women randomised to treatment with diet alone or diet and prophylactic insulin (8–12 units per day) there was no apparent difference between the two groups in blood glucose control achieved, infant weight, skin fold thickness at birth or cord blood c-peptide[157]. However, 14% of the original diet group needed insulin for blood glucose control (fasting >7.0 and postprandial 9.0 mmol/l), so this was a study of only the mildest hyperglycaemic mothers. In Uppsala, Sweden, mothers with gestational diabetes defined by an intravenous GTT or a 75 g OGTT were treated with a large dose of insulin (mean 34 units soluble and 20 units medium-acting) and showed a reduced rate of macrosomia compared with their previous pregnancies, but no control group was available[158].

A meta-analysis of insulin treatment trials showed a sharp reduction (OR: 0.35; 95% CI 0.24–0.52) in the incidence of neonatal macrosomia (birth weight >4000 g) but no reduction in Caesarean delivery rates[159].

Many of the above studies have focused on birth weight as the outcome of interest and often the only outcome responsive to insulin treatment. It is also clear that rates of fetal complications are reduced only modestly from the already low rates that occur with less intensive management. Given that fewer than 4.4% of women with untreated gestational glucose intolerance deliver infants weighing 4.5 kg (compared with 2.6% of the overall population), and that gestational glucose intolerance is implicated in the births of only 5% of all infants with birth weights of 4.5 kg or more[19], a critical question is whether it might be possible to identify which of these babies are susceptible to fetal hyperinsulinism. For many years, Weiss has performed amniocentesis as a routine procedure to allow measurement of amniotic fluid insulin, but this is unlikely to be widely accepted in a routine clinical context[159]. Buchanan *et al.*[161,162] have perhaps provided the most elegant demonstration that insulin treatment of even mild hyperglycaemia (fasting glucose less than 5.8 mmol/l) will reduce fetal macrosomia. Among Hispanic women attending Los Angeles County hospital, a subset was identified with fetal abdominal circumference greater than the 75th centile for gestational age. These mothers were randomised to diet therapy alone (29 women), or diet with twice daily insulin (30 women) (initial dose 1.2 units/kg current body weight adjusted to maintain blood glucose fasting less than 4.4 mmol/l and less than 6.1 mmol/l two hours postprandially). The 'large for gestational age' rate in the diet treated subgroup was 45%, significantly greater than the insulin treated group (13%) and the diet treated group with an initial fetal abdominal circumference <75th centile (14%). Birth weight and neonatal skinfold thickness were also significantly reduced in the insulin-treated group.

There remains the possibility of overtreatment, and there is a danger of persistent maternal hypoglycaemia producing growth-retarded babies[163]. The ability to self-monitor maternal blood glucose[164] should prevent this, and clinical management has advanced considerably since the concept of maximal tolerated insulin therapy induced by Roversi in Milan in 1980[165].

One other important randomised trial in this field is by de Veciana *et al.*[166] who compared the results of fasting and preprandial versus fasting and post-prandial monitoring of capillary glucose measurements in relation to outcome among 66 Hispanic women with GDM. The fasting glucose (7.6 ± 2.1 versus 8.0 ± 2.8 mmol/l respectively) was relatively high compared with large-scale GDM populations, especially in light of the new 7.0 mmol/l fasting glucose criterion proposed by an Expert Committee of the ADA[5]. The postprandial group had decreased risks of neonatal hypoglycaemia, macrosomia and Caesarean delivery. (Level of evidence: macrosomia I, Strength of recommendation A; Caesarean section: Level of evidence I; Strength of recommendation C.)

LONG-TERM BENEFITS

As yet, there is little evidence that the long-term incidence of postpartum diabetes or obesity can be altered through case detection during gestation and subsequent intervention with insulin therapy. It is conceivable that such benefits may be of even greater importance to health than reducing birth weight. O'Sullivan and Mahan[167] reported that gestational diabetic women randomly assigned to insulin therapy during pregnancy were no more likely to develop diabetes 16 years later than those not treated, but in subsets of insulin-treated women with a macrosomic infant, or who had a family history of diabetes, subsequent decompensated diabetes was significantly reduced. More recently, Simmons and Robertson[168] compared the adiposity of infants of mothers with past gestational diabetes when studied two years and eight months after delivery. In comparison with offspring of women treated with diet alone, offspring of women treated with insulin therapy had less subscapular (7.9 versus 5.9; p <0.05) and biceps fat (6.3 versus 5.1; p = 0.01). A criticism of the latter study was the heterogenous nature of the subjects, but the results were obtained in spite of insulin-treated mothers being more obese, older and more hyperglycaemic than those who received diet alone. (Level of evidence III; Strength of recommendation C.)

TREATMENT THRESHOLDS

There is no consensus as to when to start insulin in pregnancy (Table 10.7). The American Diabetes Association and Summary of the Third International Workshop recommended a fasting glucose of 5.8 mmol/l or 6.7 mmol/l after meals (time unspecified). Hare[169] showed that this approach leads to an excess

Table 10.7. Recommendations for commencement of insulin in pregnancy after initial dietary therapy.

	Fasting	2 h postprandial venous plasma glucose (mmol/l)
1986 Goldberg (New York)	5.3 mmol/l	
1989 Langer (San Antonio)	5.2 mmol/l	
1991 Metzger (Chicago)	5.8 mmol/l	6.7 mmol/l
1992 St Vincent Declaration	5.6 mmol/l	8.0 mmol/l
1997 British Diabetic Assoc.	6.0 mmol/l	(fasting and pre-prandial)
1999 American Diabetic Assoc.	5.3 mmo/l	6.7 mmol/l

of large-for-gestational-age infants and, as a result, several groups have explored the benefit of more aggressive treatment regimens. Langer and colleagues stratified 471 GDM patients by the level of fasting plasma glucose on the OGTT[1476]. In the group with fasting glucose <5.3 (96 mg/dl), there was no difference between diet- and insulin-treated patients. By contrast, in the intermediate group (5.3–5.8 mmol/l (96–105mg/dl)), a three-fold higher rate of larger infants was found compared with diet-treated patients (28.6% versus 10.3%) and this was observed both in obese and lean subjects[170]. Using a logistic regression model, only mean blood glucose, fasting plasma on the OGTT, gestational age at entry and previous GDM were significant. Alternatively, the policy of Jovanovic–Peterson is to screen all women with a 1 h glucose >7.8 after a 50 g glucose load and to commence women on insulin if preprandial and postprandial capillary sugars are above 5.0 mmol/l and 6.7 mmol/l respectively; LGA rates were low with this approach. Up to 10% of all pregnant women are diagnosed as having GDM, of whom some two-thirds will require insulin therapy[170]. Therapeutic approaches based on attaining good maternal glycaemia in all pregnancies can be cost-effective[171], although it remains unclear whether all women with GDM require such therapy.

Clearly, a large randomised controlled trial, possibly with different target levels, is required to examine further the question of whether insulin therapy can impact on short-term outcome. Such a study will require a consensus opinion regarding the indication for treatment, and must include adequate numbers of subjects to demonstrate a significant difference in macrosomia. Ethnic and genetic considerations should be factored into the equation[171–174] and morphological measurements may further refine the indication for the introduction of insulin. Given the experimental and epidemiological evidence that diabetes begets diabetes through an intrauterine effect on the fetal pancreas[171–177], the long-term follow-up of these offspring may be of even greater importance in the assessment of health benefit and cost-effectiveness. Outcome measures must include not only glucose and obesity but also cardiovascular risk. Agreed criteria for detection, diagnosis and treatment are vital to the performing of these studies.

SCREENING

THE CASE FOR SCREENING

A survey of clinical obstetric practice clearly reveals that the issue of screening for diabetes during pregnancy is no less confused than that of diagnosis itself[176–180]. Whether all women should be screened, by what method, and the management of those with positive results remains unclear[19,181]. Unfortunately none of the standard recommendations for screening, viz: (a) the condition is an important health problem; (b) there is a simple, safe and precise and validated screening test; (c) there should be an effective treatment; and (d) treatment benefit should outweigh the economic and social costs, can be addressed by evidence of any quality.

The concept of gestational diabetes was founded on the risk of subsequent diabetes in the mother, rather than outcome[81]. Studies of adverse outcome have largely focused on macrosomia, which affects a minority of pregnancies with gestational diabetes. While there is some evidence that treatment can reduce fetal weight[166], it is less clear whether a reduction in Caesarean section rates follows[166], as the latter seem to reflect obstetric practice and a sensitivity to the diagnostic label. There is no consensus regarding the optimal screening test. Two studies using the 75 g OGTT for epidemiological studies provide minimal estimates of incidence of 4/10 000 Europid women[58] and 18/10 000 for South Asian women[182]. There are also the psychological aspects of the acquisition of a disease label, and an increased risk of an operative delivery.

On the other hand, there is a large body of evidence to support the contention that marked maternal hyperglycaemia in the range found in patients with pre-existing diabetes mellitus can have an adverse impact on fetal growth, development and wellbeing, and the Toronto study showed a direct relationship between OGTT results and a number of adverse outcomes including Caesarean delivery, neonatal macrosomia and pre-eclampsia even when corrected for potential risk factors. Screening for gestational diabetes has the potential to detect a disease, 50% of which goes undiagnosed, and which is becoming a major health problem. In addition, knowledge of ethnicity and the degree of glucose intolerance during pregnancy and immediately postpartum identifies women at future risk for disease who can be offered dietary and physical activity prevention strategies. The impact of hyperglycaemia during pregnancy for future generations continues to be realised and will also merit public health initiatives.

SCREENING STRATEGIES

There are certain factors (such as age <25 years, normal body weight, negative family history (first-degree relative) of diabetes, ethnic/racial group with a low prevalence of diabetes) that place women at lower risk for the development of glucose intolerance during pregnancy, and to screen such patients is unlikely to be cost-effective[183–185]. The number of women, for example, affected in a White/Europid antenatal population is small (0.4%)[57,186], and the obstetric benefits are poorly validated[19,20]. It is generally agreed that the simple and traditional documentation of maternal risk factors followed by a full diagnostic test (3 h, 100 g) is only 50–70% sensitive[94,114,187]. In the USA, a 50 g 1 h challenge was first introduced by O'Sullivan in 1973 and has been well validated[113] and endorsed by the ADA. The test is administered without regard to the previous meal and positive results ($\geq$7.8 mmol/l) on this test have around a 79% sensitivity and 87% specificity for detecting pregnancy-induced glucose intolerance, which occurs at 20–28 weeks gestation. In one study, the glucose challenge test was significantly associated with fetal macrosomia even when the OGTT was negative[120]. More recently, in the Toronto Tri-Hospital Study, an abnormal glucose challenge test independently predicted macrosomia[71].

Opinions differ on the threshold values for the glucose challenge test, the range of suggested values being between 7.2–8.3 mmol/l (130–150 mg/dl)[72]. It should also be noted that until the publication of the Toronto Tri-Hospital data, no report since O'Sullivan's had administered both the glucose challenge test (GCT) and the OGTT without regard to the GCT results. There is also controversy about the impact of testing in the fasting or fed state[128]. Various studies have examined the handling of the glucose load in relation to food, and differing thresholds have been suggested to account for this. In the Toronto TriHospital Study, Naylor[69] and colleagues demonstrated that a positive result on a glucose challenge test was influenced by the length of time (one, two, or three hours) since the last meal, and proposed differing thresholds at each of these time points. These schemas, however, are complex and unlikely to be adopted in routine practice. A recent editorial stated that because of the difficulties in discerning criteria for excluding women from screening, it seemed likely that universal screening would probably be used as a matter of practical convenience[188].

Random sampling of venous[189,190], plasma[191,192] or capillary[193] blood glucose have all been proposed as screening procedures and even as a replacement for the OGTT[19]. Meal tolerance tests are conceptually appealing and have been incorporated into screening paradigms[194,195] but are difficult to standardise. The problem with many of the above studies is that they did not look at infant outcome. It should be recalled that the peak postprandial response is correlated with birth weight[166,196]. In one study of 160 pregnant women with an abnormal 50 g glucose challenge test at 24–28 weeks gestation, fasting blood glucose (r = 0.94; p <0.001) and glycosylated plasma protein values (r = 0.81, p <0.001) were significantly associated with increased infant birth weight, and a combination of the two resulted in 100% sensitivity and 93% specificity in predicting an infant weighing over 4000 g[140].

THE OFFICIAL RECOMMENDATIONS

The Second and Third International Workshop Conference on Gestational Diabetes and the American Diabetes Association recommended routine screening of all women >25 years of age using a 50 g challenge between 24 and 28 weeks of gestation[7,8]. In 1986 the American College of Obsteticians and Gynecologists (ACOG) favoured a selective screening policy of women ≥30 weeks gestation and younger women with traditional risk factors[11], but more recently noted the absence of data to support it and did not make a specific recommendation[13]. Other reports[18] also found no convincing evidence of increased fetal or maternal risk to justify a universal screening programme other than the increased risk for subsequent diabetes in the mother. A significant change in position is the recommendation by the Fourth International Workshop and the ADA in favour of a more selective screening approach focusing on gravidas at low risk of developing diabetes[9] (Table 10.8).

A much simpler and more pragmatic approach to screening has been suggested by the British Diabetic Association[197] (Table 10.8). This involves the testing of urine for glucose at each visit with the addition of a timed random laboratory plasma glucose measurement at booking, 28 weeks gestation and whenever glycosuria ≥1+ is detected. A 75 g OGTT is performed if the timed random blood glucose concentrations are (a) >6 mmol/l fasting or 2 h after food, or (b) >7 mmol/l within 2 h of food. Our practice in Belfast over many years[57], in a population with a low prevalence of GDM, has closely mirrored this protocol, only we have used a single laboratory glucose value of 6.6 mmol/l (the mean ±3 SD in this population) to indicate the need for further investigation – usually involving a glucose tolerance test.

THE POINTS TO CONSIDER

It is now accepted that a more selective screening approach is both reasonable and justified. Women at high risk of GDM should be evaluated for glucose intolerance as early in pregnancy as possible and regularly throughout pregnancy. From a pragmatic perspective, the performance of both a 50 g challenge and diagnostic OGTT is excessive. Use of the former (which was evaluated in relation to the 100 g OGTT) will be called further into question if there is universal consensus on 75 g glucose load. A random plasma glucose, which is used to screen nonpregnant subjects, deserves further evaluation in pregnancy, and may be honed by relation to time of the last meal if these figures can be made simple. Although glycosuria yields a high incidence of false-positive information, this is nonetheless the only investigation that can be performed regularly throughout pregnancy. Moreover, it is cheap, widely accepted and unlikely to miss insulin-dependent diabetes arising during pregnancy. The data available on the incidence of IGT and diabetes in women with significant glycosuria suggest that the sensitivity of glycosuria as a screening test is approximately 80%, comparable to that reported for the 50 g oral OGTT which is usually only performed once in pregnancy[60]. (Selective screening II-2; Strength of recommendation A.)

PROSPECTS FOR PROGRESS

There is universal support for the need to detect clearly abnormal degrees of hyperglycaemia during pregnancy as defined by the WHO and NDDG. The possible adverse consequences of lesser degrees of glucose intolerance (approximating the WHO class of gestational IGT and contained in the broad

Table 10.8a. Screening protocols for gestational diabetes mellitus (GDM). 50 g oral glucose challenge test as recommended by the American Diabetes Association[14] and adapted by the 4th GDM Workshop[9]

Glucose cut-point	Proportion of women with positive test%	Sensitivity for GDM%
≥7.8 mmol/l (140 mg/dl)	14–18	≅80
≥7.2 mmol/l (130 mg/dl)	20–25	≅90

Serum or plasma glucose is measured one hour after the glucose challenge which can be performed at any time of day, without regard to the time of the last meal.
  The 4th GDM workshop defined three risk categories for GDM:
  I: High risk (one or more of the following): (a) Marked obesity, (b)Diabetes in first-degree relative, (c) History of glucose intolerance, (d) Previous infant with macrosomia e) Current glycosuria.
Recommendation: Screen at initial antepartum visit or as soon as possible thereafter, and repeat at 24–28 weeks gestation if no diagnosis of GDM by that time.
  II: Intermediate risk (fitting neither the high- or low-risk profile):
Recommendation: Screen between 24 and 28 weeks gestation.
  III: Low risk (all of the following): (a) Age <25 years, (b) low-risk race or ethnic group (i.e. those other than Hispanic, black, Native American, South or East Asian, Pacific Islander or Indigenous Australian), (c) No diabetes in first-degree relatives, (d) Normal weight before pregnancy, (e) No history of abnormal glucose metabolism, (f) No history of poor obstetric outcome.
  Recommendation: No screening required.
  A positive screening test is followed by a diagnostic 100 g OGTT. In women with very high-risk clinical characteristics, diagnostic testing may be performed without prior glucose screening[9].

Table 10.8b. Screening protocol of the British Pregnancy and Neonatal Care Group[197].

1. Urine should be tested for glycosuria at every antenatal visit (preferably fasting).
2. Timed or random venous plasma glucose measurements should be made:
    (a) whenever glycosuria (1+ or more) is detected.
    (b) at the booking visit and at 28 weeks gestation.
3. A 75 g oral glucose tolerance test (OGTT) should be carried out if the blood glucose is:
    (a) 6 mmol/l or more after food.
    (b) >7 mmol/l within two hours of food.

NDDG category of gestational diabetes) is less clear and, particularly in the IGT range, factors such as maternal age, obesity and parity reduce the impact of hyperglycaemia. It is apparent that most studies concerning GDM are observational, rather than experimental, and they frequently draw on historical rather than concurrent control subjects. The evidence to date suggests that there is a continuous relationship between glycaemia (however defined) and maternal fetal outcome. This immediately poses problems for defining diagnostic categories, and much additional confusion has been generated by the evolution of methodological differences in diagnostic practice. International bodies have tended to retreat into entrenched positions or at best offer political compromise. Recent scrutiny of the usefulness of the oral glucose tolerance test in nonpregnant subjects seems to have gone largely unnoticed by international bodies deliberating on such matters in pregnancy, and there is an almost inevitable acceptance of its continued use.

... FOR DIAGNOSIS ...

Given this background and the apparently continuous nature of the glucose distribution, clear direction is needed to allow uniform standards of clinical care. Equally, it is certain that only the most rigorously conducted multicentre trial will suffice to provide definitive evidence for change. It seems inevitable that an oral glucose tolerance test, unphysiological and inconvenient as it is, will be required at least to provide some continuity with the past and settle once and for all the vexed methodological preferences which have existed between countries. That such a study has been funded and is in progress is the most encouraging development in this field for 20 years. The Hyperglycaemia and Pregnancy Outcome Study (HAPO) is a multicentre study that began in 2000 and is designed to examine the significance of impaired glucose tolerance after a 75 g OGTT. It will report in 2005. Carers will be blinded to the results unless the 2 hour postload glucose value is above 11.1 mmol/l. The study will also allow a detailed comparison of the fasting, 1 h and 2 h levels in the OGTT in relation to detailed outcome measures. Each of these time points has certain theoretical and practical advantages and reported associations with outcome. For example, the fasting value, recommended in the first international workshop, offers a stable index of basal severity, is related to outcome[68,72], and is possibly predictive of late intrauterine death[14]. Both the 1 h and 2 h postload glucose values were comparable in relation to maternal–fetal end-points in the Sacks and Toronto data and a 1 h postprandial measurement was superior to preprandial monitoring for a variety of outcomes in a study using patients' self-monitored capillary glucose readings[167]. Another major practical advantage is that use of the 75 g OGTT would allow comparison with the pregnant and non pregnant state.

... FOR SCREENING ...

Perhaps the most significant development in relation to screening has been the recent change in the ADA recommendation from a universal to a selective screening strategy at 28 weeks, based on the presence of various risk factors. Given the fact that the challenge test was largely evaluated in relation to the 100 g OGTT, its continued use will be called further into question if universal guidelines favouring the 75 g OGTT can be reached. From a pragmatic perspective, it seems unreasonable to subject pregnant women to two glucose loads when one might suffice. Our practice in Belfast of screening with a random plasma glucose at booking and again at 28 weeks, along with testing for glycosuria at every visit, has worked well, the point being that routine identification of major hyperglycaemia well before 28 weeks gestation will identify those pregnancies really at risk. Pregnant women with a plasma glucose above 6 mmol/l two hours after food (fasting above 5.5 mmol/l), or 7 mmol/l within two hours of food, should undergo a definitive 75 g OGTT. Equally, a low random plasma glucose result, e.g. below 5.5 mmol/l, would almost certainly exclude the diagnosis of gestational diabetes at that time and may obviate the need for glucose tolerance testing.

... FOR TREATMENT ...

Integral to diagnosis, and indeed providing its *raison-d'être*, is the question of whether maternal and fetal morbidity can be reversed or ameliorated with treatment. Inherent difficulties include the separation of treatment effects from obstetric practice, familial and ethnic tendencies to large birth weight and the choice of relevant end-points, given obvious advances in perinatal and obstetric care. The evidence from randomised trials to date suggest that insulin therapy is helpful, but reported benefits are largely confined to birth weight; criteria differ for the introduction of insulin; and such treatment places women in a high risk pregnancy group susceptible to a potential cascade of obstetric intervention. There is increasing recognition of the relevance of asymetrical growth patterns, rather than absolute birth weight, when assessing pregnancy outcome in diabetic women with varying degrees of glucose intolerance. The proposal of Buchanan and colleagues that women should be defined on the basis of both fetal (abdominal circumference) and maternal (fasting glucose) measurements is perhaps the most elegant demonstration of a pragmatic and selective approach which merits further exploration.

... FOR THE NEW MILLENNIUM ...

As we embark on a new millennium, there are grounds for optimism that an international consensus on diagnosing GDM is within reach. Quite simply, we need one test and one set of diagnostic criteria. If, as anticipated, there is no threshold but rather a continuum of glycaemia with outcome, then agreed guidelines will be necessary, based on such considerations as the relative costs of diagnosing or failing to diagnose subjects at substantial risk of adverse maternal–fetal outcome. The subsequent focus must inevitably shift to the level of glycaemia at which insulin or other hypoglycaemic therapy should be introduced in pregnancy and the targets for treatment, similar to the shift in focus which has occurred for cholesterol and blood pressure in nonpregnant subjects. Again, a randomised multicentre, multiethnic trial will be needed to examine the question of whether insulin therapy can reduce short-term maternal-fetal outcomes and, perhaps even more importantly, to address the longer-term health implications of diagnosis and treatment in both the mother and offspring.

Table 10.9 Summary of evidence for GDM.

Summary of evidence	Level of evidence	Strength of recommendation
Hyperglycaemia and short-term maternal/foetal outcomes	II-2	B
Hyperglycaemia and long-term maternal/foetal outcomes		
Maternal diabetes	II-2	A
Foetal outcome	II-2	B
Detection of hyperglycaemia		
100 g OGTT	II-2	B
75 g OGTT	III	C
Treatment of hyperglycaemia and reduced short-term adverse foetal outcomes		
Dietary intervention	I	B
Physical activity	I	B
Insulin therapy		
Macrosomia	I	A
Caesarean section	I	C
Treatment of hyperglycaemia and reduced long-term adverse foetal outcomes	III	C

REFERENCES

1. National Diabetes Data Group (1979) Classification and diagnosis of diabetes mellitus and other categories of glucose intolerance. *Diabetes* **28**: 1039–1057.
2. World Health Organization Expert Committee on Diabetes Mellitus (1980) Second Report. Technical Report Series No. 646. Geneva: WHO.

3. World Health Organization Study Group on Diabetes Mellitus (1985) Technical Report Series No. 727. Geneva: WHO.

4. Report of the Expert Committee on the Diagnosis and Classification of Diabetes Mellitus (1997) *Diab. Care* **7**: 1183–1197.

5. Alberti KG, Zimmett PZ (1998) Definition, diagnosis and classification of diabetes mellitus and its complications. Part 1: diagnosis and classification of diabetes mellitus provisional report of a WHO Consultation. *Diab. Med.* **15**: 539–553.

6. Freinkel N, Josimovich J (1980) Summary and recommendations of American Diabetic Association Workshop Conference on Gestational Diabetes. *Diab. Care* **3**: 499–501.

7. Summary and recommendations of the Second International Workshop-Conference on Gestational Diabetes Mellitus (1985) *Diabetes* **34 (Suppl 2)**; 123–126.

8. Metzger BE (1991) Summary and recommendations of the Third International Workshop Conference on Gestational Diabetes Mellitus. *Diabetes* **40 (Suppl 2)**: 197–201.

9. Metzger BE, Coustan DR (Eds) (1998) Summary and recommendations of the Fourth International Workshop Conference on Gestational Diabetes Mellitus. *Diab. Care* **21 (Suppl 2)**: B161–B167.

10. American Diabetes Association (1986) Position statement: Gestational Diabetes Mellitus. *Diab. Care* **9**: 430–431.

11. American College of Obstetricians and Gynecologists (1986) Management of diabetes in pregnancy. *ACOG Technical Bulletin* **92**: 1–5.

12. American Diabetes Association (1991) Position statement: Gestational Diabetes Mellitus. *Diab. Care* **14**: 5–6.

13. American College of Obstetricians and Gynecologists (1994) *Management of Diabetes Mellitus in Pregnancy*. Washington, D.C.: ACOG.

14. American Diabetes Association (1999) Gestational Diabetes Mellitus: Position Statement *Diab. Care* **22**(Suppl. 1): S74–S76.

15. Coustan DR (1991) Diagnosis of gestational diabetes. What are our objectives? *Diabetes* **40 (Suppl 2)**: 14–17.

16. Harris MI (1988) Gestational diabetes may represent discovery of preexisting glucose tolerance. *Diab. Care* **11**: 402–411.

17. Jarrett RJ (1993) Gestational diabetes: a non-entity? *Br. Med. J.* **306**: 37–38.

18. Jarrett RJ (1997) Should we screen for gestational diabetes? *Br. Med. J.* **315**: 736–737.

19. Ales KL, Santini DL (1989) Should all pregnant women be screened for gestational glucose intolerance? *Lancet* i: 1187–1191.

20. Hunter DJS, Kierse MJNC (1989) Gestational diabetes. In (eds Chalmers I, Enkin M, Keirse MJNC) *Effective Care in Pregnancy and Childbirth, Vol 1*. Oxford: Oxford University Press, pp. 403–410.

21. Naylor CD (1989) Diagnosing gestational diabetes mellitus. Is the gold standard valid? *Diab. Care* **12**: 565–572.

22. Coustan DR (1996) Management of gestational diabetes mellitus: a self-fulfilling prophecy? *JAMA* **275**: 1199–1200.

23. Pedersen J (1977) *The Pregnant Diabetic and Her Newborn: Problems and Management*, 2nd ed. Baltimore, MD: Williams and Wilkins, pp. 191–197.

24. Freinkel N, Metzger BE (1979) Pregnancy as a tissue culture experience: the critical implications of maternal metabolism for fetal development. In *Pregnancy: Metabolism, Diabetes and the Fetus*. CIBA Foundation Symposium No. 65, Amsterdam, Exerpta Medica, pp. 3–23.

25. Freinkel N (1980) The Banting Lecture 1980. Of pregnancy and progeny. *Diabetes* **29**: 1023–1035.
26. Coustan DR, Imarah J (1984) Prophylactic insulin treatment of gestational diabetes reduces the incidence of macrosomia, operative delivery and birth trauma. *Am. J. Obstet. Gynecol.* **150**: 836–842.
27. Metzger BE (1991) Biphasic effects of maternal metabolism on fetal growth. *Diabetes* **40**(Suppl. 2): 99–105.
28. Jovanovic-Peterson L, Peterson C, Reed GF, Metzger BE, Mills JL, Knopp RH, Aarons JH (1991) The National Institute of Child Health and Human Development – Diabetes in Early Pregnancy Study: maternal postprandial glucose levels and infant birth weight; the diabetes in early pregnancy study. *Am. J. Obstet. Gynecol.* **764**: 103–111.
29. Coombs CA, Gundeson E, Kitzmiller JL, Gavin LA, Main EK (1992) Relationship of fetal macrosomia to maternal postprandial glucose control during pregnancy. *Diab. Care* **15**: 1251–1257.
30. Reiher H, Fuhrmann K, Noak S, Woltanski K-P, Jutzi E, van Dorsche HH, Hahn H-J (1983) Age-dependent insulin secretion of the endocrine pancreas in vitro from fetuses of diabetic and nondiabetic patients. *Diab. Care* **6**: 446–451.
31. Ogata ES, Sabagha R, Metzger BE, Phelps RL, Depp R, Freinkel N (1980) Serial ultrasonography to assess evolving fetal macrosomia. *JAMA* **243**: 2405–2407.
32. Metzger BE, Phelps RL, Freinkel N (1980) Effects of gestational diabetes on diurnal profiles of plasma glucose, lipids and individual aminoacids. *Diab. Care* **3**: 402–409.
33. Kalhoff RK (1991) Impact of maternal fuels and nutritional state on fetal growth. *Diabetes* **40**(Suppl. 2): 61–66.
34. Knopp RH, Magee MS, Walden CE, Bonet B, Benedetti TJ (1992) Prediction of infant birth weight by GDM screening: importance of plasma triglyceride. *Diab. Care*; **15**: 1605–1613.
35. Milner RDG, Ashworth MA, Barson AJ (1972) Insulin release from human fetal pancreas in response to glucose, leucine and arginine. *J. Endocrinol.* **52**: 497–505.
36. Stoz F, Schuhmann RA, Hass B (1988) Morphometric investigations in placentas of gestational diabetes. *J. Perinat. Med.* **16**: 205–209.
37. Williams RW, Creasy RK, Cunningham GC (1982) Fetal growth and perinatal viability in California. *Obstet. Gynaecol.* **59**: 624.
38. Abrams BF, Laros RK (1986) Prepregnancy weight, weight gain and birth weight. *Am. J. Obstet. Gynecol.* **154**: 503.
39. Klebanoff MA, Mills JL, Berendes HW (1985) Mother's birth weight as a predictor of macrosomia. *Am. J. Obstet. Gynecol.* **153**: 253.
40. Dooley SL, Metzger BE, CHO N (1995) Gestational diabetes: influences of race on disease prevalence and perinatal outcome in a US population. *Diab. Care* **44**: 24–30.
41. Homoko CJ, Sivan E, Nyirjesy P (1995) The inter-relationship between ethnicity and gestational diabetes in fetal macrosomia. *Diab. Care* **18**: 1442–1445.
42. Gloria-Bottini F, Gerlin G, Lucarini N, Amante A, Lucarelli P, Borgiani P, Bottini E (1994) Both maternal and fetal genetic factors contribute to macrosomia in diabetic pregnancy. *Hum. Hered.* **44**: 24–30.
43. Barker DJP (1992) Fetal growth and adult disease. *Br. J. Obstet. Gynaecol.* **99**: 275–276.
44. McCance DR, Pettitt DJ, Hanson RL, Jacobsson LTH, Knowler WC, Bennett PH (1994) Birth weight and non-insulin dependent diabetes: thrifty genotype, thrifty phenotype or surviving small baby genotype? *Br. Med. J.* **308**: 942–945.

45. Hattersley AT, Tooke JE (1991) The fetal insulin hypothesis: an alternative explanation of the association of low birth weight with diabetes and vascular disease. *Lancet* **353**:1789–1792.
46. Hattersley AT, Beards F, Ballantyne E, Appleton M, Harvey R, Ellard S (1998) Mutations in the glucokinase gene result in reduced birth weight. *Nat. Genet.* **193**: 268–270.
47. Stride A, Shephard M, Frayling TM, Bulman MP, Ellarad S, Hattersley AT (1999) Intrauterine hyperglycaemia may alter the age of diagnosis in patients with hepatic nuclear factor 1a (HNF1a) mutations. Presented at British Diabetic Association meeting, Glasgow, April.
48. Coustan DR (1986) Hyperglycemia-hyperinsulinemia: effect on the infant of the diabetic mother. In Jovanovic L, Peterson CM, Fuhrman K (eds) *Diabetes and Pregnancy: Teratology, Toxicity and Treatment*, New York: Praeger, pp. 291–320.
49. Moss JM, Mulholland JB (1951) Diabetes and pregnancy with special reference to the prediabetic state. *Ann. Int. Med.* **34**: 678–679.
50. Du Muylder X (1984) Perinatal complications of gestational diabetes: the influence of the timing of the diagnosis. *Eur. J. Obstet. Reprod. Biol.* **18**: 35–42.
51. Cousins L (1987) Pregnancy complications among diabetic women: Review 1965–1985. *Obstet. Gynecol. Surv.* **42**: 140–149.
52. O'Sullivan JB, Mahan CM, Charles D, Dandrow RV (1973) Gestational diabetes and perinatal mortality rate. *Am. J. Obstet. Gynecol.* **116**: 901–904.
53. Oats JN, Beischer NA (1986) Gestational diabetes. *Aust. NZ J. Obstet. Gynecol.* **26**: 2–10.
54. Huddle K, England M, Nagar A (1993) Outcome of pregnancy in diabetic women in Soweto, South Africa. *Diabetic Med.* **10**: 290–294.
55. Gyves MT, Rodman HM, Little AB, Fanaroff AA, Merkatz IR (1977) A modern approach to management of pregnant diabetics: a two-year analysis of perinatal outcomes. *Am. J. Obstet. Gynecol.* **128**: 606–616.
56. Lavin JP, Lovelace DR, Miodovnik M, Knowler HC, Barden TP (1983) Clinical experience with 107 diabetic pregnancies. *Am. J. Obstet. Gynecol.* **147**: 742–752.
57. Hadden DR (1980) Screening for abnormalities of carbohydrate metabolism in pregnancy 1966–1977. The Belfast Experience. *Diab. Care* **3**: 440–446.
58. Roberts RN, Moohan JM, Foorl K, Harley JMG, Traub AI, Hadden DR (1993) Fetal outcome in mothers with impaired glucose tolerance in pregnancy. *Diabetic Med.* **10**: 438–443.
59. Philipson EH, Kalhan SC, Rosen MG, Dedlberg SC, Williams TG, Riha MM (1985) Gestational diabetes mellitus: is further improvement necessary? *Diabetes* **34**(Suppl. 2): 55–60.
60. Pettitt DJ, Knowler WC, Baird HR, Bennett PH (1980) Gestational diabetes: infant and maternal complications of pregnancy in relation to third trimester glucose tolerance in the Pima Indians. *Diab. Care* **3**: 458–464.
61. Tallarigo L, Gianpetro O, Penno G, Miccoli R, Gregori G, Navalesi R (1986) Relation of glucose tolerance to complications of pregnancy in nondiabetic women. *New Engl. J. Med.* **315**: 989–68.
62. Leiken EL, Jenkins JH, Pomerantz GA, Klein L (1987) Abnormal glucose screening tests in pregnancy: a risk factor for fetal macrosomia. *Obstet. Gynecol.* **69**: 570–573.
63. Langer O, Brustman L, Anyaegbunam A, Mazze R (1987) The significance of one abnormal glucose tolerance test value on adverse outcome in pregnancy. *Am. J. Obstet. Gynecol.* **159**: 1478–1483.
64. Lindsay MK, Graves W, Klein L (1989) The relationship of one abnormal glucose tolerance test value and pregnancy complications. *Obstet. Gynecol.* **73**: 103–106.

65. Langer O, Mazze R (1988) The relationship between large-for-gestational-age infants and glycaemic control in women with gestational diabetes. *Am. J. Obstet. Gynecol.* **159**: 1478–1483.
66. Ballard JL, Rosenn B, Khoury JC, Miodovnik M (1993) Diabetic fetal macrosomia: significance of disproportionate growth. *J. Paediatr.* **122**: 1115–1119.
67. Gillmer MDG, Beard RW, Brooke FM, Oakley NW (1975) Carbohydrate metabolism in pregnancy. *Br. Med. J.* **3**: 399–404.
68. Sacks DA, Greenspoon JS, Salim AF, Henry HM, Wolde-Tsadik G, Yao JFF (1995) Toward universal criteria for gestational diabetes: The 75-gram glucose tolerance test in pregnancy. *Am. J. Obstet. Gynecol.* **172**: 607–614.
69. Naylor CD, Sermer M, Chen E, Sykora K (1996) Cesarean delivery in relation to birth weight and gestational glucose intolerance: pathophysiology or practice style. *JAMA* **265**: 1165–1170.
70. Sermer M, Naylor CD, Gare DJ, Kenshole AB, Ritchie JWK, Farine D, Cohen HR, McArthur K, Holzapfel S, Biringer A, Chen E, Cadesky KI, Greenblatt EM, Leyland NA, Morris HS, Bloom JA, Abells YB (for the Toronto Tri-Hospital Gestational Diabetes Investigators) (1994) Impact of time since last meal on the gestational glucose challenge test. *Am. J. Obstet. Gynecol.* **171**: 607–616.
71. Sermer M, Naylor CD, Gare DJ, Kenshole AB, Ritchie JWK, Farine D, Cohen HR, McArthur K, Holzapfel S, Biringer A, Chen E, Cadesky KI, Greenblatt EM, Leyland NA, Morris HS, Bloom JA, Abells YB (1995) Impact of increasing carbohydrate intolerance on maternal fetal outcomes in 3637 women without gestational diabetes, *Am. J. Obstet. Gynecol.* **173**: 146–156.
72. Sermer M, Naylor CD, Farine D, Kenshole AB, Ritchie JWK, Gare DJ, Cohen HR, McArthur K, Holzapfel S, Biringer A (for the Toronto Tri-Hospital gestational diabetes investigators) (1998) The Toronto Tri-hospital Gestational Diabetes Project: a preliminary review. *Diab. Care* **21**(Suppl. 2): B33–B42.
73. Carpenter MW, Coustan DR (1982) Criteria for screening tests for gestational diabetes. *Am. J. Obstet. Gynecol.* **159**: 768–773.
74. Jarrett RJ (1989) Reflections on gestational diabetes mellitus. *Lancet* **2**: 1220–1222.
75. Metzger BR, Bybee DR, Freinkel N, Phelps RL, Radavny RM, Vaisrub N (1985) Gestational diabetes mellitus: correlations between the phenotypic and genotypic characteristics of the mother and abnormal glucose tolerance during the first year postpartum. *Diabetes* **34 (Suppl 2)**: 111–115.
76. Coustan DR, Nelson C, Carpenter MW, Carr Sr, Rotondo L, Widness JA (1989) Maternal age and screening for gestational diabetes: a population-based study. *Obstet. Gynecol.* **73**: 557–561.
77. Weeks, JW, Major CA, de Veciana M, Morgan MA (1994) Gestational diabetes: does the presence of risk factors influence perinatal outcome? *Am. J. Obstet. Gynecol.* **171**: 1003–1007.
78. Sepe SJ, Connell FA, Geiss LS, Teutsch SM (1985) Gestational diabetes, incidence, maternal characteristics and perinatal outcome. *Diabetes* **34**(Suppl. 2): 13–16.
79. Moses RG, Calvert D (1995) Pregnancy outcomes in women without gestational diabetes mellitus related to the maternal glucose level. Is there a continuum of risk? *Diab. Care* **12**: 1527–1533.
80. Maresh M, Beard RW, Bary CS, Elkeles RS, Wadsworth J (1989) Factors predisposing to and outcome of gestational diabetes. *Obstet. Gynecol.* **74**: 342–346.
81. Widness JA, Cowett RM, Coustan DR, Carpenter MW, Oh W (1985) Neonatal morbidities in infants of mothers with glucose glucose intolerance in pregnancy. *Diabetes* **34**(Suppl. 2): 61–65.

82. O'Sullivan JB, Mahan CM (1964) Criteria for the oral glucose tolerance test in pregnancy. *Diabetes* **13**: 278–285.
83. O'Sullivan JB (1979) Gestational diabetes: factors influencing the rates of subsequent diabetes. In: Sutherland HW, Stowers JM (eds) *Carbohydrate Metabolism in Pregnancy and the Newborn*. New York: Springer-Verlag, pp. 425–435.
84. Mestman JH (1988) Follow-up studies in women with gestational diabetes mellitus. The experience at Los Angeles County University of Southern California Medical Centre. In Weiss PA, Coustan DR (eds) *Gestational Diabetes*. New York: Springer-Verlag, pp. 191–198.
85. Henry OA, Beischer NA (1991) Long-term implications of gestational diabetes for the mother. *Ballieres Clin. Obstet. Gynaecol.* **5**: 461–483.
86. Persson B, Hanson U, Hartling SG, Binder C (1991) Follow-up of women with previous gestational diabetes mellitus: insulin, c-peptide and proinsulin responses to oral glucose load. *Diabetes* **40 (Suppl 2)**: 136–141.
87. Damm P, Kuhl C, Bertelsen A, Molsted-Pedersen L (1992) Predictive factors for the development of diabetes in females with previous gestational diabetes mellitus. *Am. J. Obstet. Gynecol.* **16**: 607–616.
88. Metzger BE, Cho NH, Roston SM, Radvany R (1993) Prepregnancy weight and antepartum insulin secretion predict glucose tolerance five years after gestational diabetes mellitus. *Diab. Care* **16**: 1598–1605.
89. Coustan Dr, Carpenter MW, O'Sullivan PS, Carr SR (1993) Gestational diabetes: predictors and subsequent disordered glucose metabolism. *Am. J. Obstet. Gynaecol.* **168**: 1139–1145.
90. Kjos SL, Peters RK, Xiang A, Henry OA, Montoro M, Buchanan TA (1995) Predicting future diabetes in Latino women with gestational diabetes. *Diabetes* **44**: 586–591.
91. Ward WK, Johnston CLW, Beard JC, Benedetti TJ, Halter JB, Porte D Jr (1985) Insulin resistance and impaired insulin secretion in subjects with histories of gestational diabetes mellitus. *Diabetes* **34**: 861–869.
92. Kjos SL, Buchanan TA, Greenspoon JS, Montoro M, Berstein FS, Mestman JH (1990) Gestational diabetes mellitus: the prevalence of glucose intolerance in the first two months post partum. *Am. J. Obstet. Gynecol.* **163**: 93–98.
93. Catalano PM, Vargo KM, Berstein JM, Amini SP (1991) Incidence and risk factors associated with abnormal postpartum glucose tolerance in females with gestational diabetes. *Amer. J. Obstet. Gynecol.* **165**: 914–919.
94. Coustan DR, Nelson C, Carpenter MW, Carr SR, Retondo L, Widness JA (1989) Maternal age and screening for gestational diabetes: a population-based study. *Obstet. Gynecol.* **73**: 557–561.
95. Peters RK, Kjos SL, Xiang A, Buchanan TA (1996) Long-term diabetogenic effect of single pregnancy in women with previous gestational diabetes mellitus. *Lancet* **347**: 227–230.
96. Anastasiou E, Lekakis JP, Alevizaks M, Papamichael CM, Megas J, Souvaatzoglou A, Stamatelopoulos SP (1998) Impaired endothelial-dependent vasodilitation in females with previous gestational diabetes mellitus. *Diab. Care* **21**: 2111–2115.
97. Vohr BR, Lipsitt LP, OH W (1980) Somatic growth of children of diabetic mothers with reference to birth size. *J. Paediatr.* **97**; 196–199.
98. Pettitt DJ, Baird HR, Aleck KA, Bennett PH, Knowler WC (1983) Excessive obesity in offspring of Pima Indian women with diabetes during pregnancy. *New Engl. J. Med.* **308**: 242–245.
99. Pettitt DJ, Aleck KA, Baird HR, Carraher MJ, Bennett PH, Knowler WC (1988) Congenital susceptibility to NIDDM: role of intra-uterine environment. *Diabetes* **37**; 622–628.

100. Pettitt DJ, Knowler WC (1998) Long-term effects of the intrauterine environment, birth weight and breast feeding in Pima Indians. *Diab. Care* **21**(Suppl. 2): B138–B141.
101. Silverman M, Metzger B, Cho N, Loeb C (1995) Impaired glucose tolerance in adolescent offspring of diabetic mothers. Relationship to fetal hyperinsulinism. *Diab. Care* **18**: 611–617.
102. Silverman B, Rizzo TA, Cho NH, Metzger BE (1998) Long-term effects of the intrauterine environment. The Northwestern University Diabetes in Pregnancy Center. *Diab. Care* **21**(Suppl. 2): B142–B149.
103. Rizzo T, Metzger BE, Burns WJ, Burns K (1991) Correlations between antepartum maternal metabolism and intelligence of offspring. *New Engl. J. Med.* **325**: 911–916.
104. Manson JE, Rimm EB, Stampfer MJ, Colditz GA, Willett WC, Krolewski AS, Rossner B, Hennekens CH, Speizer FE (1991) Physical activity and incidence of NIDDM women. *Lancet* **338**: 774–778.
105. Adler A, Turner RC (1999) The Diabetes Prevention Program. *Diab. Care* **22**: 543–545.
106. Diabetes prevention program research group (2002) Reduction in the incidence of type 2 diabetes with lifestyle intervention or metformin. *New Engl. J. Med* **346**: 393–403.
107. Duncan JM (1882) On puerperal diabetes. *Trans. Obstet. Soc. Lond.* **24**: 256–285.
108. Williams JW (1909) The clinical significance of glycosuria in pregnant women. *Am. J. Med. Sci.* **137**: 1–26.
109. Gilbert JAL, Dunlop DM (1949) Diabetic fertility, maternal mortality and fetal loss. *Br. Med. J.* **1**: 48–51.
110. Miller HC, Hurwitz D, Kuder K (1944) Fetal and neonatal mortality in pregnancies complicated by diabetes mellitus. *JAMA* **124**: 271–275.
111. Jackson WPV (1952) Studies in prediabetes. *Br. Med. J.* **2**: 690
112. Bennewitz HG (1824) Dediabete mellito, graviditatis symptomate. MD dissertation, Berlin..
113. O'Sullivan JB, Mahan CM, Charles D, Dandrow RV (1973) Screening criteria for high-risk gestational diabetic patients. *Am. J. Obstet. Gynecol.***116**: 895–900.
114. Sacks DA, Abu-Fadil S, Greenspoon JS, Fotheringham N (1989) Do the current standards for glucose tolerance in pregnancy represent a valid conversion of O'Sullivan's original criteria? *Am. J. Obstet. Gynecol.* **161**: 638–641.
115. Neiger R, Coustan DR (1991) Are the current ACOG glucose tolerance test criteria sensitive enough? *Obstet. Gynecol.* **78**: 1117–1120.
116. Pettitt DJ, Bennett PH, Hanson RL, Narayan KMV, Knowler WC (1994) Comparison of World Health Organisation and National Diabetes Data Group procedures to detect abnormalities of glucose tolerance during pregnancy. *Diab. Care* **17**: 1264–1268.
117. Deerochanawong C, Putiyanum C, Wongsuryrat M, Serirat S, Jinayon P (1996) Comparison of National Diabetes Data Group and World Health Organisation criteria for detecting gestational diabetes mellitus. *Diabetologia* **39**: 1070–1073.
118. Diabetes Pregnancy Study Group (1989) A prospective multicentre study to determine the influence of pregnancy upon the 75 g oral glucose tolerance test (OGTT). In Sutherland HN, Stowers JM, Pearson DWM (eds) *Carbohydrate Metabolism in Pregnancy and the Newborn IV*. Springer-Verlag: London, 209–226.
119. Kuhl C (1975) Glucose metabolism during and after pregnancy in normal and gestational diabetic women. Influence of normal pregnancy on serum glucose and insulin concentration during basal fasting conditions and after a challenge with glucose. *Acta Endocrinol.* **79**: 709–719.

120. Kuhl C, Andersen O (1988) Pathophysiological background for gestational diabetes. In *Gestational Diabetes*. Weiss PAM, Coustan DR (eds) Vienna: Springer-Verlag, pp. 67–71.
121. Kuhl C (1991) Insulin secretion and insulin resistance in pregnancy and GDM. Implications for diagnosis and management. *Diabetes* **40 (Suppl 2)**: 18–24.
122. Cousins L (1991) Insulin sensitivity in pregnancy. *Diabetes* **40 (Suppl 2)**: 39–43.
123. Felig P, Lynch V (1970) Starvation in human pregnancy: hypoglycemia, hypoinsulinemia and hyperketonemia. *Science* **124**: 900–902.
124. Lind T, Belewicz WZ, Brown G (1973) A serial study of changes occurring in the glucose tolerance test during pregnancy. *J. Obstet. Gynaecol. Br. Commonw.* **80**: 1033–1039.
125. Hagen A (1961) Blood sugar findings during normal and possible prediabetics. *Diabetes* **10**: 438–444.
126. Phelps RL, Metzger BE, Freinkel N (1981) Carbohydrate metabolism in pregnancy. XVII: Diurnal profiles of plasma glucose, insulin, free fatty acids, triglycerides, cholesterol and individual fatty acids. *Am. J. Obstet. Gynecol.* **140**: 730–736.
127. Forest JC, Garrido-Russo M, Lemay A, Carrier R, Dube JL (1983) Reference values for the oral glucose tolerance test at each trimester of pregnancy. *Am. J. Clin. Pathol.* **80**: 828–831.
128. Hatem M, Anthony F, Hogston P, Rowe DJF, Dennis KJ (1988) Reference values for the 75 g oral glucose tolerance test in pregnancy. *Br. Med. J.* **296**: 676–678.
129. Morris MA, Grandis AS, Litton JC (1985) Glycoslyated hemoglobin concentration in early gestation associated with neonatal outcome. *Am. J. Obstet. Gynecol.* **153**: 651–654.
130. Phelps RL, Honig G, Green D, Metzger BE, Frederiksen MC, Freinkel N (1983) Biphasic changes in haemoglobin A1c concentrations in human pregnancy. *Am. J. Obstet. Gynecol.* **147**: 651–653.
131. McDonald GWM, Fisher GF, Burnham C (1965) Reproducibility of the oral glucose tolerance test. *Diabetes* **14**: 473–480.
132. Furhman GI, Steinberg MC (1987) Diabetes screening during pregnancy. *Diabetes* **36 (Suppl 1)**: 90–94.
133. Neiger R, Coustan DR (1991) The role of repeat glucose tolerance tests in the diagnosis of gestational diabetes. *Am. J. Obstet. Gynecol.* **165**: 787–790.
134. Yudkin JS, Alberti KGMM, McLarty DG (1990) Impaired glucose tolerance: is it a fact or a diagnostic ragbag? *Br. Med. J.* **301**: 397–402.
135. Leonards JR, McCullagh EP, Christopher TC (1965) A new carbohydrate solution for testing glucose tolerance. *Diabetes* **14**: 96–99.
136. Neely RDG, Kiwanuka JB, Hadden DR (1991) Influence of sample type on the interpretation of the oral glucose test for gestational diabetes mellitus. *Diabetic Med.* **8**: 129–134.
137. Hadden DR (1985) Geographic, ethnic and racial variations in the incidence of gestational diabetes mellitus. *Diabetes* **34 (Suppl 2)**: 8–12.
138. Green JR, Pawson JG, Schumacher LB, Perry J, Kretchmer N (1990) Glucose tolerance in pregnancy: ethnic variation and influence of body habitus. *Am. J. Obstet. Gynecol.* **163**: 86–92.
139. Engelgau MM, Herman WH, Smith PJ, German RR, Aubert RE (1995) The epidemiology of diabetes and pregnancy in the US (1988). *Diab. Care* **18**: 1029–1033.
140. Bevier WC, Jovanovic-Peterson L, Peterson CM (1995) Diagnosis, management and outcome of gestational diabetes. *End. Metab. Clin. N. Amer.* **24**; 103–138.

141. Merkatz IR, Duchon MA, Yamashita TS, Houser HB (1980). A pilot community based program for gestational diabetes. *Diab. Care* **3**: 453–457.
142. Catalano PM, Tyzbir ED, Wolfe RR (1993) Carbohydrate metabolism during pregnancy in control subjects and women with gestational diabetes. *Am. J. Physiol.* **264**: E60–E67.
143. Soares JAC, Dornhorst, Beard RW (1997) The case for screening for gestational diabetes. *Br. Med. J.* **315**: 737–739.
144. Walkinshaw SA (1999) Dietary regulation for 'gestational diabetes' (Cochrane Review). In *The Cochrane Library, Issue 2.* Oxford: Update Software.
145. Li DFH, Wong VCW, O'Hoy KMKY, Yeung CY, Ma HK (1987) Is treatment needed for mild impairment of glucose tolerance in pregnancy? A randomised controlled trial. *Br. J. Obstet. Gynaecol.* **94**: 851–854.
146. Garner P, Okun N, Keely E, Wells G, Perkins S, Sylvain J, Belcher J (1997) A randomised controlled trial of strict glycaemic control and tertiary level obstetric care versus routine obstetric care in the management of gestational diabetes: a pilot study. *Am. J. Obstet. Gynecol.* **177**: 190–195.
147. Langer O (1998) Maternal glycaemic criteria for insulin therapy in gestational diabetes mellitus. Proceedings of the fourth International Workshop-Conference on Gestational Diabetes Mellitus. *Diab. Care* **21 (Suppl 2)**: B91–B98.
148. Bevier WC, Fischer R, Jovanovic L (1999) Treatment of women with an abnormal glucose challenge test (but a normal oral glucose tolerance test) decreases the prevalence of macrosomia. *Am. J. Perinatol.* **16**: 269–275.
149. Bung P, Artal R, Khodiguian N, Kjos S (1991) Exercise in gestational diabetes. An optional therapeutic approach? *Diabetes* **40 (Suppl 2)**: 182–185.
150. Jovanovic L, Durak EP, Peterson CM (1989) Randomized trial of diet versus diet plus cardiovascular conditioning on glucose levels in gestational diabetes. *Am. J. Obstet. Gynecol.* **161**: 415–419.
151. Jovanovic-Peterson L, Peterson CM (1991) Is exercise safe or useful for gestational diabetic women? *Diabetes* **40 (Suppl 1)**: 179–181.
152. O'Sullivan JB, Mahan CM, Charles D, Dandrow RV (1974) Medical treatment of the gestational diabetic. *Obstet. Gynecol.* **43**: 817–821.
153. O'Sullivan JB, Charles D, Dandrow RV (1971) Treatment of verified prediabetics in pregnancy. *J. Reprod. Med.* **7**: 21–24.
154. Coustan DR, Lewis SB (1978) Insulin therapy for gestational diabetes. *Obstet. Gynecol.* **51**: 306–310.
155. Thompson DJ, Porter KB, Gunnells DJ (1990) Prophylactic insulin in the management of gestational diabetes. *Obstet. Gynecol.* **75**: 960–964.
156. Langer O, Rodriguez DA, Xenakis EMJ, McFarland MB, Berkus MD, Arrendondo F (1994) Intensified versus conventional management of gestational diabetes. *Am. J. Obstet. Gynecol.* **170**: 1036–1047.
157. Persson B, Stangenberg M, Hansson U, Norlander E (1985) Gestational diabetes mellitus (GDM): comparative evaluation of two treatment regimens, diet versus insulin and diet. *Diabetes* **320 (Suppl 2)**: 101–105.
158. Berne C, Wibell L, Lindmark G (1995) Ten-year experience of insulin treatment in gestational diabetes. *Acta Paediatr. Scand.* **320 (Suppl 1)**: 85–93.
159. Walkinshaw SA (1993) Diet and inulin vs. diet alone for 'gestational diabetes. In: Pregnancy and Childbirth Module. (eds Enkin MW, Kierse MJNC, Renfre MJ, Neilson JP) Oxford, Update Software, Spring (Cochrane Database of Systematic Reviews), Review 06650).
160. Weiss PAM (1996) Diabetes in pregnancy: lessons from the fetus. In Dornhorst A, Hadden DR (eds) *Diabetes and Pregnancy: An International Approach to Diagnosis and Management.* John Wiley: Chichester, pp. 221–240.

161. Buchanan TA, Kjos SL, Montoro MN, Wu PV, Madilejo NG, Gonzalez M (1994) Use of fetal ultrasound to select metabolic therapy for pregnancies complicated by mild gestational diabetes. *Diab. Care* **17**: 175–183.
162. Kjos SL, Buchanan TA (1999) Gestational diabetes mellitus. *New Engl. J. Med.* **341**: 1749–1756.
163. Langer O, Brustman L, Anyaezbunam A, Merkatz R, Divon M (1989) Glycaemic control in gestational diabetes mellitus – how tight is tight enough: small for gestational age versus large for gestational age? *Am. J. Obstet. Gynecol.* **161**: 646–653.
164. Goldberg JD, Franklin B, Lasser D (1986) Gestational diabetes: impact of home glucose monitoring on neonatal birthweight. *Am. J. Obstet. Gynecol.* **154**: 546–550.
165. Roversi GD, Garginolo M,. Nicolini E, Ferrazzi E, Pedretti E, Gruft L, Tronconi G (1980) Maximal tolerated insulin therapy in gestational diabetes. *Diab. Care* **3**: 489–494.
166. De Veciana M, Major CA, Morgan MA, Asrat T, Toohey J, Lien J, Evans A (1995) Postprandial versus preprandial blood glucose monitoring in women with gestational diabetes mellitus requiring insulin therapy versus preprandial blood glucose monitoring in women with gestational diabetes mellitus requiring insulin therapy. *New Engl. J. Med.* **333**: 1237–1241.
167. O'Sullivan JB, Mahan CM (1980) Insulin treatment and high risk groups. *Diab. Care* **3**: 482–485.
168. Simmons D, Robertson S (1997) Influence of maternal insulin treatment on the infants of women with gestational diabetes. *Diabetic Med.* 14: 762–765.
169. Hare JW (1991) Gestational diabetes mellitus: levels of glycaemia as management goals. *Diabetes* **40 (Suppl 2)**: 193–196.
170. Jovanic-Peterson L, Bevier W, Peterson CM (1995) A cost-effective program to normalise birth weight by screening for and treatment of glucose intolerance of pregnancy. *Diabetes* **44**(Suppl. 1): 258A.
171. Kitzmiller JL, Elixhauser A, Carr S, Major CA, de Veciana M, Dang-kilduff L, Weschler JM (1998) Assessment of costs and benefits of management of gestational diabetes. *Diab. Care* **21**(Suppl. 2):B123–B130.
172. Aerts L, Sodoyez-Goffaux F, Sodoyez JC, Malaisse WJ, Van Assche FA (1988) The diabetic intrauterine milieu has a long-lasting effect on insulin secretion by B cells and on insulin uptake by target tissues. *Am. J. Obstet. Gynecol.* **159**: 1287–1292.
173. Alcolado JC, Alcolado R (1991) Importance of maternal history of non-insulin-dependent diabetic patients. *Br. Med. J.* 302: 1178–1180.
174. Dornhorst A, Nicholls JSD, Welch A, Ali K, Chan SP, Beard RW (1996) Correcting for ethnicity when defining large-for-gestational infants in diabetic pregnancies. *Diabetic Med.* **13**: 226–231.
175. Pettitt DJ, Knowler WC (1988) Diabetes and obesity in the Pima Indians: a cross-generational vicious cycle. *J. Obes. Weight Reg.* 7: 61–75.
176. Mazze RS, Krogh CI (1992) Gestational diabetes mellitus. Now is the the time for detection and treatment. *Mayo Clin. Proc.* **67**: 995–1002.
177. Hunter A, Doery JC, Miranda V (1990) Diagnosis of gestational diabetes in Australia: a national survey of current practice. *Med. J. Aust.* **153**: 290–292.
178. Burnett L (1990) An audit of glucose tolerance test requests. *Med. J. Aust.* 152: 607–608.
179. Nelson-Piercy C, Gale EAM (1994) Do we know how to screen for gestational diabetes? Current practice in one regional health authority. *Diabetic Med.* **11**: 493–498.

180. Landon MB, Gabbe SG, Sachs L (1990) Management of diabetes mellitus and pregnancy: a survey of obstetricians and materno-fetal specialists. *Obstet. Gynecol.* **75**: 635–640.
181. Jarrett RJ (1997) Should we screen for gestational diabetes mellitus? *Brit. Med. J.* **315**: 736–737.
182. Samanta A, Burden MI, Burden AC, Jones ER (1989) Glucose tolerance testing during pregnancy in Asian women. *Diab. Res. Clin. Pract.* **7**: 127–135.
183. Marquette GP, Klein VR, Niebyl JR (1985) Efficacy of screening for gestational diabetes. *Am. J. Perinatology* **2**: 7–14.
184. Dietrich ML, Dolnicek TF, Rayburn WR (1987) Gestational diabetes screening in a private midwestern American population. *Am. J. Obstet. Gynecol.* **156**: 1403–1408.
185. Lucas MJ, Lowe TW, Bowe L, McIntire DD (1993) Class A1 gestational diabetes: a meaningful diagnosis? *Obstet. Gynecol.* **82**: 260–265.
186. Dornhorst A, Beard RW (1993) Gestational diabetes: a challenge for the future. *Diabetic Med.* **10**: 897–905.
187. Lavin JP (1985) Screening of high-risk and general populations for gestational diabetes. *Diabetes* **34 (Suppl 2)**: 24–41.
188. Greene MF (1998) Screening for gestational diabetes mellitus. Editorial. *New Engl. J. Med.* **337**: 1625–1626.
189. Lind T, Anderson T (1984) Does random blood glucose sampling outdate testing for glycosuria in the detection of glycosuria during pregnancy? *Br. Med. J.* **289**: 1569–1571.
190. Lind T (1984) Antenatal screening for diabetes mellitus. *Br. J. Obstet. Gynaecol.* **91**: 833–834.
191. Hadden DR (1984) Random plasma glucose as a screening tool for hyperglycaemia in pregnancy. In HW Sutherland, JW Stowers (eds) *Carbohydrate Metabolism in Pregnancy and the Newborn*. Edinburgh: Churchill Livingstone, pp. 203–205.
192. Hatem M, Dennis KJ (1987) A random plasma glucose method for screening for abnormal glucose tolerance in pregnancy. *Br. J. Obstet. Gynecol.* **94**: 213–216.
193. Stangenberg M, Persson B, Norlander E (1985) Random capillary blood glucose and conventional selection criteria for glucose tolerance testing during pregnancy. *Diabetes Res.* **2**: 29–33.
194. Hadden DR (1991) Medical management of diabetes in pregnancy. *Balliere's Clin. Obstet. Gynaecol.* **5**: 369–394.
195. Sutherland HW, Pearson DWM, Lean MEJ (1989) Breakfast tolerance test in pregnancy. In Sutherland HW, Stowers JM, Person DWM (eds) *Carbohydrate Metabolism in Pregnancy and the Newborn IV*. London: Springer-Verlag, pp. 267–275.
196. Jovanovic-Peterson L, Peterson CM, Reed G, Metzger BG, Knopp RH, Mills JL, Aarous JH (1991). Postprandial blood glucose levels predict birth weight. The Diabetes in Early Pregnancy Study. *Am. J. Obstet. Gynecol.* **164**: 103.
197. Jardine-Brown C, Dawson A, Dodds R, Gamsu H, Gillmer M, Hall M, Hounsome B, Knopfler A, Ostler J, Peacock I, Rothman D, Steel J (1996) Report of the Pregnancy and Neonatal Care Group. *Diabetic Med.* **13**: S43–S53.
198. Management of Diabetes in Pregnancy (1996) A national clinical guideline recommended for use in Scotland by the Scottish Intercollegiate Guidelines Network (SIGN).

11

Gestational Diabetes Mellitus: A Commentary

THOMAS A. BUCHANAN

6602 General Hospital, Los Angeles, CA 90033, USA

ANTENATAL AND PERINATAL CONSIDERATIONS

As detailed by Dr McCance, the best (albeit suboptimal) evidence from cross-sectional studies indicates that the risk of perinatal complications increases in a gradual, continuous fashion along with increasing glucose concentrations in the maternal circulation in human pregnancies[1,2]. Thus, there does not appear to be a true biological threshold for maternal glucose that will discriminate efficiently between low-risk and high-risk pregnancies. That fact explains much of the controversy about the optimal way to diagnose gestational diabetes mellitus (GDM), as well as many of the observations about the relationship between clinically-defined glucose thresholds and perinatal outcomes that are reviewed by Dr McCance. Basically, women whose glucose levels fall above some threshold, whether on a 50 g glucose screening test, an oral glucose tolerance test or a fasting glucose determination, will have larger babies and, assuming adequate sample size, demonstrably more perinatal complications than women whose glucose levels fall below the threshold. Given this fact, two general types of approaches could be taken to detect pregnancies at risk for complications related to maternal glycemia. The more sensitive approach would set low glucose thresholds for diagnosis, identifying relatively large numbers of women as potentially at risk but including many pregnancies that will not have an adverse perinatal event. The more specific approach would set high glucose thresholds, so that 'abnormal' pregnancies would have high rates of perinatal complications but so would some of the pregnancies identified as 'normal'. No direct comparison of these two approaches has been undertaken, so no evidence-based recommendations can be made regarding the superiority of one approach over the other. The general trend in the field has been to set

The Evidence Base for Diabetes Care. Edited by R. Williams, W. Herman, A.-L. Kinmonth and N. J. Wareham.
© 2002 John Wiley & Sons, Ltd

thresholds lower and lower so as not to miss any at-risk pregnancies[3,4]. Whether this trend will decrease or increase[5] morbid events is not yet clear.

The considerations underlying the diagnosis of GDM can impact the approach to treatment once the condition is diagnosed. If diagnostic thresholds are set high, then a majority of women will be at risk and in need of treatment to lower the risk. As an example, if the diagnosis were based on a fasting serum or plasma glucose concentration >105 mg/dl (5.8 mmol/l), the risk of perinatal complications would be high and insulin treatment could reduce that risk[6]. On the other hand, if the diagnostic threshold is low (e.g. a plasma glucose concentration >140 mg/dl (7.8 mmol/l) one hour after a 50 g glucose challenge) then only a small minority of 'abnormal' women would actually have an adverse event in the absence of treatment. Other methods would be needed to identify a high-risk subset. Frequent measurement of maternal capillary blood glucose concentrations is often recommended for this purpose. Several studies in which that approach has been applied were estimated to be cost-effective in a retrospective analysis[7], despite the fact that many no-risk patients are required to perform glucose monitoring and to take insulin. Measurement of the fetal response to the maternal diabetic environment offers an alternative approach that can be combined with more simple measures of maternal glucose measurement to identify the at-risk subgroup of pregnancies[8,9]. The cost-effectiveness of this approach remains to be assessed. Additional questions that await well-designed studies to address them include: (1) What constitutes optimal dietary treatment? (2) What is the role of other non-pharmacological interventions, such as physical exercise? (3) What is the role of oral anti-diabetic agents? and (4) What is the optimal management of labor and delivery? All of these questions should be addressed in terms of optimal perinatal outcome, not in terms of the regulation of maternal glucose levels.

POSTPARTUM CONSIDERATIONS

GDM identifies mothers and offspring with an increased risk of adverse health outcomes over the long term. Dr McCance highlighted the increased risk of diabetes in women who have had GDM compared to women in the general population. The risks may come from mechanisms traditionally linked to type 1 diabetes (i.e. autoimmunity directed at pancreatic β-cells[10]) in a minority of women. Interventions to prevent diabetes in those women have not been tested. Physiological studies in patients who appear to be at risk for type 2 diabetes[11,12] reveal two fundamental defects compared to normal women: (1) reduced tissue sensitivity to insulin and (2) impaired ability of pancreatic β-cells to compensate for insulin resistance by increasing insulin secretion. Epidemiological studies[13] suggest that insulin resistance may accelerate the development of diabetes, perhaps by worsening β-cell function. Accordingly, strategies to prevent or delay the onset of diabetes by ameliorating insulin resistance are currently being tested in women with a history of GDM. The interventions include diet and exercise, biguanide therapy and thiazolidine-dione therapy. Physiological considerations suggest that at least the first of these be implemented now, pending the results of the clinical trials. However, whether the approaches will actually work remains to be determined. Likewise, the optimally type and frequency of testing for diabetes after GDM remains controversial. Oral glucose tolerance results have been shown to be superior to other clinical measures for predicting the development of diabetes in two studies[14,15]. The cost effectiveness of such tests as compared to fasting glucose determinations remains to be evaluated. Finally, family planning is logical in women with a history of GDM, to allow assessment of glycemia prior to birth and minimization of the risk of birth defects in any subsequent pregnancies[16].

Virtually nothing is known about the mechanisms for or prevention of obesity and diabetes in the offspring of women with GDM. As reviewed by Dr McCance, some of the excess risk may be related to exposure to GDM *in utero* and, theoretically, could be mitigated by excellent metabolic control during pregnancy. However, it is likely that genetic transmission of risks of obesity and diabetes plays an important role as well. In the absence of data regarding how to manage the children, close observation of growth and glycemia seem prudent, along with measures to minimize obesity. Clearly, high-quality mechanistic and interventional research is needed in this area.

SUMMARY

Maternal glucose levels during pregnancy provide clinically useful information regarding the risk of perinatal and long-term complications in mothers and their children. No clear thresholds for abnormal glucose exist. Thus, management strategies that use glucose as a screening test to separate no-risk from at-risk pregnancies should be combined with additional testing (maternal glucose levels and fetal growth during pregnancy, maternal glucose levels and childhood development thereafter) to fine-tune the assessment of risk and to direct interventions to where the risk really is. Considerable investigation is needed to allow true evidence-based recommendations in all of these areas.

REFERENCES

1. Sacks DA, Greenspoon JG, Abu-Fadil S, Herny HM, Wolde-Tsadik G, Yao JFF (1995) Toward universal criteria gestational diabetes: the 75 gram glucose tolerance test in pregnancy. *Am. J. Obstet. Gynecol.* **172**: 607–614.

2. Sermer M, Naylor CD, Gare DJ, Kenshole AB, Ritchie JWK, Farine D, Cohen HR, McArthur K, Holzapfel S, Biringer A, Chen E, Cadesky KI, Greenblatt EM, Leyland NA, Morris HS, Bloom JA, Abells YB (1995) Impact of increasing carbohydrate intolerance on maternal fetal outcomes in 3637 women without gestational diabetes. *Am. J. Obstet. Gynecol.* **173**: 146–156.
3. Metzger BE and the Conference Organizing Committee (1995) Summary and recommendations of the third international workshop-conference on gestational diabetes. *Diabetes* **40 (Suppl 2)**: 197–201.
4. Metzger BE, Coustan DM the Organizing Committee (1998) Summary and recommendations of the Fourth International Workshop-Conference on Gestational Diabetes Mellitus. *Diab. Care* **21 (Suppl 2)**: B161–B167.
5. Naylor CD, Sermer M, Chen E, Sykora K (1996) Cesarean delivery in relation to birthweight and gestational glucose tolerance: pathophysiology or practice style? *JAMA* **265**: 1165–1170.
6. Kalkhoff RK (1985) Therapeutic results of insulin therapy in gestational diabetes mellitus. *Diabetes* **34 (Suppl 2)**: 97–100.
7. Kitzmiller JL, Elixhauser A, Carr S, Major CA, DeVeciana M, Dang-Kilduff L, Weschler JM (1998) Assessment of costs and benefits of management of gestational diabetes mellitus. *Diab. Care* **21 (Suppl 2)**: B123–B130.
8. Hofmann HMH, Weiss PAM, Purstner P, Haas J, Gmoser G, Tamussino K, Schmon B. Serum fructosamine and amniotic fluid insulin levels in patients with gestational diabetes and healthy control subjects. *Am. J. Obstet. Gynecol.* **162**: 1174–1177.
9. Buchanan TA, Kjos SL, Schaefer U, Peters RK, Xiang A, Byrne J, Berkowitz K, Montoro M (1998) Utility of fetal measurements in the management of gestational diabetes. *Diab. Care* **21 (Suppl 2)**: B99–B106.
10. Mauricio D, Balsells M, Morales J, Corcoy R, Puig-Domingo M, de Levia A (1996) Islet cell autoimmunity in women with gestational diabetes and risk of progression to insulin-dependent diabetes mellitus. *Diab. Metab. Rev.* **12**: 275–285.
11. Buchanan TA, Metzger BE, Freinkel N, Bergman RN (1990) Insulin sensitivity and B-cell responsiveness to glucose during late pregnancy in lean and moderately obese women with normal glucose tolerance or mild gestational diabetes. *Am. J. Obstet. Gynecol.* **162**: 1008–1014.
12. Catalano OM, Tzyzbir ED, Wolfe RR, Cales J, Roman NM, Amini SB, Sims EAH (1993) Carbohydrate metabolism during pregnancy in control subjects and women with gestational diabetes. *Am. J. Physiol.* **264**: E60–67.
13. Peters RK, Kjos SL, Xiang A, Buchanan TA (1996) Long-term diabetogenic effect of a single pregnancy in women with prior gestational diabetes mellitus. *Lancet* **347**: 227–30.
14. Damm P, Kuhl C, Bertelsen A, Molsted-Pedersen L (1992) Predictive factors for the development of diabetes in women with previous gestational diabetes mellitus. *Am. J. Obstet. Gynecol.* **67**: 607–16.
15. Kjos SL, Peters RK, Xiang A, Henry OA, Montoro MN, Buchanan TA (1995) Predicting future diabetes in Latino women with gestational diabetes: utility of early postpartum glucose tolerance testing. *Diabetes* **44**: 586–591.
16. Kjos SL, Peters RK, Xiang A, Schaefer U, Buchanan TA (1998) Hormonal choices after gestational diabetes. *Diab. Care* **21 (Suppl 2)**: B50–B57.

Part V

GLYCAEMIC CONTROL

12

Can Intensive Glycemic Management in Type 1 Diabetes Reduce Morbidity and Mortality?

WILLIAM HERMAN

3920 Taubman Center, Ann Arbor, MI 48109, USA

INTRODUCTION

The 'glucose hypothesis' attributes the complications of diabetes to chronic hyperglycemia. It postulates that hyperglycemia causes complications, and that correction of hyperglycemia prevents them. In human subjects, numerous retrospective studies have demonstrated associations between the initial degree of maternal hyperglycemia and the incidence of major congenital malformations, and among the degree and duration of hyperglycemia and the severity of microvascular and neuropathic complications. The strong associations between hyperglycemia and diabetic complications set the stage for prospective observational studies and randomized prospective clinical trials, the most rigorous and least biased means to test the glucose hypothesis.

It was not until the late 1970s and early 1980s that the technologies necessary to conduct prospective clinical trials to test the glucose hypothesis were in place. The technologies necessary for the conduct of such trials included: (1) valid and reproducible methods to objectively assess long-term glycemic control, specifically glycosylated hemoglobin or hemoglobin A_{1c}; (2) the means to achieve near normoglycemia in type 1 diabetes including self-monitoring of blood glucose and protocols for multiple daily injections and continuous subcutaneous insulin infusion; and (3) valid and reproducible methods to assess microvascular and neuropathic outcomes including stereo fundus photography, microalbuminuria testing and standardized neurologic exams. With the availability of these technologies, it was finally possible to rigorously test the glucose hypothesis.

THE BENEFITS OF INTENSIVE GLYCEMIC MANAGEMENT: MAJOR MALFORMATIONS IN INFANTS OF DIABETIC MOTHERS

Major congenital malformations (defined as lethal malformations, those requiring surgery, or those predicted to handicap the life of the child) are the leading cause of morbidity and mortality in infants of mothers with established diabetes[1]. The organ systems most commonly affected in infants of diabetic mothers (IDM) include the central nervous system and neural tube, the cardiovascular system (especially septal and outflow tract lesions), the gastrointestinal and genitourinary systems, and the skeletal system (especially the ribs and vertebrae)[1]. The incidence of these malformations is three- to eight-times higher in IDM than in infants of non-diabetic mothers[1]. In the 1970s, it was recognized that all of these malformations occur early in gestation, by approximately five to eight weeks post-menses[2,3]. In the 1970s, Jorgen Pedersen was the first to postulate that hyperglycemia in early pregnancy might cause the increased frequency of major malformations in IDM[4]. Specifically, he noted a strong inverse correlation between insulin reactions in the first trimester and malformations. He also noted that patients with diabetic vascular disease (and presumably higher blood glucose levels) had the highest incidence of infants with malformations, but that when diabetes was well-controlled in these patients, malformations did not occur.

Development of the glycosylated hemoglobin assay, a retrospective measure of glycemic control, permitted further assessment of the relationship between hyperglycemia in pregnancy and major malformations in IDM. In 1978, Leslie and colleagues first noted an association between elevated glycosylated hemoglobin and congenital malformations[5]. Subsequently, many investigators observed that mothers with infants with major malformations had significantly higher glycosylated hemoglobin levels in the first trimester than did diabetic mothers of non-affected infants[6–15].

Numerous investigators have sought to define the degree of hyperglycemia (indicated by the level of glycosylated hemoglobin in early pregnancy) that is associated with increased risk of major malformations. Because glycosylated hemoglobin assays were not standardized and because different assay techniques were employed at different centers, investigators attempted to answer this question by defining control in terms of the number of standard deviations above the mean for a non-diabetic population for a given laboratory. When the data from seven series were pooled and analyzed by standard deviation

(SD) (Table 12.1), there was a low frequency of major malformations (2%) with moderate elevations of glycosylated hemoglobin (less than 4 to 7 SD above the mean), moderately increased risk of anomalies (9%) with elevations of glycosylated hemoglobin in the range of 4 to 12 SD above the mean, and a very high risk of major malformations (27%) with the highest glycosylated hemoglobin levels (greater than 8 to 12 SD above the mean).

With the understanding that malformations typical of IDM develop by five to eight weeks gestation, and with an awareness of the association between initial maternal glycosylated hemoglobin and the incidence of major malformations, investigators set out to test the hypothesis that intensified glycemic control before conception and during early gestation could reduce the incidence of major malformations in IDM. Initially, these studies were undertaken by Steel and co-workers in Edinburgh[16,17], Fuhrmann and colleagues in Karlsburg, Germany[18,19], and Molsted-Pedersen and Pedersen in Copenhagen[20]. The results of these and other more recent studies of intensified diabetes treatment are summarized in Table 12.2[16–29]. Although these trials employed very different methods to improve glycemic control before conception and during early gestation, most reported that >80% of subjects achieved normal glycosylated hemoglobin levels before conception, and each showed a reduction in the rate of major malformations compared with infants born to diabetic women who reported for care and intensified glycemic management when already pregnant. The National Institutes of Health (NIH)-sponsored multicenter Diabetes in Early Pregnancy Study (DIEP) was controversial by claiming a lack of relationship between glycemic control and the rate of malformations[22]. This study was unique in that it did not compare intensified treatment beginning before conception with that beginning after conception. It compared early entry diabetic women (entering the study within three weeks of conception), late entry diabetic women, and non-diabetic control women. This study reported a 4.9% incidence of major malformations in infants of early entry diabetic mothers, a 9.0% incidence in infants of late entry diabetic mothers, and a 2.1% incidence in infants of control mothers. It is noteworthy that a majority of infants with major malformations delivered to early entry diabetic women were to mothers entering the study after conception. Of these women, most had initial glycosylated hemoglobin levels above the 50th percentile for early entry diabetic women, and most had glycosylated hemoglobin levels greater than 4 SD above that for non-diabetic control subjects[22,30].

One limitation of all of these prospective observational studies is that they were not randomized. Control subjects for these studies were diabetic women who did not respond to recruitment efforts for preconception care (or in the case of the DIEP, were recruited after five weeks gestation). They often had unplanned pregnancies, with elevated glycosylated hemoglobin levels. The reason that randomized studies were not performed was that, in each instance,

Table 12.1. Association of major malformations in IDM with initial maternal glycosylated hemoglobin levels SD above normal mean elevation of glycosylated hemoglobin (malformations/infants) [% malformed]

Reference	n	Moderate	High	Highest
6	106	<7 (2/48) [4.2]	7–9.8 (8/35) [22.9]	≥10 (5/23) [21.7]
7	142	<6 (2/63) [3.2]	6–9.8 (5/62) [8.1]	≥10 (4/17) [23.5]
8	127	<6 (2/58)[3.4]	6–9.9 (5/44) [11.4]	≥10 (6/25) [24.0]
9	61	<5.8 (2/45) [4.4]	5.8–9.4 (4/13) [30.8]	≥9.5 (3/3) [100]
12	250	<6 (3/99) [3.0]	6–12 (6/123) [4.9]	≥12 (11/28) [39.3]
14	491	<6 (3/429) [0.7]	6–7.9 (2/31) [6.5]	≥8 (5/31) [16.1]
15	228	<4 (4/95) [4.2]	4–9.9 (7/121) [5.8]	≥10 (3/12) [25.0]
Total	1405	(18/837) [2.2]	(37/429) [8.6]	(37/139) [26.6]

Adapted from Kitzmiller et al.[1].

Table 12.2. Major congenital malformations in infants of diabetic mothers participating in prospective studies of preconception care.

Reference	Preconception group		Registered already pregnant	
	Infants	Anomalies	Infants	Anomalies
18, 19	184	2 (1.1)	436	22 (5.0)
21	44	0 (0.0)	31	2 (6.5)
22	347	17 (4.9)	279	25 (9.0)
23	283	7 (2.5)	148	15 (10.1)
24, 25	196	3 (1.5)	117	14 (12.0)
26	84	1 (1.2)	110	12 (10.9)
27	28	0 (0.0)	71	1 (1.4)
28	40	0 (0.0)	186	16 (8.6)
29	58	1 (1.7)	93	8 (8.6)
Total	1264	31 (2.5)	1471	115 (7.8)

Data are n or n (%). Malformations include therapeutic abortions for lethal anomalies. For Mills *et al.*[22], 14% of women did not register preconception but enrolled by three weeks postconception. Adapted from Kitzmiller *et al.*[1].

the investigators believed that it would be unethical to assign women to poor glycemic control before conception. Indeed, for most new treatments in medicine, there is a narrow window of opportunity during which randomized prospective clinical trials may be conducted. This window is between the initial retrospective or prospective demonstration of the effectiveness of the intervention and its widespread clinical acceptance and application. Thus, for ethical reasons, it is unlikely that there will be a randomized prospective clinical trial of preconception intensified glycemic control and preconception poor control. An unfortunate result of this is that it may be impossible to rigorously assess the benefits and risks of intensive preconception glycemic control.

A resultant criticism of the trials of preconception care has been that participants were well-motivated diabetic women who were already in good glycemic control, and that control women were poorly motivated, poorly controlled diabetic women who possessed additional risk factors for adverse outcomes. Because of the failure to randomize, such criticisms cannot be absolutely refuted. It has been pointed out, however, that participants in several studies had glycosylated hemoglobin levels at the time they entered the study as high as the late entry participants when they presented for care;[21,24,26] many of the participants had delivered babies with major malformations in prior pregnancies[18,24,26,27]; and only a minority of participants seeking preconception care perceived that they were in very good diabetes control in the six months prior to their enrollment[31]. Thus, the very low malformation rates observed in participants in preconception care studies are difficult to explain simply on the basis of selection bias. Nevertheless, because of the lack of a definitive randomized prospective controlled clinical trial, questions remain about the benefits and risks of such treatment.

In summary, controlled but non-randomized prospective clinical trials indicate that intensified glycemic therapy before conception and through early gestation can significantly reduce the incidence of major malformations in IDM (Level of Evidence II-1, Strength of Recommendation A).

THE BENEFITS OF INTENSIVE GLYCEMIC MANAGEMENT: MICROVASCULAR AND NEUROPATHIC COMPLICATIONS

Early randomized prospective clinical trials designed to study the relationship between glycemic control and microvascular and neuropathic complications demonstrated that intensive and conventional treatment protocols achieved different levels of glycemic control and that methods to measure the development and progression of complications were practical. However, these trials involved too few subjects and were too brief to determine whether the different treatments changed the rates of progression of complications. A meta-analysis of these small, short-term trials estimated the impact of intensive therapy on the progression of microvascular complications in type 1 diabetes[32]. A total of 16 reports (from 12 cohorts) were selected for the meta-analysis. Reports selected for the meta-analysis were published in English between January 1966 and December 1991 and were randomized, included only patients with insulin-dependent diabetes, and presented analyzable data[33–48]. The duration of follow-up ranged from eight to 60 months. Conventional therapy was accomplished by one or two injections of insulin daily, and intensive therapy was achieved, for the most part, by continuous subcutaneous insulin infusion or by multiple daily injections. In the summary estimate, glycosylated hemoglobin was significantly lower (by 1.4%) in the intensive therapy groups than in the conventionally treated groups. With intensive therapy, the risk of retinopathy progressing was slightly and non-significantly higher after six to 12 months, but significantly lower after more than two years (odds ratio (OR), 0.49; 95% confidence interval (CI), 0.28–0.85) (Figure 12.1). The risk of nephropathy progression was also significantly decreased (OR, 0.34; 95% CI, 0.20–0.58) (Figure 12.2).

Two long-term, prospective, explanatory clinical trials have now confirmed and extended the results of the meta-analysis. The Stockholm Diabetes Intervention Study (SDIS) compared the effects of intensified and standard treatment over 7.5 years in 102 type 1 diabetic patients (mean age 31 years, mean duration of diabetes 17 years at baseline) with non-proliferative retinopathy, normal serum creatinine concentrations, and 'unsatisfactory' blood glucose control[49]. Subjects were referred to the study by their personal physicians and 91% of patients who were asked to participate accepted. Intensified treatment consisted of individual education, three or more insulin injections per day, self-monitoring of blood glucose, and increased provider contacts. Standard treat-

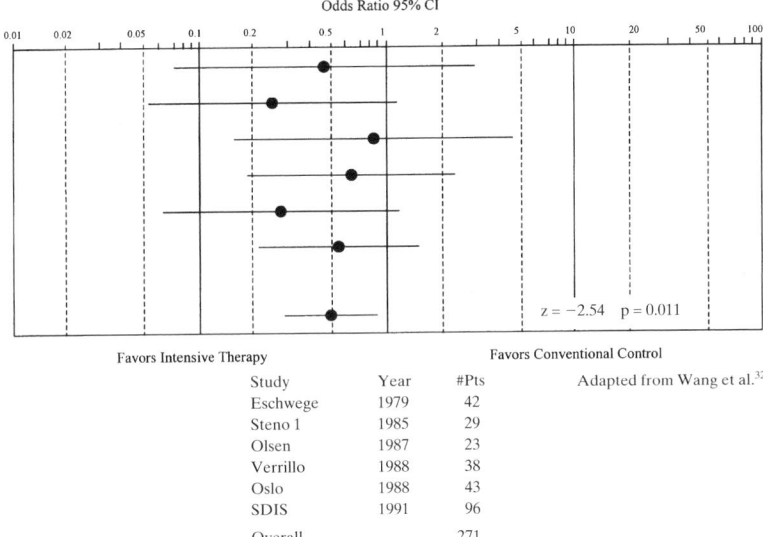

Figure 12.1. Meta-analysis of the effects of intensive glycemic control on the progression of diabetic retinopathy. Reprinted with permission from Elsevier Science[32]

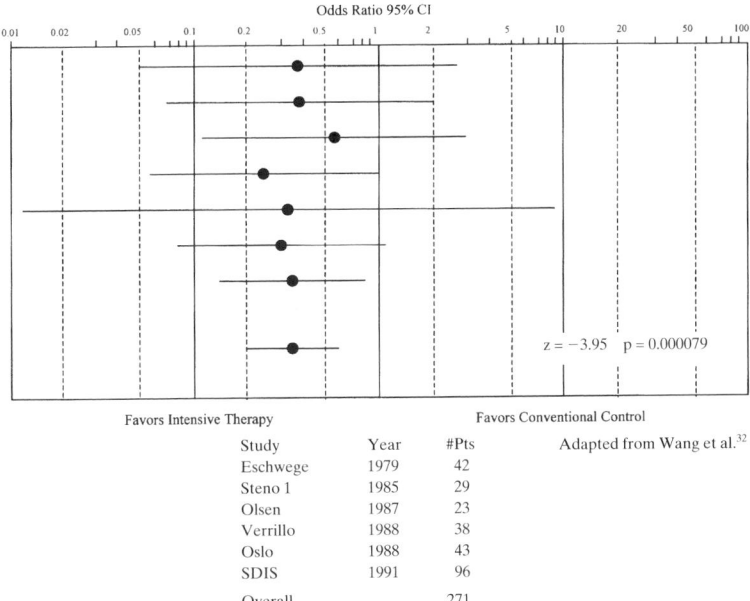

Figure 12.2. Meta-analysis of the effects of intensive glycemic control on the progression of diabetic nephropathy. Reprinted with permission from Elsevier Science[32]

ment consisted of two or three insulin injections per day and routine diabetes care with physician visits every four months. Self-monitoring of blood glucose was advised but test results were discussed only at routine visits. At entry, glycosylated hemoglobin was $9.5 \pm 1.3\%$ in the intensified treatment group and $9.4 \pm 1.4\%$ in the standard treatment group (normal range, 3.9–5.7%). The mean value for the whole study was $7.1 \pm 0.7\%$ in the intensified treatment group and $8.5 \pm 0.7\%$ in the standard treatment group (p = 0.001).

Proliferative retinopathy or clinically important macular edema requiring immediate photocoagulation developed in 27% of patients receiving intensified treatment and 52% of those receiving standard treatment (p = 0.01). Urinary albumin excretion >200 micrograms per minute developed in 2% of the intensified treatment group and 18% of the standard treatment group (p = 0.01). None of the patients in the intensified treatment group developed a glomerular filtration rate below the normal range but 12% of those in the standard treatment group did (p = 0.02). During the follow-up, deterioration in nerve conduction velocities was less in the intensive than in the standard treatment group (p $\leq$ 0.02). This study confirmed that intensive therapy significantly delays progression to proliferative retinopathy or clinically important macular edema requiring photocoagulation and to diabetic nephropathy. It also demonstrated that intensive therapy could significantly delay deterioration in nerve conduction velocities.

The Diabetes Control and Complications Trial (DCCT) confirmed and extended these findings[50]. The DCCT was a large, multicenter, randomized controlled clinical trial that compared the impact of intensive and conventional therapy on the early microvascular and neuropathic complications of type 1 diabetes. It was designed to answer two separate but related questions: (1) Could intensive therapy prevent the development of diabetic retinopathy in patients with no retinopathy (primary prevention)? 2) could intensive therapy slow the progression of early retinopathy (secondary intervention)? Subjects were recruited from 29 academic medical centers in the USA and Canada from 1983 through to 1989. A total of 1441 patients aged 13 to 39 with type 1 diabetes (726 with no retinopathy at baseline and 715 with mild retinopathy) were randomly assigned to intensive therapy administered either with an external insulin pump or by three or more daily insulin injections and guided by frequent blood glucose monitoring, or to conventional therapy with one or two daily insulin injections. Subjects were followed for up to nine years. At baseline, mean HbA_{1c} was approximately 8.9% (normal <6.05%) and did not differ between treatment groups. HbA_{1c} reached a nadir at six months in the patients receiving intensive therapy. Patients assigned to the intensive treatment group achieved and maintained HbA_{1c} values of 7.2%. Type 1 patients randomly assigned to the conventional treatment group maintained HbA_{1c} values of 9.1%.

In the primary prevention cohort, the cumulative incidence of retinopathy was similar in the two treatment groups until approximately three years, when the cumulative incidence curves began to separate. From five years onwards, the cumulative incidence of retinopathy was approximately 50% less in the intensive therapy group than in the conventional therapy group. Intensive therapy reduced the adjusted mean risk of retinopathy by 76% (95% CI, 62–85%) and the reduction in risk became more pronounced with time. In the secondary intervention cohort, patients receiving intensive therapy had a higher cumulative incidence of retinopathy during the first year than those in the conventional therapy group, but a lower cumulative incidence beginning at three years and continuing for the rest of the study. Intensive therapy reduced the average risk of progression by 54% (95% CI, 39–66%).

In the DCCT primary prevention cohort, intensive therapy also reduced the mean adjusted risk of microalbuminuria by 34% (p = 0.04). In the secondary intervention cohort, intensive therapy decreased the risk of microalbuminuria by 43% (p = 0.001) and the risk of albuminuria by 56% (p = 0.01). A post-hoc sub-group analysis of 73 type 1 diabetic patients with microalbuminuria in the DCCT failed to find an impact of intensive therapy on progression from micro-albuminuria to clinical albuminuria in patients with type 1 diabetes. Thirty-eight patients with microalbuminuria were assigned to intensive therapy and 35 to conventional therapy. In each treatment group, eight developed clinical albuminuria at one or more time-points during the course of the study (p = NS). In the same 73 subjects, the difference in mean slope of change of albumin excretion rate within intensive therapy versus conventional therapy was similar in magnitude (8.55% per year) to the difference in mean slope with intensive versus conventional therapy in the secondary cohort subjects who entered with no microalbuminuria (6.5% per year, p <0.0001). The difference was, however, not significant in subjects with baseline microalbuminuria (p = 0.09)[51].

These results were similar to those obtained by the Microalbuminuria Collaborative Study Group[52]. This group studied 70 type 1 diabetic patients with microalbuminuria but without arterial hypertension randomized to intensive (n = 36) and conventional (n = 34) therapy for a median of five years (range 2–8). A significant glycemic separation between the two groups was maintained for only three years. Progression to clinical albuminuria occurred in six patients in each group. Intensive therapy with improved glycemic control for three years had no impact on progression from microalbuminuria to albuminuria. Although both of these studies were limited by their sample size, the Microalbuminuria Collaborative Study Group concluded that the DCCT and their study together had sufficient power to detect a reduction in the risk of progression to clinical albuminuria of 33% or greater. A smaller treatment effect could not be excluded[52].

In patients in the DCCT primary intervention cohort, intensive therapy reduced the appearance of neuropathy at five years by 69% (p = 0.006) and in the secondary intervention cohort by 57% (p <0.001).

Recently, a follow-up to the DCCT demonstrated that the reduction in the risk of progressive retinopathy and nephropathy resulting from intensive therapy in patients with type 1 diabetes persists for at least four years, despite increasing hyperglycemia[53]. At the end of the DCCT, the patients in the conventional-therapy group were offered intensive therapy, and the care of all patients was transferred to their own physicians. Retinopathy was evaluated on the basis of centrally graded fundus photographs in 1208 patients during the fourth year after the DCCT ended, and nephropathy was evaluated on the basis of urine specimens obtained from 1302 patients during the third or fourth year, approximately half of whom were from each treatment group. The difference in the median glycosylated hemoglobin values between the intensive-therapy and conventional-therapy groups narrowed during follow-up (median during four years, 7.9% and 8.2%, respectively; P <0.001). Nevertheless, the proportion of patients who had worsening retinopathy, including proliferative retinopathy, macular edema and the need for laser therapy, was lower and the proportion of patients with development of new microalbuminuria (5% versus 11%, odds reduction 26–70%, p = 0.002) and development of new albuminuria (1% versus 5%, odds reduction 60–95%, p = 0.001) was significantly lower in the intensive-therapy group.

The DCCT thus demonstrated that intensive therapy could both prevent the development and delay the progression of diabetic retinopathy and nephropathy. The impact of intensive therapy on progression from microalbuminuria to clinical albuminuria is less clear. In addition, it conclusively demonstrated that intensive therapy could reduce the appearance of clinical neuropathy, not merely the electrophysiologic correlates of neuropathy. Finally, it demonstrated that these beneficial effects of intensive therapy persist for at least four years despite increasing hyperglycemia.

Table 12.3 summarizes the odds of development and progression of microvascular and neuropathic complications of type 1 diabetes with intensive therapy compared to conventional therapy. The results of a meta-analysis and two large, randomized prospective clinical trials conclusively demonstrated that intensive therapy slows the development and progression of retinopathy and nephropathy and the development of neuropathy in type 1 diabetes (Level of Evidence I, Strength of Recommendation A).

THE BENEFITS OF INTENSIVE GLYCEMIC MANAGEMENT: CARDIOVASCULAR DISEASE AND SURVIVAL

A major unresolved question is the impact of intensive therapy on cardio-vascular outcomes and survival in type 1 diabetes. None of the clinical trials cited was designed to assess the impact of therapy on macrovascular disease, and the youth of the patients and the relative shortness of follow-up made the

Table 12.3. The benefits and risks of intensive glycemic management: risk (odds ratio) of development and progression of microvascular and neuropathic complications and hypoglycemia with intensive versus conventional therapy.

Study, year (reference)	Participants	Retinopathy		Nephropathy		Neuropathy	Hypoglycemia
		Development	Progression	Development	Progression	Development	Development
Meta-analysis, 1993 (32)	12 small short-term RCTs in patients with type 1 diabetes followed for 8–60 months	—	Risk of progression halved (OR 0.5)	—	70% reduction in risk of progression (OR 0.3)	—	NS
SDIS, 1993 (49)	102 patients with type 1 diabetes followed for 7.5 yrs	—	60% reduction in risk of progression (OR 0.4)	—	90% reduction in risk of progression (OR 0.1)	—	2.8-fold increase in risk of developing severe hypoglycemia (OR 2.8)
DCCT, 1993 (50)	1441 patients with type 1 diabetes followed for 6.5 yrs	80% reduction in risk of developing retinopathy (OR 0.2)	Risk of progression halved (OR 0.5)	30% reduction in risk of developing nephropathy (OR 0.7)	60% reduction in risk of progression (OR 0.4)	60% reduction in risk of developing neuropathy (OR 0.4)	3.3-fold increase in risk of developing severe hypoglycemia (OR 3.3)
Meta-analysis, 1997 (65)	14 RCTs in patients with type 1 diabetes followed for 6–90 months	—	—	—	—	—	3.0-fold increase in risk of developing severe hypoglycemia (OR 3.0)

— not studied; NS = not significant

detection of treatment-related differences in macrovascular events unlikely. A cross-sectional analysis of the SDIS demonstrated an association between HbA_{1c}, stiffness of the carotid wall, and endothelial dysfunction in type 1 diabetic subjects[54]. The effect of long-term intensive therapy on early atherosclerosis was further examined using ultrasound to assess endothelial function, carotid intima-medial thickness and arterial stiffness[54]. Fifty-nine of the 102 original Stockholm Diabetes Intervention Study subjects were studied about 12 years after randomization to intensive or conventional therapy. Endothelial function was better and arteries were less stiff in the intensive therapy group, suggesting that intensive therapy slows atherosclerosis. When all major cardiovascular and peripheral vascular events were combined in the DCCT, intensive therapy was found to reduce the risk of macrovascular disease by 41% (from 0.8 to 0.5 events per 100 patient-years), but the difference was not significant[50]. Despite the increased incidence of overweight associated with intensive therapy, intensive therapy was associated with a small but insignificant reduction in the development of hypertension in the DCCT. In addition, intensive therapy was associated with small but significant reductions in the development of hypercholesterolemia and hypertriglyceridemia[50].

Recently, Lawson and colleagues critically reviewed randomized controlled trials of intensive insulin therapy (IIT) in type 1 diabetes, and used meta-analytical techniques to estimate the impact of IIT on the risk of developing cerebrovascular, cardiovascular and peripheral vascular complications[55]. They conducted a comprehensive literature search of articles published between January 1966 and January 1996 and selected articles if they were randomized controlled clinical trials, involved subjects with type 1 diabetes, and were of two years duration or longer. Early reports of studies were excluded if later reports were available. IIT was defined as a method of intensifying diabetes management with the goal of improving metabolic control over that achieved by conventional therapy (CT). IIT could be achieved through multiple daily injections or continuous subcutaneous insulin infusion pump, whereas CT was defined as one or two insulin injections per day. To be included, studies had to show a statistically significant difference in glycosylated hemoglobin between the IIT and CT groups. Studies were initially included regardless of whether or not data were provided on macrovascular complications, and authors were contacted to confirm outcomes and/or obtain unpublished data. The primary outcome measure was the number of major cardiovascular events. These included cerebrovascular disease (cerebrovascular accident), cardiovascular disease (angina, myocardial infarction, angioplasty, coronary artery bypass), peripheral vascular disease (intermittent claudication, peripheral artery bypass), and macrovascular death (fatal cerebrovascular accident, fatal myocardial infarction, sudden death). If a subject had different types of events, they were counted separately, even if they were within the same class. In addition to abstracting data regarding the number of events, the authors contacted the study authors to obtain data on the number of subjects having one or more macrovascular events. The authors analyzed separately the number of subjects with one or more macrovascular event and the rates of macrovascular mortality.

The initial search identified 30 studies. Six studies met all inclusion criteria and the authors were able to obtain confirmation of macrovascular outcomes. These studies are described in Table 12.4. Subject age at entry was relatively young. Duration of diabetes ranged from two to nine years. Two studies included both primary prevention and secondary intervention subjects. The remaining four studies included subjects with evidence of early microvascular complications. In each of the studies, the IIT and CT groups had similar baseline characteristics. All studies achieved a statistically significant difference in glycosylated hemoglobin levels.

IIT significantly reduced the total number of first major macrovascular events of each type: cerebrovascular, cardiovascular and peripheral vascular (OR = 0.55 [95% CI, 0.35–0.88], P = 0.015, Figure 12.3). In three of the studies, subjects had more than one event. When events within the same class (for example, angina and myocardial infarction) were counted only once, the result became non-significant. Although there was a trend toward a decrease in the number of subjects with one or more macrovascular evens with IIT, the difference between IIT and CT was not statistically significant (OR = 0.72 [95% CI, 0.44–1.17], P = 0.22). Rates of macrovascular mortality were not different between IIT and CT (OR = 0.91 [95% CI, 0.31–2.65], P = 0.93).

In summary, the meta-analysis demonstrated that IIT significantly decreased the total number of macrovascular events but had no significant effect on the number of subjects developing macrovascular disease or on macrovascular mortality. The authors speculate that IIT may stabilize macrovascular disease or prevent progression in those already at risk. Although the authors conclude that long-term prospective studies are needed to confirm these data and fully understand the effect of IIT on macrovascular disease in individuals with type 1 diabetes, they also appropriately point out that future trials of IIT versus CT would seem to be unethical in patients with type 1 diabetes, given the positive effects of IIT on microvascular complications. Thus, the answer to this question may never be more definitively answered[55].

Randomized, prospective clinical trials have also been too short to assess the impact of intensive therapy on survival. In the SDIS, 4/48 subjects (8.3%) in the intensive therapy group died as compared to 3/54 (5.6%) in the standard therapy group (p = NS)[49]. In the DCCT, 7/711 subjects (1.0%) died in the intensive therapy group and 4/730 (0.5%) died in the conventional therapy group (P = NS)[49]. In the DCCT, mortality in both groups was less than expected on the basis of population-based mortality studies, perhaps suggesting that subjects enrolled in the study were healthier than the general population with type 1 diabetes[49].

Table 12.4. Effect of intensive insulin treatment on number of macrovascular events: study characteristics.

Study	Study duration (years)	Number of patients	Age at entry (years)	Type 1 diabetes duration (years)	Mean study GHb percentage above normal	
					IIT (mean ± SD)	CT (mean ± SD)
Holman et al., UK 1983	2	74	42 ± 12	18.6 ± 6.1	123 (10.5 ± 1.4)	134 (11.4 ± 1.5)
Steno 1, Denmark, 1991	8	34	34 ± 7	19.0 ± 3.0	121 (7.6 ± 0.9)	129 (8.1 ± 1.1)
Steno 2, Denmark, 1991	5	36	18–50	5–26	125 (7.9 ± 1.1)	140 (8.8 ± 1.0)
Oslo Norway, 1992	7	45	26 ± 5	12.8 ± 3.6	121 (9.2 ± 1.3)	137 (10.4 ± 1.5)
DCCT, North America, 1993	6.5 (3–9)	Primary: 726 Secondary: 715	27 ± 8 27 ± 7	2.6 ± 1.4 8.8 ± 3.8	119 (7.2 ± 1.4)	150 (9.1 ± 1.4)
SDIS, Sweden, 1994	7.5	102	31 ± 8	17.0 ± 5.0	125 (7.1 ± 0.7)	149 (8.5 ± 0.7)

Data for age at entry and diabetes duration are means ± SD or ranges. Study duration includes intervention and follow-up. Adapted from Lawson et al.[55]

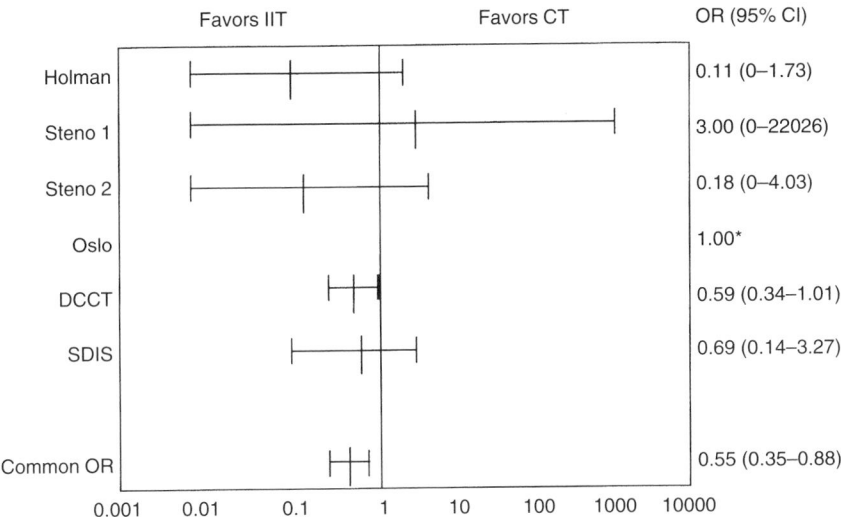

* Accurate determination of CI not possible due to zero-event rate in both groups.
Adapted from Lawson et al.[55]

Figure 12.3. Effect of intensive insulin treatment (IIT) on number of macrovascular events*.

Prospective observational studies have also suggested an association between hyperglycemia and mortality in type 1 diabetes. In the Wisconsin Epidemiologic Study of Diabetic Retinopathy, after a median follow-up of 10 years, the hazard ratio for mortality from ischemic heart disease in younger-onset (<30 years of age) insulin-treated diabetic subjects for a one-percentage-point change in glycosylated hemoglobin was 1.18 and the 95% confidence interval was 1.00–1.40[56]. Glycosylated hemoglobin was also significantly associated with all-cause mortality in younger-onset insulin-treated subjects (p <0.005)[56]. Ten-year survival in the first quartile of glycosylated hemoglobin was 96.3% compared with 93.0% in the fourth quartile[56]. After correcting for age and sex, the hazard ratio of dying for the fourth relative to the first quartile was 1.9[56]. To the extent that intensive therapy prevents the development and delays the progression of diabetic nephropathy, and to the extent that diabetic kidney disease is associated with excess mortality in type 1 diabetes, it is not unreasonable to hypothesize that intensive therapy might be associated with improved survival. Indeed, a computer simulation model developed by the DCCT Research Group to assess the long-term benefits and costs of intensive therapy suggested that intensive therapy might be associated with a 5.1-year increase in survival compared to conventional therapy[58]. This intriguing hypothesis must, however, be tested empirically.

In summary, data from these trials and prospective observational studies suggest that intensive therapy may be associated with a reduction in adverse cardiovascular outcomes and cardiovascular mortality, but these data require confirmation in either long-term follow-up studies or randomized controlled clinical trials (Level of Evidence II-3, Strength of Recommendation C).

THE RISKS OF INTENSIVE GLYCEMIC MANAGEMENT

The benefits of intensive glycemic management do not come without risks. An early concern was that maternal hypoglycemia might itself cause malformations in IDM. Although a few case reports suggested that insulin shock therapy in non-diabetic pregnant women may be associated with malformations[59,60], studies of clinical hypoglycemia in early pregnancy in insulin-treated diabetic women have failed to demonstrate an association with malformations[35,36,61–63]. Essentially all of the studies of intensive therapy for the prevention of microvascular and neuropathic complications demonstrated an increased incidence of hypoglycemia associated with intensive therapy. In the meta-analysis by Wang and colleagues, only six studies provided data on severe hypoglycemia that could be analyzed[32]. In intensively treated patients, there was a trend toward more frequent severe hypoglycemic reactions, but the difference was not statistically significant. In a more recent meta-analysis, Egger and colleagues[65] identified 14 randomized controlled trials in type 1 diabetes with at least six months of follow-up and the monitoring of glycemia by glycosylated hemoglobin[34,36,39,40,43,45,49,50,66–71]. The trials contributed 1028 subjects allocated to intensive therapy and 1039 subjects allocated to conventional therapy. Follow-up ranged from 0.5 to 7.5 years. The median incidence of severe hypoglycemia was 7.9 episodes per 100 person-years with intensive therapy and 4.6 episodes per 100 person-years with conventional therapy. The combined odds ratio (95% CI) for hypoglycemia with intensive therapy was 2.99 (2.45–3.64) (Table 12.5). The risk of severe hypoglycemia was determined by the degree of normalization of glycemia achieved. In the SDIS, there were 1.1 episodes of serious hypoglycemia (requiring help from someone else) per patient-year in the intensified-treatment group, and 0.4 such episodes per patient-year in the standard-treatment group[49]. In the DCCT, the corresponding rates were 0.62 episodes per patient-year in the intensive therapy group and 0.19 episodes per patient-year in the conventional therapy group[50].

Because of concerns that recurrent severe hypoglycemia might influence the integrity of the central nervous system and cause cognitive impairment, the SDIS and DCCT investigators performed careful measurements of neuropsychological function. Results of a three-year analysis of the SDIS showed no consistent hypoglycemia-associated cognitive impairment[72]. In the DCCT, intensive therapy did not affect neuropsychological performance[73]. In addition,

Table 12.5. Meta-analysis of the effects of intensive glycemic control on severe hypoglycemia, ketoacidosis and all-cause mortality. Reproduced by permission of Blackwell Science Ltd.[65]

Study	Year	Ref	# Pts.	Hypoglycemia OR (95% CI)	Ketoacidosis OR (95% CI)	All-cause mortality OR (95% CI)
Steno-1	1983	66	32	1.6 (0.2–11.0)	1.0 (0.1–18.0)	3.2 (0.1–84.0)
Holman	1983	34	74	1.1 (0.1–18.0)	—	1.1 (0.1–18.0)
Kroc	1984	36	70	7.1 (0.8–62.0)	22.1 (1.2–401.0)	—
Beck-Nielsen	1985	39	24	1.5 (0.3–8.8)	5.0 (0.8–33.0)	—
Oslo-MDI	1986	67	45	0.8 (0.2–3.2)	—	—
Oslo-CSII	1986	67	45	0.2 (0.1–1.1)	5.7 (0.3–130.0)	—
Steno-2	1986	40	36	1.0 (0.2–4.3)	11.5 (0.6–231.0)	1.0 (0.1–8.0)
Christensen	1987	43	24	—	3.3 (0.1–88.0)	—
Marshall	1987	68	12	2.5 (0.2–39.0)	—	—
Helve	1987	69	65	3.2 (0.1–81.0)	16.4 (0.9–305.0)	—
Verillo	1987	45	44	2.1 (0.2–25.0)	—	—
Bangstad	1992	70	30	1.0 (0.1–18.0)	5.1 (0.5–52.0)	—
SDIS	1993	49	102	2.6 (1.2–5.9)	1.1 (0.2–8.4)	1.6 (0.3–7.3)
DCCT-PP	1993	50	726	3.8 (2.8–5.2)	1.1 (0.7–1.8)	1.1 (0.2–7.8)
DCCT-SI	1993	50	715	3.1 (2.3–4.2)	1.5 (0.9–2.6)	2.4 (0.5–13.0)
MCSG	1995	71	70	0.9 (0.3–3.6)	1.5 (0.2–9.3)	0.3 (0.0–7.8)
Combined				3.0 (2.5–3.6)	1.7 (1.3–2.4)	1.4 (0.7–3.0)

MDI = multiple daily injections; CSII = continuous subcutaneous insulin infusion; PP = primary prevention; SI = secondary intervention.
Adapted from Egger et al.[65]

patients (aged 13 to 39 at baseline) who had repeated episodes of severe hypoglycemia did not have any decrease in cognitive function[74].

To compare fully the benefits and personal costs of the two treatment regimens, both diabetes-specific and generic quality-of-life assessments were included in the DCCT along with more traditional measures of disease progression[75]. All analyses of quality-of-life showed no differences between intensive and conventional therapy. In the DCCT, patients undergoing intensive therapy did not face deterioration in the quality of their lives, even while the rigor of their diabetes care was increased. The occurrence of severe hypoglycemia was not consistently associated with a subsequent increase in symptomatic distress or decline in diabetes-related quality of life. There was, however, a suggestion that in the primary prevention intensive treatment group, patients who had repeated severe hypoglycemia (three or more events resulting in coma or seizure) tended to be at increased risk of measurable symptomatic distress.

In both the SDIS and DCCT, there was also an increase in weight associated with intensive therapy. In the SDIS, weight remained stable in the conventional therapy group but body mass index increased by 5.8% in the intensive therapy group[48]. In the DCCT, intensive therapy, was associated with a 33% increase in the mean adjusted risk of becoming overweight, a condition defined as a body weight more than 120% above the ideal (12.7 cases of overweight per 100 patient-years in the intensive-therapy group versus 9.3 in the conventional-therapy group)[50].

The meta-analysis by Wang and colleagues demonstrated a significantly higher incidence of diabetic ketoacidosis (DKA) in patients treated with continuous subcutaneous insulin infusion (CSII) than in those treated conventionally[32]. Indeed, the incidence of DKA increased by 12.6 episodes per 100 person-years (95% CI, 8.7–16.5) in patients on CSII compared to those receiving conventional therapy. This finding was not confirmed by the SDIS or the DCCT. The more recent meta-analysis by Egger and colleagues which included data from the SDIS and DCCT has, however, confirmed a significantly higher incidence of DKA with CSII therapy (Table 12.4). The median incidence of DKA was 0 episodes per 100 person-years with conventional therapy and 2.9 episodes per 100 person-years with intensive therapy. The combined odds ratio (95% CI) for DKA with intensive therapy was 1.74 (1.27–2.38). With exclusive use of CSII therapy, the odds ratio for DKA (95% CI) was 7.20 (2.95–17.58). In contrast, with exclusive use of multiple daily injections (MDI), the odds ratio was 1.13 (0.15–8.35), and for trials offering a choice between CSII and MDI, the odds ratio was 1.28 (0.90–1.83).

The meta-analysis by Egger and colleagues[65] identified 26 deaths among patients with type 1 diabetes, 15 among those receiving intensive therapy and 11 among those receiving conventional therapy (OR 1.40, 95% CI 0.65–3.01) (Table 12.5). This analysis confirmed a non-significant reduction in cardiovascular mortality among intensively treated patients (OR 0.42, 95% CI

0.13–1.40). It did, however, suggest a low but increased incidence of DKA-associated mortality (five deaths versus no deaths) (p = 0.02).

In summary, intensive therapy in young adults with type 1 diabetes causes hypoglycemia and weight gain but does not appear to have an adverse impact on neuropsychological function or quality of life. Intensive therapy with CSII is, however, associated with a significantly increased incidence of DKA and, possibly, of death associated with DKA. What, then, should be recommendations for glycemic management? The answer lies in balancing the benefits and risks of intensive therapy.

THE TARGET FOR INTENSIVE GLYCEMIC MANAGEMENT

Some investigators have sought to define a glycemic threshold for microvascular complications that might minimize the incidence of severe hypoglycemia. Careful analysis of the DCCT demonstrated no HbA_{1c} threshold below which there was zero risk of the development or progression of complications[76]. In addition, although the absolute risk of severe hypoglycemia in the intensive treatment group increased as HbA_{1c} decreased, the relative risk gradient declined with decreasing HbA_{1c}[76]. Thus, in the DCCT, as HbA_{1c} was reduced, there were continuing relative reductions in the risk of complications, whereas there was a slower rate of increase in the risk of hypoglycemia. These data would support implementation of intensive therapy with the goal of achieving normal glycemia.

In the patient populations in whom prospective clinical trials were conducted (that is, willing, younger patients with type 1 diabetes with absent to moderate microvascular and neuropathic complications but without severe diabetic complications or other medical conditions) the goal of glycemic management should be to achieve a HbA_{1c} as close to the non-diabetic range as possible. Both the risks and sequelae of hypoglycemia may be greater in children under 13 years of age, in the elderly, in patients with repeated severe hypoglycemia or unawareness of hypoglycemia, and in patients with advanced diabetic complications. The risk–benefit ratio with intensive therapy may be less favorable in such patients. In such patients, the goal of glycemic management must consider both the likelihood of benefit from attaining the goal and the risks associated with the therapy required to achieve the goal. Factors limiting the benefit of intensive therapy include the existence of advanced diabetes complications, major comorbidities and limited life expectancy. Factors heightening the risk of intensive therapy include history of severe hypoglycemia or hypoglycemia unawareness, advanced autonomic neuropathy or cardiovascular disease, and factors that might impair the detection or treatment of hypoglycemia such as alterations in mental status, lack of mobility or lack of social support. In patients with substantial factors limiting the benefit or heightening the risk of intensive therapy, an individualized but less intensive goal for glycemic management is probably indicated. In addition, goal setting must consider the individual's self-determined diabetes care goal and their willingness to make the necessary lifestyle modifications.

With respect to the glycemic threshold for major malformations, the studies cited above suggest that a glycosylated hemoglobin value within or near the upper limit of normal for the laboratory or within 4 to 7 SDs of the normal mean represents an appropriate goal before conception. If glycemic control were kept within the thresholds achieved in the DCCT ($HbA_{1c} < 5$ SDs above the mean), then unplanned pregnancies might pose less of a risk to IDM. Indeed, the effects of intensive therapy on fetal outcomes were evaluated in 180 participants in the DCCT who completed 270 pregnancies[77]. Of 92 live births, with one set of twins, in the intensive therapy group, there was only one major congenital malformation (0.7%), compared with eight (5.9%) in 99 live births, with two sets of twins, in the conventionally treated group ($p = 0.06$). The good result in the intensive treatment group was obtained even though a minority of the pregnancies had been planned. These data support the conclusion that implementation of intensive glycemic management before, during and after pregnancy can prevent the excess rate of major malformations associated with type 1 diabetes, and prevent or delay microvascular and neuropathic complications.

SUMMARY OF EVIDENCE

Benefits of intensive glycemic management in type 1 diabetes:

Benefit	Level of Evidence	Strength of Recommendation
Prevention of major malformations in IDM	II-1	A
Reduction in development of retinopathy	I	A
Reduction in development of nephropathy	I	A
Reduction in development of neuropathy	I	A
Reduction in progression of retinopathy	I	A
Reduction in progression of nephropathy	I	A
Reduction in development of cardiovascular disease	II-3C	
Reduction in cardiovascular mortality	II-3	C

REFERENCES

1. Kitzmiller JL, Buchanan TA, Kjos S, Combs CA, Ratner RE (1996). Preconception care of diabetes, congenital malformations, and spontaneous abortions. *Diabetes Care* **19**: 514–541.

2. Mills JL (1972) Malformations in infants of diabetic mothers. *Teratology* **25**: 385–394.
3. Mills JL, Baker L, Goldman AS (1979) Malformations in infants of diabetic mothers occur before the seventh gestational week. *Diabetes* **28**: 292–293.
4. Pedersen J, Molsted-Pedersen L (1979) Congenital malformations: the possible role of diabetes care outside pregnancy. In *Pregnancy Metabolism, Diabetes and the Fetus*, Ciba Foundation Symposium 63 (new series). New York: Excerpta Medica, pp. 265–271.
5. Leslie RDG, Pyke DA, John PN, White JM (1978) Hemoglobin A1 in diabetic pregnancy. *Lancet* **ii**: 958–959.
6. Miller E, Hare JW, Cloherty JP, Dunn PJ, Gleason RE, Soeldner JS, Kitzmiller JL (1981) Elevated maternal hemoglobin A1 in early pregnancy and major congenital anomalies in infants of diabetic mothers. *N. Engl. J. Med.* **304**: 1331–1334.
7. Ylinen K, Aula P, Stenman UH, Kesaniemi-Kuokkanen T, Teramo K (1984) Risk of minor and major fetal malformations in diabetics with high haemoglobin A1c values in early pregnancy. *Br. Med. J.* **289**: 345–346.
8. Reid M, Hadden D, Harley JMG, Halliday HL, McClure BG (1984) Fetal malformations in diabetics with high haemoglobin A1c in early pregnancy. *Br. Med. J.* **289**: 1001.
9. Key TC, Giuffrida R, Moore TR (1987) Predictive value of early pregnancy glycohemoglobin in the insulin-treated diabetic patient. *Am. J. Obstet. Gynecol.* **156**: 1096–1100.
10. Stubbs SM, Doddridge MC, John PN, Steel JM, Wright AD (1987) Haemoglobin A1 and congenital malformation. *Diabetic Med.* **4**: 156–159.
11. Miodovnik M, Mimouni F, Dignan PSJ, Berk MA, Ballard JL, Siddiqi TA, Khoury J, Tsang RC (1988) Major malformations in infants of IDDM women: vasculopathy and early first-trimester poor glycemic control. *Diabetes Care* **11**: 713–718.
12. Greene MF, Hare JW, Cloherty JP, Benacerraf BR, Soeldner JS (1989) First-trimester hemoglobin A1 and risk for major malformation and spontaneous abortion in diabetic pregnancy. *Teratology* **39**: 225–231.
13. Lucas MJ, Leveno KJ, Williams ML, Raskin P, Whalley PJ (1989) Early pregnancy glycosylated hemoglobin, severity of diabetes, and fetal malformations. *Am. J. Obstet. Gynecol.* **161**: 426–431.
14. Hanson U, Persson B, Thunell S (1990) Relationship between haemoglobin A1c in early type 1 (insulin-dependent) diabetic pregnancy and the occurrence of spontaneous abortion and fetal malformations in Sweden. *Diabetologia* **33**: 100–104.
15. Rosenn B, Miodovnik M, Combs CA, Khoury J, Siddiqi TA (1994) Glycemic thresholds for spontaneous abortion and congenital malformations in insulin-dependent diabetes mellitus. *Obstet. Gynecol.* **84**: 515–520.
16. Steel JM, Parboosingh J, Cole RA, Duncan JP (1980) Prepregnancy counseling: a logical prelude to the management of the pregnant diabetic woman. *Diabetes Care* **3**: 371–373.
17. Steel JM, Johnstone FD, Smith AF, Duncan LPJ (1982) Five years' experience of a 'prepregnancy' clinic for insulin-dependent diabetics. *Br. Med. J.* **285**: 353–356.
18. Fuhrmann K, Reiher H, Semmler K, Fischer F, Fischer M, Glockner E (1983) Prevention of congenital malformations in infants of insulin-dependent diabetic mothers. *Diabetes Care* **6**: 219–223.
19. Fuhrmann K, Reiher H, Semmler K, Glockner E (1984) The effect of intensified conventional insulin therapy before and during pregnancy on the malformation rate in offspring of diabetic mothers. *Exp. Clin. Endocrinol.* **83**: 173–177.

20. Molsted-Pedersen L, Pedersen JF (1985) Congenital malformations in diabetic pregnancies. *Acta Pediatr. Scand.* **320(Suppl.)**: 79–84.
21. Goldman JA, Dicker D, Fedlberg D, Yeshaya A, Samuel N, Karp M (1986) Pregnancy outcome in patients with insulin-dependent diabetes mellitus with preconception diabetic control: a comparative study. *Am. J. Obstet. Gynecol.* **155**: 293–297.
22. Mills JL, Knopp RH, Simpson JL, Jovanonic-Peterson L, Metzger BE, Holmes LB, Aaron JH, Brown Z, Reed GF, Bieber FR, Van Allen M, Holzman I, Ober C, Peterson CM, Witham MJ, Duckles A, Mueller-Heubach E, Polk BF (National Institute of Child Health and Human Development Diabetes in Early Pregnancy Study) (1988) Lack of relation of increased malformation rates in infants of diabetic mothers to glycemic control during organogenesis. *N. Engl. J. Med.* **318**: 671–676.
23. Damm P, Molsted-Pedersen L (1989) Significant decrease in congenital malformations in newborn infants of an unselected population of diabetic women. *Am. J. Obstet. Gynecol.* **161**: 1163–1167.
24. Steel JM, Johnstone FD, Hepburn DA, Smith AF (1990) Can prepregnancy care of diabetic women reduce the risk of abnormal babies? *Br. Med. J.* **301**: 1070–1074.
25. Steel JM (1994) Personal experience of prepregnancy care in women with insulin-dependent diabetes. *Aust. NZ J. Obstet. Gynecol.* **34**: 135–139.
26. Kitzmiller Jl, Gavin LA, Gin GD, Jovanonic-Peterson L, Main EK, Zigrang WD (1991) Preconception care of diabetes: glycemic control prevents excess congenital malformations. *JAMA* **265**: 731–736.
27. Rosenn B, Miodovnik M, Combs CA, Khoury J, Siddiqi TA (1991) Preconception management of insulin-dependent diabetes: improvement of pregnancy outcome. *Obstet. Gynecol.* **17**: 287–294.
28. Tchobroutsky C, Vray MM, Altman JJ (1991) Risk/benefit ratio of changing late obstetrical strategies in the management of insulin-dependent diabetic pregnancies. *Diabetes Metab.* **17**: 287–294.
29. Willhoite MB, Bennert HW Jr., Palomaki GE, Zaremba MM, Herman WH, Williams JR, Spear NH (1993) The impact of preconception counseling on pregnancy outcomes. *Diabetes Care* **16**: 450–455.
30. Mills JL, Simpson JL, Driscoll SF, Jovanovic-Peterson L, Van Allen M, Aarons JH, Metzger B, Bieber FR, Knopp RH, Holmes LB, Peterson CM, Witham-Wilson M, Brown Z, Ober C, Harley E, Macpherson TA, Duckles A, Mueller-Heubach E, (National Institute of Child Health and Human Development Diabetes in Early Pregnancy Study) (1988) Incidence of spontaneous abortion among normal women and insulin-dependent diabetic women whose pregnancies were identified within 21 days of conception. *N. Engl. J. Med.* **319**: 1617–1623.
31. Janz NK, Herman WH, Becker MP, Charron-Prochownik D, Shayna VL, Lesnick TG, Jacober SJ, Fachnie JD, Druger DF, Sanfield JA, Rosenblatt SI, Lorenz RP (1995) Diabetes and pregnancy: factors associated with seeking preconception care. *Diabetes Care* **18**: 157–165.
32. Wang PH, Lau J, Chalmers TC (1993) Meta-analysis of effects of intensive blood glucose control on late complications of type 1 diabetes. *Lancet* **421**: 1306–1309.
33. Eschwege E, Job D, Guyot-Argenton C, Aubry JP, Tchobroutsky G (1979) Delayed progression of diabetic retinopathy by divided insulin administration: a further follow-up. *Diabetologia* **16**: 13–15.
34. Holman RR, Dornan TL, Mayon-White V, Howard-Williams J, Orde-Peckar C. Jenkins L, Steemson J, Rolfe R, Smith B, Barbour D, McPherson K, Poon P, Rizza C, Mann JI, Knight AH, Bron AJ, Turner RC (1983) Prevention of deterioration of

renal and sensory-nerve function by more intensive management of insulin-dependent diabetic patients. *Lancet* **i**: 204–208.

35. Deckert T, Lauritzen T, Parving HH, Christiansen JS, Steno Study Group (1984) Effect of two years of strict metabolic functions in long term insulin-dependent diabetes. *Diab. Nephropathy* **3**: 6–10.

36. The Kroc Collaborative Study Group (1984) Blood glucose control and the evolution of diabetic retinopathy and albuminuria. *N. Engl. J. Med.* **311**: 365–372.

37. Lauritzen T, Larsen KF, Larsen HW, Deckert T, Steno Study Group (1985) Two-year experience with continuous subcutaneous insulin infusion in relation to retinopathy and neuropathy. *Diabetes* **34**(S3): 74–79.

38. Wiseman MJ, Saunders AJ, Keen H, Viberti G (1985) Effect of blood glucose control on increased glomerular filtration rate and kidney size in insulin-dependent diabetes. *N. Engl. J. Med.* **312**: 617–621.

39. Beck-Nielsen H, Richelsen B, Morgensen CE, Olsen T, Ehlers N, Nielsen CB, Charles P (1985) Effect of insulin pump treatment for one year on renal function and retinal morphology in patients with IDDM. *Diabetes Care* **8**: 585–589.

40. Feldt-Rasmussen B, Mathiesen ER, Deckert T (1986) Effect of two years of strict metabolic control on progression of incipient nephropathy in insulin-dependent diabetes. *Lancet* **ii**: 1300–1304.

41. Olsen T, Richelsen B, Ehlers N, Beck-Nielsen H (1987) Diabetic retinopathy after three years' treatment with continuous subcutaneous insulin infusion (CSII). *Acta Ophthalmol.* **65**: 185–189.

42. Helve E, Laatikainen L, Merenmies L, Koivisto V (1987) Continuous insulin infusion therapy and retinopathy in patients with type 1 diabetes. *Acta Endocrinol.* **115**: 313–319.

43. Christensen CK, Christiansen JS, Schmitz A, Christensen T, Hermansen K, Mogensen CE (1987) Effect of continuous subcutaneous insulin infusion on kidney function and size in IDDM patients: a two year controlled study. *J. Diab. Compl.* **1**: 91–95.

44. Dahl-Jorgensen K, Hanssen KF, Kierulf P, Bjoro T, Sandvik L, Agenaes O (1988) Reduction of urinary albumin excretion after four years of continuous subcutaneous insulin infusion in insulin-dependent diabetes mellitus. *Acta Endocrinol.* **117**: 19–25.

45. Verrillo A, de Teresa A, Martino C, Verrillo L, di Chiara G (1988) Long-term correction of hyperglycemia and progression of retinopathy in insulin-dependent diabetes: a five-year randomized prospective study. *Diab. Res.* **8**: 71–76.

46. The Kroc Collaborative Group (1988) Diabetic retinopathy after two years of intensified insulin treatment. *JAMA* **260**: 37–41.

47. Brinchmann-Hansen O, Dahl-Jorgensen K, Hanssen KF, Sandvik L (1988) The response of diabetic retinopathy to 41 months of multiple insulin injections, insulin pumps, and conventional insulin therapy. *Arch Ophthalmol.* **106**: 1242–1246.

48. Reichard P, Berglund B, Britz A, Cars I, Nilsson BY, Rosenqvist U (1991) Intensified conventional insulin treatment retards the microvascular complications of insulin-dependent diabetes mellitus (IDDM): the Stockholm Diabetes Intervention Study (SDIS) after five years. *J. Intern. Med.* **230**: 101–108.

49. Reichard P, Nilsson BY, Rosenqvist U (1993) The effect of long-term intensified insulin treatment on the development of microvascular complications of diabetes mellitus. *N. Engl. J. Med.* **329**: 304–309.

50. The Diabetes Control and Complications Trial Research Group (1993) The effect of intensive treatment of diabetes on the development and progression of long-term complications in insulin-dependent diabetes mellitus. *N. Engl. J. Med.* **329**: 977–986.

51. The Diabetes Control and Complications Trial Research Group (1995) Effect of intensive therapy on the development and progression of diabetic nephropathy in the Diabetes Control and Complications Trial. *Kidney Intl.* **47**: 1703–1720.
52. Microalbuminuria Collaborative Study Group, UK (1995) Intensive therapy and progression to clinical albuminuria in patients with insulin-dependent diabetes mellitus and microalbuminuria. *Br. Med. J.* **311**: 973–977.
53. The Diabetes Control and Complications Trial/Epidemiology of Diabetes Interventions and Complications Research Group (2000) Retinopathy and nephropathy in patients with type 1 diabetes four years after a trial of intensive therapy. *N. Engl. J. Med.* **342**: 381–389.
54. Jensen-Urstad KJ, Reichard PG, Rosfors JS, Lindblad LEL, Jensen-Urstad MT (1996) Early atherosclerosis is retarded by improved long-term blood glucose control in patients with IDDM. *Diabetes* **45**: 1253–1258.
55. Lawson ML, Tsui E, Gerstein HC, Zinman B (1999) Effect of intensive therapy on early macrovascular disease in young individuals with type 1 diabetes – a systematic review and meta-analysis. *Diabetes Care* **22**(2): B35–B39.
56. Klein R (1995) Hyperglycemia and microvascular and macrovascular disease in diabetes. *Diabetes Care* **18**: 258–268.
57. The Diabetes Control and Complications Trial (DCCT) Research Group (1995) Effect of intensive diabetes management on macrovascular events and risk factors in the Diabetes Control and Complications Trial. *Am. J. Cardiol.* **75**: 894–903.
58. The Diabetes Control and Complications Trial (DCCT) Research Group (1996) Lifetime benefits and costs of intensive therapy as practiced in the Diabetes Control and Complications Trial. *JAMA* **276**: 1409–1415.
59. Wickes IG. Fetal defects following insulin coma in early pregnancy. *Br. Med. J.* **2**: 1029–1030.
60. Impastato DJ, Gabriel AR, Lardaro HH (1964) Electric and insulin shock therapy during pregnancy. *Dis. Nerv. Syst.* **25**: 542–546.
61. Molsted-Pedersen L, Tygstrup I, Pedersen J (1964) Congenital malformations in newborn infants of diabetic women. *Lancet* **i**: 1124–1126.
62. Lowy C, Beard RW, Goldschmidt J (1986) Congenital malformations in babies of diabetic mothers. *Diabetic. Med.* **3**: 458–462.
63. Kimmerle R, Heinemann L, Delecki A, Berger M (1992) Severe hypoglycemia: incidence and predisposing factors in 85 pregnancies of type 1 diabetic women. *Diabetes Care* **15**: 1034–1037.
64. Rosenn BM, Miodovnik M, Holeberg G, Khoury JC, Siddiqi TA (1995) Hypoglycemia: The price of intensive insulin therapy for pregnant women with insulin-dependent diabetes mellitus. *Obstet. Gynecol.* **85**: 417–422.
65. Egger M, Smith GD, Stettler C, Diem P (1997) Risk of adverse effects of intensified treatment in insulin-dependent diabetes mellitus: a meta-analysis. *Diabetic Med.* **14**: 919–928.
66. Lauritzen T, Frost-Larsen K, Larsen HW, Deckert T, Steno Study Group (1983) Effect of one year of near-normal blood glucose levels on retinopathy in insulin-dependent diabetics. *Lancet* **1**: 200–204.
67. Dahl-Jorgensen K, Brinchmann-Hanssen O, Hanssen KF, Ganes T, Kierulf P, Smeland E, Sandvik L, Aagenaes O (1986) Effect of near normoglycemia for two years on progression of early diabetic retinopathy, nephropathy, and neuropathy: the Oslo study. *Br. Med. J.* **293**: 1195–1199.
68. Marshall SM, Home PD, Taylor R, Alberti KGMM (1987) Continuous insulin infusion versus injection therapy: a randomized cross-over trial under usual diabetic clinic conditions. *Diabetic Med.* **4**: 521–525.

69. Helve E, Koivisto VA, Lehtonen A, Pelkonen R, Huttunen JK, Nikkila EA (1987) A crossover comparison of continuous insulin infusion and conventional injection treatment of type 1 diabetes. *Acta Med. Scand.* **221**: 385–393.
70. Bangstad H-J, Kofoed-Enevoldsen A, Dahl-Jorgensen K, Hanssen KF (1992) Glomerular charge selectivity and the influence of improved blood glucose control in type 1 (insulin-dependent) diabetic patients with microalbuminuria. *Diabetologia* **35**: 1165–1169.
71. Microalbuminuria Collaborative Study Group United Kingdom (1995) Intensive therapy and progression to clinical albuminuria in patients with insulin-dependent diabetes mellitus and microalbuminuria. *Br. Med. J.* **311**: 973–977.
72. Reichard P, Berglund A, Britz A, Levander S, Rosenqvist U (1991) Hypoglycemic episodes during intensified insulin treatment: increased frequency but no effect on cognitive function. *J. Int. Med.* **229**: 9–16.
73. The Diabetes Control and Complications Trial Research Group (1996) Effects of intensive diabetes therapy on neuropsychological function in adults in the Diabetes Control and Complications Trial. *Ann. Int. Med.* **124**: 379–388.
74. Austin EJ, Deary IJ (1999) Effects of repeated hypoglycemia on cognitive function: a psychometrically validated reanalysis of the Diabetes Control and Complications Trial data. *Diabetes Care* **22**: 1273–1277.
75. The Diabetes Control and Complications Trial Research Group (1996) Influence of intensive diabetes treatment on quality-of-life outcomes in the Diabetes Control and Complications Trial. *Diabetes Care* **19**: 195–203.
76. The Diabetes Control and Complications Trial Research Group (1996) The absence of a glycemic threshold for the development of long-term complications: the perspective of the Diabetes Control and Complications Trial. *Diabetes* **45**: 1289–1298.
77. The Diabetes Control and Complications Trial (1996) Pregnancy outcomes in the Diabetes Control and Complications Trial. *Am. J. Obstet. Gynecol.* **174**: 1343–1353.

13

Intensive Glycaemic Management in Type 1 Diabetes: A commentary

BRIAN M. FRIER
Department of Diabetes, Royal Infirmary, Edinburgh, Scotland

INTRODUCTION

The importance of the role of chronic hyperglycaemia in the pathogenesis of diabetic complications is now so firmly established that it is difficult to appreciate the intensity, and sometimes acrimonious nature, of the protracted debate that continued for several decades about the 'glucose hypothesis' and the development of microangiopathy[1]. In the pre-glycated haemoglobin era the large, and effectively single-handed, prospective study pursued by Pirart[2] over a 30-year period in people with type 1 diabetes, showed a definite correlation between glycaemic control, measured by blood and urinary glucose, and the development and progression of diabetic complications. A series of smaller but important studies in the 1980s (including the Kroc, Steno and Oslo studies) showed that the progression of established diabetic microangiopathy was closely related to glycaemic control, and that early microvascular disease would respond favourably to near-normal glycaemia[3]. In the 1990s, two major prospective studies in type 1 diabetes, the small Stockholm Diabetes Intervention Study (SDIS)[4], and the much larger Diabetes Control and Complications Trial (DCCT)[5], have provided definitive evidence of the benefits of achieving near-normal blood glucose in preventing and delaying the progression of diabetic complications. These studies, along with other evidence for the benefits of strict glycaemic control in the management of type 1 diabetes, were reviewed in Chapter 12.

The DCCT in North America was a massive undertaking in terms of planning, logistics and the resources required for its completion, but its clear-

The Evidence Base for Diabetes Care. Edited by R. Williams, W. Herman, A.-L. Kinmonth and N. J. Wareham.
© 2002 John Wiley & Sons, Ltd

cut conclusions have fully justified the effort and expense. This is truly a landmark study in evaluating the role of glycaemic control in the development and progression of diabetic complications of type 1 diabetes, and its influence on the modern approach to diabetes management is unquestionable. The comprehensive collection and detailed analyses of data, and the breadth of this multicentre investigation are impressive achievements, and this study has answered several important questions regarding the importance of strict glycaemic control in minimising microvascular disease and neuropathy.

What is much less clear is the feasibility of attempting to obtain strict glycaemic control, both on a daily basis and in the longer term, in the wider population of patients with insulin-treated diabetes, who encompass a wide range in age, duration of diabetes, motivation, and intellectual and practical abilities, with some already having established and advancing diabetic complications such as visual impairment from retinopathy and progressive renal impairment from nephropathy. Around 25% of the type 1 diabetic population also have impaired awareness of hypoglycaemia[6] which is a major risk factor for severe hypoglycaemia, the principal limitation to achieving good glycaemic control. Access to specialist facilities may also be variable. In this commentary, the limitations of the DCCT and other studies are examined with respect to extrapolating the results to the general population with type 1 diabetes. In addition, the feasibility of applying intensive glycaemic management is explored, with consideration of which patient groups may not be suitable for this type of treatment.

LIMITATIONS OF INTERPRETATION OF DATA IN THE DCCT

THE SELECTIVE NATURE OF THE DCCT COHORT

One insurmountable difficulty in directly extrapolating the results of the DCCT to the general population of people with type 1 diabetes is that, of necessity, the patients recruited for the DCCT comprised a self-selected and atypical group (Box 13.1). They were relatively young (mean age 27 years) had diabetes of short duration (mean 5.5 years) and were followed up for a relatively short time (average 6.5 years). They were above average in intelligence, social class and years of higher education, and were highly motivated to participate. Patients who had psychological problems or a psychiatric history, or who were unwilling to submit to the rigours of this long term study, were not recruited. Because the initial feasibility study[7] revealed an unacceptably high incidence of severe hypoglycaemia associated with intensive insulin therapy and strict glycaemic control, in the main study patients were excluded who gave a history of two or more episodes of severe hypoglycaemia or had experienced hypoglycaemic coma or convulsion, often without symptomatic warning, within the preceding two years. This effectively removed many patients with established impaired awareness of hypoglycaemia, which is known to rise in prevalence with increasing duration of diabetes[8] and is associated with a six-fold higher rate of severe hypoglycaemia than that recorded in patients with normal awareness of hypoglycaemia[9]. Patients at high risk of developing severe hypoglycaemia were excluded from the DCCT, thus introducing a further selection bias. While these selection criteria were considered to be necessary to enable the study to be performed, they must not be overlooked when interpreting the results and their clinical implications.

Box 13.1. Clinical features of diabetic patients participating in the Diabetes Control and Complications Trial

- Young adults or adolescents
- Diabetes of short duration
- No significant history of severe hypoglycaemia
- No advanced diabetic complications
- Above average intelligence
- Above average social class and years of higher education
- Highly motivated
- No history of psychiatric/psychological problems
- Willing to adhere to measures in study protocol to produce intensive therapy

---

FREQUENCY OF SEVERE HYPOGLYCAEMIA

The rates of severe hypoglycaemia (defined as any episode requiring external assistance for recovery, and not solely coma or convulsion) in the DCCT were much lower than those reported in unselected cohorts of adult patients with insulin-treated diabetes in studies from Northern Europe[8,10], and also that recorded in the intensively-treated group in the SDIS[4] (Table 13.1). A few studies of apparently unselected diabetic populations have reported much lower frequencies of severe hypoglycaemia, but these have included patients with type 2 diabetes treated with insulin, in whom the frequency of severe hypoglycaemia is often low[11]. In some studies in which patients received programmes of structured education, strict glycaemic control was obtained without a high rate of undesirable hypoglycaemia. One such example is a German study in which strict glycaemic control was associated with a low rate of severe hypoglycaemia of 0.14 episodes per patient-year[12]. Although patients who had a history of previous severe hypoglycaemia were included, the definition used for severe hypoglycaemia was more rigorous. An American study has utilised the technique of Blood Glucose Awareness Training

(BGAT) to lower the rate of severe hypoglycaemia[13]. These studies are isolated examples where strict glycaemic control was associated with a low rate of severe hypoglycaemia, principally as a consequence of the availability of resources for comprehensive education and subsequent patient support. They should not be compared with studies of unselected insulin-treated populations treated in a conventional manner[10].

Although the rate of severe hypoglycaemia was three-fold higher than in the conventionally treated group, this incidence was still considerably less that that observed in unselected diabetic populations (Table 13.1) and the overall rate of severe hypoglycaemic events declined during the course of the DCCT[14], presumably as patients and their support teams became more adept at avoiding this problem. Although it is valuable to quantitate the relative risk of intensive versus conventional therapy in increasing the frequency of severe hypoglycaemia, it is important to appreciate that the lower frequency of exposure to this metabolic insult than those recorded in unselected diabetic populations, and the relatively short duration of follow-up in the DCCT, are relevant to the evaluation of potential effects on long-term cognitive function and quality of life measures.

One other problem of intensive insulin therapy is weight gain, which can be substantial. In the intensively-treated group the mean weight gain recorded was 4.6 kg with an increased relative risk of weight gain of 1.6 compared to the conventionally treated group[5]. Many patients, particularly women, dislike this gain in weight, which is a disincentive to maintaining strict glycaemic control

EFFECTS OF HYPOGLYCAEMIA ON COGNITIVE FUNCTION

Neither the SDIS[4] nor the DCCT[15] showed any detrimental effect on cognitive function in adults as a result of recurrent exposure to severe hypoglycaemia. An independent reanalysis of the neuropsychological data from the DCCT has

Table 13.1. Incidence of severe hypoglycaemia in populations of patients with insulin-treated diabetes.

	Number of participants	Episodes per patient-year	Country
Pramming *et al.* (8)	411*	1.4	Denmark
MacLeod *et al.* (10)	600*	1.6	Scotland
Reichard *et al.* (4)			Sweden
Ter Braak *et al.* (41)	195*	1.5	Netherlands
Conventional therapy	44	0.4	
Intensive therapy	52	1.1	
DCCT(5)			USA/Canada
Conventional therapy	730	0.2	
Intensive therapy	711	0.6	

*Unselected patient populations. Severe hypoglycaemia was defined as any episode requiring external help for recovery.

confirmed this conclusion[16]. While it is reassuring that recurrent severe hypoglycaemia had no apparent effect on these study groups over the time scale (less than 10 years) of these prospective studies, this does not prove conclusively that recurrent severe hypoglycaemia does not have an effect on intellectual ability. The time scale (mean of 6.5 years in the DCCT) may be too short for any significant cognitive deficit to emerge. Furthermore, in the SDIS there was insufficient separation of the intensive and conventional treatment groups based on patients' experience of severe hypoglycaemia, and the cognitive tests employed were probably too insensitive to detect subtle cognitive changes[17]. The problem remains that the atypical nature of patients with type 1 diabetes in the DCCT makes it difficult to extrapolate this data to the wider population, over a longer time-scale. It is possible that the higher mean intellectual ability of the DCCT groups may have provided them with a greater 'intellectual reserve' to cope with any potential detrimental effect that severe hypoglycaemia might have on cognitive function. In addition, only 23 patients were exposed to five or more episodes of hypoglycaemic coma or seizure during the course of the trial[15], and the DCCT patients had little or no exposure to severe hypoglycaemia before their involvement in the study. Although apparently negative, these findings from the prospective studies must be treated with caution, and it is unsafe to generalise their conclusions to the entire population with type 1 diabetes.

Cross-sectional studies in adult patients with type 1 diabetes, using retrospective assessments of the frequency of severe hypoglycaemia, have demonstrated a direct relationship between a modest reduction in intellectual function and the rate of severe hypoglycaemia[18-21]. Anecdotal reports have highlighted individual cases where intellectual decline and altered personality appear to have been the consequences of cumulative exposure to severe hypoglycaemia[22], and patients who gave a history of severe hypoglycaemia have been noted to have evidence of intellectual impairment and symptoms consistent with chronic subclinical depression, compared to diabetic control subjects with no history of previous severe hypoglycaemia[23]. It appears that a spectrum of disability may exist in adults with type 1 diabetes; most subjects either have no, or only a mild, decrement in cognitive function, while a few individuals have evidence of severe cognitive impairment. The roles of hyperglycaemia, neuropathy, hypertension and other factors which have the potential to induce cognitive impairment remain undetermined, so any intellectual deficiency may have a multifactorial cause.

This issue continues to arouse controversy and has been reviewed in detail[17, 24, 25]. Young children are much more susceptible to the effects of severe hypoglycaemia on cerebral function, and it can definitely cause significant intellectual impairment in this age group[25]. For several reasons, young children are considered to be unsuitable for the application of therapeutic strategies that involve the imposition of strict glycaemic control.

EFFECTS OF HYPOGLYCAEMIA AND QUALITY OF LIFE ISSUES

The effect of intensive treatment schedules for type 1 diabetes on quality of life was assessed in detail annually in the DCCT[26], using measures of satisfaction of treatment, social and role functions, emotional wellbeing (psychiatric symptoms) and a record of psychosocial events that occurred during the course of the trial. No differences were shown between the intensive and conventional treatment groups, except for an adverse effect on quality of life in patients who experienced three or more hypoglycaemic episodes that had resulted in coma or seizures. This adverse effect was significant only in the intensive treatment group of the primary prevention cohort[26]. A significant effect of the frequency of severe and disabling hypoglycaemia was also noted in this sub-group on subscales of the symptom questionnaires, which measured depression, interpersonal sensitivity and paranoid ideation. The increased risk of measurable symptomatic distress was therefore limited to very few patients who had been subjected to multiple episodes of severe hypoglycaemia, and the authors of this DCCT publication suggest that the interpretation of this single positive finding should be treated with caution, implying that it is probably of very limited importance[26].

This finding, and the authors' interpretation of its importance, are remarkable in view of the recognition in clinical practice that fear of hypoglycaemia (Figure 13.1) causes considerable psychological distress and apprehension in many patients with insulin-treated diabetes[27], and also affects their relatives[28], often profoundly. Severe hypoglycaemia is stressful, unpleasant and potentially dangerous, and affects mood as well as cognitive function, so that recurrent exposure to severe hypoglycaemia can influence behaviour and modify self-management, thus limiting the quality of glycaemic control that individuals are prepared to attempt[29]. When compared to patients with no history of previous severe hypoglycaemia, diabetic patients who have been exposed to recurrent severe hypoglycaemia have increased levels of anxiety and reduced happiness as a consequence of their experience[30], and adverse psychological effects on other family members are also recognised[28, 31].

These surprising results in the DCCT can again be attributed to the selection of patients and their careful screening before inclusion in this trial. Patients were excluded who reported having experienced any problem with any aspect of the protocol, particularly in adhering to the rigorous measures required for intensive therapy, as were patients with any history of psychiatric illness or psychological disturbance. The screening procedures were designed to identify highly-motivated individuals of above average intelligence (Box 13.1)[26]. These DCCT findings should certainly be interpreted with caution as they have probably resulted from the special circumstances of the trial and the highly selective nature of the study population. The authors of the DCCT

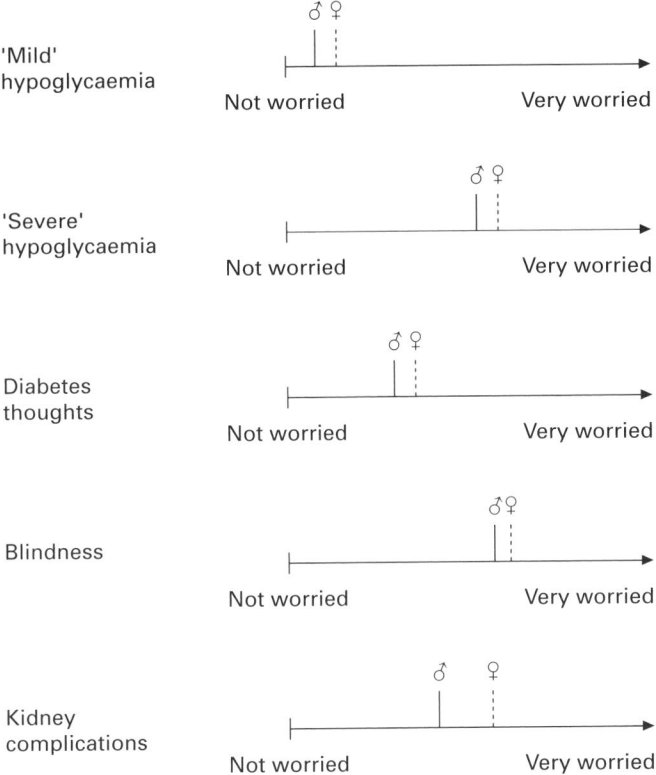

Figure 13.1. Attitudes towards different aspects of diabetes indicated by 411 patients with type 1 diabetes on a visual analogue scale[8]. In *Diabetic Medicine.* Pramming S, *et al.* 1991 **8**: 217–222. © John Wiley & Sons Limited. Reproduced with permission.

acknowledge that their volunteers might have been unusually capable of dealing with the challenges of intensive diabetes management, and were more resilient and self-sufficient than the average individual with type 1 diabetes. They therefore represent one extreme of the spectrum of human resourcefulness and ability, and are not typical of the population in general.

The likelihood that the responses to the quality of life outcomes in the DCCT are unrepresentative of the average patient is further acknowledged by the statement:

The use of intensive treatment techniques by patients who are already emotionally upset, are not fully supported by their families or healthcare providers, deny their illness, do not have adequate access to healthcare professionals, or are uncomfortable with the added demands of treatment may cause more problems with quality-of-life outcomes than were demonstrated in the DCCT[26].

Realistically, these descriptive qualifications represent a large number of people with type 1 diabetes in whom strenuous attempts to impose strict glycaemic control would inevitably induce a significant emotional burden in terms of acute and chronic psychological distress and an increased frequency of psychosocial events.

THE FEASIBILITY OF INTENSIVE GLYCAEMIC MANAGEMENT REGIMENS

THE APPLICABILITY OF THE DCCT REGIMEN FOR STRICT GLYCAEMIC CONTROL

In assessing the practical feasibility of imposing a regimen of intensive insulin therapy on patients with type 1 diabetes, it is essential to appreciate the measures applied in the DCCT, and the level and intensity of self-management to which patients had to commit themselves in attempting to achieve and sustain the required degree of strict glycaemic control. These are shown in Box 13.2, and involved the use of multiple insulin injections or Continuous Subcutaneous Insulin Infusion (CSII), frequent home blood glucose monitoring, and regular contact with the specialist team who were supervising their overall diabetes care. The personal investment in time and effort by the patient that is necessary to maintain such a regimen is substantial, notwithstanding the major resource implications for specialist support services. This approach to management is therefore extremely labour-intensive, and the continuous availability of skilled staff who have the expertise to give appropriate advice and assistance is mandatory if this is to have a reasonable prospect of success.

Many patients simply will not accept this intensity of self-management. In

---

Box 13.2. Diabetes Control and Complications Trial: measures required in intensive treatment group

- Multiple insulin injections or CSII (Continuous Subcutaneous Insulin Infusion)
- Daily blood glucose monitoring (four times or more)
- Weekly nocturnal blood glucose measurement (3 am)
- Frequent attention to diet and exercise
- Monthly (or more frequent) attendance at diabetes outpatient clinic
- Frequent telephone contact with specialist team

my clinical experience, many sensible and well-balanced patients who understand the potential long-term benefits, decline to participate in regimens for intensive glycaemic management, because of the difficulties this imposes on their lifestyles. In the UK, studies have shown that many patients who are supposed to be doing routine blood glucose monitoring are not performing the tests regularly[32] while insulin use is often less than presumed by the number of prescriptions filled, particularly in teenagers[33]. This is reflected by the rise in mean glycated haemoglobin concentration in the adolescent age group with a deterioration in glycaemic control which may persist for several years[34]. This was evident in the subgroup of 195 adolescent patients (aged 13–18) within the DCCT in whom the mean glycated haemoglobin concentrations achieved during the study remained higher than those in adults[35]. In the ordinary life of many patients, adherence to insulin therapy can be a major problem, with a linear relationship being demonstrated between reduced compliance with treatment and an elevated HbA_{1c} (Figure 13.2)[33].

It is possible to improve glycaemic control in teenagers with type 1 diabetes, albeit temporarily. This was demonstrated in a group of 69 adolescent patients (aged 12–17) with poorly controlled type 1 diabetes, who participated in a home-based intervention study in which they received the assistance of a diabetes nurse educator for six months[36]. Glycaemic control and knowledge of diabetes were improved during this period, but treatment was effective only while the intervention was maintained. Post-DCCT reports of what has happened to glycaemic control in the intensively-treated group have revealed that mean glycated haemoglobin has risen by around 1%, indicating some degree of relaxation of glycaemic control and reduced intensity of self-management by most of the participants after the study terminated[40].

Anecdotal reports have suggested that some patients were unimpressed or actively discouraged by the outcomes of the DCCT[37], and did not relish the personal commitment required. A larger systematic survey of patients' reactions to the DCCT has provided some indication of how receptive they may be to embracing the messages of this study[38]. A leaflet documenting the purpose and results of the DCCT was circulated to 771 patients (aged 15–60) with insulin-treated diabetes who were attending a diabetes clinic in Dundee, Scotland. The patients were invited to complete a questionnaire giving their responses to the DCCT and, of the 550 respondents, 60% felt that they would be prepared to improve their glycaemic control as a consequence of this study. Female patients and younger age groups (aged 15–25) were more enthusiastic about making an effort to improve glycaemic control than males or older patients, while patients with a history of severe hypoglycaemia or impaired awareness of hypoglycaemia were least likely to want to improve glycaemic control. Exposure to mild hypoglycaemia, the number of daily insulin injections and the frequency of blood glucose testing did not affect their responses, but particular concerns were expressed about the possible risk of loss of their driving licences through an increased incidence of hypoglycaemia, fear of severe hypoglycaemia and weight gain. Older patients were concerned about the life-long effort required to maintain strict glycaemic control. Relatively few patients were prepared to attend outpatient clinics more frequently, and only 11% of respondents were prepared to attend monthly, as in the DCCT.

This study[38] emphasises the importance of examining the relationship between patient characteristics and attitudes to health outcomes. With such an anonymised and cross-sectional survey, it is impossible to ascertain whether an expressed willingness to improve glycaemic control would be translated into real improvement in the long term, and the capacity of most patients to sustain protracted adherence to a demanding regimen, which requires continuous effort and commitment over many years, is unknown. While the reaction of patients to the DCCT expressed in response to this Scottish survey[38] may provide some encouragement to health care professionals in that the DCCT may have some lasting benefit on patients' behaviour and self-management, the greatest impact of the results of the DCCT has probably been on diabetes specialists and their teams. Nobody involved in the provision of diabetes care can have been left in any doubt about the importance of strict glycaemic control in minimising the development and severity of diabetic complications, even if the means of achieving this remains a formidable challenge.

HOW OFTEN WAS STRICT GLYCAEMIC CONTROL ACHIEVED IN THE DCCT?

The target HbA_{1c} in the intensively-treated group in the DCCT was below 6.05%, a value chosen because it was within two standard deviations of the non-diabetic range[14]. The implementation of the measures to attain strict glycaemic control (Box 13.2) in this group of patients was successful in producing a significantly lower mean HbA_{1c} than that observed in the conventionally-treated group (around a 2% difference in HbA_{1c}), but how effective were these policies in the intensively-treated group and were near-normal levels of HbA_{1c} sustained? In the feasibility study[7], only 17% of patients in the intensively-treated group achieved a HbA_{1c} within the non-diabetic range. In the main study, almost half the group succeeded in lowering their HbA_{1c} to the target level at some point during the trial (Box 13.3) but less than 5% of patients maintained their HbA_{1c} at this level of control[5, 14]. Throughout the study, the median HbA_{1c} was 6.7–7.2% which, although highly commendable, was above the target set by the investigators when planning the study. In retrospect, the low target level was probably too ambitious. It was certainly beyond the capability of most patients to sustain this over a prolonged period. A more suitable therapeutic option window to prevent microangiopathy, but to avoid severe hypoglycaemia, may be around 7.0–7.5% (Figure 13.3)[39], but it

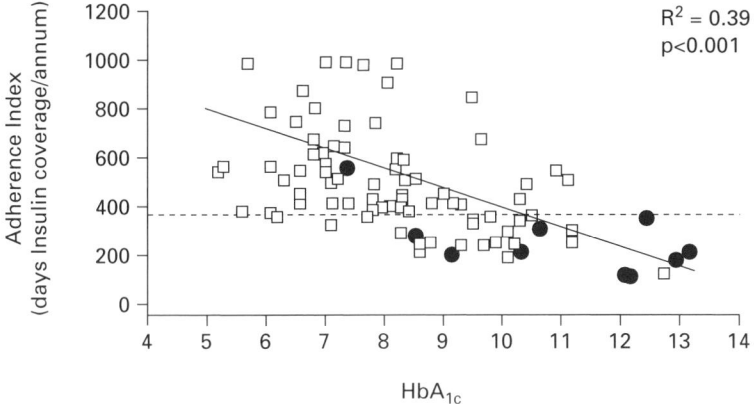

Figure 13.2. Adherence to insulin therapy as measured by an adherence index[33] showing a linear regression of the association with glycaemic control (HbA$_{1c}$) in patients with type 1 diabetes. Reproduced with permission from Elsevier Science (*The Lancet*, 1997; **350**: 1505–1510).

Box 13.3. Diabetes Control and Complications Trial: effectiveness of implementation of strict glycaemic control

- Target HbA$_{1c}$ <6.05% (within 2 SD of mean non-diabetic range)
- This was achieved at least once during the trial by 44% of intensively-treated group
- Average HbA1c was maintained by <5% of adult patients (<2% of adolescent group)
- Median HbA1c for individual patients was 6.7–7.2% throughout study (6.5 years) and was 7.9% four years after the study

---

is important to remember that any reduction in HbA$_{1c}$ is beneficial in patients with poor glycaemic control[37].

Throughout the study, the overall adherence of patients to the intensive therapy regimen was not in doubt, but the practical difficulties of maintaining such strict glycaemic control were evident, even in this highly committed, dedicated and self-selected group of patients. The immense personal effort by patients and the extensive specialist support provided were clearly major factors in achieving these outcomes. However, in most Westernised countries, where specialist diabetes services are generally well developed, this level of medical and paramedical support for patients is simply not available. In the UK, most adult patients who attend a specialist centre are seen once or twice a year for assessment of glycaemic control, therapeutic advice and screening for diabetic complications. A significant number of patients do not attend either a specialist centre or their general practitioner for diabetes management. Any attempt to promote intensive insulin therapy of sufficient degree to achieve strict glycaemic control is therefore impractical and is probably not feasible in all but a few highly motivated individuals, many of whom often succeed in maintaining strict glycaemic control irrespective of medical intervention. Some of these patients have an obsessional approach to self-management, or may participate in regular and frequent physical exercise which increases their insulin sensitivity and improves their overall glycaemic control. This is not to decry the attempts of individuals or of specialists to achieve this quality of strict glycaemic control, but it is important to acknowledge the difficulty of this task with the limitations of currently available insulins, restricted therapeutic strategies, the average level of clinical resources and the relatively modest levels of motivation and enthusiasm observed over long periods in the average patient with insulin-treated diabetes.

For most individuals, the immediacy of the risk of severe hypoglycaemia is a much greater disincentive to attempt continuous near-normoglycaemia than rational consideration of the potential, but more temporally remote, problem of eventual vascular complications. This was apparent in a Danish survey of patients with type 1 diabetes, who rated their anxiety about the development of severe hypoglycaemia as equivalent to the risk of developing serious complications of diabetes, such as sight-threatening retinopathy or renal failure from nephropathy[8], as shown in Figure 13.1.

It cannot be concluded from the DCCT that implementing intensive insulin therapy, by using either multiple insulin injections or CSII, is the only effective method of producing strict glycaemic control. If patients who are taking one or two injections of insulin per day are given the same level of supervision and support as was available in the intensive-treatment group of the DCCT, it is possible that they may also be able to achieve excellent glycaemic control. The importance of the type of therapeutic regimen employed for intensive glycaemic management was not investigated by the DCCT, and multiple insulin injection therapy or CSII may not be necessary to produce and maintain strict glycaemic control. Other approaches to management may be possible.

PATIENTS UNSUITABLE FOR STRICT GLYCAEMIC CONTROL

Some people with type 1 diabetes are not suitable for intensive insulin therapy (Box 13.4), including patients with advanced diabetic complications and those with a limited life expectancy. Many elderly patients are unlikely to benefit from strict long-term control, and in this age group, many of whom are physic-

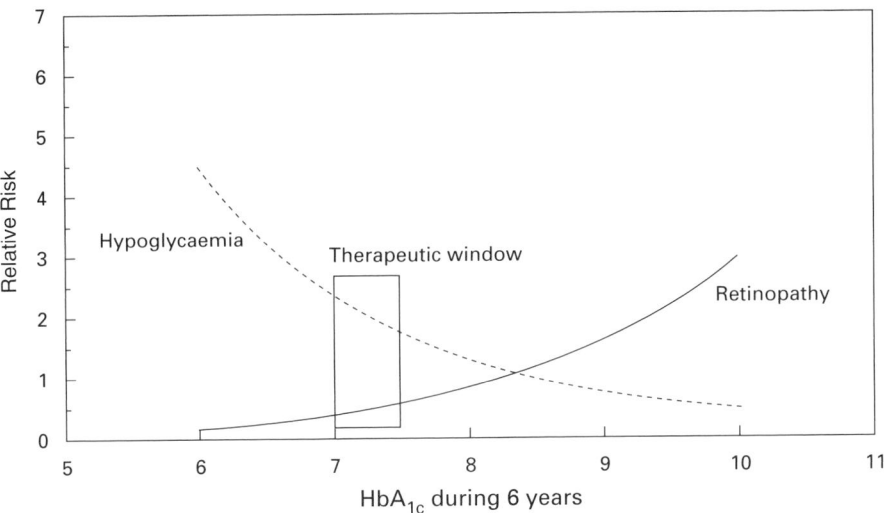

Figure 13.3. A schematic representation of the relative risk of retinopathy and severe hypoglycaemia based on several studies, with a suggested therapeutic window indicated. This graphic presentation is not intended to be an exact description of the relationship in the individual patient. From Dahl-Jorgensen *et al.*[39] *Diabetologia*, 'Blood glucose control and microvascular complications – what do we do now?' 1994; **37**: 1172–1177. Reproduced by permission of Springer–Verlag).

Box 13.4. Application of strict glycaemic control in type 1 diabetes

Caution required
- Long duration of diabetes (counter-regulatory deficiencies common)
- Impaired awareness of hypoglycaemia
- History of recurrent severe hypoglycaemia-induced convulsions or epilepsy
- Patient unwilling to do blood glucose monitoring

Contraindicated
- Extremes of age
- Advanced diabetic complications
- Limited life expectancy
- Mental subnormality; psychiatric illness
- Coronary heart disease; previous stroke or transient ischaemic attacks

---

ally frail, the potential morbidity from severe hypoglycaemia can be particularly serious. Acute vascular events such as stroke or myocardial infarction may be precipitated by severe hypoglycaemia, and fractures are more likely from resulting trauma. Patients with impaired awareness of hypoglycaemia often have co-existing counter-regulatory hormonal deficiencies, and strict glycaemic control not only increases their propensity to develop severe hypoglycaemia, which may actually worsen these acquired abnormalities, but is also associated with delayed recovery. Young children are particularly unsuitable for intensive insulin therapy. The DCCT research group have clearly stated that the risk–benefit ratio of strict glycaemic control is less favourable in specific groups, which is consistent with contraindications (Box 13.4) that are based on clinical grounds. They would discourage intensive glycaemic management in children aged less than 13, patients with coronary heart disease, cerebrovascular disease or severe complications such as end-stage renal disease, and those with impaired awareness of hypoglycaemia or a history of previous severe hypoglycaemia[5].

In conclusion, while the benefits of strict glycaemic control in reducing the microvascular complications of diabetes are evident, there is a price to pay for this. The substantial increase in the risk of severe hypoglycaemia, which carries an attendant risk of associated morbidity (and potential mortality) is unacceptable to many patients, and the risks associated with intensive glycaemic management must be explained. The targets for glycaemic control should be set for individual patients, and related to their personal circumstances. The practical difficulties of applying the methods used in the DCCT to the general population of people with type 1 diabetes must be acknowledged. This is a major consideration when considering the feasibility of this therapeutic approach in individual patients with type 1 diabetes. Many people who are willing to attempt intensive glycaemic management may be less enthusiastic when they realise the level of personal commitment required, the main side-effects (severe hypoglycaemia and significant weight gain) associated with this therapeutic regimen, and the difficulty of maintaining strict glycaemic control over several years of treatment. At present, this is the major challenge facing health care professionals providing specialist services for people with type 1 diabetes.

REFERENCES

1. Tchobroutsky G (1978) Relation of diabetic control to development of microvascular complications. *Diabetologia* **15**: 143–152.
2. Pirart J (1978) Diabetes mellitus and its degenerative complications: a prospective study of 4400 patients observed between 1947 and 1973. *Diabetes Care* **1**: 168–188
3. Hanssen KF, Dahl-Jorgensen K, Lauritzen T, Feldt-Rasmussen B, Brinchmann-Hansen O, Deckert T (1986) Diabetic control and microvascular complications: the near-normoglycaemic experience. *Diabetologia* **29**: 677–684
4. Reichard P, Phil M, Rosenqvist U, Sule J (1996) Complications in IDDM are caused by elevated blood glucose levels: The Stockholm Diabetes Intervention Study (SDIS) at 10-year follow up. *Diabetologia* **39**: 1483–1488.
5. The Diabetes Control and Complications Trial Research Group (1993) The effect of intensive treatment of diabetes on the development and progression of long-term complications in insulin-dependent diabetes mellitus. *N. Engl. J. Med.* **329**: 977–986.

6. Frier BM, Fisher BM (1999) Impaired hypoglycaemia awareness. In *Hypoglycaemia in Clinical Diabetes*. (eds BM Frier and BM Fisher). John Wiley & Sons: Chichester, pp. 111–146.
7. The DCCT Research Group (1987) Diabetes Control and Complications Trial (DCCT): results of feasibility study. *Diabetes Care* **10**: 1–19.
8. Pramming S, Thorsteinsson B, Bendtson I, Binder C (1991) Symptomatic hypoglycaemia in 411 type 1 diabetic patients. *Diabetic Med.* **8**: 217–222.
9. Gold AE, MacLeod KM, Frier BM (1994) Frequency of severe hypoglycemia in patients with type 1 diabetes with impaired awareness of hypoglycemia. *Diabetes Care* **17**: 697–703.
10. MacLeod KM, Hepburn DA, Frier BM (1993) Frequency and morbidity of severe hypoglycaemia in insulin-treated diabetic patients. *Diabetic Med.* **10**: 238–245.
11. Tattersall RB (1993) Frequency and causes of hypoglycaemia. In *Hypoglycaemia and Diabetes: Clinical and Physiological Aspects* (eds BM Frier and BM Fisher). Edward Arnold: London, pp. 176–189.
12. Jörgens V, Grüber M, Bott U, Mülhauser I, Berger M (1993) Effective and safe translation of intensified insulin therapy to general internal medicine departments. *Diabetologia* **36**: 99–105
13. Kinsley BT, Weinger K, Bajaj M, Levy CJ, Simonson DC, Quigley M, Cox DJ, Jacobson AM (1999) Blood glucose awareness training and epinephrine responses to hypoglycemia during intensive treatment in type 1 diabetes. *Diabetes Care* **22**: 1022–1028.
14. The Diabetes Control and Complications Trial Research Group (1995) Implementation of treatment protocols in the Diabetes Control and Complications Trial. *Diabetes Care* **18**: 361–376.
15. The Diabetes Control and Complications Trial Research Group (1996) Effects of intensive diabetic therapy on neuropsychological function in adults in the Diabetes Control and Complications Trial. *Ann. Int. Med.* **124**: 379–388.
16. Austin EJ, Deary IJ (1999) Effects of repeated hypoglycemia on cognitive function. A psychometrically validated reanalysis of the Diabetes Control and Complications Trial data. *Diabetes Care* **22**: 1273–1277.
17. Deary IJ, Frier BM (1996) Severe hypoglycaemia and cognitive impairment in diabetes. *Br. Med. J.* **313**: 767–768.
18. Langan SJ, Deary IJ, Hepburn DA, Frier BM (1991) Cumulative cognitive impairment following recurrent severe hypoglycaemia in adult patients with insulin-treated diabetes mellitus. *Diabetologia* **34**: 337–344.
19. Wredling R, Levander S, Adamson U, Lins PE (1990) Permanent neuropsychological impairment after recurrent episodes of severe hypoglycaemia in man. *Diabetologia* **33**: 152–157
20. Deary IJ, Crawford JR, Hepburn DA, Langan SJ, Blackmore LM, Frier BM (1993) Severe hypoglycaemia and intelligence in adult patients with insulin-treated diabetes. *Diabetes* **42**: 341–344.
21. Lincoln NB, Faleiro RM, Kelly C, Kirk BA, Jeffcoate WJ (1996) Effect of long-term glycemic control on cognitive function. *Diabetes Care* **19**: 656–658.
22. Gold AE, Deary IJ, Jones RW, O'Hare JP, Reckless JDP, Frier BM (1994) Severe deterioration in cognitive function and personality in five patients with long-standing diabetes: a complication of diabetes or a consequence of treatment? *Diabetic Med.* **11**: 499–505.
23. Strachan MWJ, Deary IJ, Ewing FME, Frier BM (2000) Recovery of cognitive function and mood after severe hypoglycemia in adults with insulin-treated diabetes. *Diabetes Care* **23**: 305–312.

24. Deary IJ (1997) Hypoglycemia-induced cognitive decrement in adults with type 1 diabetes: a case to answer? *Diabetes Spectrum* **10**: 42–47.
25. Perros P, Deary IJ (1999) Long-term effects of hypoglycaemia on cognitive function and the brain in diabetes. In *Hypoglycaemia in Clinical Diabetes* (eds BM Frier and BM Fisher). John Wiley & Sons: Chichester, pp. 187–210.
26. The Diabetes Control and Complications Trial Research Group (1996) Influence of intensive diabetes treatment on quality-of-life outcomes in the Diabetes Control and Complications Trial. *Diabetes Care* **19**: 195–203.
27. Sanders K, Mills J, Martin FIR, Horne DJD (1975)Emotional attitudes in adult insulin-dependent diabetes. *J. Psychosom. Res.* **19**: 241–246.
28. Stahl M, Berger W, Schaechinger H, Cox DJ (1998) Spouse's worries concerning diabetic partner's possible hypoglycaemia. *Diabetic Med.* **15**: 619–620 (letter).
29. Gold AE, Deary IJ, Frier BM (1997) Hypoglycaemia and non-cognitive aspects of psychological function in insulin-dependent (type 1) diabetes mellitus (IDDM). *Diabetic Med.* **14**: 111–118.
30. Wredling RAM, Theorell PGT, Roll HM, Lins PES, Adamson UKC (1992) Psychosocial state of patients with IDDM prone to recurrent episodes of severe hypoglycemia. *Diabetes Care* **15**: 518–521.
31. Frier BM (1999) Living with hypoglycaemia. In *Hypoglycaemia in Clinical Diabetes* (eds BM Frier and BM Fisher). John Wiley & Sons: Chichester, pp. 261–290.
32. Evans JMM, Newton RW, Ruta DA, MacDonald TM, Stevenson RJ, Morris AD (1999) Frequency of blood glucose monitoring in relation to glycaemic control: observational study with diabetes database. *Br. Med. J.* **319**: 83–86.
33. Morris AD, Boyle DIR, McMahon AD, Greene SA, MacDonald TM, Newton RW (for the DARTS/MEMO Collaboration) (1997) Adherence to insulin treatment, glycaemic control, and ketoacidosis in insulin-dependent diabetes mellitus. *Lancet* **350**: 1505–1510.
34. Pound N, Sturrock NDC, Jeffcoate WJ (1996) Age-related changes in glycated haemoglobin in patients with insulin dependent diabetes mellitus. *Diabetic Med.* **13**: 510–513.
35. The Diabetes Control and Complications Trial Research Group (1994) Effect of intensive diabetes treatment on the development of progression of long-term complications in adolescents with insulin dependent diabetes mellitus: Diabetes Control and Complications Trial. *J. Pediatr.* **125**: 177–188.
36. Couper JJ, Taylor J, Fotheringham, MJ, Sawyer M (1999) Failure to maintain the benefits of home-based intervention in adolescents with poorly controlled type 1 diabetes. *Diabetes Care* **22**: 1933–1937.
37. Rubin RR, Peyrot M (1994) Implications of the DCCT. Looking beyond tight control. *Diabetes Care* **17**: 235–236.
38. Thompson CJ, Cumming JFR, Chalmers J, Gould C, Newton RW (1996) How have patients reacted to the implications of the DCCT? *Diabetes Care* **19**: 876–879.
39. Dahl-Jorgensen, Brinchmann-Hansen O, Bangstad H-J, Hanssen KF (1994) Blood glucose control and microvascular complications – what do we do now? *Diabetologia* **37**: 1172–1177.
40. The Diabetes Control and Complications Trial/Epidemiology of Diabetes Interventions and Complications Research Group (2000) Retinopathy and nephropathy in patients with Type 1 diabetes four years after a trial of intensive therapy. *New Eng. J. Med.* **342**: 381–389.
41. Ter Braak EWMT, Appelman AMMF, Van de Laak MF, Stolk RP, Van Haeften, TW, Erkelens DW (2000) Clinical characteristics of Type 1 diabetic patients with and without severe hypoglycaemia. *Diabetes Care* **23**: 1467–1471.

14

Does Tight Control of Hyperglycaemia Limit Morbidity and Mortality in Type 2 Diabetes?

AMANDA ADLER

Radcliffe Infirmary, Oxford OX2 6EH, UK

There is considerable evidence demonstrating an increased risk of complications in individuals with diabetes compared to those without diabetes, and of higher risks among those with diabetes who have greater degrees of hyperglycaemia. Although hyperglycaemia defines diabetes, and is in turn associated with the risk of its complications, this is not sufficient by itself to justify the treatment of hyperglycaemia in order to avert complications. Glycaemia may be a marker for other known risk factors, or for unmeasured or unknown risk factors for complications. The justification for treating hyperglycaemia comes from trials that address whether glucose lowering lowers the risk of complications. This chapter will review the evidence from these trials with specific reference to glucose lowering in type 2 diabetes.

EVIDENCE FROM OBSERVATIONAL STUDIES

Observational epidemiological studies address whether an independent association exists between hyperglycaemia and the complications of diabetes. They also provide estimates for the risk reduction that might be expected from glucose lowering therapies. The following studies reflect examples of observational studies that have provided the background and rationale for intervention trials in type 2 diabetes, and are restricted to prospective studies since the causal

The Evidence Base for Diabetes Care. Edited by R. Williams, W. Herman, A.-L. Kinmonth and N. J. Wareham.
© 2002 John Wiley & Sons, Ltd

inference is much greater in this design, as hyperglycaemia precedes the development of complications.

DEATH

The majority of studies that have evaluated the link between blood glucose levels and mortality among the population of people with diabetes find a positive, significant association[1,2]. This association has been shown for hyperglycaemia measured by different means including fasting glucose[3], post glucose load glucose concentrations[4,5], and HbA_{1c} measured once, or multiple times during follow-up[6]. In a cohort of predominantly white individuals with type 2 diabetes in Wisconsin, hyperglycaemia as measured by HbA_{1c} was significantly associated with death from diabetic complications. This association was independent of other risk factors for death, which could reasonably be expected to be associated with hyperglycaemia[7]. The risk increase for each 1% increase in HbA_{1c} was approximately 8–20%. In the United Kingdom Prospective Diabetes Study (UKPDS), longitudinal observation of 3642 individuals for whom information on potential confounders was available showed that each 1% increase in HbA_{1c} averaged over 10 years of follow-up ($p < 0.0001$) was associated with a 16% increase in mortality due to all causes. The analyses took into account differences, by HbA_{1c} level, in age, sex, ethnicity, albuminuria, smoking, systolic blood pressure, HDL, LDL and triglycerides[6]. A significant association was seen, regardless of whether HbA_{1c} was averaged over follow-up, or on the basis of a single HbA_{1c} measured shortly after diagnosis of diabetes but before the institution of treatment. HbA_{1c} averaged over time was more highly associated with death due to specific diabetes-related complications including cardiovascular, cerebrovascular, renal, hyperglycaemic and hypoglycaemia causes than it was to all-cause mortality. Both the Wisconsin and the UKPDS participants were treated for diabetes. In the UKPDS this was done per study protocol. Observational studies that include patients not treated for hyperglycaemia would be appropriate only for patients with mild or early disease.

CARDIOVASCULAR DISEASE

Many prospective observational studies have found associations between hyperglycaemia and coronary artery disease[6–12], stroke[6,7,13,14] peripheral vascular disease[15] and lower extremity amputation[16,17,18]. Specifically, elevated fasting plasma glucose values greater than 11.5 mmol/l were associated with a nearly five-fold increase in risk for cardiovascular mortality relative to diabetic patients with lower values fasting plasma glucose[3]. Measures of glycaemia other than fasting plasma glucose, including glycohaemoglobin, have been independently associated with death from macrovascular disease[19]. The association between HbA_{1c} and complications has been observed for HbA_{1c}

when expressed as a binary variable; i.e. 'good' versus 'bad' glycaemic control. Among Finns with type 2 diabetes, poor glycaemic control as measured by an HbA_{1c} over 10.7% was associated with a greater than two-fold increase in risk of stroke, independent of other risk factors[14]. Lower cut-offs for defining poor glycaemic control have also been associated with an increased risk of cardiovascular disease[9]. Yet, glycaemia appears to have a continuous association with complications. Observational data from the UKPDS allows estimation of the magnitude of the association between HbA_{1c} as a continuous variable and the risk of cardiovascular disease in patients with newly diagnosed diabetes. Among 3642 individuals, each 1% increase in HbA_{1c} was associated with a 16 % increase in myocardial infarction (MI) (p = <0.0001). By contrast, each 1% decrement in HbA_{1c} was associated with a 43% (31–53%, p = <0.0001) reduction for fatal peripheral vascular disease and lower extremity amputation. These associations were independent of other risk factors for cardiovascular disease measured shortly after the diagnosis of type 2 diabetes. Other studies have also reported a similar magnitude of association for macrovascular disease as in the UKPDS, and have also shown a difference in effect size by site of atherosclerosis[10,20].

RETINOPATHY, NEPHROPATHY, NEUROPATHY

Observational epidemiological studies also provide evidence of an association between glycaemia and microvascular complications. Pirart described an increasing prevalence of neuropathy, nephropathy and retinopathy with 'chronic poor control' of glycaemia in a large cohort of Belgian patients with diabetes followed from 1947 [21]. In an observational analysis of UKPDS, a 1% decrease in HbA_{1c} averaged over time was associated with a 37% (33–41%) risk reduction in microvascular disease, predominantly retinopathy[6], after controlling for possible confounding factors. The degree of risk increase was similar to that for retinopathy in the Wisconsin Epidemiologic Study of Diabetic Retinopathy(WESDR)[20,22]. Hyperglycaemia has also been associated with an increased risk for proteinuria, renal decline or failure [22,23,24,25,26,27] and sensory neuropathy[22,28] in prospective analyses. Hyperglycaemia is a risk factor for death even when measured after a patient develops end-stage renal disease[29]. Although the relative risk increase for microvascular complications is greater than that for cardiovascular complications, individuals with diabetes are nonetheless at a higher absolute risk of developing cardiovascular complications[6].

EVIDENCE FROM CLINICAL TRIALS

Observational studies test whether hyperglycaemia is associated with the complications of diabetes, and experimental studies test whether treatment of the hyperglycaemia lowers the incidence of complications.

UNIVERSITY GROUP DIABETES PROGRAM (UGDP)

The University Group Diabetes Program (UGDP), was a randomised clinical trial with the aim of measuring 'the efficacy of hypoglycaemic treatments in the prevention of vascular complications in a long-term, prospective and cooperative clinical trial in type 2 diabetes'[30]. The trial was double-blinded and placebo controlled, beginning in 1961 and ending in 1975. The trial enrolled 1027 newly diagnosed individuals with type 2 diabetes, mostly female (71%) and with a mean age of 53 years. Half of the population had systolic hypertension (>140 mmHg). Diabetes was diagnosed based on the sum of the fasting, and the one-, two-, and three-hour values from an oral glucose tolerance test (OGTT). The glucose load was a function of body surface. Individuals with a sum greater than 500 mg/dl (27 mmol/l) were considered diabetic. All patients were then treated with diet alone for one month, intended to achieve normal body weight and to wash out previous therapies. After this period, treatments were added to diet. Since the trial included only those patients who finished the dietary run-in without severe or decompensated hyperglycaemia, they were possibly less ill than newly diagnosed patients in the general population.

Patients were randomised to one of essentially six treatment groups; fixed-dose insulin, variable-dose insulin, tolbutamide or its placebo and phenformin or its placebo. For the oral agents, the trial was double-blinded and placebo-controlled. Placebo injections were not used for the insulin arms of the study. Tolbutamide was dosed to approximately 2 gm per day, and phenformin dosed as 50 mg twice daily. The phenformin arm was added one and a half years into the study. In addition, all patients were assigned a diet meant to achieve and/or maintain body weight within 15% of ideal. Diet was therefore not a randomised therapy[30].

The fixed dose insulin regimen varied between individuals from 10 to 16 units of lente insulin according to body surface area. The dosage was titrated to maintain 'normal' blood glucose levels. This was defined as a fasting blood glucose level less than 110 mg/dl (6.1 mmol/l) and a level of less than 210 mg/dl (11.7 mmol/l) one hour following a 50 gm glucose load.

During the course of the study, both the tolbutamide and the phenformin arms of the study were discontinued due to the observation of an apparent increase in mortality in these groups[31]. However, the placebo group was continued and compared to the two insulin arms. Randomisation to all therapies including placebo was associated with an initial and temporary drop in fasting blood glucose ranging from a 12–25% drop from baseline. A reduction from baseline was maintained for the variable-insulin group via increasing the insulin dose, whereas all other randomised groups experienced a return to baseline fasting plasma glucose values[32]. Dosages of insulin among the patients in the variable insulin group tripled in order to maintain glycaemic control.

Despite differences in blood glucose control between the treatment groups, and fewer hospitalisations for heart disease for the variable and fixed dose insulin groups when compared to placebo, neither difference reached conventional statistical significance (p = 0.14 and p = 0.13, respectively)[32]. In addition, when compared to placebo, neither insulin regimen was associated with differences in the incidence of peripheral vascular disease or retinopathy. Fewer patients developed increased serum creatinine concentrations in the fixed dose insulin group relative to placebo (p = 0.03). There were no differences between groups with respect to cardiovascular disease, but the number of events was small. So, while the UGDP found that insulin was not associated with a lower risk for cardiovascular disease, neither was it associated with a higher risk. This was important given the prevailing theory at that time that insulin administration might be associated with an increased risk of cardiovascular disease, based on the observation that individuals with type 2 diabetes and hyperinsulinaemia also had high rates of cardiovascular disease.

In the wake of the study results, enormous controversy flared regarding multiple design issues and the potential causal role of sulphonylureas in cardiovascular disease. The logical areas of controversy surrounded the possibility that patients taking tolbutamide were, *a priori*, at higher risk for cardiovascular disease and patients taking placebo were at lower risk. Specifically, critics have suggested that hyperglycaemia accounted for the increased deaths and that the placebo group to which the tolbutamide-treated patients were compared had an implausibly low death rate[33]. Others have criticised the study because death was not a predefined end-point, randomisation failures occurred and tolbutamide was stopped prematurely[31,34,35]. The negative findings of the UGDP have been attributed to the inclusion of an insufficient number of patients to answer the research question[31]. Thus, the finding of no difference between the groups could not necessarily be interpreted as evidence that control of hyperglycaemia fails to lower the risk of cardiovascular disease.

THE KUMAMOTO STUDY

The Kumamoto Study, also prospective and randomised, was named after the Japanese city in which the study was based. The study tested whether intensive glycaemic control could prevent or slow the worsening of microvascular diabetic complications in type 2 diabetes. The study was small, with 110 patients divided into two cohorts based on prevalent albuminuria (30–300 mg/dl) or retinopathy. Fifty-five people with no retinopathy were included in the primary prevention cohort and 55 with 'simple' retinopathy were in the secondary intervention cohort. Both groups were randomised to treatment with insulin. The multiple insulin injection, intensively-treated group received insulin given by at least three injections daily of rapid-acting insulin before meals plus a once-daily injection of intermediate-acting insulin. The goal of the intensive group was to achieve blood glucose values 'as close to the normal range as possible'. The conventional group received intermediate-acting insulin once or twice daily. The groups differed, therefore, both in the frequency of injections and the types of insulin used. Fifty-five patients were assigned to each of the intensive and conventional treatment groups. These groups were split evenly between patients in the primary and secondary intervention cohorts. Patients were followed every six months for six years.

The end-points of interest were diabetic complications, including the development and progression of retinopathy, neuropathy and nephropathy. Primary development of retinopathy was defined as at least a two-stage change on the Early Treatment Diabetic Retinopathy Study classification in patients who did not have diabetic retinopathy at baseline. Progression of retinopathy was defined as a two-stage progression in patients who had evidence of diabetic retinopathy at baseline. Development of nephropathy was defined as urinary albumin >30 mg/24 h in patients who had an albumin excretion rate <30 mg/24 h at onset.

After six years, the intensively treated group had a mean HbA_{1c} value of 7.1%, and the conventional group a value of 9.4%, a difference of 2.3%. The study found that multiple injection or intensive therapy was associated with a reduced incidence and progression of retinopathy ($p = 0.039$ and $p = 0.049$). Multiple insulin injection treatment was also associated with a lower incidence and progression of nephropathy, and with lower rates of worsening of vibration perception thresholds, a measure of peripheral sensory neuropathy. A report with follow-up to eight years confirmed previous findings[36]. The trial did not address the association between intensive treatment and cardiovascular disease[37].

The study concluded that treatment of blood glucose to near normal levels lowered the risk and progression of the renal and retinal complications of diabetes. The study investigators proposed a goal of HbA_{1c} <6.5%, fasting blood glucose concentration <110 mg/dl, and 2 h postprandial blood glucose concentration <180 mg/dl as targets to prevent the complications of diabetes[36]. The results may be generalisable to non-Japanese populations, although type 2 diabetes in Japanese may be less strongly associated with insulin resistance and more with beta-cell failure than diabetes in other populations[38,39]. The Kumamoto investigators also performed economic evaluations and concluded that intensive therapy was associated with a reduction of total costs due to fewer diabetic complications[40].

VETERANS AFFAIRS COOPERATIVE STUDY IN TYPE II DIABETES (VA CSDM)

The VA CSDM study was designed as a pilot study to assess in 153 men whether a difference in HbA_{1c} of 1.5% could be maintained between a group intensively treated with insulin alone or in combination with glipizide, and a group treated in a 'standard' fashion with insulin[41]. As this study was a pilot, few patients were enrolled, diminishing the potential of the study to find differences between treatment groups, if they existed. An additional goal was to reduce blood glucose in the intensive arm to <6.1%[42]. The secondary goal was to assess whether a difference existed between the groups in the occurrence of diabetic complications including cardiovascular disease, stroke, retinopathy, neuropathy and nephropathy[41]. Participants were followed for 27 months.

The trial achieved a 2.1% difference in HbA_{1c} between 'intensive' and 'standard' groups, suggesting that improved blood glucose control could be achieved, at least over two years[42]. The intensive group had an average HbA_{1c} of 7.1%, compared to 9.2% in the standard group. Forty out of 153 patients (26.1%) had cardiovascular events during follow-up, but there was no difference in the cardiovascular event rates between the two treatment groups[43]. Only five patients in the intensive treatment group and three patients in each treatment group died from cardiovascular disease, raising questions about the power of the study. The study was also unable to confirm associations between established risk factors for cardiovascular disease and cardiovascular disease itself; e.g. blood pressure, dyslipidemia and smoking[44], nor did it show an association between intensive therapy and retinopathy[45].

UNITED KINGDOM PROSPECTIVE DIABETES STUDY

The United Kingdom Prospective Diabetes Study (UKPDS) was designed to address whether intensive (compared to conventional) control of blood glucose in individuals newly diagnosed with diabetes could lower the incidence of complications. The study was by far the largest and longest to date, starting in 1977 and ending in 1997. The study included individuals newly diagnosed with diabetes on the basis of two fasting plasma glucose (FPG) values of 6 mmol/l referred from general practitioners around the UK to 23 UKPDS clinical centres. The study recruited 5102 individuals which included 3867 individuals randomised to conventional treatment, initially with diet alone or intensive treatment, either with a sulphonylurea or insulin. Another 342 overweight (>120%) were randomised to metformin. The study was not blinded. The aim of the intensive control group was to achieve fasting plasma glucose values <6.0 mmol/l. The goal of the conventional treatment group was to achieve FPG values below 15 mmol/l. Additional pharmacological agents were added to meet these goals[46].

The UKPDS achieved a median 0.9% difference in HbA_{1c} between those subjects intensively treated and those conventionally treated. The group randomised to intensive blood glucose control had a median HbA_{1c} of 8.0% compared to the group randomised to conventional treatment, which had a median HbA_{1c} of 7.1%. Intensive therapy was associated with a 12% reduction in any diabetes-related end-point and a 6–10% non-significant reduction in diabetes-related and all-cause mortality. The occurrence of retinal photocoagulation was significantly reduced (29% risk reduction, $p = 0.0031$). Intensive treatment was associated with a lower risk of myocardial infarction (MI), the most common complication, but this was of borderline significance ($p = 0.052$). There was no difference between the incidence of MI in those patients on insulin and in those on sulphonylurea.

Overweight patients randomised to metformin had an HbA_{1c} which was 0.6% lower than patients randomised to conventional therapy (7.4% versus 8.0%). In overweight patients who received metformin compared to those who received diet fewer complications were observed, including any diabetes-related end-point, diabetes-related deaths, all-cause mortality and myocardial infarction. Indeed, the risk of myocardial infarction was reduced by 39%, with confidence intervals suggesting that the reduction could be as great as 59%, or as low as 11%. The magnitude of this risk reduction was greater than would have been anticipated, given the fairly modest difference in glycaemic control between the two groups[6]. One interpretation of this is that metformin is associated with a reduction of cardiovascular disease by means other than control of glycaemia. Of note, patients who had metformin added to sulphonylurea therapy had an increased risk of death compared to those on sulphonylureas alone. If this finding were not due to chance alone, it could represent a real increase in the rate of death amongst patients on combination therapy, or a lower risk of death in patients on sulphonylureas alone[47].

Unwelcome consequences of intensive therapy included hypoglycaemia and weight gain. The UKPDS showed that intensive therapy was associated with an increased risk of hypoglycaemia, but not with an increase in death due to hypoglycaemia. Intensive therapy was also associated with significant increases in body weight, particularly among patients randomised to insulin. Weight gain was no greater in the metformin group than in the diet-controlled group[47].

Quality of life studies performed as part of the UKPDS showed that allocation to different treatments did not in itself have an effect on quality of life. However, patients who had hypoglycaemic reactions reported a lower quality of life than those with one or fewer hypoglycaemic reactions. Quality of life was worse for people with complications relative to patients without complications[48].

Cost-effectiveness analyses supported the merits of glycaemic control in type 2 diabetes. Intensive therapy increased the cost of conventional therapy, but reduced the cost of complications. If one assumed practice visit patterns reflecting standard practice rather than in the trial setting, then intensive therapy was associated with an incremental cost of £478 (−£275 to £1232) per patient. Since the patients on intensive therapy lived, on average, 0.6 (0.12 to 1.1) years longer without complications, the incremental cost per event-free year gained was £1166, which compares favourably to other medical interventions. Hence the authors concluded that efforts aimed at improving glycaemic control were justified both on clinical and economic grounds[49].

UKPDS investigators attempted to identify a level of HbA_{1c} below which the risk of diabetic complications markedly diminished. Such a level would provide an obvious target for glycaemic control. No obvious threshold for HbA_{1c} based on observational data existed for any complication of diabetes[6]. Instead, data suggested that the nearer a patient to normoglycaemia, the better. In reality, it is difficult to obtain, let alone maintain, near-normal levels of HbA_{1c} in many patients with diabetes. Intensifying therapy by adding insulin to improve the glycaemic control achieved with oral agents may be constrained by the side-effects of hypoglycaemia or weight gain.

STUDIES WITH MULTIPLE INTERVENTIONS

Because glycaemic control in patients with type 2 diabetes frequently accompanies the treatment of other problems including hypertension, obesity and dyslipidaemia, studies which have included many interventions merit mention. The strength of these studies is their multifactorial approach, now considered standard for patients with type 2 diabetes. The weakness is that it is difficult to identify the risk reduction attributable to glycaemic control alone. Ongoing studies include among others, the ACCORD and ADDITION studies[50].

DIABETES INTERVENTION STUDY (DIS)

The DIS study enrolled 1139 subjects newly diagnosed with type 2 diabetes living in the former East Germany. The study sought to test whether interventions would alter, among other factors, the risk of myocardial infarction. This prospective intervention trial had three arms: intensified health education, intensified health education plus clofibric acid, and neither intensified health education nor clofibric acid. Health education included weight loss recommendations, a low-fat diet, increased physical activity, anti-smoking efforts, and the treatment of hypertension, if needed. All subjects initially attempted control of glycaemia with diet alone. Ultimately, patients had hypoglycaemic medication added when their hyperglycaemia exceeded fasting glucose values >11.1 mmol/l. Diabetes was diagnosed either on the basis of a fasting plasma glucose greater than 8.88 mmol/l (160 mg/dl) or, in those people with fasting values between 7.21 and 8.88 mmol/l, on the glucose concentration one and two hours following ingestion of a 50 g oral glucose load[51,52].

The investigators observed a lower death rate among patients randomised to the health intervention plus clofibrate when compared to the clofibrate group, which in turn was associated with a lower death rate than the control group. Study investigators did not report statistical analyses. However, the incidence of myocardial infarction was highest in the health intervention plus clofibric acid group, and lowest in the control group[51].

STENO TYPE 2 RANDOMISED STUDY

A multi-interventional study performed in Denmark, the Steno Type 2 Randomised Study, enrolled patients with type 2 diabetes and microalbuminuria. Patients were randomised to 'intensive treatment' which included advice (regarding diet, exercise and smoking cessation), antihypertensives, ACE-inhibition, lipid lowering, aspirin, antioxidants, hormone replacement therapy and glucose lowering. The remaining patients were randomised to 'standard treatment'. The glucose lowering target in the intensive group was an HbA_{1c} less than 6.5%, while the standard group target was 7.5%[53]. End-points of the study included the development of diabetic complications.

At baseline, the control group had a higher mean HbA_{1c}, (8.8%) relative to the intensive treatment group (8.4%). After a mean follow-up of 3.4 years, the HbA_{1c} in the standard group rose slightly, while the mean HbA_{1c} in the intensive group fell by 0.8% (p < 0.0001). In addition, patients in the intensive treatment group were significantly less likely to progress to nephropathy defined as a median albumin excretion rate greater than 300 mg per 24 hours, or to retinopathy. Patients in the intensive group were less likely to experience progression of autonomic neuropathy, but were neither more nor less likely than patients in the control group to experience progression in peripheral neuropathy. No risk reduction in any individual cardiovascular end-point (e.g. MI, stroke, lower extremity amputation) was seen. However, patients in the intensive group were less likely to have a macrovascular event (p = 0.03) if 'a substantial fall' in the ankle-arm index were included in the definition of these events[53].

As patients with diabetes require a multifactorial approach aimed at exercise, diet, blood pressure, glycaemia and lipids, a main advantage of the study is its multifactorial intervention. While all the patients were at high risk for coronary heart disease and death because of their microalbuminuria[54], there is no obvious reason why the findings would not be generalisable to type 2 diabetic patients without albuminuria. A potential shortcoming is the inclusion of therapeutic interventions, for example, antioxidants and oestrogens, which lack a substantial evidence base for their role in the prevention of heart disease in diabetes.

CONCLUSIONS

The trials reviewed in this chapter support lowering blood glucose as a means of lowering the risk of diabetic complications. The trials justify treating blood glucose as part of the overall care of patients with diabetes. Although inconsistencies exist in the results of the studies reviewed, negative results may be due to poorly powered studies. Both the Kumamoto study and the UKPDS show an impressive risk reduction for microvascular disease with improved glycaemic control. The results of the UKPDS show that intensive blood glucose control was associated with a reduction in the risk of cardiovascular disease but that the p value was 0.052. While this result is on the margin of traditional statistical threshold, the clinical significance is likely to be high, in part because the degree of risk reduction is so closely in line with what would have been expected from observational studies. Moreover, the risk reduction associated with metformin for cardiovascular disease was very impressive, possibly reflecting benefits from metformin beyond those strictly related to glucose lowering.

The concept of achieving good glycaemic control implies that there must be an accepted definition of good control. There is general agreement that the lower the blood glucose achieved, the better, with respect both to the delay or prevention of complications. However, there is no consensus about thresholds which can be used to determine 'good' as opposed to poor control. Among the key unresolved questions are whether treatment of glycaemia in the non-diabetic range by medication or lifestyle changes is associated with a reduction of cardiovascular complications. The benefits of newer hypoglycaemic medications (thiazolidinediones, postprandial glucose regulators) is also unclear and, given the evidence of UKPDS and UGDP, it would perhaps be unwise to assume that all agents which impact on blood glucose levels will have equivalent effects on outcome. Current and planned trials will provide more information about options for blood glucose lowering, and will help define the populations in which blood glucose lowering is effective and therefore merited.

REFERENCES

1. Groeneveld Y, Petri H, Hermans J, Springer M (1999) Relationship between blood glucose level and mortality in type 2 diabetes mellitus: a systematic review. *Diabetic Medicine*. 16.
2. Wild S, Dunn C, McKeigue P, Comte S (1999) Glycemic control and cardiovascular disease in type 2 diabetes: a review. *Diabetes/Metabolism Research Reviews* **15**: 197–204.
3. Wei M, Gaskill S, Haffner S, Stern M (1998) Effects of diabetes and level of glycemia on all-cause and cardiovascular mortality. The San Antonio Heart Study. *Diabetes Care* **21**: 1167 – 72.
4. Sievers M, Bennett P, Nelson R (1999) Effect of glycemia on mortality in Pima Indians with type 2 diabetes. *Diabetes* **48**: 896–902.
5. Hanefeld M, Schmechel H, Schwanebeck U, Lindner J (1997) Predictors of coronary heart disease and death in NIDDM: the Diabetes Intervention Study experience. *Diabetologia* **40**: S123–4.
6. Stratton I, Adler A, Neil H, et al. (2000) Association of glycaemia with macrovascular and microvascular complications of type 2 diabetes (UKPDS 35). *British Medical Journal* **321**: 405–11.
7. Moss S, Klein R, Klein B, Meuer S (1994) The association of glycemia and cause-specific mortality in a diabetic population. *Archives of Internal Medicine* **54**: 2473–9.
8. Lehto S, Ronnemaa T, Haffner S, Pyorala K, Kallio V, Laakso M (1997) Dyslipidemia and hyperglycemia predict coronary heart disease events in middle-aged patients with NIDDM. *Diabetes* **46**: 1354–9.
9. Kuusisto J, Mykkanen L, Pyörälä K, Laakso M (1994) NIDDM and its metabolic control predict coronary heart disease in elderly subjects. *Diabetes* **43**: 960–7I.
10. Niskanen L, Turpeinen A, Penttila I, Uusitupa M (1998) Hyperglycemia and compositional lipoprotein abnormalities as predictors of cardiovascular mortality in type 2 diabetes: a 15-year follow-up from the time of diagnosis. *Diabetes Care* **21**: 1861–9.
11. Uusitupa MI NL, Siitonen O, Voutilainen E, Pyörälä K (1993) Ten-year cardiovascular mortality in relation to risk factors and abnormalities in lipoprotein composition in type 2 (non-insulin-dependent) diabetic and non-diabetic subjects. *Diabetologia* **36**: 1175–84.
12. Adler A, Neil H, Manley S, Holman R, Turner R (1999) Hyperglycemia and hyperinsulinemia at diagnosis of diabetes and their association with subsequent cardiovascular disease in the United Kingdom Prospective Diabetes Study (UKPDS 47). *American Heart Journal* **138**: 353–9.
13. Kuusisto J, Mykkanen L, Pyörälä K, Laakso M (1994) Non-insulin-dependent diabetes and its metabolic control are important predictors of stroke in elderly subjects. *Stroke* **25**: 1157–64.
14. Lehto S, Ronnemaa T, Pyörälä K, Laakso M (1996) Predictors of stroke in middle-aged patients with non-insulin-dependent diabetes. *Stroke* **27**: 63–8.
15. Adler A, Stevens R, Neil H, Holman R, Turner R (1999) Hyperglycaemia and other potentially modificable risk factors for peripheral vascular disease in type 2 diabetes. *Diabetic Medicine* **16**: 16.
16. Lehto S, Ronnemaa T, Pyörälä K, Laakso M (1996) Risk factors predicting lower extremity amputations in patients with NIDDM. *Diabetes Care* **19**: 607–12.
17. Lee JS, Lu M, Lee VS, Russell D, Bahr C, Lee ET (1993) Lower-extermity amputation. Incidence, risk factors and mortality in the Oklahoma Indian diabetes study. *Diabetes* **42**: 876–882.

18. Humphrey A, Dowse G, Thoma K, Zimmet P (1996) Diabetes and nontraumatic lower extremity amputations. Incidence, risk factors, and prevention – a 12-year follow-up study in Nauru. *Diabetes Care* **19**: 710–4.
19. Standl E, Balletshofer B, Dahl B, et al. (1996) Predictors of 10-year macrovascular and overall mortality in patients with NIDDM: The Munich General Practitioner Project. *Diabetologia* **39**: 1540–45.
20. Klein R (1995) Hyperglycemia and microvascular and macrovascular disease in diabetes. *Diabetes Care* **18**: 258–68.
21. Pirart J (1978) Diabetes mellitus and its degenerative complications: a prospective study of 4400 patients observed between 1947 and 1973. *Diabetes Care* **1**: 168–88.
22. Klein R, Klein B, Moss S (1996) Relation of glycemic control to diabetic microvascular complications in diabetes mellitus. *Annals of Internal Medicine* 90–6.
23. Ballard DJ, Humphrey LL, III LJM, et al. (1978) Epidemiology of persistent proteinuria in type II diabetes mellitus: population-based study in Rochester, Minnesota. *Diabetes* **37**: 405–12.
24. Ravid M, Brosh D, Ravid-Safran D, Levy Z, Rachmani R (1998) Main risk factors for nephropathy in type 2 diabetes mellitus are plasma cholesterol levels, mean blood pressure, and hyperglycemia. *Archives of Internal Medicine* **158**: 998–1004.
25. Lee ET, Lee VS, Lu M, Lee JS, Russell D, Yeh J (1994) Incidence of renal failure in NIDDM. *Diabetes* **43**: 572–9.
26. Yokoyama H, Okudaira M, Otani T, et al. (1998) High incidence of diabetic nephropathy in early-onset Japanese NIDDM patients. *Diabetes Care* **21**: 1080–5I.
27. Gall AM, Hougaard P, Borch-Johnsen K, Parving HH (1997) Risk factors for development of incipient and overt diabetic nephropathy in patients with non-insulin dependent diabetes mellitus: prospective, observational study. *British Medical Journal* **314**: 783–88.
28. Adler AI, Ahroni AJ (1996) A prospective study of distal sensory neuropathy: the Seattle Diabetic Foot Study.
29. Morioka T, Emoto M, Tabata T, et al. (2001) Glycemic control is a predictor of survival for diabetic patients on hemodialysis. *Diabetes Care* **24**: 909–13.
30. University Group Diabetes Program (1970) A study of the effects of hypoglycemic agents on vascular complications in patients with adult-onset diabetes. *Diabetes* **19**: 789–830.
31. Feinglos M, Bethel M (1999) Therapy of type 2 diabetes, cardiovascular death, and the UGDP. *American Heart Journal* **138**: 346–52.
32. Knatterud G, Klimt C, Levin M, Jacobson M, Goldner M (1978) Effects of hypoglycemic agents on vascular complications in patients with adult-onset diabetes. VII. Mortality and selected nonfatal events with insulin treatment. *JAMA* **240**: 37–42.
33. Kilo C, Miller J, Williamson J (1980) The Achilles heel of the University Group Diabetes Program. *JAMA* **243**: 450–7.
34. Feinstein A (1971) Clinical biostatistics. 8. An analytic appraisal of the University Group Diabetes Program (UGDP) study. *Clinical Pharmacology and Therapeutics* **12**: 167–91.
35. Report of the Committee for the Assessment of Biometric Aspects of Controlled Trials of Hypoglycemic Agents (1975) *JAMA* **231**: 583–608.
36. Shichiri M, Kishikawa H, Ohkubo Y, Wake N (2000) Long-term results of the Kumamoto Study on optimal diabetes control in type 2 diabetic patients. *Diabetes Care* **23 (Suppl 2)**: B21–9.
37. Ohkubo Y, Kishikawa H, Araki E, et al. (1995) Intensive insulin therapy prevents the progression of diabetic microvascular complications in Japanese patients with

non-insulin-dependent diabetes mellitus: a randomized prospective six-year study. *Diabetes Research and Clinical Practice* **28**: 103–17.

38. Chen K, Boyko E, Bergstrom R, et al. (1995) Earlier appearance of impaired insulin secretion than of visceral adiposity in the pathogenesis of NIDDM. Five-year follow-up of initially nondiabetic Japanese–American men. *Diabetes Care* **18**: 747–53.

39. Yoshinaga H, Kosaka K (1999) Heterogeneous relationship of early insulin response and fasting insulin level with development of non-insulin-dependent diabetes mellitus in non-diabetic Japanese subjects with or without obesity. *Diabetes Research Clinical Practice* **44**: 129–36.

40. Wake N, Hisashige A, Katayama T, et al. (2000) Cost-effectiveness of intensive insulin therapy for type 2 diabetes: a 10-year follow-up of the Kumamoto study. *Diabetes Research Clinical Practice* **48**: 201–10.

41. Abraira C, Colwell J, Nuttall F, et al. (1995) Veterans Affairs Cooperative Study on glycemic control and complications in type II diabetes (VA CSDM). Results of the feasibility trial. Veterans Affairs Cooperative Study in Type II Diabetes. *Diabetes Care* **18**: 1113–23.

42. Abraira C, McGuire D (1999) Intensive insulin therapy in patients with type 2 diabetes: implications of the Veterans Affairs (VA CSDM) feasibility trial. *American Heart Journal* 138.

43. Colwell J (1996) Intensive insulin therapy in type II diabetes. Rationale and collaborative clinical trial results. *Diabetes* **45**: S87–S90.

44. Abraira C, Colwell J, Nuttall F, et al. (1997) Cardiovascular events and correlates in the Veterans Affairs Diabetes Feasibility Trial. Veterans Affairs Cooperative Study on Glycemic Control and Complications in Type II Diabetes. *Archives of Internal Medicine* **157**: 181–8.

45. Emanuele N, Klein R, Abraira C, Colwell J, Comstock J, Henderson W G, Levin S, Nuttall F, Sawin C, Silbert C, Lee H S, Johnson-Nagel N (1996) Evaluations of retinopathy in the VA Cooperative Study on Glycemic Control and Complications in Type II Diabetes (VA CSDM). A feasibility study. *Diabetes Care* **19**: 1375–81.

46. UKPDS Group (1998) Intensive blood glucose control with sulphonylureas or insulin compared with conventional treatment and risk of complications in patients with type 2 diabetes (UKPDS 33). *Lancet* **352**: 837–53.

47. UKPDS Group (1998) Effect of intensive blood-glucose control with metformin on complications in overweight patients with type 2 diabetes (UKPDS 34). *Lancet* **352**: 854–65.

48. UKPDS Group (1999) Quality of life in type 2 diabetic patients is affected by complications but not by intensive policies to improve blood glucose or blood pressure control (UKPDS 37). *Diabetes Care* **22**: 1125–36.

49. Gray A, Raikou M, McGuire A, et al. (2000) Cost-effectiveness of an intensive blood glucose control policy in patients with type 2 diabetes (UKPDS 41). *British Medical Journal* **320**: 1373–8.

50. Lauritzen T, Griffin S, Borch-Johnsen K, Wareham N, Wolffenbuttel B, Rutten G (2000) The ADDITION study: proposed trial of the cost-effectiveness of an intensive multifactorial intervention on morbidity and mortality among people with type 2 diabetes detected by screening. *International Journal of Obesity and Related Metabolic Disorders* **24 (Suppl 3S)**: 6–11.

51. Hanefeld M, Fischer S, Schmechel H, et al. (1991) Diabetes Intervention Study. Multi-intervention trial in newly diagnosed NIDDM. *Diabetes Care* **14**: 308–17.

52. Hanefeld M, Fischer S, Julius U, et al. (1996) Risk factors for myocardial infarction and death in newly detected NIDDM: the Diabetes Intervention Study, 11-year follow-up. *Diabetologia* **39**: 1577–83.
53. Gaede P, Vedel P, Parving H, Pedersen O (1999) Intensified multifactorial intervention in patients with type 2 diabetes mellitus and microalbuminuria: the Steno type 2 randomised study. *Lancet* **353**: 617–22.
54. Dinneen S, Gerstein H. (1997) The association of microalbuminuria and mortality in non-insulin-dependent diabetes mellitus. A systematic overview of the literature. *Archives of Internal Medicine* **157**.

15

Does Tight Control of Hyperglycaemia Limit Mortality in Type 2 Diabetes?: A Commentary

R. JOHN JARRETT

Bishopthorpe Road, London, SE26 4PA, UK

Dr Adler reviews the evidence for the relationship between measures of glycaemia and subsequent cardiovascular disease in type 2 diabetes mellitus. Undoubtedly there is an association, but is it one of cause and effect? Despite there being potential biological processes, in particular glycation of proteins, which *could* explain the association, there is still doubt, at least in some minds, whether glycaemia *is* a determinant.

There are two observations which lead to doubt. First, while observational studies in type 2 diabetes mellitus consistently find diabetes duration to be a strong, or the strongest, predictor of microvascular complications, a similar association with cardiovascular disease is inconsistently observed[1]. If glycaemia were a substantial independent determinant, then a consistent relationship with duration would be expected. Second, the association extends below those levels of glycaemia regarded as diagnostic of type 2 diabetes. In the UKPDS the association extended down to the group with maintained levels of glycated Hb below 6%, i.e. below the authors' upper limit of normal (for the general population) of 6.2%[2]. In the EPIC Study of non-diabetics, the association of glycated Hb and mortality did not have a threshold level[3]. Similarly, for fasting blood glucose, the association with cardiovascular disease either shows no threshold or has one apparently well below the diagnostic level for type 2 diabetes mellitus[4]. It is difficult to believe that glycaemia at these levels is a

The Evidence Base for Diabetes Care. Edited by R. Williams, W. Herman, A.-L. Kinmonth and N. J. Wareham.
© 2002 John Wiley & Sons, Ltd

motive force for disordered metabolism leading to atherogenesis or other progenitors of clinical disease. One immediately thinks of confounding.

This is reinforced by the findings of the DECODE Study in over 26 000 individuals, all of whom had an oral GTT (glucose tolerance test) with measurements of fasting and 2 h blood glucose levels[5]. Here both fasting and 2 h post-load levels were significantly associated with subsequent cardio-vascular disease across the non-diabetic range, but fasting levels became non-significant when adjusted for 2 h levels. In other words, the association appears to be with glucose tolerance rather than with prevalent glycaemia. Hence the confounding factors may be those which are *responsible* for the glucose intolerance, or which are associated determinants of cardiovascular disease. Indeed, it may be in context that two clinical trials of secondary prevention of CV disease, one using ramipril[6] and one using pravastatin[7], have reported a reduction in the incidence of type 2 diabetes mellitus in the actively treated groups.

The other part of the debate concerns clinical trials of hypoglycaemic therapy, which Dr Adler has also reviewed. Only two provide relevant data concerning cardiovascular disease and/or overall mortality – the UGDP and the UKPDS. Because of the withdrawal of the groups treated with tolbutamide and phen-formin, respectively, the comparison in the UGDP rests with individualised insulin therapy and standard insulin therapy compared with placebo. Although numbers were small – approximately 200 in each group – the trial lasted for 13 years. Despite clear separation of mean fasting blood glucose levels in the intensively treated group, by intention to treat analyses the incidence of cardiovascular endpoints was similar and not significantly different between groups[8]. In the UKPDS, by intention to treat analysis there were no significant differences between intensively treated and control groups in any end-point, through when fatal and non-fatal myocardial infarctions were combined, the difference approached conventional significance ($p = 0.052$)[9]. Only in separate analyses relating prevalent levels of glycated Hb to end-points[2] was there a clear association between glycated Hb and cardiovascular endpoints[2]. Any resolution between intention to treat and observational analyses has to be sub-jective, so the question remains of whether the association is due to a reduction in glycaemia or to an association with other factors, independently related to glycaemia and perhaps even determining its level.

There can only be speculation about the interpretation of the apparently different results of UGDP and UKPDS, which means that the truth is not yet evident. Perhaps the debate has been overtaken, at least in pragmatic, if not scientific terms, by the positive and substantial results of treatment with such agents as ramipril[6], the statins[10] and aspirin and hypotensive drugs[11] in second-ary prevention trials which include subjects with type 2 diabetes. Currently there are several primary prevention trials, using various agents, in progress and if they reproduce the results of secondary prevention trials the debate about glycaemia and cardiovascular disease may become redundant. However, control of glycaemia will remain of importance in the relief of symptoms and the prevention of microvascular disease.

REFERENCES

1. Jarrett RJ (1984) Type 2 (non-insulin-dependent) diabetes mellitus and coronary heart disease – chicken, egg or neither? *Diabetologia* **26**: 99–102.
2. Stratton IM, Adler AI, Neil HAW, Matthews DR, Manley SE, Cull CA, Hadden D, Turner RC, Holman RR (2000) Association of glycaemia with macrovascular and microvascular complications of Type 2 diabetes (UKPDS 35): prospective observational study. *BMJ* **321**: 405–19.
3. Khaw K T, Wareham N, Luben R, Bingham S, Oakes S, Welch A, Day N (2001) Glycated haemoglobin, diabetes and mortality in men in Norfolk cohort of European Prospective Investigation of Cancer and Nutrition (EPIC- NORFOLK). *BMJ* **322**: 15–18.
4. Charles M A, Balkau B, Vauzel-Kervroeden F, Thibult N (1996) Revision of diagnostic criteria for diabetes. *Diabetes Care* **348**: 1657.
5. The DECODE Study Group (1999) Glucose tolerance and mortality: comparison of WHO and American Diabetes Association diagnostic criteria. *Lancet* **354**: 617–21.
6. Heart Outcomes Prevention Evaluation (HOPE) Study Investigation. (2000) Effects of ramipril on cardiovascular and microvascular outcomes in people with diabetes mellitus: results of the HOPE study and MICRO-Hope substudy. *Lancet* **355**: 253–9.
7. Freeman DJ, Norrie J, Sattar N, Neely DG. Cobbe SM, Ford I, Isles C, Lorimer AR, Macfarlane PW, McKillop JH, Packard CJ, Shepherd J, Gaw A (2001) Pravastatin and the development of diabetes mellitus. *Circulation* **103**: 357–62.
8. Knatterud GL, Klimt CR, Levin E, Jacobson ME, Goldner MG (1978) Effects of hypoglycemic agents on vascular complications in patients with adult-onset diabetes VII. Mortality and selected nonfatal events with insulin treatment. *JAMA* **240**: 37–42.
9. UK Prospective Diabetes Study (UKPDS) Group. (1998) Intensive blood-glucose control with sulponylureas or insulin compared with conventional treatment and risk of complications in patients with type 2 diabetes (UKPDS 33). *Lancet* **352**: 837–53.
10. Pyorala K, Pedersen TP, Kjekshus J, Faergeman O, Olsson AG, Thorgeirsson G (1997) Cholesterol lowering with simvastatin improves prognosis of diabetic patients with coronary disease: a subgroup analysis of the Scandinavian Simvastatin Survival Study (4S). *Diabetes Care* **20**: 614–20.
11. Hansson L, Zanchetti A, Carruthers SG, Dahlof B, Elmfeldt D, Julius S, Menard J, Rahn KH, Wedel H, Westerling S (1998) Effects of intensive blood pressure lowering and low-dose aspirin in patients with hypertension: principal results of the Hypertension Optimal Treatment (HOT) randomised trial. *Lancet* **351**: 1755–62.

Part VI

PREVENTION OF COMPLICATIONS

16

The Effectiveness of Interventions Aimed at Weight Loss, and other Effects of Diet and Physical Activity in Achieving Control of Diabetes and Preventing its Complications

NICHOLAS J. WAREHAM

University Forvie Site, Cambridge CB2 2SR, UK

This chapter reviews the evidence of the effectiveness of interventions aimed at achieving weight loss and other effects of changing diet and physical activity in individuals with established diabetes. The overall effectiveness of these interventions is a product of the efficacy of individual behaviour change interventions and the impact that this behaviour change has on individual risk. Sometimes it is difficult to separate these issues. Many of the studies described have had to assume that changes in these behaviours have been achieved, either because they have not been measured or because they have been poorly measured. Thus an important distinction has been made between studies which have measured the effectiveness of interventions *aimed* at changing physical activity and diet and those which have, more directly, assessed the effectiveness of behaviour change. This chapter is most concerned with the former, and therefore the interventions described are mostly 'black box'. One can state what the interventions were designed to affect, but very little inference can be made about the mechanisms by which an effect was achieved, nor which component of the intervention was most effective in achieving it. Some of the issues concerned with opening up this 'black box' are described

The Evidence Base for Diabetes Care. Edited by R. Williams, W. Herman, A.-L. Kinmonth and N. J. Wareham.
© 2002 John Wiley & Sons, Ltd

by Roter and Kinmonth in Chapter 30 of this book and by Goldstein in Chapter 31.

When reviewing the evidence from various studies, one would like, as with pharmacological interventions, to identify randomised controlled clinical trials restricted to people with diabetes in which the primary endpoint was one of the key health outcomes related to diabetes such as mortality, incident heart disease or retinopathy. Few such studies exist and, therefore, the bulk of the available evidence comes from short-term studies in which the endpoints are intermediate factors such as weight, blood glucose, lipids, insulin or blood pressure which have been demonstrated in other studies to be associated with the long-term complications of diabetes. This chapter reviews this evidence and considers possible explanations for the absence of long-term health endpoint trials of behavioural interventions.

WHAT IS THE EVIDENCE OF THE EFFECTIVENESS OF WEIGHT REDUCTION IN REDUCING THE RISK OF THE COMPLICATIONS OF DIABETES?

As Hamman has reviewed in Chapter 6, the evidence from longitudinal observational studies on the association between obesity and type 2 diabetes is strong, and weight loss is widely considered to be one of the cornerstones of diabetic therapy. This chapter focuses on trials of the effectiveness of weight reduction in people with diabetes, which may be designed to address several different questions:

• Is weight loss effective in reducing the risks of the complications of diabetes?
• Is weight loss effective in improving glycaemia?
• What are the most effective approaches for achieving weight loss in people with diabetes?

IS WEIGHT LOSS EFFECTIVE IN REDUCING THE RISKS OF THE COMPLICATIONS OF DIABETES?

There are no randomised controlled trials of treatments aimed at weight reduction in people with diabetes where the outcome is a health-related event. Non-experimental evidence from prospective population-based studies is available, but may be limited by problems of confounding and reverse causality, as it is difficult to separate intentional and disease-related weight loss[1]. For example, in the WHO multinational study of vascular disease in diabetes[2], baseline body mass index (BMI) was positively associated with mortality in European men. There was a U-shaped relationship in Native

American men and East Asians and an inverted U-shape in European women and Native American women. In general, lean patients had had diabetes longer, were more likely to be receiving insulin therapy, and had a higher prevalence of retinopathy. Even when adjusted for confounding, no clear relationship between body mass index and mortality was observed. Weight loss in people who had a body mass index less than 29 kg/m^2 at baseline was associated with two- to three-fold increase in risk of mortality compared to people whose weight was stable. This study illustrates the difficulty of determining the effectiveness of weight loss on health endpoints from observational studies.

In order to address some of these limitations of observational evidence, a randomised controlled trial, provisionally entitled SHOW (the Study of Outcomes of Weight Loss) was proposed in the USA to investigate two primary research questions: (1) Do interventions designed to produce sustained weight loss in obese individuals with type 2 diabetes mellitus improve health, and (2) How do the benefits and risks of interventions designed to produce weight loss compare with the benefits and risks related to treatment of obesity-related comorbid conditions in the absence of weight-loss interventions? Initial planning suggested that such a trial would need to enrol at least 6000 obese people with type 2 diabetes and follow them for four to seven years. Even a trial of this magnitude and duration would not have been powered to have a health event as the main outcome, the proposed primary outcome at that stage being progression of atherosclerosis as measured by carotid ultrasound. However, the SHOW design has now evolved into the Look AHEAD Trial, a multicentre randomised clinical trial aimed at examining the effects of lifestyle intervention designed to achieve and maintain weight loss over the long term through decreased caloric intake and increased exercise. This trial, which is mainly funded by the US National Institute of Diabetes, Digestive and Kidney Diseases, has cardiovascular disease-related outcomes (heart attack, stroke and cardiovascular death) as its main outcome. In order to achieve sufficient power, it will recruit 5000 obese patients with type 2 diabetes over a 2.5 year period and randomise them to one of two interventions, the Lifestyle Intervention or Diabetes Support and Education, and will follow them for up to 11.5 years.

IS WEIGHT LOSS EFFECTIVE IN IMPROVING GLYCAEMIA?

The absence of randomised controlled trial evidence concerning the efficacy of weight loss on health events in people with diabetes leads to greater emphasis on studies where the impact of weight loss on glycaemic control is evaluated. The largest observational study is the United Kingdom Prospective Diabetes Study (UKPDS)[3], described in detail by Adler in Chapter 14, in which 3044 patients were advised to follow the British Diabetic Association recommendation of a diet containing 50% carbohydrate, 30% fat and 20% protein. Suggested energy intake was related to the degree of overweight, so that for someone greater than 150% ideal body weight, the recommended energy intake was 4.6 MJ per day, whereas for patients less than 110% ideal body weight, the recommendation was 7 MJ per day. Fifteen per cent of this population were considered to have shown 'primary diet failure' in that, despite a prescription of recommended dietary change, their fasting glucose remained greater than 15 mmol/L or they had symptoms of hyperglycaemia. In the 2597 patients in the UKPDS who were recommended to follow the dietary treatment for three months only, the reduction in fasting glucose, adjusted for initial level, was significantly related to the degree of attained weight loss. The authors noted that the overall weight loss by centre was proportional to the availability of dietetic advice[3]. Four hundred and eighty-two (16%) of the patients achieved a fasting glucose <6 mmol/L after three months on diet alone, and these patients were more likely to have a lesser degree of hyperglycaemia at presentation. The average weight loss overall was 7% ideal body weight. It was estimated that, on average, patients needed to lose 30% ideal body weight to achieve a fasting glucose <6 mmol/l at three months.

IS THERE A GROUP OF PATIENTS WITH TYPE 2 DIABETES WHO DO NOT RESPOND TO DIET?

In the UKPDS[3], 15% of patients were deemed to have been 'primary diet failures' at three months (see previous section for a description of this group). This group included more patients who were not overweight, giving rise to speculation that the underlying pathophysiology of diabetes in these individuals may be different and may influence their response to diet therapy. Other groups have shown in cohort studies that the effect of dietary prescription on glycaemic control is minimal in people with diabetes who are not overweight[4]. Studies have suggested that the distribution of the glucose response to weight loss is bimodal, indicating possible separation into responder and non-responder groups[5]. Comparison of these two apparently distinct groups suggests that they do not differ in terms of age, the proportion of women, initial fasting glucose or initial body weight. Whether groups of responders and non-responders differ in other pathophysiological characteristics that may be related to weight loss such as insulin sensitivity or secretion remains to be determined[5].

WHAT ARE THE MOST EFFECTIVE APPROACHES FOR ACHIEVING WEIGHT LOSS IN PEOPLE WITH DIABETES?

The question of the most effective strategy for achieving weight loss has been considered in previous reviews of the management of obesity. The main conclusions are summarised here as findings in general populations of people with obesity are likely to be generalisable to the sub-group of people who also have diabetes[7-9]. This assumption may not, however, be correct, as there is some suggestion that people with diabetes find it harder to lose weight than non-diabetics[10] and pharmacological therapy for diabetes may promote weight gain. Where possible, therefore, studies specifically aimed at the population of people with diabetes have been described in more detail.

Weight loss interventions may be categorised as being:

- focused on diet alone;
- aimed at diet and exercise;
- pharmacological; or
- surgical.

HOW EFFECTIVE ARE DIETARY INTERVENTIONS ON WEIGHT LOSS?

A review for the Effective Health Care series in the UK[7] describes 12 studies[11-22], five of which were restricted to individuals with type 2 diabetes. In one of these, Pascale *et al.*[12] recruited 44 obese women with type 2 diabetes and randomly assigned them either to calorie restriction or to calorie restriction combined with fat restriction. Patients in the calorie restriction group were advised to consume 1000–1500 Kcal/day and were given general information about healthy eating and encouraged to keep their fat intake <30% of total energy. Those in the low calorie/low fat group were given similar calorie targets, but were also given specific instructions on how to reduce fat intake to 20% of total calories. Both groups also participated in a 16-week 'behavioural weight loss' programme. The loss in weight over the 16-week programme and at the one-year follow-up was greater in subjects in the low calorie–low fat group (5.2 kg $\pm$ 7.3) compared to those in the calorie restriction only group (0.96 kg $\pm$ 3.7, p < 0.05). However, in this study there were no detectable differences in glucose, HbA_{1c} or lipids between treatment groups either at 16 weeks or at one year.

An alternative approach to a continued low calorie diet is the use of intermittent very low calorie diets. The effectiveness of these two approaches was compared in a study by Wing and colleagues[13] who randomised 93 individuals with type 2 diabetes to one or other treatment. A similar number of individuals in each group completed the one-year assessments and, although there was greater weight loss in the intermittent very low calorie diet group (14.2 $\pm$ 10.3 kg) the difference when compared to the low calorie group was non-significant (10.5 $\pm$ 11.6 kg, p = 0.06). A sub-analysis stratifying by sex showed that the between-treatment group differences were significant in women only (14.1 kg versus 8.6 kg, p = 0.02). Differences in responses to weight control programmes have also been observed between black and white individuals with diabetes. Wing and Anglin reported[23] that black individuals randomly assigned to either a low calorie diet or an intermittent very low calorie diet had a greater degree of weight regain between six months and one year than an equivalent group of white individuals. The extent to which differences in response are attributable to differences in adherence or physiology are unknown. The benefits of low calorie diets in people with type 2 diabetes may extend beyond their effect on weight. Wing and colleagues have speculated that the benefits on glucose control and insulin sensitivity of calorie restriction in obese patients with type 2 diabetes are independent of the effect on weight[24–25].

In a meta-analysis of studies aimed at promoting weight loss in type 2 diabetes, Brown *et al.*[26] identified 89 studies involving 1800 subjects. This meta-analysis did not restrict its attention to randomised controlled trials, nor did it limit its attention to studies with a particular duration of follow up. seventy two per cent of the studies included used a one-group pre-test/post-test comparison. Overall effect sizes were at least two-fold greater in the non-randomised studies. The authors scored each study for methodological quality and the average score (out of a possible total of 21) was 10. Studies that scored badly tended to lack key attributes such as randomisation, a clear description of the intervention and direct longitudinal measures of outcome. In only four of the 89 studies was a double-blind design used. Brown *et al.* concluded that, apart from the surgically treated individuals, the largest change in body weight occurred in the people treated through dietary means[26].

A similar review by Ciliska *et al.* identified 19 weight loss studies in obese people with type 2 diabetes where a comparison group was included, of which only six were rated as being methodologically strong on the basis of an assessment of sample size, study design, allocation method, outcome and follow-up[27]. All six of the studies compared different diet interventions or diet against diet plus exercise. None involved an attention-only control group, perhaps illustrating the conviction that dietary therapy is such a key element of diabetes care that a no-diet control group would be unethical.

Table 16.1, which summarises the data from this section, includes only the evidence from randomised controlled trials of dietary approaches to weight loss in people with diabetes. It includes studies where the primary outcome was weight loss, and different dietary approaches are compared or where a standard care control group was employed.

HOW EFFECTIVE ARE COMBINED DIET AND PHYSICAL ACTIVITY INTERVENTIONS ON WEIGHT LOSS?

The UK Effective Health Care review[7] identified four trials which evaluated exercise in combination with a dietary weight loss programme[28–31]. Overall, the combination of diet and exercise appeared to be more beneficial for weight

Table 16.1. Effectiveness of programmes aimed at weight reduction in patients with diabetes through changes in diet.

Reference	Study year	n	Population	Duration – intervention/ follow-up	Intervention	Primary outcome: effect on weight	Secondary outcome: effect on metabolic parameters
Wing et al.[11]	RCT 1985	53	Obese patients with type 2 diabetes	16 week intervention/ 16 month follow-up	Three groups receiving behaviour modification, nutrition education or standard care	Behaviour modification group lost more weight. No treatment effect on weight loss at 16 months	No maintenance of improved HbA_{1c}
Heitzman et al.[151]	RCT 1987	55	Obese patients with type 2 diabetes	18 months	Behaviour, cognitive modification or both, relaxation control	Behaviour modification group had greatest decrease in weight	Non-significant effect on HbA_{1c}
Wing et al.[14]	RCT 1991	36	Obese patients with type 2 diabetes	One year	Behavioural therapy compared with behavioural therapy plus eight weeks of VLCD (very low eight calorie diet)	No significant difference in weight loss at one year	No difference in fasting glucose levels. Short-term improvement in HbA_{1c} in behaviour modification group but increase over pre-treatment level at one year
d'Eramo-Melkus et al.[152]	RCT 1992	82	Obese patients with type 2 diabetes	Six months	Three intervention groups receiving (a) single individual education session, (b) a 12-week behavioural education and weight control group intervention or (c) the group intervention with six individual follow-up sessions	All three groups experienced significant weight loss	Fasting glucose improved in the two group interventions but HbA_{1c} was not affected
Milne et al.[153]	RCT 1994	64	Overweight individuals with type 2 diabetes (mean age 59 years)	18 month intervention/ 27 month follow-up	Three dietary prescriptions; 'weight management', high carbohydrate/fibre, modified lipid	No significant difference between diets in weight change. No overall effect on weight	No difference between groups on HbA_{1c}. Overall decline in HbA_{1c} in all groups combined. Improvement maintained at 27 months in 43 participants who completed follow-up

Table 16.1. contd.

Agurs-Collins et al.[154]	RCT 1997	64	Overweight African Americans (age 55–79) with type 2 diabetes	Six month intervention follow-up at six months	Group education aimed at 55–60∞ energy from carbohydrate, 12–20∞ protein,<30% fat, with weight loss at a rate of 0.9 kg per week. Control group – usual care	Six-month change from baseline in intervention group –1.3 kg, control group +1.1 kg, difference 2.4 kg (0.5–4.3), p = 0.006	Significant reduction in HbA$_{1c}$ in intervention group (–1.1%) compared to control (1.3%), difference 2.4% (0.6–4.2∞, p <0.01. No significant differences in lipids or systolic blood pressure
Manning et al.[155]	RCT 1998	147	Patients with type 1 or type 2 diabetes aged 16–70 with a BMI 28–45 kg/m	One year intervention/ follow-up at four years	Four groups: (1) clinic-based individual dietetic consultation every six weeks for six months and two monthly thereafter, (2) group behavioural therapy fortnightly for three months and two-monthly thereafter,(3) as per group one plus dexfenfluramine, (4) home and clinic-based dietetic consultation every six weeks for six months and two-monthly thereafter	Intention to treat analysis showed that only the dexfenfluramine group showed significant weight loss after four years	No effect on HbA$_{1c}$ either in intention to treat analysis or completion basis

loss than simply diet by itself. The benefits of combined interventions may result from the effects of exercise in reducing the loss of lean body mass and the reduction in basal metabolic rate that may occur with weight loss[32]. A review by King and Tribble of studies with a follow-up of at least six months found that the average weight loss was 4.0 kg in four diet-only programmes, 4.9 kg in five exercise-only programmes and 7.2 kg in three combined diet and exercise programmes[33].

Only one of the four trials was specifically focused on people with diabetes. Wing and colleagues[31] randomised 25 obese individuals with type 2 diabetes to diet therapy plus moderate exercise or diet plus 'placebo' exercise. A second group of 30 similar individuals were randomly assigned to diet only or diet plus exercise. In the first study, volunteers in both groups exercised twice a week as a group and once a week on their own, with each exercise session lasting one hour. The intervention exercise mostly consisted of walking, with individuals asked to increase their speed and distance until they were walking three miles within the hour-long session. The 'placebo' exercise was light callisthenics and flexibility exercises set to music. The intention was to control for the non-specific social and psychological aspects of exercise. Weight loss during the initial 10-week programme was not statistically different between the groups; 8.5 kg $\pm$ 0.8 kg in the exercise group compared to 7.3 kg $\pm$ 0.7 kg in those who were randomised to the placebo exercise. Nor was there a significant difference at one year. The authors postulated that the lack of difference between the treatment groups could be attributable to the absence of a difference in activity levels. Thus in the second study the emphasis was on obtaining greater differences in activity levels between the groups by removing the attention control. This was achieved and those subjects in the diet plus exercise group lost significantly more weight than those in the diet only group. The emphasis of this section of the chapter is on weight loss as the primary outcome. However, it is important to note that, in this trial, the diet plus exercise group had reduced medications to a greater extent than the diet only group at the one-year follow-up (83% versus 38%). There was, however, no significant between-group difference in glycated haemoglobin at one year. The effects of interventions aimed at increasing physical activity on metabolic parameters are considered in a separate section of this chapter and are summarised in Table 16.2.

In a trial not included in the UK Effective Health Care review, Blonk *et al.*[34] randomised 60 obese patients with type 2 diabetes (40 women and 20 men) to either a conventional or comprehensive approach to weight reduction. The main outcome in this trial was change in body weight measured at two years, by which time seven patients (12%) had dropped out. The patients in the conventional programme visited the outpatient clinic at two-monthly intervals and were seen by the same physician and dietician on each visit. The comprehensive programme included the same basic items as the conventional programme, plus two extra sessions on behavioural modification strategies

Table 16.2. Effectiveness of interventions aimed at changing physical activity on glycaemia and other outcomes in patients with diabetes.

Reference	Study and year	n	Population	Duration/follow-up	Intervention	Primary outcome: effect on glycaemia	Secondary outcome: effect on weight and other metabolic parameters
Yamanouchi et al.[156]	CT – no evidence of random allocation. 1995	24	Obese patients with type 2 diabetes aged 23–59	6-8 week intervention /follow-up at 6-8 weeks	Two groups both receiving diet controlled by supervision within hospital. One group also participated in walking to achieve minimum of 10 000 steps per day	No difference between groups in fasting glucose levels. Walking group had greater reduction in insulin resistance	Body weight declined in both groups, but the reduction was greater in the walking group
Verity and Ismail[157]	RCT: 1989	10	Overweight women with type 2 diabetes aged 50–70	4 month intervention and follow-up	Individualised exercise prescription aimed at 65–80% of predicted cardiac reserve compared to controls	No change in glucose or HbA$_{1c}$	No statistically significant change in body weight or fat percentage. Intervention group showed improvement in VO$_2$ max
Wing et al.[31]	RCT: 1988. Two studies reported in one paper	(a) 25 (b) 30	Obese patients with type 2 diabetes, age 30–65	(a) Six- month intervention /follow-up (b) One-year intervention /follow-up	(a) Diet plus moderate exercise compared to diet plus placebo (b) Diet plus exercise (walking) compared with diet alone	No between-group difference in HbA$_{1c}$ in either study (a) or (b)	Study (b) demonstrated significantly greater reduction in weight in those in the diet plus exercise group
Vanninen et al.[158]	RCT: 1992	78	Patients with newly diagnosed type 2 diabetes	12-month intervention and follow-up	Diet and exercise intervention compared with standard care. Exercise advice aimed at achieving 3–4 sessions per week lasting 30–60 minutes. The diet intervention was intensified, and education	Significant reduction in HbA$_{1c}$ among women in the intervention group compared to control	No change in VO$_2$ max. Reduction in BMI in both groups initially with greater rebound in conventionally

Table 16.2. contd.

Study	Design; year	n	Population	Duration	Intervention	Outcome	Outcome
Stratton et al.[159]	RCT; 1987	16	Adolescents with type 1 diabetes, mean age 15 years	8-week intervention /8-week follow-up	aimed at energy resolution, reduction in total fat. Supervised exercise 30–45 mins on three days per week for eight weeks. Control group – usual activity	No difference in men. No significant difference in glycosylated haemoglobin or fasting glucose	treated group. Significant reduction in insulin requirement in exercising group
Dunstan et al.[101]	RCT; 1997	55	Sedentary non-smoking people with type 2 diabetes aged 30–65	4-week baseline period, 8 week intervention /follow-up at 8 weeks	Two-way factorial design trial with individuals randomised to low-fat diet with or without one fish meal daily, and also randomised to moderate or light exercise programme. Moderate exercise 30 mins three times per week on bicycle ergometer at 55–65% VO_2 max. Light exercise – cycling with no workload for 10 mins plus stretching/ flexibility exercises for 30 mins, three times per week	Significant reduction in fasting glucose (1.2 mmol/1, p = 0.01) and HbA_{1c} (0.34%, p = 0.07) in moderate exercise group compared to light exercise	Significantly greater reduction in weight in moderate exercise group (1.3 kg) than light exercise group. Significant increase in cardiovascular fitness in moderate exercise group
Samaras et al.[160]	RCT; 1997	26	People with type 2 diabetes aged 40–70. NB marked difference in mean weight at baseline between two groups (15.2 kg)	6-month intervention /12 month follow-up	Exercise Support Group Programme using precede-proceed model of health promotion.	Greater rise in HbA_{1c} in the control group compared to intervention group at six months. No difference at 12 months	Non-significant trend for weight stabilisation in intervention group
Mourier et al.[161]	RCT; 1997	24	Patients with type 2 diabetes, mean age 45	10-week intervention /follow-up	Factorial design: training with and without dietary supplementation with branched-chain amino acids compared to placebo	Significant reduction in HbA_{1c} in training group (−2.3%) compared to control (+0.3%)	Significant reduction in visceral obesity in training group

Table 16.2. contd.

Raz et al.[162]	RCT; 1994	40	Patients with type 2 diabetes aged 50–70 with persistent hyperglycaemia on diet and oral hypoglycaemic agents	12 week intervention and follow-up	Exercise programme three times per week ~45 minutes at 65% of VO$_2$ max compared to control	Reduction of 0.8% in mean HbA$_{1c}$ in exercise group compared to an increase of 0.5% in control group	Exercise group improved maximal work capacity. No change in BMI in either group.
Tessier et al.[163]	RCT; 2000	45	Elderly patients with type 2 diabetes aged >65 years who were reported to be otherwise free of medical illnesses in the six months prior to the study and to be on stable pharmacological therapy	16 week intervention and follow-up	Exercise group trained three times per week for one hour at 50–74% VO$_2$ max. Patients in the control group 'received instructions to continue with their usual activity regimen'	No significant difference in change in HbA$_{1c}$ or fasting glycaemia. Significant reduction in total area under the curve for glucose in oral glucose tolerance in exercise group	No significant difference in BMI between groups. Significant increase in treadmill time in exercise group

and exercise training. Mean weight loss at six months was 2.9 kg in the comprehensive programme versus 1.2 kg in the conventional. There was no overall difference between the programmes over the two years of the trial. An initial reduction in HbA_{1c} in the comprehensive programme was observed (-1.0% at six months). There was no change in the conventional group (-0.1%). This trial is not included in Table 16.1 as the combination of approaches to weight reduction does not allow the effectiveness of the dietary component to be isolated.

DOES PHYSICAL ACTIVITY AID IN THE PREVENTION OF WEIGHT GAIN IN PEOPLE WITH DIABETES?

Weight gain is a consequence of intensified insulin therapy in individuals with type 1 diabetes[35] and type 2 diabetes[3]. Although it is likely that increased physical activity would attenuate this weight gain, there have been few systematic studies. Beyond the specific context of diabetes, there have been few studies that have analysed the role of physical activity in the prevention of weight gain. Indeed one systematic review only identified a handful of trials that have evaluated the effectiveness of any interventions aimed at preventing weight gain[36], a marked difference to the number of trials of interventions aimed at treating obesity or preventing weight regain in people who have successfully lost weight.

HOW EFFECTIVE ARE PHARMACOLOGICAL INTERVENTIONS ON WEIGHT LOSS?

An increasing number of pharmacological therapies are being developed for the treatment of obesity. A pooled analysis of the results of four RCTs of dexfenfluramine suggested that use of the drug was associated with significantly greater weight loss at one year (2.6 kg, 95% confidence interval, 1.3–3.8 kg) than placebo therapy. However, this drug and the related compound, fenfluramine, have been withdrawn following reports of valvular heart disease associated with their use[37]. The intestinal lipase inhibitor Orlistat has been shown to reduce weight in randomised controlled trials[38–39]. The use of this drug in these trials was carefully controlled. Whether the benefits demonstrated in this context can be generalised to use in routine care is uncertain. The long-term results of treatment with sibutramine, a serotonin and noradrenalin reuptake inhibitor, are awaited but early data indicate that it is likely to be effective in diabetic individuals, at least in the short term[40].

HOW EFFECTIVE ARE SURGICAL INTERVENTIONS ON WEIGHT LOSS?

The UK Effective Health Care review[7] identified 15 studies of surgery for obesity. Jejunoileal bypass, vertical banded gastroplasty and gastric bypass all produced significant weight loss. Six of the seven RCTs that allowed comparison showed that gastric bypass resulted in more weight loss than gastroplasty.

WHAT IS THE EVIDENCE OF THE EFFECTIVENESS OF PHYSICAL ACTIVITY IN MODIFYING THE LONG-TERM RISKS OF THE MACROVASCULAR COMPLICATIONS OF DIABETES?

As with weight loss, there are no trials in which the impact of physical activity on the long-term complications of diabetes has been demonstrated. The evidence supporting physical activity as a means of reducing CHD risk in diabetic populations comes from the observational relative risk reduction of activity in the general population, and the effects of activity on known cardiovascular risk factors in people with diabetes.

The epidemiological evidence of the association between physical inactivity and coronary heart disease (CHD) has previously been reviewed by Powell *et al.*[41], and Berlin and Colditz[42]. These studies indicate a relative risk (RR) of future CHD in sedentary individuals of 1.9 (95%, confidence interval (CI) 1.6–2.2) compared to those with active occupations and an RR of 1.6 (95%, CI 1.2–2.2) compared to individuals who are recreationally active. Many of the studies reviewed in these meta-analyses were characterised by the use of summary indices of activity which may be prone to error and bias, the introduction of surrogate markers of activity and unresolved questions of confounding. The type of physical activity that is most likely to be beneficial to long-term risk and the amount of activity that is required to have a health benefit remain unresolved. These issues arise from the difficulty of measuring physical activity in free-living populations[43] problems that are relevant not only to the analysis of cohort studies, but also to the evaluation of intervention programmes where the goal is to measure change in physical activity[44].

There are no epidemiological data on the magnitude of the relative risk for CHD of physical inactivity specifically for populations with diabetes. However, there is no reason to expect that the relative risk reduction from activity would be any less than for the general population. Although supportive, this evidence is not strong and the inference involves the extrapolation of observational evidence from a general population to allow estimation of the benefits of intervention in a diabetic population. However, it may be unreasonable and premature to anticipate RCT-level evidence since the major question may not be whether physical activity can be beneficial to people with diabetes, but rather how individual physical activity change can be supported and maintained.

ARE THERE ANY SPECIFIC METABOLIC EFFECTS OF PHYSICAL ACTIVITY OVER AND ABOVE AN EFFECT ON WEIGHT CONTROL?

Physical activity has a series of direct effects that impact on metabolic control independently of weight. Exercise in people with type 2 diabetes is particularly relevant because of the central role of insulin resistance in the pathogenesis of this disorder[45]. In overweight type 2 patients, glucose is lowered during activity because of increased glucose utilisation and lowered hepatic glucose production[46,47]. Exercise also increases insulin sensitivity at the liver and skeletal muscle[48]. Improvements in insulin sensitivity with exercise are also demonstrable in patients with type 1 diabetes[49,50].

In a review published in 1992, Zierath and Wallberg-Henriksson[51] described 14 studies of the long-term effects of physical training in people with type 2 diabetes. There was considerable heterogeneity in the study designs, with seven being uncontrolled and two using non-diabetic controls. Four of the six trials that reported an effect on glycated haemoglobin showed a significant reduction in HbA_{1c} in those randomised to physical activity. These and other trials published more recently are summarised in Table 16.2 which includes trials with a physical activity component compared with placebo, usual care or dietary controls. The primary outcome considered in this table is the effect on glycaemic control. A trial by Wing and colleagues, described in the above section on weight loss, is included in this table as it analysed the attention of exercise to a dietary programme and included glycaemia as an outcome. The table does not include the effects of exercise on other important metabolic parameters relevant to risk of complications in people with diabetes, blood pressure problems and dyslipidaemia, factors which are considered in more detail in Chapters 17 and 18.

IS THERE ANY EVIDENCE TO INDICATE WHAT TYPE AND INTENSITY OF EXERCISE IS NEEDED?

Epidemiological studies which have relied solely on self-reported measures of activity are unlikely to be able to separate the aetiological effects of different types of activity, nor will they be able to accurately quantify their importance. By contrast, studies which have incorporated objective measures of activity with knowledge of measurement error can determine the relative importance of different types of activity. These studies suggest that increasing overall energy expenditure has beneficial effects on the 2 h post-glucose load glucose concentration[52] and other features of the insulin resistance syndrome[53,54] independently of the degree of obesity and cardio-respiratory fitness. These results may be of importance in translating findings into preventive action, as they suggest that approaches aimed at increasing overall energy expenditure through whatever means will have benefits, and that interventions need not necessarily be of the intensity required to increase cardio-respiratory fitness. Some experimental support for this conclusion is derived from studies such as that by Oshida *et al.*[55] who measured the effects of low intensity activity on insulin sensitivity. In this study an improvement in insulin sensitivity was observed at one year, even though there was no change in body mass index or fitness.

No similar long-term studies have been conducted in people with diabetes. However, in a study of six obese men with type 2 diabetes, Kang *et al.*[56] examined the effect of one week of low intensity exercise compared to shorter, more intense activity providing equivalent energy expenditure. The exercise interventions consisted of two seven-day blocks of daily sessions. In the low-intensity activity, individuals exercised at 50% of maximum oxygen uptake (VO_2 max), whereas in high intensity activity they aimed at 70% of VO_2 max. After seven days of exercise the area under the plasma insulin response curve during an oral glucose tolerance test was reduced in those exercising at the higher intensity only. Neither group showed a change in plasma glucose concentrations. A different conclusion was reached by Braun *et al.* who showed that high intensity activity and low-intensity exercise had comparable effects on insulin sensitivity in women with type 2 diabetes[57]. Short-term improvements in glycaemic control have been demonstrated in patients with type 1 diabetes who undergo resistance training either by itself[58] or in combination with aerobic activity[59,60].

IS EXERCISE ASSOCIATED WITH ADVERSE EFFECTS ON THE COMPLICATIONS OF DIABETES?

Epidemiological evidence of the magnitude of the risks of activity is difficult to acquire, because of the heterogeneity of physical activity behaviour patterns. Few diabetes-specific studies exist, particularly for mortality, and thus most authorities generalise from studies of the general population. Although it is possible that silent coronary heart disease may be more prevalent in the population of people with diabetes, the absolute risk of harm even for vigorous activity is low[61,62]. The presence of autonomic neuropathy, in particular QT interval lengthening, may increase the risk of the adverse effects of activity, but few data are available to quantify these risks[63,67].

Epidemiological studies of the risk of diabetic eye disease in individuals who undertake increased physical activity suggest that activity has little role in promoting the development of proliferative retinopathy[68,71]. Although it is plausible that exercise may increase the risk of vitreous haemorrhage or retinal detachment in people with pre-existing proliferative retinopathy either through the mechanical effects of movement or through rises in systolic blood pressure, systematic quantification of the magnitude of this risk has not been undertaken[72–73].

In people with type 1 diabetes who are free of renal disease, the effects of exercise on glomerular filtration rate (GFR) and renal plasma flow (RPF) are similar to those in non-diabetic individuals in that exercise causes a reduction in both GFR and RPF[75]. However, there are no data beyond small case series[76] to indicate whether such short-term changes are associated with long-term adverse effects on renal function. The extent of the exercise-induced albuminuria is related to the level of blood pressure increase[77] and also to the degree of glycaemic control. It may be reduced by intensified therapy[78•80]. Although less frequently studied, the effects in type 2 diabetes may be similar[81].

IS EXERCISE ASSOCIATED WITH ADVERSE EFFECTS ON METABOLIC CONTROL IN PEOPLE WITH DIABETES?

In people with type 1 diabetes, the increase in glucose release from the liver and non-esterified fatty acids (NEFAs) from adipose tissue that normally occur with exercise are inhibited. Muscle glucose utilisation increases with exercise and, therefore, the limitation on hepatic glucose production can lead to falls in circulating glucose. Thus in a person with well treated type 1 diabetes, the risk of hypoglycaemia during periods of exercise is significant. This is a manageable problem if the person with diabetes can adjust the dose of insulin to account for periods of activity. However, if that exercise is episodic or unpredictable, or if no adjustment to insulin is made, hypoglycaemia may result. Not only is this a problem during the period of activity, but because the exercise-induced increase in insulin action persists when the exercise in terminated, the risk of hypoglycaemia may also persist for several hours[82,83]. The risks of hypoglycaemia are compounded by an acceleration in the absorption of insulin from subcutaneous tissues during exercise[84]. This effect is exacerbated if insulin is accidentally injected intramuscularly[85], suggesting the need for extra caution in injection prior to exercise.

The metabolic effects of physical activity in patients with poorly controlled type 1 diabetes are somewhat different. In a study comparing the effects of a three-hour moderate exercise intervention in patients with type 1 diabetes with differing degrees of baseline control, Berger *et al.* demonstrated that people with poor control showed worsening of hyperglycaemia and ketosis in contrast to those with reasonable control in whom glucose levels fell[86].

There are a variety of different approaches to dealing with the immediate metabolic consequences of exercise in type 1 diabetes. None have been submitted to the rigour of a randomised controlled trial. Individuals differ in their metabolic response to activity[87,88] and each individual may participate in a variety of activities of differing intensity and duration. Such variations create difficulties in making uniform recommendations for adjustment to insulin dosage or carbohydrate intake[89] and therefore in providing a clear evidence base for management. It is probably more prudent to base individual recommendations on physiological knowledge of the general effects of activity on glucose control in type 1 diabetes, and to advocate careful individual blood glucose monitoring.

ARE THERE ANY SPECIFIC EFFECTS OF NUTRITIONAL MANIPULATION OVER AND ABOVE AN EFFECT ON WEIGHT?

In the same way that physical activity plays a role in the treatment of diabetes independently of its effect on weight, nutritional factors may impact on metabolic control through non-weight-related pathways. This section considers the evidence for these effects.

ALTERING THE COMPOSITION OF THE FAT CONTENT OF THE DIET

Monounsaturated fats

In a meta-analysis of the effects of prescribing high monosaturated (MS) fat diets to people with type 2 diabetes, Garg identified nine randomised, crossover design trials which contrasted the effects of isoenergetic, weight maintaining diets which were high in MS or high in carbohydrate. The primary outcome was the mean difference between dietary groups in changes in blood glucose and lipids. The overall effect of diets rich in monosaturated fat compared to those high in carbohydrate was a significant reduction in fasting triglyceride, total cholesterol and VLDL cholesterol and an increase in HDL cholesterol. The effect on fasting glucose was a reduction of 0.23 mmol/l, with no detectable difference in insulin concentration. Only three of the studies assessed glycated haemoglobin, which was not affected by diet group. However, all of the studies considered were probably of too short a duration to impact on long-term measures of glycaemic control[90]. The question of whether the metabolic effects were independent of weight loss was studied by Low and colleagues[91] who investigated 17 obese patients with type 2 diabetes before and after dieting for six weeks with a formula diet enriched with monounsaturated fatty acids (MUFA) or carbohydrates (CHO). There was no evidence of random allocation in this trial. Weight loss was comparable in the two groups but fasting glucose decreased significantly more in the MUFA group (-4.6 mmol/l) than in the CHO group (-2.4 mmol/l, $p < 0.05$)

Fish oil supplementation

Epidemiological data suggest that fish intake is inversely associated with the incidence of cardiovascular disease and the prevalence of type 2 diabetes[92–93]. These observations have given rise to considerable interest in the possible benefits of fish-derived oils, particularly n-3 fatty acids[95–97]. A large number of clinical trials have evaluated the effects of fish oil supplementation in people with diabetes, and these have been subjected to a meta-analysis[98] and a recent systematic review[99]. Both reviews come to broadly similar conclusions. Montori *et al.*, in their quantitative systematic review, identified 18 trials, seven with a parallel group design and 11 crossover studies. The duration of study was from two to 24 weeks. Twelve of the studies reported fasting glucose results in a way that allowed pooling of the data. The pooled weighted mean difference for fasting glucose was 0.26 mmol/l with 95% confidence intervals of −0.08 to 0.60, suggesting no overall significant effect on glycaemia. The equivalent figures for HbA_{1c} were 0.15% (95% CI, −0.08–0.37). By contrast, the overall effect of fish oil on triglyceride, reported in 14 trials, was beneficial, with a pooled weighted mean difference of −0.56 mmol/l (95% CI, −0.71 to −0.41). From these results, the authors concluded that in people with type 2 diabetes who have normal triglyceride levels, fish-oil supplementation leads to a modest lowering of triglyceride without an adverse effect on glycaemia, a conclusion similar to that reached by the authors of the previous meta-analysis[98]. The Gruppo Italiano per lo Studio della Soprarvivenza nell'Infarto Miocardio (GISSI) trial, published after this review was completed, suggests that fish oil supplementation may be of benefit to people after a myocardial infarction[100]. The combined effects of dietary fish intake and exercise may be greater than either separately[101].

Altering the nature of the carbohydrate content of the diet

Daly and colleagues undertook a review of the effects of different types of carbohydrate on insulin sensitivity[102]. They identified 12 trials in which sugars had been compared with starch. All of these trials were of relatively short duration (ranging between one week to three months), and five were specifically focussed on people with diabetes. Overall in these studies there was no significant effect of type of carbohydrate on insulin sensitivity. A non-systematic review of the effects of sucrose on glycaemia was included in the American Diabetes Association technical review of nutritional principles for the management of diabetes[103]. Ten studies were described. Five assessed the effects of single meals containing between 12–25% of calories as sucrose. These studies found no adverse effect on glycaemic control. Five longer-term studies lasting from two days to four weeks with 7–38% of calories from sucrose found no adverse effects on glycaemia. The authors of this review concluded that 'restriction of sucrose in the diabetic diet because of concern about adverse effects on glycaemia cannot be justified.' Studies of the effect of fructose, in particular, have been reviewed by Henry *et al.*[104]. They identified seven studies in which the effects of fructose on glycaemic control and insulin levels were assessed. None of these studies demonstrated adverse effects on glucose and insulin, but variation in experimental design and duration of study preclude more definitive conclusions. In isolation fructose has been shown to produce a relatively low postprandial glucose response[105].

The differing effects of foods on glycaemic response has led to the notion of the glycaemic index, reflecting the rate at which carbohydrate is digested and absorbed. It has been suggested that classifying foods on the basis of this glycaemic index may be a useful addition in the management of diabetes over and above knowledge of the overall nutritional content of the diet[106]. Epidemiological data suggest that the glycaemic index of an individual's diet is associated with metabolic abnormalities[107]. In a small randomised crossover dietary study (n = 6), Wolever *et al.* showed[108] that although there was a significant reduction in fructosuria when subjects were on a low glycaemic index diet compared to one with a high index, weight loss and fall in fasting glucose were similar on both diets. These two diets were of similar macronutrient context (57% carbohydrate, 23% fat, 20% protein) and had a similar fibre content.

The final element of carbohydrate intake that may be modulated is fibre intake. At least eight trials have addressed the impact of increasing the fibre content of the diet by adding soluble fibre supplements. Five of these trials were in patients with type 2 diabetes[109–113] and three involved people with type 1 diabetes[114–116]. All of these studies were of short duration (3-20 weeks) and only one demonstrated a significant reduction in HbA_{1c} in those receiving the supplement[117]. However, the effect of additional fibre as part of dietary intake rather than as a supplement may be more promising. In a random order crossover trial, Kinmonth *et al.* compared a low-fibre, refined carbohydrate diet with a high-fibre one which contained three times as much dietary fibre. Ten children with type 1 diabetes ate both diets for six weeks each. Glycaemic control significantly improved on the high-fibre diet[117]. Similar results have been observed in trials in adults[118,119].

Changing the protein content of the diet

The major interest in protein intake in people with diabetes has been in relation to the effect of protein restriction on the progression of diabetic renal disease[120]. Although the Modification of Diet in Renal Disease Study (MDRD) did not show any significant effect of lowering protein intake on the rate of decline of glomerular filtration rate (GFR) in non-diabetics[121], the effect may be different in people with diabetes[122]. A review for the Cochrane Collaboration by Waugh and Robertson[123] focused on trials which included at least a four-month protein restriction diet in people with type 1 diabetes. The outcomes were expressed in terms of change in GFR rather than clinical outcome. Overall the authors concluded that protein restriction was associated with slowing of progression of diabetic nephropathy.

Alcohol

The specific effects of alcohol in people with diabetes include a potential increased risk of hypoglycaemia, especially when alcohol is consumed without food[124]. Although epidemiological data may suggest an association between increased alcohol intake and improved glycaemic control, it is difficult to separate the specific effects of alcohol from other related lifestyles including the pattern of food intake that occurs with alcohol consumption[125].

Other forms of dietary supplementation

The final group of dietary interventions includes vitamins, micronutrients and minerals. Observational epidemiological evidence indicates that low levels of the antioxidant vitamins C and E are associated with worse glucose tolerance[126,127], observations supported both by *in vitro* evidence of the effects of antioxidants on insulin action[128,129] and by associations between diabetes and consumption of diets low in fresh fruit and vegetables[130,131], the major source of dietary vitamin C. The clinical trial evidence of the benefits of these two antioxidants is less conclusive. The possibility of a major benefit of vitamin E seems unlikely given the results of the HOPE study, in which the benefits of vitamin E and Ramipril were compared in a factorial design RCT[132]. There was no effect of vitamin E on cardiovascular outcome. Although vitamin D levels have been reported to have effects on insulin secretion and are associated with diabetes in some[133] but not all studies[134], there are no trials of supplementation in people with diabetes.

Chromium has been reported to have effects on insulin resistance[135] and severe chromium deficiency has been associated with glucose intolerance[136]. Although some small chromium intervention studies have suggested that supplementation may result in improved glucose control[137] or insulin secretion[138], others have been inconclusive[135]. No formal meta-analysis has been published. It would be interesting to observe if the number of small studies demonstrating beneficial effects is balanced by an equivalent number of studies in which the effect was in the opposite direction, or if the funnel plot of effect size and study size indicates publication bias.

Magnesium levels in people with diabetes have been investigated because of evidence of a potential role of magnesium in insulin action[139]. Mather *et al.*[140] measured plasma magnesium in 582 patients with diabetes attending a hospital diabetes clinic and 140 controls selected from apparently healthy blood donors and people attending day centres for the elderly. Mean plasma magnesium concentrations were significantly lower in the diabetic group, and within the diabetic population there was a significant negative correlation with clinic blood glucose. On the basis of this and other similar observations, Paolisso *et al.* measured insulin action before and after dietary supplementation with 2 g/day of magnesium, demonstrating a decrease in fasting glucose on magnesium compared to placebo[141]. The net increase in acute insulin response and insulin sensitivity were correlated with the increase in erythrocyte magnesium levels. A trial by De Lourdes Lima *et al.*[142] demonstrated a fall in fructosamine in people on magnesium supplementation for one month, but no fall in Hba_{1c} or fasting glucose.

A possible role for salt in the aetiology of insulin resistance has been proposed[143] but there are no trials of the glycaemic benefits of salt restriction, although the effects on blood pressure may be more important[144]. Another micronutrient that has been proposed as being of benefit to people with diabetes is taurine. Although some biological activities of taurine on insulin sensitivity and glucose intolerance have been reported[145,146], there are no reports of trials in people with type 2 diabetes[135]. Reports of the benefits of vanadium[147] are not supported by randomised controlled trials[148,149]. A systematic review of the efficacy of ginseng concluded that there was no strong evidence of a benefit to people with type 2 diabetes[150]. Supplementation with other minerals (zinc, copper) or vitamins (A, B flavenoids) is not supported by clinical trial evidence[143].

WHY HAVE FEW LONG-TERM OUTCOME TRIALS OF LIFESTYLE INTERVENTIONS BEEN UNDERTAKEN IN PEOPLE WITH ESTABLISHED DIABETES?

As interventions aimed at altering diet and physical activity are central to diabetes care, it is perhaps surprising that long-term randomised controlled studies have not been undertaken to evaluate the impact of these interventions on the complications of this disorder. One possible explanation could be that as the provision of some form of dietary and physical activity advice is so widely accepted as part of routine diabetes care, randomisation is considered inappropriate. Alternatively, as these behavioural interventions are seldom sufficient to limit progression of the disorder without pharmacological therapy, some may feel that they are not worth evaluating separately. The evaluation of complex lifestyle interventions is difficult, as maintaining the distinction between intervention groups in longer trials is hard. Trials of this type have also been affected by high dropout rates. The measurement of the effect of any intervention on diet and physical activity is difficult because the behaviours are not easy to measure. Intervention trials which have used subjective self-report measures are likely to be affected by recall bias in which participants randomised to the intervention arm report greater activity or dietary change solely by virtue of being allocated to that group rather than as a result of true behaviour change[44]. Although the use of objective biomarkers of activity and diet would be preferable, these have rarely been included in such studies. Probably the most important reason for the absence of long term studies is that the time necessary to produce an impact on health endpoints makes them expensive and consequently unattractive to potential funders. Overall, given the available data, this chapter demonstrates that diet and physical activity interventions are effective in short, explanatory trials among people with diabetes in achieving weight loss and glycaemic control. Their added contribution to medication strategies now deserves evaluation in longer-term pragmatic studies.

SUMMARY OF THE EVIDENCE PROVIDED IN THIS CHAPTER

Area of interest	Strength of recommendation	Quality of the evidence
Weight reduction is effective in reducing risks of the complications of diabetes	B	II-2
Weight loss is effective in improving glycaemia	A	I
Dietary interventions in people with diabetes are effective in producing weight loss	A	I
Combined diet and physical activity interventions are effective in people with diabetes in producing weight loss	A	I
Increasing physical activity is effective in the prevention of weight gain in people with diabetes	B	II-2
Pharmacological interventions are effective in producing weight loss in people with diabetes	A	I
Surgical interventions are effective in producing weight loss in people with diabetes	A	I
Increasing physical activity results in a reduction of the long-term risks of the complications of diabetes	B	II-2
Increasing physical activity has beneficial effects on metabolic control over and above the effect on weight	A	I

Area of interest	Strength of recommendation	Quality of the evidence
Altering the composition of the fat content of the diet has beneficial effects on glycaemia	**B**	**II-1**
Fish-oil supplementation has a beneficial effect on triglyceride concentrations	**A**	**I**
Altering the nature of the carbohydrate content of the diet, to include high-fibre foods, has beneficial effects on glycaemic control	**A**	**I**
Calorie restriction plus reduction in fat has no detectable effect on glycaemia over and above the effect on weight loss	**A**	**I**
Protein restriction is effective in reducing the rate of progression of diabetic nephropathy	**A**	**I**
Antioxidant supplementation is effective in improving glycaemia	**B**	**II-2**
Chromium supplementation has beneficial effects on glycaemic control	**C**	**II-3**
Magnesium supplementation is effective in improving glycaemic control	**C**	**II-3**

REFERENCES

1. Pi-Sunyer FX. Weight and non-insulin-dependent diabetes mellitus. *American Journal of Clinical Nutrition* 1996; **63**: 426S–429S.
2. Chaturvedi N, Fuller JH. The WHO Multinational Study Group. Mortality risk by body weight and weight change in people with NIDDM. *Diabetes Care* 1995; **18**: 766–774.
3. UKPDS Group. UK Prospective Diabetes Study 7: Response of fasting plasma glucose to diet therapy in newly presenting type II diabetic patients. *Metabolism* 1990; **39**: 905–912.
4. Wolffenbuttel BHR, Weber RFA, Van Koestsveld PM, Verschoor L. Limitations of diet therapy in patients with non-insulin-dependent diabetes mellitus. *International Journal of Obesity* 1989; **13**: 173–182.
5. Watts NB, Spanheimer RG, DiGirolamo M, Gebhart SSP, Murey V, Khalid Siddiq Y. Phillips LS. Prediction of glucose response to weight loss in patients with non-insulin-dependent diabetes mellitus. *Archives of Internal Medicine* 1990; **150**: 803–806.
6. Bosello O, Armellini F, Zamboni M, Fitchet M. The benefits of modest weight loss in type II diabetes. *International Journal of Obesity* 1997; **21**: S10–S13.
7. Anon. The prevention and treatment of obesity. *Effective Health Care* 1997; **3**: 1–11.
8. British Nutrition Foundation. *Obesity: The Report of the BNF Taskforce.* Oxford, UK: Blackwell Sciences; 1999.
9. World Health Organization. Obesity: Preventing and managing the global epidemic. Geneva: World Health Organization; 1997.

10. Guare JC, Wing RR, Grant A. Comparison of obese NIDDM and nondiabetic women: short and long-term weight loss. *Obesity Research* 1995; **3**: 329–335.
11. Wing RR, Epstein LH, Nowalk MP, Koeske R, Hagg S. Behaviour change, weight loss improvements in type 2 diabetes. *Journal of Consultant Clinical Psychology* 1985; **53**: 111–122.
12. Pascale RW, Wing RR, Butler BA, Mullen M, Bononi P. Effects of a behavioural weight loss programme stressing calorie restriction versus calorie plus fat restriction in obese individuals with NIDDM or a family history of diabetes. *Diabetes Care* 1995; **18**: 1241–1248.
13. Wing RR, Blair E, Marcus M, Epstein LH, Harvey J. Year-long weight loss treatment for obese patients with type II diabetes: does including an intermittent very-low-calorie diet improve outcome? *American Journal of Medicine* 1994; **97**: 354–362.
14. Wing RR, Marcus MD, Epstein LH, Jawad A. A family-based approach to the treatment of obese type 2 diabetic patients. *Journal Consultant Clinical Psychology* 1991; **59**: 156–162.
15. Anderson JW, Brinkman-Kaplan V, Hamilton CC, Logan JE, Collins RW, Gustafson NJ. Food containing hypocaloric diets are as effective as liquid-supplement diets for obese individuals with NIDDM. *Diabetes Care* 1994; **17**: 602–604.
16. Wadden TA, Stunkard AJ. Controlled trial of very-low calorie diet, behaviour therapy, and their combination in the treatment of obesity. *Journal Consultant Clinical Psychology* 1986; **54**: 482–488.
17. Wadden TA, Sternberg JA, Letizia, KA, Stunkard AJ, Foster GD. Treatment of obesity by very low fat diet, behaviour therapy and their combination: a five-year perspective. *International Journal of Obesity* 1989; **13**: 39–46.
18. Schlundt DG, Hill JO, Pope-Cordle J, Arnold D, Virts KL, Katahn M. Randomised evaluation of a low calorie ad libitum carbohydrate diet for weight reduction. *International Journal of Obesity* 1993; **17**: 623–629.
19. Jeffery RW, Hellerstedt WL, French SA, Baxter JE. A randomised trial of counselling for fat restriction v calorie restriction in the treatment of obesity. *International Journal of Obesity* 1995; **19**: 132–137.
20. Jeffery RW, Wing RR, Thorson C, Burton LR, Raether C, Harbey J, Mullen M. Strengthening behavioural interventions for weight loss: a randomised trial of food provision and monetary incentives. *Clinical Psychology* 1993; **61**: 1038–1045.
21. Wing RR, Jeffery RW, Burton LR, Thorson C, Nissinoff KS, Baxter JE. Food provision versus structured meal plans in the behavioural treatment of obesity. *International Journal of Obesity* 1996; **20**: 56–62.
22. Hakala P. Weight reduction programmes at a rehabilitation centre and a health centre based on group counselling and individual support: short- and long-term follow up study. *International Journal of Obesity* 1994; **18**: 483–489.
23. Wing RR, Anglin K. Effectiveness of a behavioural weight control programme for blacks and whites with NIDDM. *Diabetes Care* 1996; **19**: 409–13.
24. Wing RR, Blair EH, Bononi P, Marcus MD, Watanabe R, Bergman RN. Calorie restriction per se is a significant factor in improvements in glycemic control and insulin sensitivity during weight loss in obese NIDDM patients. *Diabetes Care* 1994; **17**: 30–36.
25. Kelley DE, Wing R, Buonocore C, Sturis J, Polonsky K, Fitzsimmons M. Relative effects of calorie restriction and weight loss in noninsulin-dependent diabetes mellitus. *Journal of Clinical Endocrinology and Metabolism* 1993; **77**: 1287–93.

26. Brown SA, Upchurch S, Anding R, Winter M, Ramirez G. Promoting weight loss in type II diabetes. *Diabetes Care* 1996; **19**: 613–624.

27. Ciliska D, Kelly C, Petrov N, Chalmers J. A review of weight loss interventions for obese people with non-insulin-dependent diabetes mellitus. *Canadian Journal of Diabetes Care* 1995; **19**: 10–15.

28. Bertram SR, Venter I, Stewart RI. Weight loss in obese women - exercise versus dietary education. *South African Medical Journal* 1990; **78**: 15–18.

29. Johnson WG, Stalonas PM, Christ MA, Wing RR, Jeffery RW, Burton LR, Thorson C, Nissinoff KS, Baxter JE The development and evaluation of a behavioral weight reduction program. *International Journal of Obesity* 1979; **3**: 229–238.

30. Pavlou KN, Krey S, Steffee WP. Exercise as an adjunct to weight loss and maintenance in moderately obese subjects. *American Journal of Clinical Nutrition* 1989; **49**: 1115–1123.

31. Wing RR, Epstein LH, Paternostro-Bayles M, Kriska A, Nowalk MP, Gooding W. Exercise in a behavioral weight control programme for obese patients with type 2 (non-insulin-dependent) diabetes. *Diabetologia* 1988; **31**: 902–909.

32. Bouchard C, Despres J-P, Tremblay A. Exercise and obesity. *Obesity Research* 1993; **1**: 133–147.

33. King AC, Tribble DL. The role of exercise in weight regulation in nonathletes. *Sports Medicine* 1991; **11**: 331–349.

34. Blonk MC, Jacobs MA, Biesheuvel EH, Weeda-Mannak WL, Heine RJ. Influences on weight loss in type 2 diabetic patients: little long-term benefit from group behaviour therapy and exercise training. *Diabetic Medicine* 1994; **11**: 449–457.

35. Carlson MG, Campbell PJ. Intensive insulin therapy and weight gain in IDDM. *Diabetes* 1993; **42**: 1700–1707.

36. Hardeman W, Griffin S, Johnston M, Kinmonth AL, Wareham NJ. Interventions to prevent weight gain: a systematic review of psychological models and behaviour change methods. *International Journal of Obesity* 2000; **24**: 131–143.

37. Gardin JM, Schumacher D, Constantine G, David KD, Leung C, Reid CL. Valvular abnormalities and cardiovascular status following exposure to dexfenfluramine or phentermine/fenfluramine. Journal of the American Medical Association 2000; **283**: 1703–1709.

38. Sjostrom L, Rissanen A, Andersen T, Boldrin M, Golay A, Koppeschaar HP, Krempf M. Weight loss and prevention of weight regain in obese patients: a two year European randomised trial of Orlistat. *Lancet* 1988; **352**: 167–172.

39. Davidson MH, Hauptman J, DiGirolamo M, Foreyt JP, Halsted CH, Heber D, Heimburger DC, Lucas CP, Robbins DC, Chung J, Heymsfield SB. Weight control and risk factor reduction in obese subjects treated for two years with Orlistat – a randomised controlled trial. Journal of the American Medical Association 1999; **281**: 235–242.

40. Heath MJ, Chang E, Weimstein SP, Seaton TB. Sibutramine enhances weight loss and improves glycemic control and plasma lipid profile in obese patients with type 2 diabetes mellitus. *Diabetes* 1999; **48**: 1346.

41. Powell KE, Thompson PD, Caspersen CJ, Kendrick JS. Physical activity and the incidence of coronary heart disease. *Annual Reviews of Public Health* 1987; **8**: 253–287.

42. Berlin JA, Colditz GA. A meta-analysis of physical activity in the prevention of coronary heart disease. *American Journal of Epidemiology* 1990; **132**: 612–628.

43. Rennie KL, Wareham NJ. The validation of physical activity instruments for

measuring energy expenditure: problems and pitfalls. *Public Health Nutrition* 1998; **1**: 265–271.

44. Wareham N, Rennie K. The assessment of physical activity in individuals and populations: Why try to be more precise about how physical activity is assessed? *International Journal of Obesity* 1998; **22**: S30–S38.

45. Reaven GM. Role of insulin resistance in human disease. *Diabetes* 1988; **37**: 1595–1607.

46. Minuk HL, Vranic M, Marliss EB, Hanna AK, Albisser AM, Zinman B. Glucoregulatory and metabolic response to exercise in obese noninsulin-dependent diabetes. *American Journal of Physiology* 1981; **240**: E458–E464.

47. Jenkins AB, Furler SM, Bruce DG, Chisholm DJ. Regulation of hepatic glucose output during moderate exercise in non-insulin-dependent diabetes. *Metabolism* 1988; **37**: 966–972.

48. Devlin J, Hirshman M, Horton E. Enhanced peripheral and splanchnic insulin sensitivity in NIDDM men after a single bout of exercise. *Diabetes* 1987; **36**: 434–439.

49. Landt KW, Campaigne BN, James FW, Sperling MA. Effects of exercise training on insulin sensitivity in adolescents with type 1 diabetes. *Diabetes Care* 1985; **8**: 461–65.

50. Wallberg-Henriksson H, Gunnarsson R, Henriksson J, DeFronzo R, Felig P, Ostman J, Wahren J. Increased peripheral insulin sensitivity and muscle mitochondrial enzymes but unchanged blood glucose control in type 1 diabetics after physical training. *Diabetes* 1982; **31**: 1044–1050.

51. Zierath JR, Wallberg-Henriksson H. Exercise training in obese diabetic patients: special considerations. *Sports Medicine* 1992; **14**: 171–189.

52. Wareham NJ, Wong M-Y, Day NE. Glucose intolerance and physical inactivity: the relative importance of low habitual energy expenditure and cardiorespiratory fitness. *American Journal of Epidemiology* 2000; **152**: 132–139.

53. Wareham NJ, Wong M-Y, Hennings S, Mitchell J, Rennie K, Cruickshank K, Day NE. Quantifying the association between habitual energy expenditure and blood pressure. *International Journal of Epidemiology* 2000; **29**: 655–660.

54. Wareham NJ, Hennings SJ, Byrne CD, Hales CN, Prentice AM, Day NE. A quantitative analysis of the relationship between habitual energy expenditure, fitness and the Metabolic Cardiovascular Syndrome. *British Journal of Nutrition* 1998; **80**: 235–241.

55. Oshida Y, Yamanouchi K, Hayamizu S, Sato Y. Long-term mild jogging increases insulin action despite no influence on body mass index or VO2 max. *Journal of Applied Physiology*. 1989; **66**: 2206–2210.

56. Kang J, Robertson RJ, Hagberg JM, Kelley DE, Goss FL, DaSilva SG, Suminski RR, Utter AC. Effect of exercise intensity on glucose and insulin metabolism in obese individuals and obese NIDDM patients. *Diabetes Care* 1996; **19**: 341–349.

57. Braun B, Zimmermann MB, Kretchmer N. Effects of exercise intensity on insulin sensitivity in women with non-insulin dependent diabetes mellitus. *Journal of Applied Physiology* 1995; **78**: 300–306.

58. Durak EP, Jovanovic-Peterson L, Peterson CM. Randomized crossover study of effect of resistance training on glycemic control, muscular strength, and cholesterol in type 1 diabetic men. *Diabetes Care* 1990; **13**: 1039–43.

59. Peterson CM, Jones RL, Dupuis A, Levine BS, Bernstein R, O'Shea M. Feasibility of improved blood glucose control in patients with insulin-dependent diabetes mellitus. *Diabetes Care* 1979; **2**: 329–335.

60. Miller WJ, Sherman WM, Ivy JL. Effect of strength training on glucose tolerance and post-glucose insulin response. *Medicine and Science in Sports and Exercise* 1984; **16**: 539–543.

61. Siscovick DS, Weiss NS, Fletcher RH, Lasky T. The incidence of primary cardiac arrest during vigorous exercise. *N Engl J Med* 1984; **311**: 874–7.

62. Kohl HW 3rd, Powell KE, Gordon NF, Blair SN, Paffenbarger JRS. Physical activity, physical fitness, and sudden cardiac death. *Epidemiological Reviews* 1992; **14**: 37–58.

63. Hilsted J, Galbo H, Christensen NJ. Impaired cardiovascular responses to graded exercise in diabetic autonomic neuropathy. *Diabetes* 1979; **28**: 313–319.

64. Kahn JK, Sisson JC, Vinik A. QT Interval Prolongation and Sudden cardiac death in diabetic autonomic neuropathy. *Journal of Clinical and Endocrinal Metabolism* 1987; **64**: 751–754.

65. Kahn JK, Sisson JC, Vinik AI. Prediction of sudden cardiac death in diabetic autonomic neuropathy. *Journal of Nuclear Medicine* 1988; **29**: 1605–6.

66. Ewing DJ, Boland O, Neilson JMM, Cho CG, Clarke BF. Autonomic neuropathy, QT interval lengthening, and unexpected deaths in male diabetic patients. *Diabetologia* 1991; **34**: 182–185.

67. Zola BE, Vinik AI. Effects of autonomic neuropathy associated with diabetes mellitus on cardiovasular function. *Current Science* 1992; **3**: 33–41.

68. Cruikshanks KJ, Moss SE, Klein R, Klein BEK. Physical activity and proliferate retinopathy in people diagnosed with diabetes before age 30 yr. *Diabetes Care* 1992; **15**: 1267–1272.

69. La Porte RE, Dorman JS, Tajima N, Cruickshanks KJ, Orchard TJ, Cavender DE, Becker DJ, Drash AL. Pittsburgh insulin-dependent diabetes and mortality study: physical activity and diabetic complications. *Pediatrics* 1986; **78**: 1027–1033.

70. Kriska AM, LaPorte RE, Patrick SL, Kuller LH, Orchard TJ. The association of physical activity and diabetic complications in individuals with insulin-dependent diabetes mellitus: The epidemiology of diabetes complications study-VII. *Journal of Clinical Epidemiology* 1991; **44**: 1207–1214.

71. Orchard TJ, Dorman JS, Maser RE, Becker DJ, Ellis D, LaPorte RE, Kuller LH, Wolfson SK, Drash AL. Factors associated with avoidance of severe complications after 25 yr of IDDM. *Diabetes Care* 1990; **13**: 741–47.

72. Anderson B. Activity and diabetic vitreous haemorrhages. *Ophthalmology* 1980; **87**: 173–175.

73. Graham C, Lasko-McCarthey P. Exercise options for people with diabetic complications. *Diabetes Educator* 1990; **16**: 212–220.

74. Bernbaum M, Albert SG, Cohen JD. Exercise training in individuals with diabetic retinopathy and blindness. *Archives of Physical and Medical Rehabilitation* 1989; **70**: 605–611.

75. Vittinghus E, Mogensen CE. Albumin excretion and renal haemodynamic response to physical exercise in normal and diabetic man. *Scandinavian Journal of Clinical Laboratory Investigations* 1981; **41**: 627–632.

76. Matsuoka N, Nakao T, Takekoshi H. Exercise regimen for patients with diabetic retinopathy. *Journal of Diabetic Complications* 1991; **5**: 98–100.

77. Christensen CK. Abnormal albuminuria and blood pressure rise in incipient diabetic nephropathy induced by exercise. *Kidney International* 1984; **25**: 819–823.

78. Viberti G, Pickup JC, Bilous RW, Keen H, Mackintosh D. Correction of exercise-induced microalbuminuria in insulin-dependent diabetics After 3 weeks of subcutaneous insulin infusion. *Diabetes* 1981; **30**: 818–823.

79. Koivisto VA, Huttunen N-P, Vierikko P. Continuous subcutaneous insulin

infusion corrects exercise-induced albuminuria in juvenile diabetes. *British Medical Journal* 1981; **282**: 778–779.

80. Vittinghus E, Mogensen CE. Graded exercise and protein excretion in diabetic man and the effect of insulin treatment. *Kidney International* 1982;**21**: 725–729.

81. Mohamed A, Wilkin T, Leatherdale BA, Rowe D. Response of urinary albumin to submaximal exercise in newly diagnosed non-insulin dependent diabetes. *British Medical Journal* 1984; **288**: 1342–1343.

82. Bogardus C, Thuillez P, Ravussin E, Vasquez B, Narimiga M, Azhar S. Effect of muscle glycogen depletion on in vivo insulin action in man. *Journal of Clinical Investigation* 1983; **72**: 1605–1610.

83. MacDonald MJ. Postexercise late-onset hypoglycemia in insulin-dependent diabetic patients. *Diabetes Care* 1987; **10**: 584–588.

84. Zinman B, Murray FT, Vranic M, Albisser AM, Leibel BS, McClean PA, Marliss EB. Glucoregulation During moderate exercise in insulin treated diabetics. *Journal of Clinical and Endocrinal Metabolism* 1977; **45**: 641–652.

85. Frid A, Östman J, Linde B. Hypoglycemia risk during exercise after intramuscular injection of insulin in thigh in IDDM. *Diabetes Care* 1990; **13**: 473–477.

86. Berger M, Berchtold P, Cuppers HJ, Drost H, Kley HK, Muller WA, Wiegelmann W, Zimmerman-Telschow H, Gries FA, Kruskemper HL, Zimmermann H. Metabolic and hormonal effects of muscular exercise in juvenile type diabetics. *Diabetologia* 1977; **13**: 355–365.

87. Caron D, Poussier P, Marliss EB, Zinman B. The effect of postprandial exercise on meal-related glucose intolerance in insulin-dependent diabetic individuals. *Diabetes Care* 1982; **5**: 364–369.

88. Campaigne BN, Wallberg-Henriksson H, Gunnarsson R. Glucose and insulin responses in relation to insulin dose and caloric intake 12h after acute physical exercise in men with IDDM. *Diabetes Care* 1987; **10**: 716–21.

89. Horton ES. Role and management of exercise in diabetes mellitus. *Diabetes Care* 1988; **11**: 201–11.

90. Garg A. High monosaturated fat diets for people with diabetes mellitus: a meta-analysis. *American Journal of Clinical Nutrition* 1998; **67**: 577s–582s.

91. Low CC, Grossman EB, Gumbiner B. Potentiation of effects of weight loss by mono-unsaturated fatty acids in obese NIDDM patients. *Diabetes* 1996; **45**: 569–575.

92. Kromhout D, Bosschieter EB, De Lezenn Coulander C. The inverse relation between fish consumption and 20-year mortality from coronary heart disease. *New Engl J Med* 1985; **312**: 1205–1209.

93. Mouratoff GF, Carroll NV, Scott EM. Diabetes mellitus in Athabaskan Indians in Alaska. *Diabetes* 1969; **18**: 29–32.

94. Feskens EJM, Bowles CH, Kromhout D. Inverse association between fish intake and risk of glucose intolerance in normoglycemic elderly men and women. *Diabetes Care* 1991; **14**: 939–941.

95. Heine RJ. Dietary fish oils and insulin action in humans. *Annals of the New York Academy of Sciences* 1993; **683**: 110–121.

96. Hannah JS, Howard BV. Dietary fats, insulin resistance, and diabetes. *Journal of Cardiovascular Risk* 1994; **1**: 31–37.

97. Malasanos TH, Stacpoole PW. Biological effects of ω-3 fatty acids in diabetes mellitus. *Diabetes Care* 1991; **14**: 1160–1179.

98. Friedberg CE, Janssen MJFM, Heine RJ, Grobbee DE. Fish oil and glycemic control in diabetes. *Diabetes Care* 1998; **21**: 494–500.

99. Montori VM, Farmer A, Wollan PC, Dinneen SF. Fish oil supplementation in type 2 diabetes. *Diabetes Care* 2000; **23**: 1407–1415.

100. ISSI-Prevenzione Investigators. Dietary supplementation with n-3 polyunsaturated fatty acids and vitamin E after myocardial infarction: results of the GISSI-Prevenzione trial. *Lancet* 1999; **354**: 447–455.
101. Dunstan DW, Mori TA, Puddey IB, Beilin LJ, Burke V, Morton AR, Stanton KG. The independent and combined effects of aerobic exercise and dietary fish intake on serum lipids and glycemic control in NIDDM. *Diabetes Care* 1997; **20**: 913–921.
102. Daly ME, Vale C, Walker M, Alberti KG, Mathers JC. Dietary carbohydrates and insulin sensitivity: a review of the evidence and clinical implications. *American Journal of Clinical Nutrition* 1997; **66**: 1072–1085.
103. Franz MJ, Horton ES, Bantle JP, Beebe CA, Brunzell JD, Coulston AM, Henry RR, Hoogwerf BJ, Stacpoole PW. Nutrition principles for the management of diabetes and related complications. *Diabetes Care* 1994; **17**: 490–518.
104. Henry RR, Crapo PA. Current issues in fructose metabolism. *Annual Review of Nutrition* 1991; **11**: 21–39.
105. Crapo PA, Kolterman OG, Olefsky JM. Effects of oral glucose in normal, diabetic, and impaired glucose tolerance subjects. *Diabetes Care* 1980; **3**: 575–582.
106. Jenkins DJA, Wolever TMS, Jenkins AL. Starchy foods and the glycemic index. *Diabetes Care* 1988; **11**: 149–159.
107. Frost G, Leeds AA, Doré CJ, Maldeiros S, Brading S, Dornhorst A. Glycaemic index as a determinant of serum HDL-cholesterol concentration. *Lancet* 1999; **353**: 1045–1048.
108. Wolever TMS, Jenkins DJA, Vuskan V, Jenkins AL, Wong GS, Josse RG. Beneficial effect of low-glycemic index diet in overweight NIDDM subjects. *Diabetes Care* 1992; **15**(4): 562–564.
109. Vuksan V, Jenkins DJ, Spadafora P, Sievenpiper JL, Owen R, Vidgen E, Brighenti F, Josse R, Leiter LA, Bruce-Thompson C. Konjac-mannan (glucomannan) improves glycemia and other associated risk factors for coronary heart disease in type 2 diabetes. A randomized controlled metabolic trial. *Diabetes Care* 1999; **22**: 913–919.
110. Anderson JW, Allgood LD, Turner J, Oeltgen PR, Daggy BP. Effects of psyllium on glucose and serum lipid responses in men with type 2 diabetes and hypercholesterolemia. *American Journal of Clinical Nutrition* 1999; **70**: 466–473.
111. Lalor BC, Bhatnagar D, Winocour PH, Ishola M, Arrol S, Brading M, Durrington PN. Placebo-controlled trial of the effects of guar gum and metformin on fasting blood glucose and serum lipids in obese, type 2 diabetic patients. *Diabetic Medicine* 1990; **7**: 242–245.
112. Beattie VA, Edwards CA, Hosker JP, Cullen DR, Ward JD, Read NW. Does adding fibre to a low energy, high carbohydrate, low fat diet confer any benefit to the management of newly diagnosed overweight type II diabetics ? *British Medical Journal* 1988; **296**: 1147–1149.
113. Holman RR, Steemson J, Darling P, Turner RC. No glycemic benefit from guar administration in NIDDM. *Diabetes Care* 1987; **10**: 68–71.
114. Lafrance L, Rabasa Lhoret R, Poisson D, Ducros F, Chiasson JL. Effects of different glycaemic index foods and dietary fibre intake on glycaemic control in type 1 diabetic patients on intensive insulin therapy. *Diabetic Medicine* 1998; **15**: 972–978.
115. Vaaler S, Hanssen KF, Dahl Jorgensen K, Frolich W, Aaseth J, Odegaard B, Aagenaes O. Diabetic control is improved by guar gum and wheat bran supplementation. *Diabetic Medicine* 1986; **3**: 230–233.

116. Sharma RD, Raghuram TC, Rao NS. Effect of fenugreek seeds on blood glucose and serum lipids in type I diabetes. *European Journal of Clinical Nutrition* 1990; **44**: 301–306.
117. Kinmonth AL, Angus RM, Jenkins PA, Smith MA, Baum JD. Whole foods and increased dietary fibre improve blood glucose control in diabetic children. *Archives of Diseases of the Child* 1982; **57**: 187–194.
118. Simpson RW, Mann JI, Eaton J, Carter RD, Hockaday TDR. High-carbohydrate diets and insulin-dependent diabetics. *British Medical Journal* 1979; **2**: 523–525.
119. Simpson HCR, Lousley S, Geekie M, Simpson RW, Carter RD, Hockaday TDR. A high-carbohydrate leguminous fibre diet improves all aspects of diabetic control. *Lancet* 1981; **1**: 1–5.
120. Brenner BM, Meyer TW, Hostetter TH. Dietary protein intake and the progressive nature of kidney disease: the role of hemodynamically mediated glomerular injury in the pathogenesis of progressive glomerular sclerosis in aging, renal ablation and intrinsic renal disease. *The New England Journal of Medicine* 1982; **307**: 652–659.
121. Klahr S, Levey AS, Beck GJ, Caggiula AW, Hunsicker L, Kusek JW, Striker G. The effects of dietary protein restriction and blood-pressure control on the progression of chronic renal disease. *New England Journal of Medicine* 1994; **330**: 877–884.
122. Friedman EA. Diabetic nephropathy: Strategies in prevention and management. *Kidney International* 1982; **21**: 780–791.
123. Waugh NR, Robertson AM. Protein restriction for diabetic renal disease. *Cochrane Database Systems Review* 2000(2): Cd002181.
124. Lieber CS. Alcohol and the liver: 1994 update. *Gastroenterology* 1994; **106**: 1085–105.
125. Harding AH, Sargeant LA, Khaw KT, Welch A, Oakes S, Luben RN, Bingham S, Day NE, Wareham NJ. Cross-sectional association between total level and type of alcohol consumption and glycosylated haemoglobin level: the EPIC-Norfolk study. *European Journal of Clinical Nutrition* 2002: in press.
126. Sargeant LA, Wareham NJ, Bingham S, Day NE, Luben RN, Oakes S, Welch A, Khaw K-T Vitamin C and Hyperglycemia in the European Prospective Investigation Into Cancer-Norfolk (EPIC-Norfolk) Study. *Diabetes Care* 2000; **23**: 726–732.
127. Salonen JT, Nyyssonen K, Tuomainen TP, Maenpaa PH, Korpela H, Kaplan GA, Lynch J, Helmrich SP, Salonen R. Increased risk of non-insulin dependent diabetes mellitus at low plasma vitamin E concentrations: a four year follow up study in men. *British Medical Journal* 1995; **311**: 1124–1127.
128. Paolisso G, D'Amore A, Giugliano D, Pharmacologic doses of vitamin E improve insulin action in healthy subjects and non-insulin-dependent diabetic patients. *American Journal of Clinical Nutrition* 1993; **57**: 650–656.
129. Paolisso G, D'Amore A, Balbi V, Volpe C, Galzerano D, Giugliano D, Sgambato S, Varricchio M, D'Onofrio F. Plasma vitamin C affects glucose homeostasis in healthy subjects and in non-insulin dependent diabetics. *American Journal of Physiology* 1994; **266**: E261–E268.
130. Sargeant LA, Khaw KT, Bingham S, Day NE, Luben RN, Oakes S, Welch A, Wareham NJ. Fruit and vegetable intake and population glycosylated haemoglobin levels: the EPIC-Norfok Study. *European Journal of Clinical Nutrition* 2001; **55**: 342–348.
131. Williams DEM, Wareham NJ, Cox BD, Byrne CD, Hales CN, Day NE. Frequent

salad vegetable consumption is associated with a reduction in the risk of diabetes mellitus. *J Clin Epidemiol* 1999; **52**: 329–335.

132. HOPE Study Investigators. Effects of ramipril on cardiovascular and microvascular outcomes in people with diabetes mellitus: results of the HOPE study and MICRO-HOPE substudy. *Lancet* 2000; **355**: 253–259.

133. Boucher BJ, Mannan N, Noonan K, Hales CN, Evans SJW. Glucose intolerance and impairment of insulin secretion in relation to vitamin D deficiency in East London Asians. *Diabetologia* 1995; **38**: 1239–1245.

134. Wareham NJ, Byrne CD, Carr C, Day NE, Boucher BJ, Hales CN. Glucose intolerance is associated with altered calcium homeostasis: a possible link between increased serum calcium concentrations and cardiovascular disease mortality. *Metabolism* 1997; **46**: 1171–1177.

135. McCarty MF. Exploiting complementary therapeutic strategies for the treatment of type II diabetes and prevention of its complications. *Medical Hypotheses* 1997; **49**: 143–152.

136. Jeejeebhoy KN, Chu RC, Marliss EB, Greenberg GR, Bruce-Robertson A. Chromium deficiency, glucose intolerance, and neuropathy reversed by chromium supplementation in a patient receiving long-term parenteral nutrition. *American Journal of Clinical Nutrition* 1977; **30**: 531–538.

137. Anderson, RA, Cheng N, Bryden NA, Polansky MM, Cheng N, Chi J. Feng J. Elevated intakes of supplemental chromium improve glucose and insulin variables in individuals with type 2 diabetes. *Diabetes* 1997: 1786–1791.

138. Grant KE, Chandler RM, Castle AL, Ivy JL. Chromium and exercise training: effect on obese women. *Medicine & Science in Sports and Exercise* 1997; **29**: 992–998.

139. ADA Consensus Conference. Magnesium supplementation in the treatment of diabetes mellitus. *Diabetes Care* 1993; **16**(S2): 1065–1067.

140. Mather HM, Nisbet JA, Burton GH, Poston GJ, Bland JM, Bailey PA, Pilkington TR. Hypomagnesaemia in Diabetes. *Clinica Chimica Acta* 1979; **95**: 235–242.

141. Paolisso G, Sgambato S, Pizza G, Passariello N, Varricchio M, D'Onofrio F. Improved insulin response and action by chronic magnesium administration in aged NIDDM subjects. *Diabetes Care* 1989; **12**: 265–269.

142. Lima M-de-L, Cruz T, Pousada JC, Rodrigues LE, Barbosa K, Cangucu V. The effect of magnesium supplementation in increasing doses on the control of type 2 diabetes. *Diabetes Care* 1998; **21**: 682–686.

143. Ha TK, Lean ME. Recommendations for the nutritional management of patients with diabetes mellitus. *European Journal of Clinical Nutrition* 1998; **52**: 467–481.

144. Intersalt Co-operative Research Group. Intersalt: an international study of elecrode excretion and blood pressure. Results for 24-hour urinary sodium and potassium excretion. *Br Med J* 1988; **297**: 319–328.

145. Lampson WG, Kramer JH, Schaffer SW. Potentiation of the actions of insulin by taurine. *Canadian Journal of Physiology and Pharmacology* 1983; **61**: 457–463.

146. Kulakowski EC, Maturo J. Hypoglycemic properties of taurine: not mediated by enhanced insulin release. *Biochemistry and Pharmacology* 1984; **33**:2835–2838.

147. Shechter Y. Insulin-mimetic effects of vanadate. Possible implications for future treatment of diabetes. *Diabetes* 1990; **39**: 1–5.

148. Halberstam M, Cohen N, Shlimovich P, Rossetti L, Shamoon H. Oral vanadyl sulfate improves insulin sensitivity in NIDDM but not in obese nondiabetic subjects. *Diabetes* 1996; **45**: 659–666.

149. Boden G, Chen X, Ruiz J, van Rossum GD, Turco S. Effects of vanadyl sulfate on

carbohydrate and lipid metabolism in patients with non-insulin-dependent diabetes mellitus. *Metabolism* 1996; **45**: 1130–1135.

150. Vogler BK, Pittler MH, Ernst E. The efficacy of ginseng. A systematic review of randomised clinical trials. *Eur J Clin Pharmacol* 1999; **55**: 567–575.

151. Heitzman CA, Kaplan RM, Wilson DK, Sandre J. Sex difference in weight loss among adults with Type II diabetes Mellitus. *Journal of Behavioural Medicine* 1987; **10**: 197–211.

152. D'Eramo-Melkus GA, Wylie-Rosett J, Hagan JA. Metabolic impact of education in NIDDM. *Diabetes Care* 1992; **15**: 864–869.

153. Milne RM, Mann JI, Chisholm AW, Williams SM. Long-term comparison of three dietary prescriptions in the treatment of NIDDM. *Diabetes Care* 1994; **17**: 74–80.

154. Agurs-Collins TD, Kumanyika SK, Ten Have TR, Adams-Campbell LL. A randomized controlled trial of weight reduction and exercise for diabetes management in older African-American subjects. *Diabetes Care* 1997; **20**: 1503–1511.

155. Manning RM, Jung RT, Leese GP, Newton RW. The comparison of four weight reduction strategies aimed at overweight patients with diabetes mellitus: four-year follow-up. *Diabetic Medicine* 1998; **15**: 497–502.

156. Yamanouchi K, Shinozaki T, Chikada K, Nishikawa T, Ito K, Shimizu S, Ozawa N, Suzuki Y, Maeno H, Kato K, Oshida Y, Sato Y. Daily walking combined with diet therapy is a useful means for obese NIDDM patients not only to reduce body weight but also to improve insulin sensitivity. *Diabetes Care* 1995; **18**: 775–778.

157. Verity LS, Ismail AH. Effects of exercise on cardiovascular disease risk in women with NIDDM. *Diabetes Research and Clinical Practice* 1989; **6**: 27–35.

158. Vanninen E, Uusitupa M, Siitonene O, Laitinen J, Lansimies E. Habitual physical activity, aerobic capacity and metabolic control in patients with newly-diagnosed type 2 (non-insulin dependent) diabetes mellitus: effect of one-year diet and exercise intervention. *Diabetologia* 1992; **35**: 340–346.

159. Stratton R, Wilson DP, Endres RK, Goldstein DE. Improved glycemic control after supervised 8-wk exercise program in insulin-dependent diabetic adolescents. *Diabetes Care* 1987; **10**: 589–593.

160. Samaras K, Aswell S, Mackintosh A-M, Fleury AC, Campbell LV, Chisholm DJ. Will older sedentary people with non-insulin-dependent diabetes mellitus start exercising? A health promotion model. *Diabetes Research and Clinical Practice* 1997; **37**: 121–128.

161. Mourier A, Gautier JF, De-Kerviler E, Bigard AX, Villette JM, Garnier JP, Duvallet A, Guezennec CY, Cathelineau G. Mobilization of visceral adipose tissue related to the improvement in insulin sensitivity in response to physical training in NIDDM. *Diabetes Care* 1997; **20**: 385–391.

162. Raz I, Hauser E, Bursztyn M. Moderate exercise improves glucose metabolism in uncontrolled elderly patients with non-insulin-dependent diabetes mellitus. *Israel Journal of Medical Science* 1994; **30**: 766–770.

163. Tessier D, Ménard J, Fülöp T, Ardilouze JL, Roy MA, Duuc N, Dubois MF, Gauthier P. Effects of aerobic physical exercise in the elderly with type 2 diabetes mellitus. *Archives of Gerontology and Geriatrics*. 2000; **31**: 121–132.

17

Prevention of Hypertension

JOHN FULLER

University of London, London WC1E 6BT, UK

INTRODUCTION

Type 2 (non-insulin dependent) diabetes mellitus is approaching epidemic proportions worldwide[1], mainly as a consequence of an ageing and increasingly obese population. The incidence of the less common type 1 (insulin-dependent) diabetes is also increasing worldwide[2]. The associated macrovascular, microvascular and neurological complications account for much of the severe morbidity and premature mortality occurring in people with both types of diabetes. There is increasing epidemiological evidence that raised arterial pressure ranks alongside hyperglycaemia itself as being a major modifiable risk factor for these chronic diabetic complications. There is considerable evidence that the prevalence of hypertension is increased in type 2 diabetes and is often present at diagnosis or even earlier in the pre-diabetic phase of glucose intolerance associated with insulin resistance[3]. On the other hand, the incidence of diabetes is increased 2.5 times in hypertensive compared with normotensive individuals[4]. These two common conditions therefore frequently co-exist. This chapter will review the relationship of raised blood pressure (BP) to diabetic complications and assess the evidence for the efficacy of antihypertensive therapy for their prevention.

HYPERTENSION AND CARDIOVASCULAR DISEASE IN DIABETES

EPIDEMIOLOGY

Several large prospective studies of diabetic subjects have shown that, as in the general population, raised blood pressure, both systolic and diastolic, is a

The Evidence Base for Diabetes Care. Edited by R. Williams, W. Herman, A.-L. Kinmonth and N. J. Wareham.
© 2002 John Wiley & Sons, Ltd

strong graded risk factor of the development of coronary heart disease (CHD) and stroke[5-9]. This relationship is demonstrated in subjects with both type 1 and type 2 diabetes and in men and women[9]. It is independent of other potential confounding factors such as age, duration of diabetes, glycaemic control, dyslipidaemia or proteinuria[9].

The WHO Multinational Study of Vascular Disease in Diabetes (MSVDD) was a prospective study of median duration 12 years in 1260 type 1 and 3483 type 2 diabetic patients from 10 centres throughout the world[10]. It showed a strong positive, graded relationship between raised BP and both CHD and stroke in men and women with type 1 and type 2 diabetes, with no suggestion of a J-shaped relationship[11]. The WHO MSVDD also showed a strong interaction between hypertension and proteinuria in predicting excess mortality in the diabetic cohorts compared with their respective local populations [12].

CLINICAL TRIALS

A list of the completed trials of the effects of antihypertensive therapy on CVD outcomes in diabetic subjects is given in Table 17.1. Before the publication in 1998 of the results of the UK Prospective Diabetes Study (UKPDS), information from clinical trials on the efficacy of blood pressure lowering for the prevention of cardiovascular outcomes in diabetes was extremely sparse. Up to that date only two intervention trials, using mainly diuretic-based regimes, had reported results in their respective diabetic sub-groups. These were the Hypertension Detection and Follow-up Programme (HDFP) and the Systolic Hypertension in the Elderly Program (SHEP). Since the UKPDS publication, the results of a further nine trials with diabetic sub-groups have been pub-

Table 17.1. Names and acronyms of completed randomised controlled trials evaluating the effect of antihypertensive therapy on cardiovascular outcomes in type 2 diabetes (to 2001).

Acronym	Trial name
ABCD[28]	Appropriate Blood Pressure Control in Diabetes
CAPPP[25]	Captopril Prevention Project
FACET[27]	Fosinopril versus Amlodipine Cardiovascular Events Randomised Trial
HDFP[13]	Hypertension Detection and Follow-up Program
HOPE[23]	Heart Outcomes Prevention Evaluation Study
HOT[21]	Hypertension Optimal Treatment Trial
NORDIL[33]	Nordic Diltiazem Study
SHEP[16]	Systolic Hypertension in the Elderly Program
STOP-2[34]	Swedish Trial in Old Patients with Hypertension
SYST-EUR[19]	Systolic Hypertension in Europe Trial
SYST-CHINA[20]	Systolic Hypertension in China
UKPDS[18,24]	United Kingdom Prospective Diabetes Study

lished. All the trials have been divided into two categories: those comparing active treatment with a placebo or less actively treated group (Table 17.2a) and those comparing active treatments (Table 17.3a).

COMPARISON OF ACTIVE TREATMENT WITH A PLACEBO OR LESS ACTIVELY TREATED GROUP

HDFP compared stepped-care with referred-care regimes in 10 940 hypertensive individuals [13]. In 722 subjects who had a history of clinically diagnosed diabetes, the CVD mortality rate five-years afterwards was significantly reduced in the stepped-care group, with an absolute risk reduction of $16.3/10^3$ person-year (pyr)[14] (Table 17.3a).

In SHEP, 4736 men and women aged 60 years or more with isolated systolic hypertension were randomised initially to the thiazide diuretic chlorthalidone 12.5 mg/d or placebo, with a stepped-care treatment programme thereafter using atenolol or reserpine to achieve a goal blood pressure[15]. The five-year major CVD rate was 34% lower in active compared with placebo-treated groups for the 583 diabetic patients (absolute risk reduction $15.0/10^3$ pyr)[16]. Other outcomes including non-fatal MI and fatal CHD were also significantly reduced in the diabetic sub-group (Table 17.3a). A meta-analysis of these two studies of diabetic sub-groups[17] showed a significant treatment effect on CVD mortality and morbidity with an odds ratio (OR) of 0.64 (95% CI: 0.50,0.82). There was a non-significant reduction in all-cause mortality in this meta-analysis: OR 0.85 (0.62,1.17).

The UKPDS was a randomised controlled trial comparing tight BP control, aiming at a BP of <150/85 Hg (using the ACE inhibitor (ACEI) captopril or the β-blocker atenolol as the main treatment) with less tight control aiming at a BP of <180/105 mmHg[18]. Of the 1148 type 2 patients with hypertension, 36% were already on treatment at trial entry, 758 were allocated to tight BP control and 390 to less tight control, with a median follow-up of 8.4 years. The mean blood pressure during follow-up was significantly reduced in the group assigned to tight control (144/82 mmHg) compared with the group assigned to less tight control (154/87 mmHg).

A total of 21 clinical end-points were predefined in this study. These were used to define three primary outcomes:-

1. A first clinical end-point related to diabetes (sudden death, death from hyperglycaemia or hypoglycaemia, fatal or non-fatal MI, angina, heart failure, stroke, renal failure, amputation, vitreous haemorrhage, retinal photo-coagulation, blindness in one eye or cataract extraction).
2. Death related to diabetes (death due to MI, sudden death, stroke, peripheral vascular disease, renal disease, hyper- or hypoglycaemia).
3. Death from all causes.

Table 17.2a. Studies of antihypertensive therapies in type 2 diabetes: comparisons of active treatments with a placebo or less actively treated group

Study	Year	Total sample size	Diabetes sample size	Age range (years)	Entry criteria	Intervention (first step)	Duration (years) (median/mean)
HDFP[14,17]	1979	10940	772	30–69	Diast. BP ≥90 mmHg	Stepped care versus referred care	5
SHEP[16]	1996	4736	583	60+	Syst. BP ≥160 mmHg and Diast. BP <90mmHg	Chlorthalidone versus placebo	4.5
UKPDS[18]	1998	1148	1148	25–65	BP ≥160/90 mmHg or BP ≥150/85 mmHg on treatment	Tight versus less tight BP control	8.4
HOT[21]	1998	18790	1501	50–80	Diast. BP 100–115 mmHg	Felodipine + other agents. Target Diast BP ≤90, ≤85, ≤80 mmHg	3.8
SYST-EUR[19]	1999	4695	492	60+	Syst. BP 160–219 mmHg and Diast. BP <95 mmHg	Nitrendipine versus placebo	2
SYST-CHINA[20]	2000	2394	98	60+	Syst. BP 160–219 mmHg and Diast. BP <95 mmHg	Nitrendipine versus placebo	3
HOPE[23]	2000	9297	3577	55+	History of CVD or diabetes plus one other cardiovascular risk factor	Ramipril versus placebo	4.5

Table 17.2b. Studies of antihypertensive therapies in type 2 diabetes: comparisons of active treatments.

Study	Year	Total sample size	Diabetes sample size	Age range (years)	Entry criteria	Intervention (first step)	Duration (years) (median/mean)
ABCD[28]	1998	470	470	47–74	Diast. BP ≥90 mmHg	Enalapril versus Nisoldipine	5
FACET[27]	1998	380	380	mean 63	BP >140/90 mmHg	Fosinopril versus Amlodipine	3.5
UKPDS[24]	1998	758	758	25–65	BP ≥160/90 mmHg or BP ≥150/85 mmHg on treatment	Captopril versus Atenolol	8.4
CAPPP[25]	1999	10985	572	25–66	Diast. BP ≥100 mmHg	Captopril versus Conv*.	6.1
STOP-2[34]	1999	6614	719	70–84	BP ≥180/105 mmHg	ACEI vs CCB versus Conv.	4
NORDIL[33]	2000	10916	727	50–74	Diast. BP ≥100 mmHg	Diltiazem versus Conv.	4.5

*Conv. = β-blocker/diuretic

Table 17.3a. Studies of antihypertensive therapies in type 2 diabetes: Comparisons of active treatment with a placebo or less active treatment.

Study	End-points	Event rates(/10^3 pyr)		Absolute risk reduction*/(10^3 pyr)	Relative risk reduction* (95% CI)
		Active treatment	Less active treatment		
HDFP[14,17]	Total CVD	35.2	51.2	16.3	0.62 (0.44–0.57)
	Total mortality	22.0	25.0	3.0	0.86 (0.56–1.34)
SHEP[16]	MI	12.8	22.7	9.9	0.46 (0.24–0.88)
	Stroke	17.7	24.0	6.3	0.78 (0.45–1.34)
	Total CVD	40.3	55.3	15.0	0.66 (0.46–0.94)
	Total mortality	27.6	32.0	4.4	0.84 (0.53–1.32)
UKPDS[18]	MI	18.6	23.5	0.59 p = 0.13	0.79 (0.59–1.07)
	Stroke	6.5	11.6	0.59 p = 0.013	0.56 (0.35–0.89)
	Total mortality	22.4	27.2	4.8 p = 0.17	0.82 (0.63–1.08)
HOT[21]	MI	NA	NA	NA	**0.50 (NS)
	Stroke	NA	NA	NA	**0.70 (NS)
	Total CVD	NA	NA	NA	**0.50 (p = 0.04)
SYST-EUR[19]	MI	11.7	27.1	15.4 p = 0.06	†0.37 (p = 0.12)
	Stroke	8.3	26.6	18.3 p = 0.02	†0.27 (p = 0.13)
	Total CVD	22.0	57.6	35.6 p = 0.002	†0.31 (p = 0.01)
	Total mortality	26.4	45.1	18.7 p = 0.09	†0.45 (p = 0.04)
SYST-CHINA[20]	Cardiac (MI, heart failure or sudden death)	NA	NA	NA	0.90 (p = 0.08)
	Stroke	NA	NA	NA	0.45 (p = 0.42)
	Total CVD	32.1	76.4	NA	0.74 (p = 0.03)
	Total mortality	NA	NA	NA	0.59 (p = 0.15)
HOPE[23]	MI	NA	NA	NA	0.88 (0.64–0.94)
	Stroke	NA	NA	NA	0.67 (0.50–0.90)
	Total CVD	NA	NA	NA	0.75 (0.64–0.88)
	Total mortality	NA	NA	NA	0.76 (0.63–0.92)

*Active versus untreated or less actively treated group   **Approximate risk reductions for target groups ≤80 mmHg versus ≤90 mmHg.
†Adjusted relative hazards. P values are for the interaction between treatment and diabetes.
NA = not available.   NS = not significant.

Tight BP control was associated with a 24% reduction in the risk of developing any end-point related to diabetes (p = 0.0046). There was a 32% reduction in diabetes-related deaths (p = 0.019) but all-cause mortality was not significantly reduced (Table 17.3a). There was a non-significant reduction of 21% in the risk of fatal or non-fatal MI or sudden death. The risk of fatal or non-fatal stroke was reduced by 44% (p = 0.013) with an absolute risk reduction of $4.9/10^3$ pyr, but amputations were not significantly reduced. In the tight BP control group, 29% of patients required three or more hypertensive treatments.

Several trials comparing a calcium channel blocker (CCB) with placebo as the first intervention step have diabetic sub-groups of varying sizes. Post-hoc analysis of the 492 diabetic participants in the SYST-EUR trial of CCB-based antihypertensive therapy in older patients with isolated systolic hypertension showed benefits in a number of cardiovascular end-points for active first-time treatment with nitrendipine versus placebo (Table 17.3a)[19]. The companion SYST-CHINA trial whose design was similar to that of SYST-EUR had only 98 diabetic subjects out of a total sample of 2394 participants[20]. However, the benefit of treatment with nitrendipine was particularly evident in the diabetic patients, with active treatment reducing all-cause mortality by 55%, stroke by 73% and all cardiovascular events by 69% (Table 17.3a).

In the Hypertension Optimal Treatment (HOT) trial[21], the hypertensive diabetic subgroup (n = 1501) experienced a 50% lower risk of major cardio-vascular events for those in the lowest target level (diastolic BP ≤80 mmHg) compared with those in the highest target level (diastolic BP ≤90 mmHg) (Table 17.3a). In this trial the baseline therapy was the CCB felodipine with the addition of other agents according to a five-step regimen.

The Heart Outcomes Prevention Evaluation (HOPE) study was a random-ised placebo controlled trial of the ACE-inhibitor ramipril in 9297 high-risk patients, aged 55 years or more, who had evidence of vascular disease or diabetes plus one other cardiovascular risk factor (total cholesterol >5.5 mmol/L, HDL cholesterol ≤0.9 mmol/L, hypertension, known micro-albuminuria or current smoking)[22]. The primary outcome was a composite of MI, stroke or death from cardiovascular causes. The ramipril or placebo was added to current therapy. The 3577 diabetic patients enrolled in HOPE were analysed separately in a sub-study of microalbuminuria, cardiovascular and renal outcomes (MICRO-HOPE)[23] (Table 17.2a).

The study was stopped six months early (after 4.5 years) because a consistent benefit of ramipril compared with placebo was found. In keeping with the findings of the main study, the primary outcome in the diabetic sub-group was reduced by 25% (Table17.3a). The secondary outcomes of total mortality and need for revascularisation, as well as MI and stroke, were also significantly reduced in the ramipril group compared with placebo. These large reductions in risk associated with ramipril therapy were achieved in spite of comparatively small changes in systolic (2.4 mmHg) and diastolic (1.0 mmHg) blood pressures.

In the interpretation of the HOPE results in diabetic subjects it should be noted that at baseline 70% had a history of cardiovascular disease and 56% had a history of hypertension. A sub-group analysis showed that the reduction in the primary outcome in those 1119 subjects without cardiovascular disease was not significant[23]. However, the study was not designed to examine the treatment effect in sub-groups such as those with or without cardiovascular disease or hypertension, and probably lacked the statistical power to do so.

COMPARISONS OF ACTIVE TREATMENTS

In the UKPDS, captopril and atenolol gave similar blood pressure reductions to a mean of 144/83 mmHg and 143/81 mmHg respectively. The two drugs were equally effective at reducing the risk of macrovascular end-points[24] (Table 17.3b). In contrast to these UKPDS findings, a possible beneficial effect of the ACE-inhibitor captopril in preventing cardiovascular morbidity and mortality has been shown in the hypertensive diabetic sub-group (n = 572) of the Captopril Prevention Project (CAPP)[25]. In this open label study, captopril was compared with conventional antihypertensive therapy with diuretics, β-blockers or both and was associated with a 66% lower rate of total and non-total MI (Table 17.3b). However, in the group as a whole (n = 10 955), captopril and conventional treatment did not differ in efficacy.

Several recent studies have examined the effects of calcium channel blockers (CCBs) in comparison with other therapies in hypertensive patients with type 2 diabetes[19,21,26,27]. The Appropriate Blood Pressure Control in Diabetes (ABCD) trial is comparing the effects of intensive with moderate BP control on the progression of diabetic nephropathy, retinopathy, cardiovascular disease and neuropathy in subjects with type 2 diabetes[26]. It is also comparing the efficacy of the CCB nisoldipine with that of the ACE-inhibitor enalapril as a first-line antihypertensive agent. There are two populations in the study, a hypertensive one (diastolic BP ≥ 90 mmHg) and a normotensive one (diastolic BP 80–89 mmHg) with 470 and 480 participants respectively. In 1998, after five years' follow-up, the investigators reported[28] that in the hypertensive group, nisoldipine was associated with a higher incidence of fatal and non-fatal myocardial infarction (total 25) than enalapril (total 5) (risk ratio 9.5; 95% CI: 2.3–21.4). On the basis of this finding, the Data and Safety Monitoring Committee recommended the discontinuation of nisoldipine in the hypertensive group. A difference in cardiovascular events between treatments was not found in the normotensive patients who are continuing on randomised therapy.

The Fosinopril Amlodipine Cardiovascular Events Trial (FACET)[27] was an open-label randomised trial in 380 hypertensive type 2 diabetic patients (systolic BP >140 mmHg or diastolic BP >90 mmHg) comparing the ACE-inhibitor fosinopril with the CCB amlodipine over a 3.5 year follow-up. Its primary aim was to assess treatment-related differences in serum lipids and

Table 17.3b. Studies of antihypertensive therapies in type 2 diabetes: Comparisons of active treatment with a placebo or less active treatment.

Study	End-points	Event rates (/10³ pyr)		Absolute risk reduction* (/10³ pyr)	Relative risk reduction* (95% CI)
		Newer treatment	Comparison treatment		
ABCD[28]	MI	NA	NA	NA	0.18 (0.07–0.48)
	Stroke	NA	NA	NA	0.63 (0.24–1.67)
	Total CVD	NA	NA	NA	0.50 (0.16–1.43)
	Total mortality	NA	NA	NA	0.77 (0.36–1.67)
FACET[27]	MI	NA	NA	NA	0.77 (0.34–1.75)
	Stroke	NA	NA	NA	0.39 (0.12–1.23)
	Total CVD	NA	NA	NA	0.49 (0.26–0.95)
	Total mortality	NA	NA	NA	0.81 (0.22–3.02)
UKPDS[24]	MI	20.2	16.9	−3.3 p = 0.35	1.20 (0.82–1.76)
	Stroke	6.8	6.1	−0.7 p = 0.74	1.12 (0.59–2.12)
	Total mortality	23.8	20.8	−3.0 p = 0.44	1.14 (0.81–1.61)
CAPP[25]	MI	NA	NA	NA	0.34 (0.17–067)
	Stroke	NA	NA	NA	1.02 (0.55–1.88)
	Fatal CVD	NA	NA	NA	0.48 (0.21–1.10)
	Total mortality	NA	NA	NA	0.54 (0.31–0.96)
STOP-2[34]	Fatal CVD	NA	NA	NA	(No significant differences)
NORDIL[33]	MI	11.2	11.1	−0.1 p = 0.99	0.99 (0.51–1.94)
	Stroke	13.3	12.3	−1.0 p = 0.92	0.97 (0.52–1.81)
	Total CVD	29.8	27.7	−2.1 p = 0.98	1.01 (0.66–1.53)
	Total mortality	18.1	15.6	−2.5 p = 0.80	1.07 (0.63–1.84)

*ACEI versus comparison treatment except CCB versus comparison treatment in NORDIL.
NA = not available

diabetes control. Both treatments were effective in lowering blood pressure. The fosinopril-treated group had a significantly lower risk of the combined outcome of acute MI, stroke or hospitalised angina than the amlodipine group (14/189 versus 27/191; hazards ratio = 0.49; 95% CI: 0.26–0.95).

A possible explanation for the findings of these CCB trials has been suggested by the FACET investigators[29]. They argue that 'the changes in the composition of cellular membranes resulting from diabetes increase the binding of lipophilic drugs such as amlodipine, so diabetic patients may be vulnerable to adverse effects of high doses of calcium antagonists'. However, the findings of these studies should be treated with caution since cardiovascular outcomes were not the primary outcome measures of the studies and the results are based on multiple post-hoc sub-group analyses, often with small sample sizes. Furthermore in the ABCD study, patients assigned to enalapril were more likely to receive additional drugs, particularly diuretics and β-blockers, with known cardioprotective effects[30-32].

The large NORDIL study in 10 891 hypertensive patients compared the effect of the non-dihydropyridine CCB diltiazem with that of conventional therapy (diuretics, β-blockers or both) on cardiovascular morbidity and mortality[33]. For the total sample, diltiazem was as effective as conventional therapy in preventing the primary end-point of all stroke, MI and other cardio-vascular death. The same results were obtained in a sub-group analysis of the 727 diabetic participants in the trial (Table 17.3b). Similar results were obtained in the 721 diabetic participants in the STOP-2 trial where newer antihyper-tensives (ACE-inhibitor's and CCBs) were compared with conventional therapy in elderly hypertensive patients (Table 17.3b)[34].

This controversy concerning the possible reduced benefit for cardiovascular outcomes in diabetic subjects associated with CCB therapy may not be resolved until the results of ongoing studies such as the Antihypertensive and Lipid-Lowering treatment to prevent Heart Attack Trial (ALLHAT)[35] become available.

ALLHAT is a double-blind randomised trial in 42 448 high-risk hyper-tensive subjects, aged ≥55 years, assessing whether the rate of cardiovascular events differs between diuretic treatment (chlorthalidone) and three altern-ative therapies: a CCB (amlodipine), an ACE-inhibitor (lisinopril), and an α-blocker (doxazosin). There are 15 297 diabetic participants in the trial, which is planned to be completed in March 2002 [36]. In 2000, the ALLHAT investigators reported that the doxazosin arm of the trial had been discontinued, since a significantly higher incidence of combined CVD events and congestive heart failure (CHF) had been found in the doxazosin group compared with the chlorthalidone group. Rates for the primary CHD outcome and total mortality were essentially the same in the two groups[37]. Information on the comparative efficacy and safety of the newer drugs versus conventional therapy (diuretics/β-blockers) will also be forthcoming from several other large ongoing trials including diabetic sub-groups such as the Anglo-Scandinavian Cardiac Outcome Trial (ASCOT)[38.]

HYPERTENSION AND DIABETIC RETINOPATHY

EPIDEMIOLOGY

Diabetic retinopathy is the most common health-threatening complication of diabetes and is a major cause of vision loss and blindness in the working population[39,40]. Poor long-term glycaemic control is now established as the major risk factor for the development and progression of diabetic retinopathy[41,42]. Indeed, therapeutic interventions to improve glycaemic control have convincingly been shown to improve significantly the rate of progression of retinopathy in both type 1[43] and type 2[44] diabetes.

Most of the epidemiological studies of the relation between raised BP and diabetic retinopathy have been cross-sectional in design with small sample sizes giving rise to inconsistent results. The few prospective studies in type 1 diabetes have shown that systolic, but not diastolic, BP predicts the development of retinopathy[45,46], with these associations becoming non-significant after adjustment for duration of diabetes and glycated haemoglobin. On the other hand, diastolic BP is consistently related to the progression of retinopathy, but more weakly so after adjustment for confounding factors[41,45-47].

In a study of 534 Swiss diabetic patients, mainly with type 2 diabetes, Teuscher *et al*[48] found that the incidence of non-proliferative retinopathy was significantly related to systolic BP. This Swiss study was part of the larger WHO Multinational Study of Vascular Disease in Diabetes (MVSDD) in which 2877 subjects from 10 centres, about three-quarters of whom had type 2 diabetes, were studied prospectively over 8.5 years for the progression of retinopathy. For all centres, systolic BP was significantly associated with the incidence of retinopathy, but diastolic BP was a significant risk factor for the progression to proliferative retinopathy[49]. A significant relationship of systolic BP to the incidence but not the progression of retinopathy was found in the UKPDS[50]. Thus for both type 1 and type 2 diabetes, epidemiological evidence seems to suggest that a raised systolic BP is important in the development of diabetic retinopathy, whereas an increased diastolic BP has a more substantial role in the progression of this complication.

CLINICAL TRIALS

Until recently, there has been very little evidence from RCTs that blood pressure control in diabetic subjects will reduce the rate of progression of retinopathy. However, the situation has now changed with the recent publication of trials in both type 1 and type 2 diabetes. The UKPDS has shown that in hypertensive type 2 diabetic patients tight control of blood pressure can reduce the rate of progression of retinopathy by 34% after nine years of follow-up[18]. Treatment was also associated with a 47% reduction in the deterioration of visual activity, which suggested that tight BP control also prevented the development of diabetic maculopathy. In the UKPDS, anti-hypertensive treatment with a β-blocker (atenolol) was as effective as ACE-inhibitor therapy (captopril) in the prevention of microvascular end-points which mainly comprised retinal photocoagulation[24].

A much smaller study in normotensive type 2 patients showed a non-significant beneficial effect of ACE-inhibitors on retinopathy[51]. In normotensive type 1 diabetic subjects, the largest trial so far has been the EUCLID study which showed that the ACE-inhibitor lisinopril reduced the progression of retinopathy by one grading level by 50% over a two year period[52]. Lisinopril also significantly reduced the progression by two or more levels and progression to proliferative retinopathy. Active therapy reduced retinopathy incidence by 31%, but this was not statistically significant. Two much smaller studies in normotensive type 1 subjects also showed beneficial, but non-significant, effects of ACE-inhibitors on progression of retinopathy [53,54]. A meta-analysis of all four ACE-inhibitor studies in normotensive diabetic subjects gave P^2 for heterogeneity between studies of 0.59 (p >0.5), with a combined odds ratio (95% CI) of 0.49 (0.30–0.79) for treatment effect on the progression of retinopathy[52]. It has been suggested that ACE-inhibitors may have an effect on retinal angiogenesis, independent of their BP-lowering effect, by inhibiting production of angiotensin II which is a potent stimulus for the production of vascular endothelial growth factor (VEGF), itself thought to be involved in the pathogenesis of diabetic neovascularisation[55].

Larger clinical trials are needed, in both type 1 and type 2 diabetes, possibly using the newer angiotensin Il type 1 (AT_1) receptor blockers, to confirm these findings before changes in clinical practice are recommended. Such a trial, the Diabetic REtinopathy Cardesartan Trial (DIRECT), is now in progress.

HYPERTENSION AND DIABETIC NEUROPATHY

EPIDEMIOLOGY

Diabetic polyneuropathy is a major cause of morbidity in diabetic patients, being an important risk factor for foot ulceration and subsequent lower-extremity amputation[56]. Several epidemiological studies, both cross-sectional and prospective, have shown that the major risk factors for diabetic neuropathy are age, duration of diabetes and poor glycaemic control[43,57-59]. In the EURODIAB IDDM Complications Study diastolic, but not systolic, BP was significantly related to the prevalence of neuropathy in 3250 type 1 diabetic subjects[59]. In the prospective Epidemiology of Diabetes Complications (EDC) Study, hypertension was found to be a significant independent predictor of the development of distal symmetrical polyneuropathy in type 1 patients[60].

CLINICAL TRIALS

A randomised, double-blind, placebo-controlled trial using the ACE-inhibitor trandolapril in 41 normotensive patients with type 1 diabetes and type 2 diabetes with mild neuropathy indicated that this therapy may be associated with improvements in nerve conduction velocities[61]. However, vibration-perception threshold, autonomic function and the neuropathy symptom and deficit score showed no improvement. It is postulated that the mode of action of these drugs may be via an improvement in nerve blood flow. These potentially important findings need to be confirmed in larger studies using agents which block the action of angiotensin II.

HYPERTENSION AND DIABETIC NEPHROPATHY

EPIDEMIOLOGY

Diabetic nephropathy (DN) is now the leading cause of end-stage renal failure in the Western world[62]. In the USA in 1991, the cost of treating diabetic patients with renal replacement therapy exceeded $2 billion[63]. In type 1 diabetic subjects, DN is characterised by persistent albuminuria, a fall in glomerular filtration rate (GFR) and an increase in blood pressure[64]. Apart from raised BP, longer duration of diabetes and poor glycaemic control are also related to development of DN. In type 1 diabetes, DN occurs in only about one-third of patients, and there is evidence for familial clustering of this complication[65]. Several studies have shown that parental hypertension is associated with renal disease in offspring with type 1 diabetes[66-68]. This has led to a search for the susceptibility genes for DN which are likely to be linked to those for hypertension in general, and possibly for the renin-angiotensin system in particular[69].

CLINICAL TRIALS

The history of the treatment of hypertension in diabetic nephropathy has recently been reviewed by Mogensen[70]. He points out that about 40 years ago some physicians warned against antihypertensive treatment in renal disease, believing that the failing kidney needed a certain perfusion pressure to function and survive. In the early 1980s, however, Mogensen[71] and Parving[72] showed in uncontrolled trials that antihypertensive treatment, mainly with β-blockers and diuretics, was effective in preserving GFR and improving renal prognosis[73].

The largest randomised controlled trial in hypertensive type 1 patients with nephropathy indicated that ACE-inhibitors (in this case enalapril) might have a renal protective effect beyond their antihypertensive function[74]. The advantage of ACE-inhibitors over other antihypertensives in the reduction of proteinuria and preservation of GFR has been supported by several meta-analyses[75-77].

There has been much recent research as to whether ACE-inhibitors may be of benefit in preventing the progression of microalbuminuria to macro-albuminuria in normotensive diabetic subjects. In type 1 diabetes there have been at least 12 such randomised controlled trials, often with relatively small sample sizes, which have tended to support this hypothesis[78-89]. A meta-analysis of these 12 studies, using patient-specific data for 698 subjects, showed that ACE-inhibitor therapy reduced progression from microalbuminuria to macroalbuminuria by 62% (odds ratio 0.38, 95% CI 0.25, 0.57). Regression to normoalbuminuria was also increased significantly by ACE-inhibitor therapy[90]. Studies of ACE inhibition in non-European type 2 normotensive microalbu-minuric patients have also shown a benefit in terms of reduced progression of albuminuria[51,91-93].

There have been several recent reports[101-103] from trials using the newer AT_1-receptor blockers at various stages of diabetic nephropathy. The IRMA-A (Irbesartan MicroAlbuminuria) study group has examined the effect of two doses of the AT_1-receptor blocker irbesartan compared to placebo on the progression to nephropathy in hypertensive type 2 patients with persistant microalbuminuria[101]. With the high dose of the drug (300 mg) progression to nephropathy was reduced by 70%. The same drug has been used in the IDNT (Irbesartan Diabetic Nephropathy Trial) in hypertensive type 2 patients with proteinuria[102]. This trial compared the effect of irbesartan, the CCB amlo-dipine and placebo on the primary end-point which was a doubling of serum creatinine, end-stage renal failure (ESRF) or death. Patients had their blood pressure controlled with other antihypertensives where necessary. After an average follow-up of 2.6 years, irbesartan had produced a 33% reduction in the time to doubling of serum creatinine, but there was no difference in the time to all-cause mortality. Similar results were obtained in RENAAL (Reduction of End-points in Non-insulin dependent diabetes mellitus with the Angiotensin-II receptor Antagonist Losartan[103]). This was also a study in hypertensive type 2 patients with proteinuria. In addition to receiving conventional anti-hypertensives, patients were randomised to either losartan or placebo. After a mean follow-up of 3.4 years, the composite end-point of doubling of serum creatinine, ESRF or death was reduced by 16% (p = 0.024) in the losartan-treated group. The risk of progression to ESRD was reduced by 28% (p = 0.002). It has been estimated that in these patients treatment with losartan plus conventional blood pressure therapy would reduce the number of days with ESRF by 32%.

GUIDELINES FOR THE TREATMENT OF HYPERTENSION IN DIABETIC PATIENTS

Between 1992 and 1996, at least nine sets of guidelines had been published which generally recommended target BP levels of below 140/90 mmHg for the treatment of hypertension in diabetic subjects. Since 1996 three sets of guidelines have suggested that the target BP for diabetic subjects should be lower, at 130/85 mmHg[94-96] (see Table 17.4). The results of the HOT study and the UKPDS were cited as providing evidence for a reduction in cardiovascular risk with reduction in BP to these levels in diabetic subjects. The Joint National Committee (JNC) VI report[95] suggested that for diabetic subjects with proteinuria >1 g/24hr a treatment goal of below 125/75 mmHg was recommended.

Following the publication of these various guidelines, several studies have examined the extent of awareness, treatment and control of hypertension in samples of diabetic subjects. In the EURODIAB IDDM complications study, 3250 type 1 diabetic subjects were studied in 31 diabetes centres in 16 European countries[97]. Hypertension was defined as a systolic BP $\geq$140 mmHg or diastolic BP $\geq$90 mmHg or current use of antihypertensives. Control was defined as a BP <130/85 mmHg. The findings were that 24% of subjects had hypertension, of whom less than one-half (48%) were aware of a previous diagnosis and of whom 42% were currently on treatment. Only 11.3% of those with hypertension were both treated and controlled. The majority (81%) of those treated were on a single drug, most commonly an ACE-inhibitor (47%).

Two population-based studies in the USA[98] and England[99] have provided data on the extent of under-diagnosis and under-treatment of hypertension in type 2 diabetic subjects. The National Health and Nutrition Examination Surveys (NHANES) carried out in 1976–1980 in the USA used the older WHO definition of hypertension ($\geq$160/95 mmHg) and the JNC V definition of ($\geq$140/90 mmHg). Using the WHO definition, 63% of persons with type 2 diabetes had hypertension, of whom 45% were uncontrolled. With the JNC V definition, these figures were 74% and 67% respectively. In the Health Surveys for England (1991–94), 51% of those with diabetes had hypertension

Table 17.4. Guidelines on management of hypertension in diabetes.

	Year	Intervention threshold	Target BP
American Diabetes Association[94]	1996	140/90	$\leq$130/85
Joint National Committee-VI[95]	1997	130/85	$\leq$130/85
Proteinuria >1 g/24h		130/85	$\leq$125/75
British Hypertension Society[100]	1999	140/90	<140/80
World Health Organisation/International Society for Hypertension[96]	1999	140/90	<130/85

($\geq$160/90 mmHg or on treatment). One-third of these were untreated and less than one-half of those on treatment had BP <160/95 mmHg.

CONCLUSIONS

Recent years have seen a rapid accumulation of epidemiological evidence that raised arterial pressure is an important, and potentially modifiable, contributor to increased risk of the major diabetic complications. Completed and ongoing clinical trials are clarifying the threshold levels of blood pressure above which antihypertensive treatment is of benefit. However, there are also indications that the awareness, treatment and control of hypertension in diabetic populations is far from satisfactory in many parts of the world. This raises an important challenge for those involved in the planning and implementation of diabetes care programmes in primary and secondary care settings.

ACKNOWLEDGEMENTS

The skilled assistance provided by Tara and Ashley West in the preparation of this chapter is gratefully acknowledged.

REFERENCES

1. Amos AF, McCarty DJ, Zimmet P (1997) The rising global burden of diabetes and its complications: estimates and projections to the year 2010. *Diabetic Med.* **14 (Suppl 5)**: S1–S85.
2. Bingley PJ, Gale EAM (1989) Rising incidence of IDDM in Europe. *Diabetes Care* **12**: 289–95.
3. Colhoun HM, Fuller JH (2000) Blood pressure and diabetes mellitus. In Bulpitt CJ, (ed.) *Handbook of Hypertension*, Amsterdam: Elsevier, pp. 489–508.
4. Gress TW, Nieto FJ, Shahar E, Wofford MR, Brancati FL (Atherosclerosis Risk in Communities Study Investigators) (2000) Hypertension and antihypertensive therapy as risk factors for type 2 diabetes mellitus. *New Engl. J. Med.* **342**: 905–12.
5. Hanefeld M, Fischer S, Julius U, Schulze J, Schwanebeck U, Schmechel H, Ziegelasch HJ, Linder J (1996) Risk factors for myocardial infarction and death in newly detected NIDDM: the Diabetes Intervention Study, 11-year follow-up. *Diabetologia* **39**: 1577–83.
6. Stamler J, Vaccaro O, Neaton JD, Wentworth D (Multiple Risk Factor Intervention Trial Research Group) (1993) Diabetes, other risk factors, and 12-year cardiovascular mortality for men screened in the multiple risk factor intervention trial. *Diab. Care* **16**: 434–44.
7. Manson JE, Colditz GA, Stampfer MJ, Willett WC, Krolewski AS, Rosner B, Arky RA, Speizer FE, Hennekens CH (1991) A prospective study of maturity-onset

diabetes mellitus and risk of coronary heart disease and stroke in women. *Arch. Intern. Med.* **151**: 1141–7.

8. Turner RC, Millns H, Neil HAW, Stratton IM, Manley SE, Matthews DR, Holman RR (1998) Risk factors for coronary artery disease in non-insulin dependent diabetes mellitus: United Kingdom Prospective Diabetes Study (UKPDS: 23). *BMJ* **316**: 823–8.

9. Fuller JH, Stevens LK, Wang S-L, and the WHO Multinational Study Group (2001) Risk factors for cardiovascular disease in diabetes mellitus: the WHO multinational study of vascular diseases in diabetes. *Diabetologia* **44 (Suppl 2)**: S54–S64.

10. Lee ET, Keen H, Bennett PH, Fuller JH, Lu M, and the WHO Multinational Study Group (2001) Follow-up of the WHO Multinational Study of Vascular Disease in Diabetes: general description and morbidity. *Diabetologia* **44**(Suppl. 2): S3–S13.

11. Fuller JH, Stevens LK (1991) Epidemiology of hypertension in diabetic patients and implications for treatment. *Diab. Care* **14 (Suppl 4)**: 8–12.

12. Wang S-L, Head J, Stevens L, Fuller JH (WHO Multinational Study Group) (1996) Excess mortality and its relation to hypertension and proteinuria in diabetic patients: the WHO Multinational Study of Vascular Disease in Diabetes. *Diab. Care* **19**: 305–12.

13. Hypertension Detection and Follow-up Program Cooperative Group (1979) Five-year findings of the hypertension detection and follow-up Program. 1. Reduction in mortality of persons with high blood pressure, including mild hypertension. *JAMA* **242**: 2562–71.

14. The Hypertension Detection and Follow-up Program Cooperative Research Group (1985) Mortality findings for stepped-care and referred-care participants in the hypertension detection and follow-up program, stratified by other risk factors. The Hypertension Detection and Follow-up Program Cooperative Research Group. *Prevent. Med.* **14**: 312–35.

15. SHEP Cooperative Research Group (1991) Prevention of stroke by antihypertensive drug treatment in older persons with isolated systolic hypertension. Final results of the systolic hypertension in the elderly program (SHEP). *JAMA* **265**: 3255–64.

16. Curb JD, Pressel SL, Cutler JA, Savage PJ, Applegate WB. Camel G, Davis BR, Frost PH, Gonzalez N, Gutnrie G, Oberman A, Rutan GH, Stamler J (1996) Effect of diuretic-based antihypertensive treatment on cardiovascular disease risk in older diabetic patients with isolated systolic hypertension. *JAMA* **276**: 1886–92.

17. Fuller J, Stevens LK, Chaturvedi N, Holloway JF (1999) Antihypertensive therapy in diabetes mellitus (Cochrane Review). *The Cochrane Library* 1–13.

18. UK Prospective Diabetes Study Group (1998) Tight blood pressure control and risk of macrovascular and microvascular complications in type 2 diabetes: UKPDS 38. *BMJ* **317**: 703–13.

19. Tuomilehto J, Rastenyte D, Birkenhager WH, Thijs L, Antikainen R, Bulpitt CJ, Fletcher AE, Forette F, Goldhaber A, Palatini P, Sarti C, Fagard R, for the Systolic Hypertension in Europe Trial Investigators (1999) Effects of calcium-channel blockade in older patients with diabetes and systolic hypertension. *New Engl. J. Med.* **340**: 677–84.

20. Wang JG, Staessen JA, Gong L, Liu L (2000) Chinese trial on isolated systolic hypertension in the elderly. Systolic Hypertension in China (Syst-China) Collaborative Group. *Arch. Intern. Med.* **160**: 211–20.

21. Hansson L, Zanchetti A, Carruthers SG, Dahlof D, Julius S, Menard J *et al.* (1998) Effects of intensive blood-pressure lowering and low dose aspirin in patients with

hypertension: prinicipal results of the Hypertension Optimal Treatment (HOT) randomised trial. *Lancet* **351**: 1755–62.

22. The Heart Outcomes Prevention Evaluation Study Investigators (2000) Effects of an angiotensin-converting-enzyme inhibitor, ramipril, on cardiovascular events in high-risk patients. *New Eng. J. Med.* **342**: 145–53.

23. Heart Outcomes Prevention Evaluation (HOPE) Study Investigators (2000) Effects of ramipril on cardiovascular and microvascular outcomes in people with diabetes mellitus: results of the HOPE study and MICRO-HOPE substudy. *Lancet* **355**: 253–9.

24. UK Prospective Diabetes Study Group (1998) Efficacy of atenolol and captopril in reducing risk of macrovascular and microvascular complications in type 2 diabetes: UKPDS 39. *BMJ* **317**: 713–20.

25. Hansson L, Lindholm LH, Niskanen L, Lanke J, Hedner T, Niklason A, Luomanmaki K, Dahlof B, de Faire U, Morlin C, Karlberg BE, Wester PO, Bjorck J-E, for the Captopril Prevention Project (CAPP) Study Group (1999) Effect of angiotensin-converting-enzyme inhibition compared with conventional therapy on cardiovascular morbidity and mortality in hypertension: the Captopril Prevention Project (CAPP) randomised trial. *Lancet* **353**: 611–6.

26. Estacio RO, Savage S, Nagel NJ, Schrier RW (1996) Baseline characteristics of participants in the Appropriate Blood Pressure Control in Diabetes trial. *Control. Clin. Trials* **17**: 242–57.

27. Tatti P, Pahor M, Byington RP, Di Mauro P, Guarisco R, Strollo F (1998) Outcome results of the Fosinopril versus Amlodipine Cardiovascular Events Randomised Trial (FACET) in patients with hypertension and NIDDM. *Diab. Care* **21**: 597–603.

28. Estacio RO, Jeffers BW, Hiatt WR, Biggerstaff SL, Gifford N, Schrier RW (1998) The effect of nisoldipine as compared with enalapril on cardiovascular outcomes in patients with non-insulin-dependent diabetes and hypertension. *New Engl. J. Med.* **338**: 645–52.

29. Pahor M, Psaty BM, Furberg CD (1998) Treatment of hypertensive patients with diabetes. *Lancet* **351**: 689–90.

30. Hebert PR, Manson JE, Hennekens CH (1992) Pharmacologic therapy of mild to moderate hypertension: possible generalizability to diabetics [Review]. *J. Am. Soc. Nephrology* **3**: S135–9.

31. Staessen JA, Birkenhäger WH, Fagard RH (2000) Dihydropyridine calcium-channel blockers for the treatment of hypertensive diabetic patients. *Europ. Heart. J.* **21**: 2–7.

32. Cutler JA (1998) Calcium-channel-blockers for hypertension—uncertainty continues. *New Engl. J. Med.* **338**: 679–81.

33. Hansson L, Hedner T, Lund-Johansen P, Kjeldsen SE, Lindholm LH, Syvertsen JO, Lanke J. de Faire U, Dahlof B, Karlberg BE (2000) Randomised trial of effects of calcium antagonists compared with diuretics and β-blockers on cardiovascular morbidity and mortality in hypertension: the Nordic Diltiazem (NORDIL) study. *Lancet* **356**: 359–65.

34. Hansson L, Lindholm LH, Ekbom T, Dahlöf B, Lanke J, Scherstén B, Wester P-O, Hedner T, de Faire U, for the STOP-Hypertension-2 Study Group (1999) Randomised trial of old and new antihypertensive drugs in elderly patients: cardiovascular mortality and morbidity. The Swedish Trial in Old Patients with Hypertension-2 study. *Lancet* **354**: 1751–6.

35. Davis BR, Cutler JA, Gordon DJ, Furberg CD, Wright JT Jr., Cushman WC, Grimm RH, LaRosa J, Whelton PK, Perry HM, Alderman MH, Ford CE, Oparil S,

Francis C, Proschan M, Pressel S, Black HR, Hawkins CM (1996) Rationale and design for the Antihypertensive and Lipid Lowering Treatment to Prevent Heart Attack Trial (ALLHAT). ALLHAT Research Group. *Am. J. Hypertens.* **9**: 342–60.

36. Barzilay JI, Jones CL, Davis BR, Basile JN, Goff DC Jr., Ciocon JO *et al.* (2001) Baseline characteristics of the diabetic participants in the antihypertensive and lipid-lowering treatment to prevent heart attack trial (ALLHAT). ALLHAT Collaborative Research Group. *Diab. Care* **24**: 654–8.

37. The ALLHAT Officers and Coordinators for the ALLHAT Collaborative Research Group (2000) Major cardiovascular events in hypertensive patients randomized to doxazosin vs. chlorthalidone. The Antihypertensive and Lipid-Lowering Treatment to Prevent Heart Attack Trial (ALLHAT). *JAMA* **283**: 1967–75.

38. Sever PS, Mackay JA (1996) The hypertension trials. *J. Hypertens. Suppl* **14**: S29–S33.

39. Klein R, Klein BEK (1997) Diabetic eye disease. *Lancet* **350**: 197–204.

40. Sjolie AK (1994) Eye diseases. In Williams DRR, Papoz L, Fuller JH (eds) *Diabetes in Europe*, London: John Libbey, pp. 61–71.

41. Janka HU, Warram JH, Rand LI, Krolewski AS (1989) Risk factors for progression of background retinopathy in long-standing IDDM. *Diabetes* **38**: 460–4.

42. Klein R (1995) Hyperglycemia and microvascular and macrovascular disease in diabetes. *Diab. Care* **18**: 258–68.

43. The Diabetes Control and Complications Trial Research Group (1993) The effect of intensive treatment of diabetes on the development and progression of long-term complications in insulin-dependent diabetes mellitus. *New Engl. J Med.* **329**: 977–86.

44. UK Prospective Diabetes Study Group (1998) Intensive blood-glucose control with sulphonylureas or insulin compared with conventional treatment and risk of complications in patients with type 2 diabetes (UKPDS 33). *Lancet* **352**: 837–53.

45. Klein R, Klein BEK, Moss SE, Davis MD, DeMets DL (1989) Is blood pressure a predictor of the incidence or progression of diabetic retinopathy? *Arch. Intern. Med.* **149**: 2427–32.

46. Orchard TJ (1994) From diagnosis and classification to complications and therapy. *Diab. Care* **17**: 326–38.

47. Sjolie AK, Stephenson J, Aldington S, Kohner E, Janka H, Stevens L, Fuller JH, The EURODIAB IDDM Complications Study Group (1997) Retinopathy and vision loss in insulin-dependent diabetes in Europe. *Ophthalmology* **104**: 252–60.

48. Teuscher A, Schnell H, Wilson PWF (1998) Incidence of diabetic retinopathy and relationship to baseline plasma glucose and blood pressure. *Diabetes Care* **11**: 246–51.

49. Keen H, Lee ET, Russell D, Miki E, Bennett PH, Lu M, and the WHO Multinational Study Group (2001)The appearance of retinopathy and progression to prolferative retinopathy: the WHO Multinational Study of Vascular Disease in Diabetes. *Diabetologia* **44 (Suppl 2)**: 522–530.

50. Stratton IM, Kohner EM, Aldington SJ, Turner RC, Holman RR, Manley SE, Matthews DR, UK Prospective Diabetes Study Group (2001) UKPDS 50: Risk factors for incidence and progression of retinopathy in type 2 diabetes over six years from diagnosis. *Diabetologia* **44**: 156–63.

51. Ravid M, Savin H, Jutrin I, Bental T, Katz B, Lishner M (1993) Long-term stabilizing effect of angiotensin-converting enzyme inhibition on plasma creatinine and on proteinuria in normotensive type II diabetic patients. *Ann. Intern. Med.* **118**: 577–81.

52. Chaturvedi N, Sjolie A-K, Stephenson JM, Abrahamian H, Keipes M, Castellarin A, Rogulja-Pepeonik Z, Fuller JH, and the EUCLID Study Group (1998) Effect of lisinopril on progression of retinopathy in normotensive people with type 1 diabetes. *Lancet* **351**: 28–31.
53. Chase HP, Garg SK, Harris S, Hoops S, Jackson WE, Holmes DL (1993) Angiotensin-converting enzyme inhibitor treatment for young normotensive diabetic subjects: a two-year trial. *Ann. Ophthalmol.* **25**: 284–9.
54. Larsen M, Hommel E, Parving H-H, Lund-Andersen H (1990) Protective effect of captopril on the blood-retina barrier in normotensive insulin-dependent diabetic patients with nephropathy and backgroung retinopathy. *Graefe's Arch. Clin. Exp. Ophthalmol.* **228**: 505–9.
55. Williams B, Baker AQ, Gallacher B, Lodwick D (1995) Angiotensin II increases vascular permeability factor gene expression by human vascular smooth muscle cells. *Hypertension* **25**: 913–7.
56. Ward JD (1994) Diabetic neuropathy. In Williams DRR, Papoz L, Fuller JH (eds) *Diabetes in Europe*, London: John Libbey, pp. 72–7.
57. Maser RE, Steenkiste AR, Dorman JS, Nielsen VK, Bass EB, Drash AL, Becker DJ, Kuller LH, Greene DA, Orchard TJ (1989) Epidemiological correlates of diabetic neuropathy. Report from Pittsburgh Epidemiology of Diabetes Complications Study. *Diabetes* **38**: 1456–61.
58. Franklin GM, Shetterly SM, Cohen JA, Baxter J, Hamman RF (1994) Risk factors for distal symmetric neuropathy in NIDDM. The San Luis Valley Diabetes Study. *Diab. Care* **17**: 1172–7.
59. Tesfaye S, Stevens LK, Stephenson JM, Fuller JH, Plater M, Ionescu-Tirgoviste C, Nuber A, Pozza G, Ward JD, EURODIAB IDDM Study Group (1996) Prevalence of diabetic peripheral neuropathy and its relation to glycaemic control and potential risk factors: the EURODIAB IDDM Complications Study. *Diabetologia* **39**: 1377–84.
60. Forrest KYZ, Maser RE, Pambianco G, Becker DJ, Orchard TJ (1997) Hypertension as a risk factor for diabetic neuropathy. A prospective study. *Diabetes* **46**: 665–70.
61. Malik RA, Williamson S, Abbott C, Carrington AL, Iqbal J, Schady W, Boulton AJ (1998) Effect of angiotensin-converting-enzyme (ACE) inhibitor trandolapril on human diabetic neuropathy: randomised double- blind controlled trial. *Lancet* **352**: 1978–81.
62. Raine AEG (1997) Evolution worldwide of the treatment of patients with advanced diabetic nephropathy by renal replacement therapy. In Mogensen CE (ed.) *The Kidney and Hypertension in Diabetes Mellitus*, Boston: Kluwer Academic Publishers, pp. 473–80.
63. Nelson RG, Knowler WC, Pettitt DJ, Bennett PH (1999) Kidney diseases in diabetes. In Harris MI, Cowie CC, Stern MP, Boyko EJ, Reiber GE, Bennett PH (eds) *Diabetes in America*, National Institutes of Health, pp. 349–400.
64. Parving H-H, Smidt UM, Friisberg B, Bonnevie-Nielsen V, Andersen AR (1981) A prospective study of glomerular filtration rate and arterial blood pressure in insulin-dependent diabetics with diabetic nephropathy. *Diabetologia* **20**: 457–61.
65. Krolewski AS, Fogarty DG, Warram JH (1998) Hypertension and nephropathy in diabetes mellitus: what is inherited and what is acquired? *Diabetes Res. Clin. Pract.* **39 (Suppl)** S1–14.
66. Viberti GC, Keen H, Wiseman MJ (1987) Raised arterial pressure in parents of proteinuric insulin dependent diabetics. *Br. Med. J.* **295**: 515–7.

67. Fagerudd JA, Tarnow L, Jacobsen P, Stenman S, Nielsen FS, Pettersson-Fernholm KJ, Gronhagen-Riska C, Parving H-H, Groop P-H (1998) Predisposition to essential hypertension and development of diabetic nephropathy in IDDM patients. *Diabetes* **47**: 439–44.
68. Roglic G, Colhoun HM, Stevens LK, Lemkes HH, Manes C, Fuller JH, and the EURODIAB IDDM Complications Study Group (1998) Parental history of hypertension and parental history of diabetes and microvascular complications in insulin-dependent diabetes mellitus: the EURODIAB IDDM complications study. *Diabetic Med.* **15**: 418–26.
69. Moczulski DK, Rogus JJ, Antonellis A, Warram JH, Krolewski AS (1998) Major susceptibility locus for nephropathy in type 1 diabetes on chromosome 3q. Results of novel discordant sib-pair analysis. *Diabetes* **47**: 1164–9.
70. Mogensen CE (1995) Diabetic renal disease: The quest for normotension – and beyond. *Diabetic Med.* **12**: 756–69.
71. Mogensen CE (1982) Long-term antihypertensive treatment inhibiting progression of diabetic nephropathy. *B. Med. J.* **285**: 685–8.
72. Parving H-H, Smidt UM, Andersen AR, Svendsen PA (1983) Early aggressive antihypertensive treatment reduces rate of decline in kidney function in diabetic nephropathy. *Lancet* **28**: 1175–9.
73. Mogensen CE (1999) Microalbuminuria, blood pressure and diabetic renal disease: origin and development of ideas. *Diabetologia* **42**: 263–85.
74. Lewis EJ, Hunsicker LG, Bain RP, Rohde RD, and the Collaborative Study Group (1993) The effect of angiotensin-converting-enzyme inhibition on diabetic nephropathy. *New Engl. J. Med.* **329**: 1456–62.
75. Kasiske BL, Kalil RSN, Ma JZ, Liao M, Keane WF (1993) Effect of antihypertensive therapy on the kidney in patients with diabetes: a meta-regression analysis. *Annals of Internal Medicine* **118**: 129–38.
76. Gansevoort RT, Sluiter WJ, Hemmelder MH, de Zeeuw D, de Jong PE (1995) Antiproteinuric effect of blood-pressure-lowering agents: a meta-analysis of comparative trials. *Nephrol. Dial. Transplant* **10**: 1963–74.
77. Weidmann P, Schneider M, Bohlen L (1995) Therapeutic efficacy of different antihypertensive drugs in human diabetic nephropathy: an updated meta-analysis. *Nephrol. Dial. Transplant* **10(Suppl. 9)**: 39–45.
78. Mathiesen ER, Hommel E, Giese J, Parving H-H (1991) Efficacy of captopril in postponing nephropathy in normotensive insulin dependent diabetic patients with microalbuminuria. *Br. Med. J.* **303**: 81–7.
79. Marre M, Chatellier G, Leblanc H, Guyene TT, Menard J, Passa P (1988) Prevention of diabetic nephropathy with enalapril in normotensive diabetics with microalbuminuria. *Br. Med .J.* **297**: 1092–5.
80. O'Donnell MJ, Rowe BR, Lawson N, Horton A, Gyde OH, Barnett AH (1993) Placebo-controlled trial of lisinopril in normotensive diabetic patients with incipient nephropathy. *J. Human Hypertens.* **7**: 327–32.
81. Viberti G, Mogensen CE, Groop LC, Pauls JF (1994) Effect of captopril on progression to clinical proteinuria in patients with insulin-dependent diabetes mellitus and microalbuminuria. *JAMA* **271**: 275–9.
82. Laffel LMB, McGill JB, Gans DJ (1995) The beneficial effect of angiotensin-converting enzyme inhibition with captopril on diabetic nephropathy in normotensive IDDM patients with microalbuminuria. *Am. J. Med.* **99**: 497–504.
83. The EUCLID Study Group (1997) Randomised placebo-controlled trial of lisinopril in normotensive patients with insulin-dependent diabetes and normo-albuminuria or microalbuminuria. *Lancet* **349**: 1787–92.

84. Crepaldi G, Carta Q, Deferrari G, Mangili R, Navalesi R, Santeusanio F, Spalluto A, Vanasia A, Marco Villa G, Nosadini R, the Italian Microalbuminuria Study Group (1998) Effects of lisinopril and nifedipine on the progression to overt albuminuria in IDDM patients with incipient nephropathy and normal blood pressure. *Diab. Care* **21**: 104–10.
85. Melbourne Diabetic Nephropathy Study Group (1991) Comparison between perindopril and nifedipine in hypertensive and normotensive diabetic patients with microalbuminuria. *Br. Med. J.* **302**: 210–15.
86. Ebbehoj E, Poulsen PL, Nosadini R, Fioretto P, Crepaldi G, and Mogensen CE (1998) Early ACE-I intervention in microalbuminuria: 24h BP, renal function, and exercise changes. *Diabetologia* **41 (Suppl 1)**, A5.
87. Bojestig,M, Karlberg BE, and the PRIMA study group (1997) ACE-inhibition during two years did not improve U-AER in normotensive microalbuminuric IDDM patients. *Diabetologia* **40 (Suppl 1)**, A544.
88. The Atlantis Study Group (2000) Low-dose ramipril reduces microalbuminuria in type 1 diabetic patients without hypertension. *Diab. Care* **23**: 1823–9.
89. The European Study for the Prevention of Renal Disease in Type 1 Diabetes (ESPRIT) (2001) Effect of three years of antihypertensive therapy on renal structure in type 1 diabetic patients with albuminuria *Diabetes* **50**: 843–50.
90. The ACE Inhibitors in Diabetic Nephropathy Trialist Group (2001) Should all patients with type 1 diabetes mellitus and microalbuminuria receive angiotensin-converting enzyme inhibitors? *Ann. Intern. Med.* **134**: 370–9.
91. Ravid M, Lang R, Rachmani R, Lishner M (1996) Long-term renoprotective effect of angiotensin-converting enzyme inhibition in non-insulin-dependent diabetes mellitus. A seven-year follow-up study. *Arch. Intern. Med.* **156**: 286–9.
92. Sano T, Kawamura T, Matsumae H, Sasaki H, Nakayama M, Hara T, Matsuo S, Hotta N, Sakamoto N (1994) Effects of long-term enalapril treatment on persistant microalbuminuria in well-controlled hypertensive and normotensive NIDDM patients. *Diab. Care* **17**: 420–4.
93. Ahmad J, Siddiqui MA, Ahmad H (1997) Effective postponement of diabetic nephropathy with enalapril in normotensive type 2 diabetic patients with microalbuminuria. *Diab. Care* **20**: 1576–81.
94. Consensus Statement (1996) Treatment of hypertension in diabetes. *Diab. Care* **19 (Suppl 2)**: S107–S113.
95. Joint National Committee on Prevention, Detection, Evaluation and Treatment of High Blood Pressure (1997) Sixth Report. *Arch. Intern. Med.* **157**: 2413–46.
96. Guidelines Subcommittee (1999) World Health Organization – International Society of Hypertension guidelines for the management of hypertension. *J. Hypertens.* **17**: 151–83.
97. Collado-Mesa F, Colhoun HM, Stevens LK, Boavida J, Ferriss JB, Kempler P, Michel G, Roglic G, Fuller JH, and the EURODIAB IDDM Complications Study Group (1999) Prevalence and management of hypertension in type 1 diabetes mellitus in Europe: the EURODIAB IDDM complications study. *Diabetic Med.* **16**: 1–9.
98. Cowie CC, Harris MI (1995) Physical and metabolic characteristics of persons with diabetes. In Harris MI, Cowie CC, Stern MP, Boyko EJ, Reiber GE, Bennett PH, (eds) *Diabetes in America*, National Institutes of Health, pp. 117–64.
99. Colhoun HM, Dong W, Barakatt MT, Mather HM, Poulter NR (1999) The scope for cardiovascular disease risk factor intervention among people with diabetes mellitus in England: a population-based analysis from the Health Surveys for England 1991–94. *Diabetic Med.* **16**: 35–40.

100. British Hypertension Society (1999) Guidelines for management of hypertension: report of the third working party. *J. Human. Hypertens.* **13**: 570–92.

101. Parving HH, Lehnert H, Brochner-Mortensen J, Gomis R, Andersen S, Arner P (2001) The effect of Irbesartan on the development of diabetic nephropathy in patients with type 2 diabetes. *New Engl. J. Med.* **345**: 870–878.

102. Lewis EJ, Hunsicker LG, Clarke WR, Berl T, Pohl MA, Lewis JB, Ritz E, Atkins RC, Rohde R, Raz I (2001) Renoproctive effect of the angiotensin-receptor antagonist ibersartan in patients with nephropathy due to type 2 diabetes. *New Engl. J. Med.* **345**: 851–860.

103. Brenner BM, Cooper ME, de Zeeuw D, Keane WF, Mitch WE, Parving HH, Remuzzi G, Snipinn SM, Zhang Z, Shahinfar S (2001) Effects of losartan on renal and cardiovascular outcomes in patients with type 2 diabetes and nephropathy. *New Eng. J. Med.* **345**: 861–869.

18

Prevention of Hyperlipidaemia

TREVOR J. ORCHARD AND LINDA FRIED

Epidemiology and Medicine, Univ. of Pittsburgh, Pittsburgh, PA 15213, USA

INTRODUCTION

The effect of improving the lipoprotein profile on complication outcomes in diabetic subjects is critical, for diabetes is clearly more than a 'sugar' disease alone. In this chapter, we will discuss the evidence for lipid modulation in terms of both micro- and macrovascular outcomes. The first two sections will briefly review the background to a lipid/lipoprotein connection and then present the current state of the art. In the conclusion an assessment of the extent to which current interventions are evidence-based, and the studies that need to be done in order to fill the gaps, will be made. Interested readers should contact Trevor Orchard for a copy of the search strategy used for this chapter.

BACKGROUND

Classical diabetic dyslipidaemia is characterized by high serum triglycerides and low HDL cholesterol concentrations. These result from the overproduction and/or impaired clearance of VLDL particles (processes linked to insulin resistance) which are the key lipid metabolic abnormalities seen in type 2 diabetes[1]. Associated with the decreased VLDL catabolism is a partially consequential reduction of HDLc. It should be noted that total and LDL cholesterol concentrations are not greatly altered in moderately well controlled type 2 diabetes. Another characteristic lipid abnormality seen in type 2 diabetes and insulin resistance is a shift in density of the LDL particle to the more dense, or type B, particle[2]. This change is thought to enhance the atherogenecity of LDL[3] and is correlated with triglycerides and, in women, with postmenopausal status. These multiple, interrelated changes make it difficult to identify exactly which component of the lipid profile is pathologically related

The Evidence Base for Diabetes Care. Edited by R. Williams, W. Herman, A.-L. Kinmonth and N. J. Wareham.
© 2002 John Wiley & Sons, Ltd

to disease. From a clinical (and trial evidence based) standpoint, we are, however, essentially limited to the three main measures: LDLc, HDLc and triglycerides.

Interestingly, in moderately well controlled type 1 diabetes, absolute concentrations are not greatly disturbed[1]; indeed, HDL cholesterol is often a little above normal[4]. Lipoprotein concentration, therefore, accounts for little of the excess cardiovascular disease (CVD) risk seen in type 1 diabetes. This has led to an increased focus on lipoprotein composition, and a number of differences have been identified, including triglyceride enrichment of LDL/HDL[5] and a disordered, reverse cholesterol transport system[6]. Recent work has also suggested LDL oxidation and immune complex formation may be particularly important risk factors[7]. Further study is needed to determine if interventions directed at improving these compositional changes or oxidative properties will result in a reduction in CVD events.

MACROVASCULAR COMPLICATIONS

Many studies have demonstrated the predictive power of cholesterol, both LDL (directly) and HDL (indirectly) for CVD in type 2 diabetes from early Framingham[8] data to the more recent follow-ups of men screened for the Multiple Risk Factor Intervention Trial (MRFIT) trial[9], and women in the Nurses Health Study[10]. Also apparent in diabetes is the greater predictive power of triglycerides[11,12], which probably reflects a different VLDL (and remnant) particle distribution. Our knowledge of lipid/CVD relationships in type 1 diabetes is more limited. However, in general terms, similar relationships to the general population appear to be present from the Pittsburgh and Eurodiab studies with, as in type 2, a suggestion that triglycerides may play a greater role[13-15].

Unfortunately, most of the early prevention trials with CVD outcomes ignored or excluded patients with diabetes. Thus, there has been until recently an incomplete evidence base on which to build therapeutic recommendations. Nonetheless, in the USA, the third report of the National Cholesterol Education Programme (NCEP)[16] Adult Treatment Panel (ATP) in 2001 and previously the American Diabetes Association (ADA)[17] in 1998 have made such recommendations, which apply primarily to type 2 subjects. They are summarized in Table 18.1 along with the less aggressive European and UK recommendations, which do not specifically focus on diabetes. The equivalence of the NCEP III and ADA goal for LDLc for diabetic subjects without coronary artery disease (CAD) (100 mg/dl; 2.6 mmol/L) to the NCEP III goal for general subjects with CAD (also 100 mg/dl; 2.6 mmol/L) is supported by the recent demonstration by Haffner that, at least in Finland, these two subject groups are at similar risk for future events[18]. NCEP ATP III also focuses on the metabolic syndrome (insulin resistance) as a secondary target for intervention.

Table 18.1. NCEP-III, ADA and BHL Guidelines – Cholesterol Goal + Intervention Levels (mg/dl: mmol/L)[5]

	NCEP-II[16]			ADA[17]		BHL[ILS]	
	CAD+	No CAD+ 2 RF	No CAD <2 RF[1]	CAD+	CAD-	CAD+	No CAD + RF[4]
LDL-c goal	100 (2.6)	130[2] (3.4)	160[2] (4.1)	100 (2.6)	100 (2.6)	132 (3.4)	159 (4.1)
Diet initiation level	100 (2.6)	130[2] (3.4)	160[2] (4.1)	100 (2.6)	100 (2.6)	132 (3.4)	159 (4.1)
Drug initiation level	130 (2.6)	160[2] (3.4)	190[2] (4.9)	100 (2.6)	100–130[3] (2.6–3.4)	132 (3.4)	193 (5.0)

NCEP = National Cholesterol Education Programme. ADA = American Diabetes Association. BHL = British Hyperlipidaemia Association. RF = risk factors.
[1] As diabetes is one risk factor, all male diabetic persons aged 45 years or over or females aged 55 years or over, qualify as having two risk factors irrespective of their other risk factor status (HDL, hypertension, smoking).
[2] Statement in text adds 'Because of the high risk for CHD resulting from non-insulin-dependent diabetes mellitus, aggressive lowering of LDL cholesterol levels, similar to that recommended for established CHD, can be applied to diabetic patients'.
[3] Statement in text adds 'For diabetic patients with multiple CHD risk factors some authorities recommend initiation of drug therapy when LDL levels are between 100–130 m/dl'.
[4] No specific recommendations are made for those with diabetes.
[5] A Task Force of the European Society of Cardiology, European Atherosclerosis Society, and European Society of Hypertension recommends intervention based on 20%, 10-year risk of CAD with no specific recommendation for those with diabetes except '…the threshold for the reduction of these other risk factors has to be lower in diabetic patients'.[116]

In the next two sections, we will review the data on which such recommendations are based by summarizing the major trials that have included (or focused on) diabetic participants. We divide these according to whether the participants have known cardiovascular disease (secondary prevention) or not (primary prevention). These trials predominantly feature type 2 diabetic participants. With the exception of three fibrate trials (Helsinki, VA-HIT and BIP; see below), the primary lipid fraction targeted was LDL cholesterol, while the outcomes in all trials were generally based on clinical events. Measures of lesion progression or regression were studied, however, only one major study, which has recently reported exclusively studied diabetic subjects[39].

PRIMARY PREVENTION

Table 18.2 presents data from the three primary prevention trials with data involving diabetic participants. While the majority of the early primary lipid lowering trials systematically excluded those with diabetes (e.g. Lipid Research Clinic Trial (LRC)[19] and the Multiple Risk Factor Intervention Trial (MRFIT)[20]), one of them, the Helsinki Heart Study[21], did include a small group of type 2 diabetic patients. This remains one of only three fully described studies of lipid modulation in diabetes by drugs in the primary setting. In general, this study, using a fibric acid, gemfibrozil (whose principal action is to enhance VLDL catabolism through stimulation of lipoprotein lipase) was remarkably successful, yielding a 34% fall in the primary end-point, CHD death or MI[21]. The trial was initially conceived as an HDLc-raising trial, but was later reformatted so that the entry criteria was a non-HDL cholesterol >5.2 mmol/L (200 mg/dl). The mean LDLc, 5.2 mmol/L (200 mg/dl) was a little lower (p = 0.03), and triglycerides a little higher, 2.7 mmol/L (239 mg/dl) in the 135 type 2 subjects compared to the 3946 non-diabetic subjects (5.3 and 2.0 mmol/L (205 and 177 mg/dl) respectively)[22]. HDLc was also lower in the type 2 diabetic subjects, 1.18 versus 1.26 mmol/L (45–49 mg/dl), p = 0.001. Gemfibrozil had similar lipid altering effects in the diabetic subjects, although each effect was slightly less than that seen overall (exact reductions not reported). Although gemfibrozil was associated with a 68% relative reduction in the incidence of CHD death/MI (7.1% absolute reduction), since only 10 subjects with type 2 had an end-point, this was not significant, despite the risk reduction being greater than in the main trial. Of particular importance and relevance to diabetes is the subsequent demonstration that the bulk of the benefit in the Helsinki Heart Study was seen in subjects with a mixed dyslipidaemia, i.e. raised LDLc (>175 mg/dl; >45 mmol/L), triglyceride (>200 mg/dl; >2.25 mmol/L), and lowered HDL (<35 mg/dl; <0.9 mmol/L), the so-called triopathy[23]. As gemfibrozil is predominantly a triglyceride-lowering agent (it may even raise LDL cholesterol in some subjects), this is not surprising. It is clearly a useful agent for the patient with increased triglycerides and LDLc, but is not suitable for

Table 18.2. Lipid modulation trials including diabetic participants: primary CHD prevention.

Author/Trial name	Year	# Diabetic participants	Intervention	Entry criteria	Dur	End-point	Rx incidence	Control incidence	Crude risk reduction % (abs %)	Reported adjustment in relative risk (95 CI)
Koskinen et al.R 'Helsinki HS'	1992	135 type 2 No CAD men only	Gemfibrozil 600 mg bid	Non HDLc >5.2 mmol/L	5 yr	CHD death/MI	3.4%	10.5%	68% (7.1) p=0.19	NA
Elkeles et al. SENDCAP	1998	164 No CAD	Bezafibrate 400 mg/day	Total c ≥5.2 mmol/L[1] or Trig ≥1.8 mmol/L[1] or HDL ≤1.1mmol/L[1] Total to HDLc ratio >4.7	37 yr	Carotid IMT; Arterial ultrasound score;	n/a n/a	n/a n/a	NS NS	67% (NR)
						MI/probable ischemia	6.2%	19.3%	68% (13.1) p<0.01	
AFCAPS TexCAPS	1998	155 diagnosed type 2 No CAD Men and women (84 FBG >126 mg/dl)	Lovastatin 20–40 mg/day	TC 180–264 mg/dl LDLc 130–190 mg/dl[2] HDLc <45 mg/dl men HDLc <47 mg/dl women Trig<400 mg/dl	5.2 y	MI (fatal or non-fatal) or sudden cardiac death or unstable angina	5.6%	7.1% (7.5%)	21.1%	n/a

mmol/L cholesterol = 38.6 mg/dl; mmol/L triglyceride = 88.6 mg/dl: NS = p >0.05. Rx incidence = incidence of cardiovascular events in treated group.
[1] Excluded if TC or Trig >8.0 mmol/L and TC:HDL ratio ≥7.2.
[2] Subjects were also included with LDLc 125-129 mg/dl if TC/HDLc ratio >6.0.

isolated LDL cholesterol alone. Although outside the remit of this chapter, the use of fibric acids was heavily questioned as a result of the WHO Clofibrate Trial[24]. However, the main concerns in that trial, an excess of cancer and gall stones in the treated group, do not appear to be a problem with gemfibrozil. A lack of effect on blood sugar levels is also encouraging as there have been occasional reports of worsening glycaemic control[25,26], though this is not a universal finding[22,28]. The representativeness of the diabetes subgroup is also questionable for not only were women and type 1 subjects excluded, but the 135 type 2 subjects included represented less than 3.5% of the population, far less than the 14+% that would be expected for this age group.

The second primary prevention trial in diabetes (SENDCAP) also used a fibric acid – this time Bezafibrate[29]. This is the only primary prevention study to report to date with complication outcomes that was focused on diabetic subjects. In this UK study, 164 type 2 diabetic subjects were randomized to either Bezafibrate (400 mg daily) or placebo. Subjects were excluded if total cholesterol or triglycerides were over 8.0 mmol/L (310 and 709 mg/dl respectively), Total:HDLc ratio was ≥7.2 or, if severely hypertensive (≥180/110). Intervention caused a 36% fall (placebo corrected) in triglycerides, an 11.5% fall in non-HDL cholesterol, and an 8.4% increase in HDL cholesterol. The primary end-points were carotid intimal wall thickness and arterial ultrasound score – a summation of plaque formation from both carotid and femoral arteries. These were not affected by the intervention (p = 0.4–0.9). However, a composite secondary end-point of definite CHD events (MI and probable ECG ischaemia, i.e. Q waves or LBBB; left bundle branch block) was reduced (p <0.01). Other secondary end-points showed non-significant results, including a trend in the opposite direction for angina and 'possible' ECG ischaemia.

The third and most recent primary prevention trial used lovastatin (the first HMG CoA reductase inhibitor to be used in the USA) in subjects with average cholesterol levels (LDLc 130–190 mg/dl; 3.4–4.9 mmol/L) and low HDLc (men: <45mg/dl; 1.1 mmol/L; women: <47mg/dl; 1.2 mmol/L). This study, called AFCAPS/TexCAPS[30], has not as yet fully reported analyses of the prespecified subgroups which did include 155 type 2 diabetic subjects. These formed only 3% of the total population, and diabetic subjects in poor control (HbA$_{1c}$ >20% above normal) were excluded, as were those on insulin. Thus again only a select group was studied. The primary outcome variable was a major coronary event defined as fatal or non-fatal myocardial infarction (MI), unstable angina or sudden cardiac death. Only 10 events were seen in those with diabetes. Though the relative risk reduction (21%) was comparable, the small number of events prohibits any firm conclusions. For completeness, two further primary prevention studies should be mentioned. First, the West of Scotland Coronary Prevention Study (WOSCOPS) study included 75 diabetic subjects (out of 6595) and used pravastatin but did not (understandably) report separate data for this small subgroup. Finally, a small 12-month trial of 40 asymptomatic type 2 diabetic subjects showed a significant reduction in the progression of carotid intimal medial wall thickness in the 20 patients treated with gemfibrozil (900 mg/day) compared to the 20 treated with diet alone[31].

SECONDARY PREVENTION

In terms of secondary prevention (Table 18.3), the first to report was the 4S Study[32] which was also the first of the new generation of 'statin' trials using the HMG CoA reductase inhibitors, powerful LDLc-lowering drugs. This Scandinavian Secondary Prevention Trial involved 4444 men with stable angina or MI, and moderately high cholesterol, 5.5 to 8.0 mmol/L (213–309 mg/dl) and triglycerides below 2.5 mmol/L (221 mg/dl). This latter restriction, plus the exclusion of conditions likely to reduce life expectancy, probably explains why only 4.5% of the trial population (202) had diabetes, almost certainly type 2 for the majority of cases. Overall, the trial reported a 35% fall in LDL cholesterol, accompanied by a 30% fall in total mortality (the primary outcome), a 42% fall in CHD mortality, a 34% fall in major CHD events and a 26% fall in any atherosclerotic event – all highly significant. In the 202 diabetic subjects[33], a 36% fall in LDLc was seen, along with a Cox regression adjusted 43% fall in total mortality (p = 0.09), a 36% fall in CHD mortality (p = 0.24) and a 55% fall in major CHD events (p = 0.002). In addition, all atherosclerotic events were reduced by 37% (p = 0.02). Results for the diabetic subgroup thus parallel those for the main study population, and for major CHD events and indeed any atherosclerotic event, showed a greater overall benefit. The medication was well tolerated and also had no apparent effect on fasting blood sugar levels. While very encouraging, particularly in conjunction with the Helsinski Heart Study, both studies need to be seen as post-hoc subgroup analyses of non-representative groups of diabetic subjects, most of whom appear to have relatively mild glucose disturbance. Fifty per cent of 4S patients with diabetes were diet-controlled, as were 71% of Helsinski Heart Study participants. While it is possible, even likely, that similar benefits will accrue from treatment of the more metabolically disturbed patients with advanced complications, especially renal disease, this has not been clearly demonstrated and, thus, whether intensive (or even more intensive than general) treatment of these high-risk subjects is justified is still open for debate and investigation.

The second 'statin' trial to report data concerning diabetes, the CARE Study[34], involved a more representative diabetic group[35] that totalled 588, 14% of all subjects. Though severe hyperglycaemia (fasting glucose >220 mg/dl; 12.21 mmol/L), severe hypertriglyceridaemia (>350 mg/dl; >4.0 mmol/L) and/or those with heart failure were still excluded, the majority of the diabetic group was drug treated, with only 10% untreated and 30% treated with diet alone. The CARE Study focused on subjects with modest, not severe, cholesterol elevation, i.e. total cholesterol <240 mg/dl (6.2 mmol/L), and LDL cholesterol between 115 and 174 mg/dl (3.0–4.5 mmol/L). Thus, a somewhat more typical diabetic dyslipidaemic patient group was studied which had lower LDL cholesterol than seen in the 4S Study (138 versus 187 mg/dl; 3.6 versus 4.8 mmol/L) and higher triglycerides (164 versus 152 mg/dl; 1.8 versus 1.7 mmol/L), reflecting the differing selection criteria. Importantly, while the CARE diabetic subjects also had a lower LDL cholesterol and higher triglyceride than the CARE non-diabetic subjects (LDLc = 139 mg/dl; 3.6 mmol/L and triglycerides 154 mg/dl; 1.7 mmol/L), they experienced almost identical LDLc lowering as the non-diabetic subjects (27% versus 28%). Unfortunately, the reduction in the primary end-point (CHD death plus non-fatal MI) was only about half that seen in the non-diabetic group (13 versus 26%) and for a variety of other end-points the difference was not significant. The difference in effect size reflects a lack of reduction of CHD mortality in the diabetic group. Nonetheless, the reduction (25%) in an expanded end-point was similar to that seen in the non-diabetic group. This was seen as a result of a significant reduction (p = 0.04) in revascularization in those diabetic subjects treated with pravastatin. There is no obvious explanation for why pravastatin had only a weak effect on CHD mortality in the CARE Study in the diabetic subgroup, although it is possible that the more severe patient population studied in CARE (compared to 4S) was a contributory factor. It is encouraging that overall CHD events were reduced in CARE to a similar degree to that seen in the non-diabetic population. Finally, CARE did include a small group of post-menopausal women (20% of the sample). Therefore, these data further extend the results from the all-male 4S. Like 4S, diabetes in CARE was not a primary stratification variable before randomization, nor a prespecified subgroup, therefore, the results have to be treated cautiously as 'post hoc'.

The third secondary prevention statin trial also used pravastatin. This was an Australian-based study (LIPID) of 9014 patients with a past history of MI or hospitalized unstable angina[36]. A somewhat broader range of cholesterol (total 155–271 mg/dl; 4.0–7.0 mmol/L) and fasting triglycerides (<445 mg/dl; 5.0 mmol/L) were allowed compared to either CARE or 4S, while the primary outcome was CHD death. Nine per cent (782) of the cohort had diabetes, a lower than expected frequency of diabetes in such a CHD-based population, but nonetheless this study has the largest diabetic population studied to date. Reported data concerning the diabetic subjects is limited at the time of writing, but as they formed a prespecified subgroup and were sizable, the results are perhaps the most definitive to date. The relative risk reduction was 15.8% (crude) or 19% (Cox model adjusted), which however was not significant (95% CI−10 to +41), but comparable to the 25% reduction seen in the non-diabetic population. These positive results extend the pool of 'indicated' patients overall to include women and those with unstable angina. However, the relatively low number of women (17%) precludes any firm conclusions for the few with diabetes.

In late 1999, the VA-HIT trial reported their findings[37]. This study used gemfibrozil and involved men aged less than 75 years who had a history of CAD, and a low HDLc (≤40 mg; 1.04 mmol/L). Significant elevations of LDL cholesterol (>140 mg/dl; >3.6 mmol/L) or triglycerides (>300 mg/dl; >3.4 mmol/L) were exclusion criteria. Six hundred and twenty-seven diabetic patients (by history) were included, which made up 24.8% of the total trial population. Clearly, this is a relatively high proportion, and thus likely to be quite representative, especially considering the relatively high triglyceride exclusion criterion. The primary outcome was MI or CHD death, and those with diabetes experienced the same benefit (24% reduction) as those without. This trial was designed to focus particularly on the benefits of raising HDLc, which it did by 6%. It also lowered triglycerides by 31% but did not, as anticipated, lower LDLc.

These results contrast with the Bezafibrate Infarction Prevention (BIP) study, which showed little benefit from HDL-raising in subjects with a history of MI or angina[38]. Ten per cent of subjects had type 2 diabetes (309 subjects), however, results have not so far been published separately for this subgroup. As the overall results showed no effect on clinical outcome despite an 18% increase in HDLc, one may suspect that the much smaller diabetic subgroup would likewise show no effect. However, it should be noted that the contrasting VA-HIT gemfibrozil study which, as discussed, was positive, had proportionally 2.5 times as many subjects with diabetes and, overall, the subjects had a more 'diabetic type' dyslipidaemia (high triglyceride, low HDL) than seen in BIP, suggesting the possibility that fibrates may be more effective in individuals with this lipid profile. This speculation is supported by a post-hoc subgroup analysis in BIP which showed a positive effect on clinical events for those with a baseline triglyceride above 200 mg/dl (2.3 mmol/L). Thus, while the role of bezafibrate itself in coronary prevention in diabetes is unclear, the evidence in favour of fibrates generally is persuasive. It rests on the results of the Helsinki and VA-HIT trials as well as those from the first major trial on coronary prevention that focused entirely on diabetic subjects, called the Diabetes Atherosclerosis Intervention Study (DAIS)[39]. This trial examined the effect of fenofibrate on the progression of coronary atherosclerotic lesions in type 2 diabetic subjects with minimal coronary atherosclerosis. Almost half, however, had prior clinical coronary artery disease and 30% had undergone prior revascularization. The fenofibrate had a profound (35%) triglyceride lowering effect with smaller effects on LDLc (10% lowering) and HDLc (5% raising). These effects were associated with a significant reduction in both the minimal lumen diameter (p = 0.024) and mean percentage stenosis (p = 0.020) although the third end-point, mean segmental diameter, did not differ between the groups at follow-up (p = 0.171). Though not powered to show differences in clinical events, an encouraging (but non-significant) 23% reduction was noted.

This trial thus gives major encouragement that specifically correcting diabetic dyslipidaemia is of benefit.

For completeness, mention should be made of three further trials with angiographic end-points. The Canadian Coronary Atherosclerosis Intervention Trial (CCAIT) used titrated doses of lovastatin in subjects with CAD and included 46 diabetic patients (14% of the total). While separate diabetes data are not reported, it is noted that, in women, lovastatin appeared to eliminate the predictive power of diabetes for progression seen in the placebo group[40]. Another trial, the Post Coronary Artery Bypass Graft Trial[41] included 116 subjects with, and 1235 without, diabetes. Interventions comprised aggressive cholesterol lowering (with lovastatin and cholestyramine) to a goal LDLc of 60–85 mg/dl (1.55–2.20 mmol/L) and low dose warfarin in a 2 × 2 factorial design. Cholesterol lowering was associated with a slightly greater risk reduction of both 'substantial progression' and 'occlusion' of saphenous vein grafts in those with diabetes although, because of the much smaller sample size, this was not, unlike the overall results, significant. Warfarin had no benefit. Finally, a study of coronary atherosclerosis called HATS examined the effects of combined niacin and simvastatin therapy with and without antioxidants [42]. Twenty-five subjects had diabetes and 15 had impaired fasting glucose (IFG: 110–125 mg/dl; 6.1–7.0 mmol/L). As in the overall results, those with diabetes or IFG who received combined niacin/simvastatin showed significantly less progression than those given placebo (p <0.05).

These studies (Tables 18.2 and 18.3), thus, comprise our evidence-based data set in terms of lipid modulation in diabetes with clinical macrovascular outcomes. It should be noted that we have no separate 'diabetic' data on women (except for DAIS; Diabetes Atherosclerosis Intervention Study), or on stroke (apart from a non-significant 18% reduction in the CARE study [34]) or amputation as macrovascular outcomes. Five studies appear to have been 'post hoc' analyses, and most have yet to report their diabetes data in any detail. Hence, in the strictest sense, we have little 'hard' evidence to date. Furthermore, three studies included only men, while the three smaller trials were in a primary prevention setting, yielding a total sample of less than 500, while for secondary prevention interventions, even when fully reported, the current data will include fewer than 3000 diabetic subjects.

CONCLUSIONS

It is clear that more data are needed before an adequate evidence base is available. In particular, as far as secondary prevention is concerned, the benefits of lipid modulation in diabetic women are poorly studied. In terms of primary prevention, although the Helsinki Heart Study post hoc analysis[22] and the SENDCAPS[29] and AFCAPS/TEXCAPS[30] studies are encouraging, more

Table 18.3. Lipid modulation trials including diabetic subjects: secondary CHD prevention.

Author	Year	# Diabetic subjects	Intervention	Entry criteria	Dur	End-point	Rx incid.	Control incidence	Crude risk reduction % (abs %)	Reported Adj. RR↓ (95 CI)
Pyörälä et al.[33] '4S'	1997	202 type 2 Prior MI	Simvastatin 20–40 mg/day	Total chol 5.5–8.0 mmol/L Triglycerides ≤2.5 mmol/L	5.4 yr	Total mortality CHD (MI/CHD death)	14.3% 22.8%	24.7% 45.4%	42% (10.4) 50% (22.6)	43% p=0.09 (−8 to 70) 55% p=0.002 (26 to 73)
Goldberg et al.[35] 'CARE'	1998	586 type 2 Post-MI 342 IFG 110–125 mg/dl Fasting glucose	Pravastatin 40 mg/day	Total chol <240 mg/dl LDLc 115–174 mg/dl Trig < 350 mg/dl	5 yr	CHD death/ MI; expanded CHD (CHD death/MI CABG/ PTCA)	17.7% 28.7% ?	20.4% (2.7) 36.8% ?	13% (NR) 22% (8.1) 23% (?)	13% NS 25% p=0.05 (NR)
Lipid Study Group[36] [41] 'LIPID'	1998	782 type 2 MI or unstable angina	Pravastatin 40 mg/day	Total chol 155–271 mg/dl Trig <445 mg/dl	6.1 yr	CHD death	19.2%	22.8%	15.8% (3.6%)	19% (NR) (−10 to
Rubins et al.[39] VA-HIT [43] Study	1999	627 unspecified type; history of MI, angina or stenosis >50%	Gemfibrozil 1200 mg/day	HDLc ≤140 mg/dl LDLc ≤140 mg/dl Trig ≤300 mg/dl	5.1 yr	MI or CHD death	28.5%	36.5%	21.9% (8.0%)	24% (−0.1 to

mmol/L cholesterol = 38.6 mg/dl; mmol/L triglyceride = 88.6 mg/dl definitive data on larger sample sizes are needed before any conclusions can be drawn. Nonetheless, fairly vigorous lipid intervention would seem appropriate, given the high risks. The limited evidence available supports more aggressive interpretations of the current guidelines, especially in individuals with existing CHD (Table 18.1).

Finally, although epidemiological evidence suggests a strong lipid role, particularly for hypertriglyceridaaemia, it must be stressed that no lipid-lowering CHD prevention trials in type 1 diabetes have been reported. This is a major deficit in our evidence base for both primary and secondary prevention of CHD.

FUTURE STUDIES

A number of studies currently underway, or planned, may answer some of the remaining questions. First, another trial with micronized fenofibrate will provide further data on type 2 diabetes subjects with clinical events (FIELD). A particularly relevant study in the UK, the Lipid Diabetes Study, involves a 2×2 factorial design comparing cerivastatin and fenofibrate in CHD patients*, while a further UK study similarly examines simvastatin and/or an antioxidant 'cocktail'**. Another trial, based in Europe, will report in 2004. This study, called CARDS, is studying the effect of atorvastatin on CAD risk in type 2 diabetes without CAD but with an LDLc of <4.2 mmol/L.

In the USA, the National Heart, Lung and Blood Institute is undertaking an intervention trial in high CVD risk diabetic subjects which is planned to compare, in one dimension, intensive glycaemic control with a conventional glycaemic control group, and in additional dimensions, very intensive lipid and blood pressure interventions including combined statin and fibrate therapy versus standard risk factor control. A different glycaemic approach (insulin resistance lowering drugs versus insulin secretion drugs) is being tested by the Bypass Angioplasty Revascularisation Initiative (BARI) group of investigators, who also propose to study early revascularization in diabetic subjects (see later section). Finally, the National Institute for Diabetes, Digestive Disorders and Kidney Disease is conducting a 'weight control in diabetes' study with a variety of subclinical and clinical atherosclerotic outcomes. The many unanswered questions concerning women with diabetes and primary prevention thus, may, in time, be answered.

MICROVASCULAR COMPLICATIONS

The effect of lipid reduction on the microvascular complications of diabetes (retinopathy, nephropathy and neuropathy) has likewise not been extensively

---

* Trial stopped due to withdrawal from market in 2001.
** Preliminary reports of Heart Protection Study showed substantial benefit in person with diabetes with or without prior CAD.

studied, and much of the evidence linking hyperlipidaemia and diabetic complications relies on observational and analytic epidemiological studies and not on trials. Analyses are complicated by the interrelationships between risk factors.

The sections below summarize the evidence for the role of lipids and the effect of lipid reduction on the development and progression of diabetic retinopathy, nephropathy and neuropathy. Only published English language studies are included. Treatments that affect lipids but are not focused on lipid lowering, such as fish oil and linoleic acid supplementation, are not considered as these have multiple effects on other variables including arachidonic acid metabolism and platelet aggregation.

RETINOPATHY

Early diabetic retinopathy is characterized by increased capillary permeability. At later stages, damage to the retinal vessels produces microaneurysms, haemorrhages and exudates of plasma proteins and lipids. Severe non-proliferative retinopathy is characterized by vessel closure, with resulting ischaemia. Proliferative retinopathy, which is sight-threatening, is characterized by neovascularization[43]. Many studies have reported an association between hyperlipidaemia and the presence and severity of diabetic retinopathy[44–55]. For some of the studies, the association with lipid values was seen in univariate but not multivariate analyses[44–46]. In a number of cross-sectional or case-control studies, the association appeared stronger with triglycerides or HDL cholesterol than with total or LDL cholesterol[47,48]. However, these studies are hampered by the inability to completely adjust for prior glycaemic control. Current HbA_{1c} and duration of diabetes were mainly used for adjustment. In a cross-sectional analysis of 650 participants in the Wisconsin Epidemiologic Study of Diabetic Retinopathy, total blood cholesterol was a predictor of the severity of hard exudates but not of retinopathy as defined by the Arlie House Classification Scheme[50]. The association appeared to depend on the type of diabetes (OR 1.50–1.65 for type 1 and insulin-requiring type 2, not significant for non-insulin-requiring type 2). However, there was a correlation of cholesterol levels with duration of diabetes (r = 0.26), which might explain the differences in the type of diabetes.

A number of cohort studies have been performed (Table 18.4). The results from these studies are mixed. An association of serum cholesterol with the development of hard exudates was seen in the Early Treatment of Diabetic Retinopathy Study (ETDRS) (OR 1.54 for cholesterol >240 mg/dl; 6.21 mmol/L versus <200 mg/dl; 5.17 mmol/L) in which 84% of subjects used insulin[51]. In addition, an elevated cholesterol at baseline was associated with an increased risk of vision loss, as defined by doubling of the visual angle (OR 1.5 cholesterol >240 mg/dl; 6.21 mmol/L versus <200 mg/dl; 5.17 mmol/L). In a separate

Table 18.4. Cohort studies examining the relationship between hyperlipidemia and diabetic retinopathy.

Reference	Study duration	Number of subjects	Study purpose	Study results with Regards to Risk Factors[a]
ETDRS 1996[51]	7 years	2709 60% Type 2	To examine the relationship between serum lipid levels, retinal hard exudate and visual acuity in a cohort of diabetics	Controlled for age, HbA_{1c}, baseline retinopathy severity and extent of retinal thickening, diabetes duration. Higher total cholesterol or LDL cholesterol were associated with development of hard exudates
ETDRS 1998 (Davis et al.)[52]	5 years	2654	To identify risk factors for the development of high-risk proliferative retinopathy	Controlled for type and duration of diabetes, HbA_{1c}, percentage of desired weight, visual acuity and macular oedema at baseline. age, gender and race/ethnicity; serum triglycerides (age-based definition) were a predictor of the development of retinopathy. Other predictors were baseline severity of retinopathy, decreased visual acuity or extent of macular oedema, neuropathy, lower haematocrit, lower serum albumin and, in persons with mild to moderate non-proliferative retinopathy, younger age of onset of type 1 diabetes. LDL and total cholesterol were not significant
EDC 1995[54]	2-year follow-up	496 type 1	To examine risk factors for the incidence and progression of retinopathy in a cohort of type 1 diabetics	Baseline diastolic blood pressure was the only significant predictor of the development of retinopathy. In univariate analysis (controlling for diabetes duration), LDL cholesterol, fibrinogen, glycohaemoglobin,

Table 18.4. contd.

Lee *et al.* 1992[55]	Mean 12.7 years (9.8–16.2)	354 type 2	To determine the incidence of and risk factors for the development and progression of proliferative retinopathy in American Indians with type 2 diabetes	triglycerides and diastolic blood pressure were significant predictors of progression of retinopathy. LDL and triglycerides were not significant predictors in the multivariate analyses. The significant predictors in the multivariate analysis were diabetes duration, baseline retinopathy severity and glycohaemoglobin.
Araki *et al.* 1993[56]	7.9±2.6 years	110 type 2	To determine the risk factors for the development of retinopathy in Japanese diabetic patients over the age of 60 years	In univariate analysis, significant predictors for the development of proliferative retinopathy were duration of diabetes, fasting plasma glucose, systolic blood pressure, therapeutic regimen (diet, oral agent, insulin) total cholesterol, and triglycerides. In multivariate analysis, the significant predictors were fasting glucose and diabetes duration, with a trend for total cholesterol (p = 0.052) Initial fasting glucose (or HbA₁), diabetes duration and the presence of proteinuria at baseline were significant predictors. Total serum cholesterol and triglycerides were not
Chen *et al.* 1995[57]	4 years	344 type 2	To assess the incidence and progression of diabetic retinopathy and the risk factors associated with them	In univariate analysis, significant risk factors for the development of retinopathy were insulin use, duration of diabetes, poorer control, proteinuria, and residential area (rural). Total cholesterol and

Table 18.4. contd.

Study	Duration	Sample	Objective	Results
Kim et al. 1998[58]	5.3±1.0 years	186 type 2	To determine the incidence and risk factors for the development and progression of diabetic retinopathy in a Korean cohort of type 2 diabetics	triglycerides were not. The significant predictors in univariate analysis for progression were proteinuria and fasting blood glucose. In multivariate analysis the only significant predictor for development or progression was mean HbA_1. Total cholesterol, HDL and triglycerides were not predictors of either outcome in the univariate analyses
Tudor et al. 1998[59]	Median 4.8 years (2.0-6.6)	169 type 2 65.3% Hispanic	To determine if Hispanic people with type 2 diabetes have a higher incidence and/or rate of progression of retinopathy and to explore risk factors associated with retinopathy	The significant predictors for the development of retinopathy were the use of insulin and systolic blood pressure, with a trend for glycohemoglobin. Total cholesterol, triglycerides and HDL were not
EURODIAB Prospective Complications Study 2001 (Chaturvedi et al.)	Mean 7.3 years	764 type 1	To determine risk factors for the development of retinopathy in diabetics without retinopathy at baseline	In the univariate analysis, significant predictors were albumin excretion rate, total cholesterol, triglycerides, fibrinogen, von Willebrand factor, γGGT, waist-to-hip ratio, insulin dose, HbA_{1c} and diabetes duration. In the multivariate analysis, significant risk factors were fasting triglyceride level, waist-to-hip ratio, diabetes duration and HbA_{1c}.

aMultivariate analysis unless otherwise stated

follow-up study of the ETDRS examining risk factors for the development of high-risk proliferative diabetic retinopathy, a higher triglyceride level (age-based definition) was associated with a greater risk at five years[52]. In contrast to the previous report, total and LDL cholesterol were only of borderline significance. The EURODIAB Prospective Complications Study examined 764 individuals with type 1 diabetes and no retinopathy at baseline[53]. They found that markers of insulin resistance, including serum triglyceride levels, predicted the development of retinopathy (RR 1.24 for log-transformed tri-glycerides). Total cholesterol was a risk factor in univariate but not multi-variate analysis. Two other cohorts, the Pittsburgh Epidemiology of Diabetes Complications Study (EDC) and a cohort of diabetic American Indians found only a weak association between total blood cholesterol and the development of retinopathy[54,55]. Other smaller longitudinal studies did not find a relation-ship between hyperlipidaemia and the development or progression of retin-opathy[56–59]. In the cohort studies, the duration of diabetes, glycaemic control and perhaps hypertension were the strong risk factors for retinopathy develop-ment, and the smaller studies may have lacked sufficient power to assess a weaker association with lipid levels.

In the 1960s, a number of uncontrolled intervention studies of the effect of lipid-lowering diets on retinopathy were published[60–62]. These trials found an improvement in retinal exudates, but no effect on visual acuity. This led to a number of small controlled trials of lipid-lowering medication[63–66]. The results are summarized in Table 18.5. The four studies were randomized and all used clofibrate. None of the publications gave complete details of cholesterol and triglyceride levels during the study. In all four studies, the results were con-sistent and similar to the uncontrolled trials. There was an improvement in the extent or severity of hard exudates, but no difference was seen in visual acuity. Harrold *et al.*[65] found a trend toward improvement in haemorrhages, but the results were not significant. In addition, this trial was analysed by eyes, as opposed to the number of individuals treated (which would double-count most individuals), so the p value, it may be argued, would be decreased inappro-priately. Figure 18.1 shows the results of a meta-analysis of randomized con-trolled trials of lipid-lowering therapy on exudative retinopathy. Treatment decreases the risk of worsening exudates (OR 0.20, 95% CI 0.11; 0.39) and improves existing exudative retinopathy (OR 5.16, 95% CI 2.91; 9.14), although the confidence intervals would be wider if we could analyse the Harrold *et al.* data by individual[65].

There are few data on the effect of lipid lowering agents, other than clofibrate, on lipid reduction and retinopathy. It is therefore difficult to assess whether greater degrees of lipid reduction, such as with a HMG-CoA reduct-ase inhibitor would show a greater benefit. One small series in six subjects using pravastatin found an improvement in microaneurysms in four[67]. We recently completed a pilot study of the effect of simvastatin on microvascular

Table 18.5. Controlled trials of lipid reduction in diabetic retinopathy.

Reference	Study Design	Study duration	Number of subjects	Purpose of study	Study results
Duncan et al. 1968[63]	Randomized controlled trial	3 years	48	To study patients with exudative retinopathy to determine whether lipid reduction with clofibrate improved retinal lesions	Exudate: Control: 20% improved 44% worse Treated: 65% improved 5% worse No difference in incidence of neovascularization or haemorrhage. No difference visual acuity
Houtsmuller 1968[64]	Randomized controlled trial	2 years	30	To study patients with exudative retinopathy to determine whether lipid reduction with clofibrate improved retinal lesions	Control: 23% improved 41% worse Treated: 30% improved 23% worse No change in visual acuity
Harrold et al. 1969[65a]	Randomized controlled trial	1 year	63 entered/56 completed	To study patients with retinopathy to see if lipid reduction with clofibrate improved retinopathy	Exudate: Control: 13% improved 21% worse Treated: 43% improved 6% worse

Table 18.5. Controlled trials of lipid reduction in diabetic retinopathy.

Cullen *et al.* 1974[66b]	Randomized controlled trial	2 years	40 entered/32 completed	To study patients with early exudative retinopathy to determine whether lipid reduction with clofibrate improved retinopathy	Haemorrhage: Control: 13% improved 17% worse Treated: 22% improved 12% worse Exudate: Control: 33% improved 56% worse Treated: 76% improved 24% worse No difference in incidence of neovascularization or haemorrhage. No difference visual acuity
Fried *et al.* 2001[68]	Randomized controlled trial	1 year for retinopathy outcome	27 without proliferative retinopathy at baseline (out of 39 in study). type 1	Pilot study to determine the effect of lipid lowering with simvastatin on microvascular outcomes	At one year, one in the treated and two in the placebo group had progression in retinopathy grade (not significant)

[a] Analyszed in terms of number of eyes, not subjects. treated.
[b] Three of the subjects were removed for worsening retinopathy; they were added back for the calculation of results in the table.

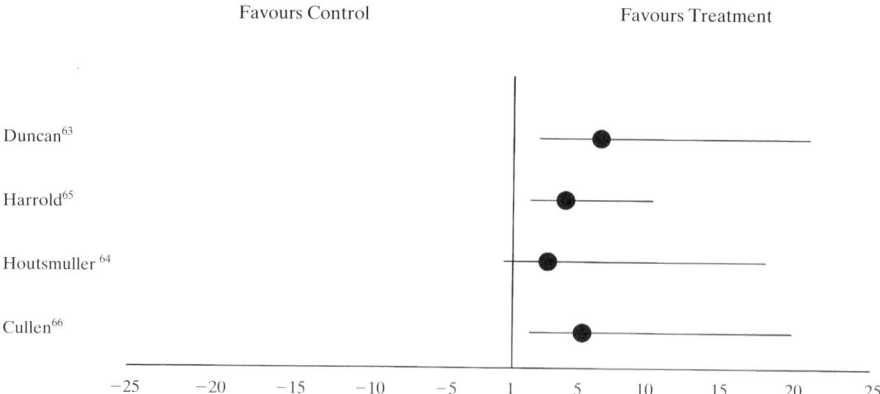

Figure 18.1. Lipid modulation trials with exudative retinopathy as end-point. Odds ratios and 95% confidence intervals. See text and tables 18.5 for details.

complications in 39 individuals with type 1 diabetes[68]. At baseline 12 patients had proliferative retinopathy (seven in simvastatin group, five in placebo). We did not find a difference in the development of proliferative retinopathy, although only three patients had progressed at one year to proliferative retinopathy (one simvastatin, two placebo). In summary, the data appears to support a relationship between treatment of hyperlipidaemia and improvement in retinal hard exudates. However, it has not been shown that lipid reduction improves sight-threatening retinopathy. Further large-scale studies are needed. (Strength of recommendation B; Level of evidence I.)

NEPHROPATHY

Diabetic nephropathy progresses through several recognizable stages[69]. The earliest subclinical stage is characterized by hyperfiltration and an elevated glomerular filtration rate. As the disease progresses, structural changes in the kidney develop, with an increase in basement membrane thickness and mesangial expansion. Initially, albumin excretion rate is normal, but microalbuminuria subsequently develops. Patients with persistent microalbuminuria are at increased risk for progressing to overt nephropathy, and the risk of progression is greater with higher levels of albuminuria. Overt nephropathy is characterized by proteinuria on routine urinalysis. Over time without intervention, the proteinuria increases to the nephrotic range and the glomerular filtration rate declines until end-stage renal disease is reached.

The majority of patients with proteinuria have hyperlipidaemia, characterized by high total cholesterol, LDL cholesterol, Lp(a) and triglycerides[70]. The degree of hyperlipidaemia correlates with the degree of proteinuria and hypoalbuminaemia[71,72]. The actual mechanism leading to the hyperlipidaemia is unclear, but appears to be related to both increased hepatic synthesis of lipoproteins and impaired clearance of circulating lipoproteins[71]. It has been postulated that glomerulosclerosis and atherosclerosis result from similar pathological mechanisms[73,74]. This had led investigators to theorize that hyperlipidaemia not only results from renal disease, but also contributes to its progression[75–77]. Renal mesangial cells, which resemble smooth muscle cells, bind LDL and this leads to cell proliferation, increased cytokine production and increased mesangial matrix production in *in vitro* models[78–80]. In animal models of type 2 diabetes, treatment of hyperlipidaemia reduces glomerular injury[81]. Data in humans with diabetes are not as strong.

Cross-sectional studies finding a relationship between hyperlipidaemia and progression of diabetic nephropathy are difficult to interpret, as nephropathy produces hyperlipidaemia. This criticism is also true about cohorts of patients that start with subjects who already have nephropathy, although most of these studies showed a faster rate of progression in those with hyperlipidaemia[82–84]. A few cohort studies have examined risk factors for the development and progression of renal disease in subjects without nephropathy at baseline. In an analysis of data from the Epidemiology of Diabetes Complications Study, a cohort of type 1 diabetic subjects, Coonrod *et al.*[85], found that higher LDL and triglycerides predicted the development of microalbuminuria two years later, after controlling for blood pressure and glycaemic control. The relative risks found were 2.47 for LDL ≥ 2.59 versus <2.59 mmol/L; 100 mg/dl and 3.14 for triglyceride level ≥ 1.13 versus <1.13 mmol/L; 100mg/dl. A subsequent analysis after six years examined the risk factors for progression to overt nephropathy found that LDL was a risk factor in females but not in males[86]. Ravid *et al.*[87], in a nine-year cohort of individuals with type 2 diabetes, found that total cholesterol and HDL were predictors of the development of microalbuminuria. The high correlation found between HbA_{1c} and cholesterol ($r = 0.62$), makes it difficult to separate the two effects. Three other smaller cohorts of type 2 diabetic individuals also found, in multivariate analyses, that increased total cholesterol or high triglyceride/HDL levels were associated with progression of nephropathy[88–90]. The Atherosclerosis Risk in Communities (ARIC) study recently reported an analysis of the association of lipids with the loss of renal function, as characterized by a rise in serum creatinine of 0.4 mg/dl or greater[91]. This population-based study examined 12 728 individuals, of which 10% were diabetic. They found that hypertriglyceridaemia was associated with a higher risk of developing renal impairment. The relative risk was greater for diabetics than for non-diabetics (RR 2.44 for diabetics versus 1.48 for nondiabetics for each three-fold higher baseline triglyceride level, after adjusting for gender, race, age, antihypertensive medications, baseline serum creatinine and systolic blood pressure). After further adjustment for baseline glucose level, the relative risk drops to 1.88 for the diabetics and the p value became borderline (p = 0.07). An inverse, though not statistically significant, relationship was found for HDL cholesterol and the risk of developing a rise in creatinine in diabetics (RR = 0.39 for 30 mg/dl higher HDL level, p = 0.11). Total and LDL cholesterol were not associated with a rise in creatinine.

A number of small, relatively short-term controlled studies have been performed to examine the effect of lipid reduction on diabetic nephropathy. These are summarized in Table 18.6. Eight of the nine trials utilized HMG-CoA reductase inhibitors and showed a 20–40% decline in LDL cholesterol[68,92–99]. Smulders *et al.*[99] utilized gemfibrozil and found a 33% reduction in triglycerides and a 16% reduction in total cholesterol. None of the trials had long enough follow-up to see a difference in progression to renal failure, i.e. dialysis. They all utilized surrogate markers – albumin excretion and glomerular filtration rate. Lam *et al.*, in a two year study, showed a difference in decline of glomerular filtration rate (84.3 to 74 ml/min in control versus 83.1 to 82 ml/min in the treated), but this was not seen in the other trials[96]. There was a trend for the longer-term studies (at least one year duration) to show a decreased progression or actual reduction in albuminuria. It is not clear from these trials whether the decline in albuminuria would translate into delayed progression to renal failure, if the studies were longer-term. The degree of proteinuria has been found to be a risk factor for renal failure[100]. Spontaneous remission or a decline in proteinuria with treatment of hypertension has been associated with better renal outcomes in other studies[100,101].

In summary, epidemiological and animal data suggest a role of lipids in the progression of diabetic nephropathy. However, short-term (less than two-year) trials of lipid lowering did not find a difference in speed of decline of glomerular filtration rate. Further large-scale, longer-term trials are needed. However, this may be ethically impossible as it would expose the untreated group to prolonged hyperlipidaemia. (Strength of recommendation C; Quality of evidence II-2.)

NEUROPATHY

The aetiology of distal, symmetric diabetic polyneuropathy is controversial and it is unclear whether it should be considered a microvascular complication. Focal motor forms, such as mononeuritis multiplex, are thought to be ischaemic. Some authors advocate a vascular etiology for the distal neuropathy and point to decreased sural nerve hypoxia, seen in diabetics with neuropathy[102,103]. Others suggest that it is a metabolic disorder, though both processes may be active[103,104].

There are few studies examining the microvascular hypothesis and the data examining the role of lipids are sparse (Table 18.7). The epidemiological data

Table 18.6. Controlled trials of lipid reduction in diabetic nephropathy.

Reference	Study design	Study duration	Number of subjects	Purpose of study	Study results[a]
Hommel et al 1992 (84)	Randomized controlled trial	12 weeks	26 type 1 overt nephropathy	To assess the effect of simvastatin on lipoproteins and renal function in hyperlipidemic type 1 diabetics with nephropathy	GFR: Control: 72±23 ml/min start 74±23 ml/min end Treated: 64±30 ml/min start 63±29 ml/min end UAE Control: 481 μg/min (1.62) start 368 μg/min (1.78) end Treated: 458 μg/min (1.58) start 393 μg/min (1.61) end
Zhang *et al.* 1995[93]	Crossover	12 weeks each arm	20 type 1 microalbuminuria	To evaluate the effect of pravastatin on plasma lipids, *in vitro* oxidizability of non-HDL fraction, metabolic control and UAE in type 1 subjects with incipient nephropathy	UAE: Start 65±37 μg/min End placebo 54±64 μg/min End treatment 49±66 μg/min
Nielsen *et al.* 1993[94]	Randomized controlled trial	36 weeks	18 type 2 microalbuminuria	To assess the effect of simvastatin on renal function. UAE and insulin sensitivity	GFR (ml/min): Control: 97.1±6.7 start 88.8±6 end Treated: 96.6±8 start 96±5.7 end UAE (μg/min) Control: 33.1 (1.3) start 42.7 (1.3) end Treated: 18.4 (1.3) start 16.2 (1.2) end

Table 18.6. contd.

Bazzato et al. 1992[95b]	Randomized trial	1 year	12 overt nephropathy	To evaluate the effect of simvastatin on rate of decline of GFR	GFR rate of decline: Control: −0.25 ml/min/month Treated −0.21
Lam et al. 1995[96c]	Randomized controlled trial	2 years	34 type 2 overt nephropathy	To assess the effect of cholesterol-lowering therapy with lovastatin on progression of diabetic nephropathy	GFR (ml/min) Control: 84.3±21.6 start 74±25 end Treated: 83.1±38 start 82±28 end UAE (μg/min) Control: 791.7±884 start 1319±442 end Treated: 562.5±472 start 833±556 end
Tonolo et al. 1995[97]	Cross-over	1 year each arm	19 type 2 microalbuminuria	To assess the effect of simvastatin on UAE in patients with type 2, microalbuminuria and hypercholesterolemia	GFR^d : (ml/min) Control: Group A: 97±6 start 97±6 end Group B: 97±7 start 90±6 end Treated: Group A: 101±8 start 97±6 end Group B: 90±6 start 90±6 end UAE (mg/day) Control: Group A: 48 (17–88) start 60 (21 to 100) end Group B: 70 (36–98) start 81 (41–94 end) Treated: Group A: 73 (36–104) start 48 (17–88) end Group B: 81 (41–94) start 46 (22–68 end)

Table 18.6. contd.

Mori *et al.* 1992[98]	Randomized controlled trial	18 months	33 type 2 microalbuminuria	To evaluate the effect of pravastatin on microalbuminuria in patients with type 2 diabetes	UAE (mg/g creatine): Control: 114.9±112.8 start 113.3±108.8 end Treated: 129.3±86.1 start 71.6±63.4 end
Smulders *et al.* 1997[99]	Randomized controlled trial	1 year	15 type 2 microalbuminuria	To investigate whether reduction in hypertriglyceridemia with gemfibrozil is associated with slower rate of progression of microalbuminuria	UAE (mg/mmol creatinine): Control: 14.5±6.8 start 21.3±15.8 end Treated: 9.4±6.8 start 17.1±23.4 end
Fried *et al.* 2001[68]	Randomized controlled trial	18 months (designed as a 2-year study but stopped early when the ADA lipid treatment guidelines for diabetes were changed)	39 type 1 with normal or microalbuminuria: 39 completed six months, 36 completed one year, 17 completed 18 months	Pilot study to determine the effect of lipid lowering with simvastatin on urinary albumin excretion rate	Change in UAE compared to baseline (% change/month): Control: 0.77 (−1.71, 4.74) Treated: 0.0805 (−1.93, 3.69)

[a] GFR = glomerular filtration rate; UAE = urinary albumin excretion, for Nielsen and Hommel expressed as geometric mean and anti-log of standard error, Tonolo as median and range Fried as median and interquartile range, otherwise as mean and standard deviation.
[b] Published in abstract form.
[c] Final results read off a figure.
[d] Group A: simvastatin for 12 months then placebo for 12 months. Group B: placebo for 12 months then simvastatin for 12 months.

Table 18.7. Studies examining the relationship of lipids on diabetic neuropathy.

Reference	Study design	Number of subjects	Study purpose	Study results
Lithner et al. 1995[105]	Observational, Cross-sectional	239	To assess the association between serum lipid levels and abnormalities in the fibrinolytic system on sensory thresholds in Type 1 diabetes	Significant associations with sensory thresholds in multivariate analysis for age, duration of diabetes, height and triglycerides
Matsumoto et al. 1994[106]	Observational, cross-sectional	742	To examine the association between neuropathy and clinical variables in a group of type 2 diabetic subjects with diabetes less than 5 years duration	Significant associations between neuropathy and fasting glucose, duration of diabetes and maximal body mass index. Non-significant association with total cholesterol
Maser et al. 1996[107]	Observational, cross-sectional	91	To assess the association between neuropathy by vibratory thresholds and various lipid parameters	Significant associations with age, height and duration of diabetes but not lipid parameters
EDC 1989[108]	Observational, cross-sectional	400	To examine the associations between possible correlates of distal polyneuropathy in type 1 diabetic subjects	Significant associations in multivariate analysis with duration of diabetes, HbA$_1$, HDL, smoking and presence of macrovascular disease.
EDC 1990[109]	Observational, cross-sectional	168	To examine the associations between autonomic neuropathy and cardiovascular risk factors in type 1 diabetic subjects	Significant associations of autonomic neuropathy with hypertension, LDL, HDL and female gender

Table 18.7. contd.

EDC 1997[110]	Observational, cohort	463	To examine the risk factors for the development of distal polyneuropathy in type 1 diabetic subjects	Independent risk factors for the development of neuropathy were age, body height and duration of diabetes. Lipid parameters were not
Dyck et al. 1999[112]	Observational, cohort	264	To examine the predictors of the severity of diabetic neuropathy	Independent predictors of the severity of neuropathy were the presence/severity of other microvascular disease, diabetes duration, mean glycohaemoglobin and type 1 diabetes. Lipid or lipoprotein concentrations were not
Bereyni et al. 1971[114]	Randomized controlled trial	22 enrolled, 15 completed	To examine the effect of the lipid-lowering agent clofibrate in diabetic neuropathy	Clinical improvement in: 7/9 treated with clofibrate; 1/6 treated with placebo. No significant change in conduction velocity
Fried et al. 2001[68]	Randomized controlled trial	39 enrolled, 36 completed one-year follow up	Pilot study to determine the effect of lipid lowering with simvastatin on microvascular outcomes	There was a trend towards a lower rate of change in vibratory threshold: Control: 0.94 (interquartile range 2.1) Treated: 0.03 (interquartile range 1.49). No subject had autonomic neuropathy at baseline. There was no change in RR variation or blood pressure/heart rate response to standing in either group

are mixed. Lithner *et al.*, in a cross-sectional study of type 1 diabetics, found that triglycerides and Lp(a) levels were associated with increased vibratory thresholds[105]. Total cholesterol was not associated with sensory thresholds in the multivariate analysis. Matsumoto *et al.*[106], in another cross-sectional study, did not find an association of increased cholesterol with polyneuropathy, but only examined total cholesterol. In a smaller cross-sectional study of type 2 diabetics, Maser[107] examined the association of Lp(a), HDL, LDL and triglycerides with vibratory thresholds. A significant relationship was not found.

The Epidemiology of Diabetes Complications study examined risk factors for the development of neuropathy in type 1 diabetes. In the initial, cross-sectional baseline analysis, a lower HDL concentration was associated with distal symmetric polyneuropathy, although elevated Lp(a) was not[108,109]. Elevated triglycerides and lower HDL or increased LDL (depending on the model), were also associated cross-sectionally with autonomic neuropathy[110]. A subsequent analysis of the longitudinal data showed that increased LDL was a predictor in the univariate, but not multivariate, analysis[111]. (The predictors of neuropathy were diabetes duration, height, HbA_{1c}, smoking and hypertension.) In a recent report by the Rochester Diabetic Neuropathy Study, Dyck *et al.* analysed predictors of the severity of diabetic neuropathy, as measured by a composite score based on electromyographic data, vibratory and temperature thresholds, heart-rate variability and clinical exam data[112]. In this study, the presence and increased severity of other microvascular disease (retinopathy or nephropathy) predicted the severity of diabetic neuropathy. Other important risk factors were glycohaemoglobin, diabetes duration and type 1 diabetes. Total cholesterol, HDL, triglycerides and Lp(a) were not predictors.

Duncan *et al.*[113] published case reports of patients with dramatic clinical improvement in diabetic neuropathy, who were started on clofibrate for hyperlipidaaemia. This led to a small controlled trial. Berenyi *et al.*[114] studied clofibrate versus placebo in a one-year double-blind study (nine clofibrate, six placebo). Triglycerides declined in the treated subjects (13% decrease versus 22% increase in untreated), though there was not a significant change in the total cholesterol (1% decline in treated, 13% increase in controls). Seven out of nine clofibrate patients versus one out of six placebo patients improved clinically (decreased pain and paresthesias). Nerve conduction velocity did not significantly change. In another small study in 39 type 1 diabetic individuals, there was a trend towards a slower rate of progression of vibratory threshold in those treated with simvastatin (median change 0.03 versus 0.94, p = 0.07)[68]. In summary, the evidence for the role of lipid reduction in diabetic neuropathy is weak, but the early results of the intervention studies suggest that a full-scale study is warranted. (Strength of recommendation C; Quality of evidence II-3.)

REFERENCES

1. Orchard TJ (1990) Dyslipoproteinaemia and diabetes. *Endocrinology and Metabolism Clinics of North America* **19**: 361–380.
2. Feingold KR, Grunfeld C, Pang M, Doerrler W, Krauss RM (1992) LDL subclass phenotypes and triglyceride metabolism in non-insulin-dependent diabetes. *Arteriosclerosis and Thrombosis* **12**: 1496–1502.
3. Krauss RM. Relationship of intermediate and low-density lipoprotein subspecies to risk of coronary artery disease (1987) *American Heart Journal* **113**: 578–582.
4. Nikkilä EA, Hormila P (1978) Serum lipids and lipoproteins in insulin-treated diabetes. Demonstration of increased high density lipoprotein concentrations. *Diabetes* **27**: 1078–1086.
5. Oberman A, Kreisberg RA, Henkin Y (eds) *Principles and management of lipid disorders. A primary care approach.* Baltimore: Williams & Williams, pp. 157–160.
6. Bagdade JD, Subbaiah PV (1989) Abnormal high-density lipoprotein composition in women with insulin-dependent diabetes. *Journal of Laboratory and Clinical Medicine* **113**: 235–240.
7. Orchard TJ, Virella G, Forrest KY-Z, Evans RW, Becker DJ, Lopes-Virella MF (1999) Antibodies to oxidized LDL predict CAD in type 1 diabetes: a nested case control study from the Pittsburgh Epidemiology of Diabetes Complication Study. *Diabetes* **48**: 1454–1458.
8. Kannel WB, McGee DL (1999) Diabetes and cardiovascular risk factors: the Framingham Study. *Circulation* **59**: 8–13.
9. van Essen GG, Rensma PL, de Zeeuw D, Sluiter WJ, Scheffer H, Apperloo AJ, de Jong PE (1996) Association between angiotensin-converting-enzyme gene polymorphism and failure of renoprotective therapy. *Lancet* **347**: 94–95.
10. Manson JE, Colditz GA, Stampfer MJ, Willett WC, Królewski AS, Rosner B, *et al.* A prospective study of maturity-onset diabetes mellitus and risk of coronary heart disease and stroke in women. *Archives of Internal Medicine* **151**: 1141–1147.
11. West KM, Ahuja MMS, Bennett PH, Czyzyk A, De Acosta OM, Fuller JH, *et al.* (1983) The role of circulating glucose and triglyceride concentrations and their interactions with other 'risk factors' as determinants of arterial disease in nine diabetic population samples from the WHO multinational study. *Diabetes Care* **6**: 361–369.
12. Gordon T, Castelli WP, Hjortland MC, Kannel WB, Dawber TR (1977) Diabetes, blood lipids, and the role of obesity in coronary heart disease risk for women. *Annals of Internal Medicine* **87**: 393–397.
13. Lloyd CE, Kuller LH, Becker DJ, Ellis D, Wing RR, Orchard TJ (1996) Coronary artery disease in IDDM: Gender differences in risk factors, but not risk. *Arteriosclerosis, Thrombosis and Vascular Biology* **16**: 720–726.
14. Maser RE, Wolfson SK, Stein EA, Drash AL, Becker DJ, Dorman JS, *et al.* (1991) Cardiovascular disease and arterial calcification in insulin-dependent diabetes mellitus: Interrelationships and risk factor profiles. Pittsburgh Epidemiology of Diabetes Complications Study – VI. *Arteriosclerosis and Thrombosis* **11**: 958–965.
15. Orchard TJ, Stevens LK, Forrest KY-Z, Fuller JH (1983) Cardiovascular disease in IDDM: similar rates, but different risk factors in the United States compared with Europe. *International Journal of Epidemiology* **27**: 976–983.
16. Expert Panel (2001) Executive summary on the Third Report of the National Cholesterol Education Program (NCEP) expert panel on detection, evaluation, and treatment of high blood cholesterol in adults (Adult Treatment Panel III). *Journal of American Medical Association* **285**: 2486–2497.

17. American Diabetes Association (1999) Management of dyslipidaemia in adults with diabetes. *Diabetes Care* **22**(1): s56–s61
18. Haffner SM, Lehto S, Rönnemaa T, Pyörälä K, Laakso M (1998) Coronary heart disease mortality in type 2 diabetic and non-diabetic subjects with and without previous myocardial infarction. *New England Journal of Medicine* **339**(4): 229–234.
19. Lipid Research Clinic Trial (LRC).
20. MRFIT trial.
21. Frick MH, Elo O, Haapa K, Heinonen OP, Heinsalmi P, Helo P, *et al.* (1987) Helsinki Heart Study: primary prevention trial with gemfibrozil in middle-aged men with dyslipidaemia: safety of treatment, changes in risk factors, and incidence of coronary heart disease. *New England Journal of Medicine* **317**: 1237–1245.
22. Koskinen P, Mänttäri M, Manninen V, Huttunen JK, Heinonen OP, Frick MH (1992) Coronary heart disease incidence in NIDDM patients in the Helsinski Heart Study. *Diabetes Care* **15**: 820–825.
23. Manninen V, Elo O, Frick MH, Haapa K, Heinonen OP, Heinsalmi P, *et al.* (1988) Lipid alterations and decline in the incidence of coronary heart disease in the Helsinki Heart Study. *Journal of American Medical Association* **260**: 641–651.
24. Oliver MF, Heady JA, Morris JN, Cooper J (1984) WHO cooperative trial on primary prevention of ischaemic heart disease with clofibrate to lower serum cholesterol: final mortality follow-up. *Lancet* **2**(8403): 600–604.
25. Hulley SB, Rosenman RH, Bawol RD, Brand RJ (1980) Epidemiology as a guide to clinical decision. The association between triglyceride and coronary heart disease. *N Engl J Med* **302**(25): 1383–1389.
26. Marks J, Howard AN (1982) A comparative study of gemfibrozil and clofibrate in the treatment of hyperlipidaemia in patients with maturity-onset diabetes. *Res Clin Forums* **4**: 95–103.
27. Goldberg R, LaBelle P, Zupkis R, Ronca P (1990) Comparison of the effects of lovastatin and gemfibrozil on lipids and glucose control in non-insulin-dependent diabetes mellitus. *American Journal of Cardiology* **66**: 16B–21B.
28. Lintott CJ, Scott RS, Sutherland WHF, Bremer JM, Shand BI, Frampton CM (1992) Comparison of simvastatin vs. gemfibrozil therapy on lipid, glycaemic and haemorheological parameters in type II diabetes mellitus. *Diab.Nutr.Metab*. **5**: 183–189.
29. Elkeles RS, Diamond JR, Poulter C, Dhanjil S, Nicolaides AN, Mahmood S, *et al.* (1998) Cardiovascular outcomes in type 2 diabetes. A double-blind placebo-controlled study of bezafibrate: the St. Mary's Ealing, Northwick Park Diabetes Cardiovascular Disease Prevention (SENDCAP) Study. *Diabetes Care* **21**(4): 641–648.
30. Downs JR, Clearfield M, Weis S, Whitney E, Shapiro DR, Beere PA, *et al.* (1998) Primary prevention of acute coronary events with lovastatin in men and women with average cholesterol levels: Results of AFCAPS/TexCAPS. *Journal of the American Medical Association* **279**(20): 1615–1622.
31. Migdalis IN, Kozanidou GB, Voudouris G, Hatzigakis SM, Petropoulos A (1997) Effect of gemfibrozil on early carotid atherosclerosis in diabetic patients with hyperlipidaaemia. *International Angiology* **16**(4): 258–261.
32. Scandinavian Simvastatin Survival Group (1994) Randomised trial of cholesterol lowering in 4444 patients with coronary heart disease: The Scandinavian Simvastatin Survival Study (4S). *Lancet* **344**: 1383–1389.
33. Pyörälä K, Pedersen TR, Kjekshus J, Faergeman O, Olsson AG, Thorgeirsson G, *et al.* (1997) Cholesterol lowering with simvastatin improves prognosis of diabetic patients with coronary heart disease. *Diabetes Care* **20**(4): 614–620.

34. Plehn JF, Davis BR, Sacks FM, Rouleau JL , Pfeffer MA, Bernstein V, *et al.* (1999) Reduction of stroke incidence after myocardial infarction with pravastatin. The Cholesterol and Recurrent Events (CARE) Study. *Circulation* **99**: 216–223.
35. Goldberg RB, Mellies MJ, Sacks FM, Moyé LA, Howard BV, Howard WJ, *et al.* (1998) Cardiovascular events and their reduction with pravastatin in diabetic and glucose-intolerant myocardial infarction survivors with average cholesterol levels. Subgroup analyses in the Cholesterol and Recurrent Events (CARE) Trial. *Circulation* **98**: 2513–2519.
36. The Long-Term Intervention with Pravastatin in Ischaemic Disease (LIPID) Study Group (1998) Prevention of cardiovascular events and death with pravastatin in patients with coronary heart disease and a broad range of initial cholesterol levels. *New England Journal of Medicine* **339**(19): 1349–1357.
37. Rubins HB, Robins SJ, Fye CL, Anderson JW, Elam MB, Faas FH, Linares E, Schaefer EJ, Schechtman G, Wilt TJ, Wittes J (1999) Gemfirbrozil for the secondary prevention of coronorary heart disease in men with low levels of high-density lipoprotein cholesterol. Veterans Affairs High-Density Lipoprotein Cholesterol Intervention Trial Study Group. *New England Journal of Medicine* **341**: 410–418
38. The BIP Study Group (Behar S) (2000) Secondary prevention by raising HDL cholesterol and reducing triglycerides in patients with coronary artery disease: The Bezafibrate Infarction Prevention (BIP) Study. *Circulation* **102**: 21–27.
39. Diabetes Atherosclerosis Intervention Study Investigators (Steiner G) (2001) Effect of fenofibrate on progression of coronary artery disease in type 2 diabetes: the Diabetes Invervention Study, a randomized study. *Lancet* **357**: 905–910.
40. Waters D, Higginson L, Gladstone P, Boccuzzi SJ, Cook T, Lespérance J (1995) Effects of cholesterol lowering on the progression of coronary atherosclerosis in women: A Canadian coronary atherosclerosis intervention trial (CCAIT) substudy. *Circulation* **92**: 2404–2410.
41. Hoogwerf B, Waness A, Cressman M, Canner J, Campeau L, Domanski M, *et al.* (1999) Effects of aggressive cholesterol lowering and low-dose anticoagulation on clinical and angiographic outcomes in patients with diabetes. The Post Coronary Artery Bypass Graft Trial. *Diabetes* **48**: 1289–1294.
42. HATS study.
43. Aiello LP, Gardner TW, King GL, Blankenship G, Cavallerano JD, Ferris FL, Klein R (1998) Diabetic Retinopathy: Technical Review. *Diabetes Care* **21**: 143–56.
44. Vallalpando MEG, Martinez DR, Villalpando CG, Klein R, Pérez BA, Haffner SM, Díaz SVM, Stern MP, Mitchell B (1997) Moderate-to-severe diabetic retinopathy is more prevalent in Mexico City than in San Antonio, Texas. *Diabetes Care* **20**: 773–777.
45. Nagia DK, Pettitt DJ, Bennett PH, Klein R, Knowler WC (1997) Diabetic retinopathy assessed by fundus photography in Pima Indians with impaired glucose tolerance and NIDDM. *Diabetic Medicine* **14**: 449–456.
46. Kordonouri O, Danne T, Hopfenmüller W, Enders I, Hövener G, Weber B (1996) Lipid profiles and blood pressure: are they risk factors for the development of early background retinopathy and incipient nephropathy in children with insulin-dependent diabetes mellitus. *Acta Paediatrics* **85**: 43–48.
47. Sjølie AK, Stephenson J, Aldington S, Kohner E, Janka H, Stevens L, Fuller J (the EURODIAB IDDM Complications Study Group) (1997) Retinopathy and vision loss in insulin-dependent diabetes in Europe. *Ophthalmology* **104**: 252–260.
48. Sakene N, Yoshida T, Yoshioka K, Nakamura Y, Umekawa T, Kogure A, Takakura Y, Kondo M (1997) ß3-adrenoreceptor gene polymorphism: a newly identified risk factor for proliferative retinopathy in NIDDM patients. *Diabetes* **46**: 1633–1636.

49. Mouton DP, Gill AJ (1988) Prevalence of diabetic retinopathy and evaluation of risk factors: a review of 1005 diabetic clinic patients. *South African Medical Journal* **74**: 399–402.
50. Klein BEK, Moss SE, Klein R, Surawicz TS (1991) The Wisconsin Epidemiologic Study of Diabetic Retinopathy: XIII relationship of serum cholesterol to retinopathy and hard exudate. *Ophthalmology* **98**: 1261–1265.
51. Chew EY, Klein ML, Ferris FL, Remaley NA, Murphy RP, Chantry K, Hoogwerf BJ, Miller D (for the ETDRS Research Group) (1996) Association of elevated serum lipid levels with retinal hard exudate in diabetic retinopathy: Early Treatment Diabetic Retinopathy Study (ETDRS) Report 22. Archives of Ophthamology **114**: 1079–1084.
52. Davis MD, Fisher MR, Gangnon RE, Barton F, Aiello LM, Chew EY, Ferris FL, Knatterud GL, for the Early Treatment Diabetic Retinopathy Study Research Group (1998) Risk factors for high-risk proliferative retinopathy and severe visual loss: Early Treatment Diabetic Retinopathy Study report #18. Investigative Ophthalmology & Visual Science **39**: 233–252.
53. Chaturvedi N, Sjoelie AK, Porta M, Aldington SJ, Fuller JH, Songini M, Kohner EM (2001) Markers of insulin resistance are strong risk factors for retinopathy incidence in type 1 diabetes: for the EURODIAB Prospective Complications Study. *Diabetes Care* **24**: 284–289.
54. Lloyd CE, Klein R, Maser RE, Kuller LH, Becker DJ, Orchard TJ (1995) The progression of retinopathy over two years: The Pittsburgh Epidemiology of Diabetes Complications (EDC) Study. Journal of Diabetes and its complications **9**: 140–148.
55. Lee ET, Lee VS, Lu M, Russell D (1992) Development of proliferative retinopathy in NIDDM: a follow-up study of American Indians in Oklahoma. *Diabetes* **41**: 359–367.
56. Araki A, Sato T, Ito H, Shiraki M, Hattori A, Orimo H, Inoue J (1993) Risk factors for the development of retinopathy in elderly Japanese patients with diabetes mellitus. *Diabetes Care* **16**: 1184–1186.
57. Chen MS, Kao CS, Fu CC, Chen CJ, Tai TY (1995) Incidence and progression of diabetic retinopathy among non-insulin-dependent diabetic subjects: a four-year follow-up. International Journal of Epidemiology **24**: 787–795.
58. Kim HK, Hing SK, Kim CH, Yoon YH, Kim SW, Lee KU, Park JY (1998) Development and progression of diabetic retinopathy in Koreans with NIDDM. *Diabetes Care* **21**: 134–138.
59. Tudor SM, Johnson DW, Hamman RF, Shetterly SM, Baron A (1998) Incidence and progression of diabetic retinopathy in Hispanics and non-Hispanic whites with type 2 diabetes: San Luis Valley Diabetes Study, Colorado. *Diabetes Care* **21**: 53–61.
60. Van Eck WF (1959) The effect of a low fat diet on the serum lipids in diabetes and its significance in diabetic retinopathy. American Journal of Medicine **27**: 196–211.
61. King RC, Dobree JH, Kok DA, Foulds WS, Dangerfield WG (1963) Exudative diabetic retinopathy: spontaneous changes and effects of a corn oil diet. *British Journal of Ophthalmology* **47**: 666–672.
62. Ernest I, Linnér E, Svanborg A (1965) Carbohydrate-rich, fat-poor diet in diabetes. *American Journal of Medicine* **39**: 594–600.
63. Duncan LJP, Cullen JF, Ireland JT, Nolan J, Clarke BF, Oliver MF (1968) A three-year trial of atromid therapy in exudative diabetic retinopathy. *Diabetes* **17**: 458–467.

64. Houtsmuller AJ (1968) Treatment of exudative diabetic retinopathy with atromid-S. *Ophthalmologica* **156**: 2–5.
65. Harrold BP, Marmion VJ, Gough KR (1969) A double-blind controlled trial of clofibrate in the treatment of diabetic retinopathy. *Diabetes* **18**: 285–291.
66. Cullen JF, Town SM, Campbell CJ (1974) Double-blind trial of atromid-S in exudative diabetic retinopathy. *Transactions of the UK Ophthalmology Society* **94**: 554–562.
67. Gordon B, Chang S, Kavanagh M, Berrocal M, Yannuzzi L, Robertson C, Drexler A (1991) The effects of lipid lowering on diabetic retinopathy. *American Journal of Ophthalmology* **112**: 385–391.
68. Fried LF, Forrest KYZ, Ellis D, Chang Y, Silvers N, Orchard TJ (2001) Lipid modulation in insulin dependent diabetes mellitus: effect on microvascular outcomes. Journal of Diabetes and its Complications **15**: 113–119.
69. Mauer SM, Mogensen CE, Kjellstrand CM (1993) Diabetic nephropathy. In Schrier RW, Gottschalk CW (eds) *Diseases of the Kidney*, 5th edn. Little, Brown: Boston, pp. 2153–2188.
70. Levey AS, Beto JA, Coronado BE, Eknoyan G, Foley RN, Kasiske BK, *et al.* (1998) Controlling the epidemic of cardiovascular disease in chronic renal disease: What do we know? What do we need to learn? Where do we go from here? *American Journal of Kidney Disease* **32**: 853–906.
71. Kasiske BL (1998) Hyperlipidaemia in patients with chronic renal disease. *American Journal of Kidney Disease* **32**(Suppl. 3): S142–S156.
72. Appel G (1991) Lipid abnormalities in renal disease. *Kidney International* **39**: 169–83.
73. Keane WF, Kasiske BL, O'Donnell MP (1988) Lipids and progressive glomerulosclerosis: a model analogous to atherosclerosis. *American Journal of Nephrology* **8**: 261–271.
74. Diamond JR (1991) Analogous pathobiologic mechanisms in glomerulosclerosis and atherosclerosis. *Kidney International* **39**(Suppl. 31): S29–S34.
75. Moorhead JF (1991) Lipids and the pathogenesis of kidney disease. *American Journal of Kidney Disease* **17**(Suppl. 1): 65–70.
76. Keane WF, Mulcahy WS, Kasiske BL, Kim Y, O'Donnell MP (1991) Hyperlipidaemia and progressive renal disease. *Kidney International* **39**(Suppl. 31): S41–S48.
77. Remuzzi G, Bertani T (1990) Is glomerulosclerosis a consequence of altered glomerular permeability to macromolecules? *Kidney International* **38**: 384–394.
78. Rovin BH, Tan LC (1993) LDL stimulates mesangial fibronectin production and chemoattractant expression. *Kidney International* **43**: 218–225.
79. Nishida Y, Yorioka N, Oda H, Yamakido M (1997) Effect of lipoproteins on cultured human mesangial cells. *American Journal of Kidney Disease* **29**: 919–930.
80. Schlondorff D (1993) Cellular mechanisms of lipid injury in the glomerulus. *American Journal of Kidney Disease* **22**: 72–82.
81. Kasiske BL, O'Donnell MP, Cleary MP, Keane WF (1988) Treatment of hyperlipidaemia reduces glomerular injury in obese Zucker rats. *Kidney International* **33**: 667–672.
82. Hasslacher C, Bostedt-Kiesel A, Kempe HP, Wahl P (1993) Effect of metabolic factors and blood pressure on kidney function in proteinuric type 2 (non-insulin-dependent) diabetic patients. *Diabetologia* **36**: 1051–1056.
83. UK Prospective Diabetes Study Group (1993) UK Prospective Diabetes Study (UKPDS): X. Urinary albumin excretion over three years in diet-treated type 2

(non-insulin-dependent) diabetic patients, and association with hypertension, hyperglycaemia and hypertriglyceridaemia. *Diabetologia* **36**: 1021–1029.

84. Krolewski AS, Warram JH, Christlieb AR (1994) Hypercholesterolaemia-a determinant of renal function loss and deaths in IDDM patients with nephropathy. *Kidney International* **45 (Suppl 45)**: S125–S131.

85. Coonrod BA, Ellis D, Becker DJ, Bunker CH, Kelsey SF, Lloyd CE, Drash AL, Kuller LH, Orchard TJ (1993) Predictors of microalbuminuria in individuals with IDDM: Pittsburgh Epidemiology of Diabetes Complications Study. *Diabetes Care* **16**: 1276–1383.

86. Norwalk MP, Stuhldreher WL, Becker D, Ellis D, Caggiula AW, Orchard TJ (1996) The relationship of protein intake to changes in renal function in an adult population with insulin-dependent diabetes mellitus. *Diabetes, Nutrition & Metabolism* **9**: 247–257.

87. Ravid M, Brosh D, Ravid-Safran D, Levy Z, Rachmani R (1998) Main risk factors for nephropathy in type 2 diabetes mellitus are plasma cholesterol levels, mean blood pressure, and hyperglycaemia. *Archives Internal Medicine* **158**: 998–1004.

88. Gall MA, Hougaard P, Borch-Johnsen K, Parving HH (1997) Risk factors for development of incipient and overt diabetic nephropathy in patients with non-insulin dependent diabetes mellitus: a prospective, observational study. *British Medical Journal* **314**: 783–788.

89. Wirta O, Pasternack A, Laippala P, Turjanmaa V (1996) Glomerular filtration rate and kidney size after six years disease duration in non-insulin-dependent diabetic subjects. *Clinical Nephrology* **45**: 10–17.

90. Smulders YM, Weijers RNM, Rakic M, Slaats EH, Stehouwer CDA, Silberbusch J (1997) Determinants of progression of microalbuminuria in patients with NIDDM. *Diabetes Care* **20**: 999–1005.

91. Muntner P, Coresh J, Smith JC, Exkfeldt J, Klag MJ (2000) Plasma lipids and the risk of developing renal dysfunction: The Atherosclerosis Risk in Communities Study. *Kidney International* **58**:293–301.

92. Hommel E, Anderson P, Gall MA, Nielsen F, Jensen B, Rossing P, Dyerberg J, Parving HH (1992) Plasma lipoproteins and renal function during simvastatin treatment in diabetic nephropathy. *Diabetologia* **35**: 447–451.

93. Zhang A, Vertommer J, Van Gaal L, De Leeuw I (1995) Effects of pravastatin on lipid levels, in vitro oxidizability on non-HDL lipoproteins and microalbuminuria in IDDM patients. *Diabetes Research in Clinical Practice* **29**: 189–194.

94. Nielsen S, Schmitz O, Moller N, Porksen N, Klausen IC, Alberti KGMM, Mogensen CE (1993) Renal function and insulin sensitivity during simvastatin treatment in type 2 (non-insulin-dependent) diabetic patients with micro-albuminuria. *Diabetologia* **36**: 1079–1086.

95. Bazzato G, Fracasso A, Scanferla F (1992) Risk factors on the progression of diabetic nephropathy. Role of hyperlipidaemia and its correction. *Nephrology, Dialysis, Transplantation* **7**: 710(abstract).

96. Lam KSL, Cheng IKP, Janus ED, Pang RWC (1995) Cholesterol-lowering therapy may retard the progression of diabetic nephropathy. *Diabetologia* **38**: 604–609.

97. Tonolo G, Ciccarese M, Brizzi P, Puddu L, Secchi G, Calvia P, Atzeni MM, Melis MG, Maioli M (1997) Reduction in albumin excretion rate in normotensive microalbuminuric type 2 diabetic patients during long-term simvastatin therapy. *Diabetes Care* **20**: 1891–1895.

98. Mori Y, Yokoyama J, Tsuruoka A, Ikeda Y (1992) Effect of pravastatin on microalbuminuria in patients with non-insulin dependent diabetes mellitus: a randomized control study. *Jikeikai Medical Journal* **39**: 341–348.

99. Smulders YM, Van Eeden AE, Stehouwer CDA, Weijers RNM, Slaats EH, Silberbusch J (1997) Can reduction of hypertriglyceridaaemia slow progression of microalbuminuria in patients with non-insulin-dependent diabetes mellitus? *European Journal of Clinical Investigation* **27**: 997–1002.

100. Hunt LP, Short CD, Mallick NP (1988) Prognostic indicators in patients presenting with the nephrotic syndrome. *Kidney International* **34**: 382–388.

101. Rossing P, Hommel E, Smidt UM, Parving HH (1994) Reduction in albuminuria predicts diminished progression in diabetic nephropathy. *Kidney International* **45 (Suppl 45)**: S145–S149.

102. Newrick PG, Wilson AJ, Jakubowski J, Boulton AJM, Ward JD (1986) Sural nerve oxygen tension in diabetes. *British Medical Journal* **293**: 1053–1054.

103. Johnson PC, Doll SC, Cromey DW (1986) Pathogenesis of diabetic neuropathy. *Annals of Neurology* **19**: 450–457.

104. Greene DA, Lattimer SA, Sima AAF (1987) Sorbitol, phosphoinositides and sodium-potassium-ATPase in the pathogenesis of diabetic complications. *New England Journal of Medicine* **316**: 599–606.

105. Lithner F, Bergenheim T, Borssén B, Dahlén G, Nilsson TK (1995) The association of fibrinolysis and hyperlipidaaemia with quantitative sensory tests in an epidemiological study of Swedish type 1 diabetic patients. *Diabetic Medicine* **12**: 590–594.

106. Matsumoto T, Ohashi Y, Yamada N, Kikuchi M (1994) Hyperglycaemia as a major determinant of distal polyneuropathy independent of age and diabetes duration in patients with recently diagnosed diabetes. *Diabetes Research in Clinical Practice* **26**: 109–113.

107. Maser RE, Usher DC, DeCherney CG (1996) Little association of lipid parameters and large sensory nerve fiber function in diabetes mellitus. *Journal of Diabetes Complications* **10**: 54–59.

108. Maser RE, Steenkiste AR, Dorman JS, Nielsen VK, Bass EB, Manjoo Q, Drash AL, Becker DJ, Kuller LH, Greene DA, Orchard TJ (1989) Epidemiological correlates of diabetic neuropathy: report from Pittsburgh Epidemiology of Diabetes Complications Study. *Diabetes* **38**: 1456–1461.

109. Maser RE, Usher D, Becker DJ, Drash AL, Kuller LH, Orchard TJ (1993) Lipoprotein(a) concentration shows little relationship to IDDM complications in the Pittsburgh Epidemiology of Diabetes Complications Study cohort. *Diabetes Care* **16**: 755–758.

110. Maser RE, Pfeifer MA, Dorman JS, Kuller LH, Becker DJ, Orchard TJ (1990) Diabetic autonomic neuropathy and cardiovascular risk: Pittsburgh Epidemiology of Diabetes Complications Study III. *Archives of Internal Medicine* **150**: 1218–1222.

111. Forrest KYZ, Maser RE, Pambianco G, Becker DJ, Orchard TJ (1997) Hypertension as a risk factor for diabetic neuropathy: a prospective study. *Diabetes* **46**: 665–670.

112. Dyck PJ, Service FJ, Daview JL, Melton LJ, Wilson DM, O'Brien PC (1999) Risk factors for severity of diabetic polyneuropathy: intensive longitudinal assessment of the Rochester Diabetic Neuropathy Study Cohort. *Diabetes Care* **22**: 1479–1486.

113. Duncan GC, Elliott FA, Duncan TG, Schatanoff J (1968) Some clinical potentials of chlorphenoxyisobutyrate (clofibrate) therapy (hyperlipidaemia-angina pectoris-blood sludging-diabetic neuropathy). *Metabolism: clinical and experimental* **17**: 457–473.

114. Berenyi MR, Straus B, Miglietta OE (1971) Treatment of diabetic neuropathy with clofibrate. Journal of American Geriatrics Society **19**: 763–772.

115. Betteridge DJ, Dodson PM, Durrington PN, Hughes EA, Laker MF, Nicholls DP, *et al.* (1993) Management of hyperlipidaaemia: guidelines of the British Hyperlipidaaemia Association. *Postgraduate Medical Journal* **69**: 359–369.
116. Pyorala K, Backer GD, Graham I, Poole-Wilson P, Wood D (1994) Prevention of coronary heart disease in clinical practice; Recommendations of the Task Force of the European Society of Cardiology, European Atherosclerosis Society and European Society of Hypertension. *European Heart Journal* **15**: 1300–1331.

19

What is the Evidence that Changing Tobacco Use Reduces the Incidence of Diabetic Complications?

DEBORAH L. WINGARD, ELIZABETH BARRETT-CONNOR
AND NICOLE WEDICK

University of California, San Diego,
9500 Gilman Drive, La Jolla, CA 92093-0607

INTRODUCTION

Diabetes is associated with the development of numerous complications, including nephropathy, neuropathy, retinopathy and heart disease. Smoking is also associated with the development of heart disease, as well as cancer, stroke and lung disease[1]. Smoking may also be associated with the development of other complications of diabetes[2–6]. Unfortunately, the prevalence of smoking appears to be essentially the same for individuals with and without diabetes[2,4,5]. Based on this information the American Diabetes Association recently issued a position statement that prevention or cessation of tobacco use is an important component of clinical diabetes care[7]. This chapter reviews current evidence that changing tobacco use could reduce the incidence of diabetic complications.

POSSIBLE MECHANISMS

Smoking could increase the risk of complications in individuals with diabetes, if smoking interferes with metabolic control. Several studies have demonstrated that metabolic control is worse in smoking compared with non-smoking diabetic

The Evidence Base for Diabetes Care. Edited by R. Williams, W. Herman, A.-L. Kinmonth and N. J. Wareham.
© 2002 John Wiley & Sons, Ltd

patients, the smokers having increased blood glucose concentrations and increased levels of glycosylated haemoglobin[3,8–10]. Smoking has also been shown to increase the secretion of catecholamines, growth hormone and cortisol[10–13], hormones which counteract insulin action and could lead to an increased insulin requirement in diabetic patients. Targher and colleagues[14] found that insulin resistance was markedly worse among individuals with type 2 diabetes who smoked. However, Hleve and colleagues[15] found that neither acute nor habitual smoking caused substantial changes in insulin sensitivity in type 1 diabetic patients.

Smoking could also increase the risk of complications in individuals with diabetes, if smoking influences other risk factors for those complications. For example, research has demonstrated that smoking is associated with higher serum concentrations of cholesterol, triglycerides, very-low-density lipoprotein (VLDL) cholesterol, and low density lipoprotein (LDL) cholesterol and lower serum concentrations of high-density lipoprotein (HDL) cholesterol and apolipoprotein A1[16–19]. These associations could lead to the development of heart disease.

In clinical trials, smoking has been shown to acutely raise blood pressure[20] and reduce retinal blood flow[21], while the vasoconstriction caused by nicotine induces a transient rise in pulse rate[11], effects that could potentially affect kidney function and cause retinal disease. As reviewed by Christen and colleagues, smoking also increases carboxyhemoglobin and platelet adhesiveness, and causes vasoconstriction of peripheral arteries[22]. These changes could lead to tissue hypoxia and possibly the peripheral nerve abnormalities seen in individuals with diabetes.

Alternatively, smoking may not directly or indirectly increase the risk of complications in individuals with diabetes, but rather may serve as a marker for other aspects of lifestyle that influence complication rates. For example, individuals who smoke cigarettes are more likely to drink alcohol and eat a high-fat diet, while being less likely to exercise, behaviors shown to influence the risk of heart disease. Smoking may also serve as a marker for socio-economic status and access to medical care, which may in turn influence risk of complications. If smoking helps the diabetic individual maintain weight control, smoking could prevent complications; however, several studies indicate that smoking is associated with increased visceral adiposity, a stronger risk factor for coronary heart disease than body mass index[25–27].

PREVALENCE OF SMOKING AMONG ADULTS WITH DIABETES

Despite substantial evidence of the harmful effects of smoking, approximately 25% of adults in the USA continue to report smoking cigarettes[23,24], while even higher rates are reported by adults in other countries[28]. In these surveys, smoking is generally reported more frequently by men than women, and in the USA by African–Americans than Caucasians[23,24,28]. The prevalence of smoking among adults with diabetes appears to reflect these same geographic, gender and racial trends[23,24,28]. Moreover, as summarized in Table 19.1, most of the studies that compared the prevalence of smoking among adults with and without diabetes found few differences[23,24,30-38]. The notable exception was among black men in the USA, where 40% of black men with diabetes in the 1989 National Health Interview Study reported smoking compared to 34% of those without diabetes[23]. Similarly, 55% of black men with diabetes in the 1988 Behavioral Risk Factor Survey reported smoking, compared to 31% of those without diabetes[24]. No differences in rates of smoking were seen among black women with and without diabetes, or among white men or women with and without diabetes.

Reports based on the US National Health Interview Study[23] and the London data from the WHO Multinational Study of Vascular Disease in Diabetes[39] found similar smoking rates for those with type 1 and type 2 diabetes. This is consistent with the Whitehall Study from England, which found no difference in smoking prevalence between individuals with diabetes treated or not treated with insulin[37]. In contrast, a study from Sweden[40] found a higher rate of smoking among those with type 1 compared to type 2 diabetes, 26% and 20% respectively, while a study from Wisconsin[41] found a lower rate of smoking among those with type 1 compared to type 2 diabetes, 14% and 20% respectively. (Three of these studies did not present data on a comparison group of individuals without diabetes[39-41], and are therefore not included in Table 19.1.)

Among those with diabetes, the prevalence of smoking decreased with increasing duration of disease[23]. This may be due to increased mortality associated with the combination of smoking and diabetes.

Virtually all of the foregoing studies rely on self-reported smoking status, and many also rely on self-reported diabetes status. While these self-reports may be underestimates, the data suggest that individuals with diabetes smoke at rates equivalent to the general population.

DIABETIC COMPLICATIONS IN SMOKERS VERSUS NONSMOKERS

Diabetes is associated with the development of numerous complications, the primary ones being nephropathy, neuropathy, retinopathy and cardiovascular disease. The following section reviews evidence that smoking is associated with the risk of developing each of these complications.

Table 19.1. Prevalence of smoking in diabetic compared to nondiabetic adults.

Study	Participants	'Current smoker' prevalence	
		Diabetes	No diabetes
Cross-sectional			
Ford et al. United States 1994[23]	1989 National Health Interview Survey (NHIS) 2405 individuals with self-reported diabetes (94% type 2) and 20131 individuals without diabetes aged ≥ 18 years	*Age-adjusted:* Black men = 40.5% White men = 30.7% Hispanic men = 36.6% Black women = 22.1% White women = 24.4% Hispanic women = 17.6% Total = 27.3% type 1 = 30.2% type 2 = 28.6%	*Age-adjusted:* Black men = 33.8% White men = 27.4% Hispanic men = 23.8% Black women = 24.5% White women = 25.3% Hispanic women = 19.8% Total = 25.9%
Gay et al. Colorado, USA 1992[29]	Colorado IDDM Registry 241 individuals with type 1 diabetes and 5876 controls from the 1985 NHIS aged 18–28 years	Non-Hispanic white men and women = 22.4%	Non-Hispanic white men and women = 33.2%
Ford and Newman 37 states, USA 1991[24]	1988 Behavioral Risk Factor Surveillance System (BRFSS) Survey 3006 individuals with diabetes and 52 750 without diabetes aged ≥ 18 years	*Age-adjusted:* Black men = 54.8% White men = 23.9% Black women = 20.0% White women = 25.7% Total = 26.0%	*Age-adjusted:* Black men = 30.9% White men = 26.7% Black women = 23.1% White women = 25.9% Total = 25.5%
Songer Pennsylvania, USA 1988[30]	Pittsburgh IDDM Registry 158 sibling pairs (type 1) mean age = 33 years	*Age- and sex-matched:* Total = 34.0%	*Age- and sex-matched:* Total = 33.3%
Schumacher and Smith Utah, USA 1988[31]	1986 Telephone Survey of Utah 255 individuals with type 2 diabetes and 622 matched controls aged 20–79 years	*Age, sex- and county-matched:* Total = 9.8%	*Age, sex- and county-matched:* Total = 12.5%

Table 19.1. contd.

Kesson and Slater West of Scotland 1979[32]	914 patients from 2 diabetes clinics and 1080 controls from dermatology clinics	Men = 17.7% Women = 15.5%	Men = 24.6% Women = 23.7%
Cyzyk and Krolewski Warsaw, Poland 1976[33]	4530 patients from 4 diabetes clinics and controls from population survey aged 18–68 years	Men = 43.9% Women = 16.1%	Men = 49.2% Women = 22.4%
Cohort (baseline data)			
Ford and DeStefano United States 1991[34]	NHANES I Epidemiologic Follow-Up Study 602 individuals with diabetes and 12 562 without diabetes aged 25–74 years	*Age, sex- and race-adjusted:* Total = 19.6%	*Age, sex- and race-adjusted:* Total = 18.2%
Manson *et al.* 11 states, USA 1991[35]	Nurses Health Study 1483 female nurses with type 2 diabetes and 114694 without diabetes aged 30–55 years	*Age-adjusted:* Women = 30.6%	*Age-adjusted:* Women = 33.3%
Brand *et al.* Framingham, MA USA 1989[36]	Framingham Study 644 individuals with diabetes and 3673 s without diabetes aged 30+ year	*Age-adjusted:* Men = 35.6% Women = 32.3%	*Age-adjusted:* Men = 43.0% Women = 33.6%
Jarrett and Shipley London, England 1985[37]	Whitehall Study 168 male civil servants with diabetes and 18 229 without diabetes aged 40–64 years	*Age-adjusted:* Men = 39.3% Insulin treated = 39.5% Not insulin treated = 41.1%	*Age-adjusted:* Men = 41.4%
Suarez, Barrett-Connor Rancho Bernardo, CA USA 1984[38]	Rancho Bernardo Study 229 individuals with type 2 diabetes and 2391 without diabetes aged 60–79 years	White men = 15.0% White women = 25.8%	White men = 16.7% White women = 19.8%

NEPHROPATHY

There is consistent and diverse evidence that smoking increases the risk of the development and progression of nephropathy, defined variously as microalbuminuria, albuminuria and proteinuria, in individuals with diabetes[6,41–44,46–53,56] (see Table 19.2). Among individuals with type 1 diabetes, the EURODIAB Study found an association between smoking and prevalence of albuminuria in both men and women[50], while two out of three prospective studies found an association between smoking and incidence of nephropathy[48,56] (one including children[48]) and three out of four with progression of nephropathy[47,49,53]. Among individuals with type 2 diabetes, four studies found an association between smoking and prevalence of nephropathy[42,46,51,52], while three out of four found an association between smoking and incidence[41,43] or progression[44] of nephropathy. Only one patient series from Denmark[45] failed to identify an association between smoking and the development of nephropathy among patients with type 2 diabetes. However, over 70% of these patients reported smoking cigarettes at baseline, possibly obscuring the possibility of detecting an association. The foregoing represent data from over 10 separate countries, including clinical trial participants and several population-based cohorts.

NEUROPATHY

As shown in Table 19.3, smoking was significantly associated with neuropathy prevalence in three cross-sectional studies of patients with type 1 diabetes[57–59]. All studies identified a two- to three-fold increase after multivariate adjustment. One of the cross-sectional studies[57] identified a significant dose–response relationship, such that the prevalence of neuropathy increased with increasing number of pack-years smoked (p <0.001). Baseline data from the DCCT failed to identify an association with mild neuropathy; however, those with renal impairment and severe neuropathy had been excluded[60]. Two prospective studies identified a significant association with distal symmetric polyneuropathy incidence, after multivariate adjustment[22,61], but the Stockholm Diabetes Intervention Study did not find an association with progression of neuropathy[54].

Among individuals with type 2 diabetes, one cross-sectional study did not find an association between smoking and neuropathy[57], however the prospective San Luis Valley Diabetes Study identified a two-fold increased risk for individuals with type 2 diabetes followed for an average of 4.7 years[62]. This cohort study also identified a possible dose–response relationship; incidence of distal symmetric sensory neuropathy was greater in those with more than 10 pack-years compared to those with 1–10 pack-years, after multivariate adjustment which included duration of diabetes.

Table 19.2. Risk of development and progression of nephropathy in diabetic smokers versus nonsmokers.

Study	Participants	Nephropathy	
		Development	Progression
Patient series			
Pijls *et al.* Netherlands 2001[42]	270 patients with type 2 diabetes, mean age = 64 years cross-sectional data	Smoking associated with micro/macro albuminuria prevalence OR current = 4.89, ns OR past = 2.36, p <0.05 (multivariate)	—
Forsblom *et al.* Finland 1998[43]	108 patients with type 2 diabetes and normoalbuminuria followed 9 years	Smoking associated with micro/macroalbuminuria incidence, p = 0.011	—
Biesenbach *et al.* Austria 1997[44]	36 patients with type 2 diabetes and nephropathy followed 6 years	—	Smoking promoted progression p <0.025
Gall *et al.* Denmark 1997[45]	191 patients with type 2 diabetes and normoalbuminuria aged <66 years median follow-up = 5.8 years	Smoking not associated with nephropathy incidence	—
Ikeda *et al.* Japan 1997[46]	148 patients with type 2 diabetes, cross-sectional data	Smoking associated with micro/macro albuminuria prevalence OR current = 4.5, p = 0.001 OR past = 2.0, ns	—
Sawicki *et al.* Germany 1994[47]	93 patients with type 1 diabetes, hypertension, and nephropathy mean age ≈ 36 years followed one year	—	Smoking associated with nephropathy progression OR per 10 pack-years = 2.74 p = 0.0004 (multivariate)

Table 19.2. contd.

Couper et al. South Australia 1994[48]	169 children with type 1 diabetes mean age = 12.4 years followed 2 years	Smoking associated with microalbuminuria incidence p <0.003	—
Chase et al. Colorado, USA 1991[49]	359 patients with type 1 diabetes mean age ≈ 20 years mean follow-up = 2.4 years	—	Smoking associated with progression of albuminuria p = 0.03
Cross-sectional Chaturvedi et al. Europe 1995[50]	EURODIAB IDDM Complications Study 3250 individuals with type 1 diabetes from 31 centers in 16 countries aged 15–60 years	Smoking associated with albuminuria prevalence Men OR current = 1.65, p <0.01 OR past = 1.51, p <0.05 Women OR current = 1.48, p <0.05 OR past = 1.52, ns (multivariate)	—
Haffner et al. Texas, USA 1993[51]	San Antonio Heart Study 234 individuals with type 2 diabetes aged 25–64 years cross-sectional data	Smoking associated with microalbuminuria prevalence OR ever = 1.60, p = 0.74 (multivariate)	—
Trial participants Mehler et al. Colorado, USA 1998[52]	Appropriate Blood Pressure Control in Diabetes Trial 904 participants with type 2 diabetes mean age = 58 years cross-sectional data	Smoking associated with nephropathy prevalence OR ever = 1.61, p = 0.046 (multivariate)	—

Table 19.2. contd.

Study	Description	Outcome	Nephropathy
Mühlhauser et al. Germany 1995[53]	Trial of Intensive Insulin Therapy 601 participants with type 1 diabetes mean age = 27 years followed 6 years	—	Smoking associated with 'development and/or progression' of nephropathy OR = 1.27, p = 0.049 (per 10 pack-years, multivariate)
Reichard et al. Stockholm, Sweden 1991[54]	Stockholm Diabetes Intervention Study 96 participants with type 1 diabetes and non-proliferative retinopathy mean age = 30 years followed 5 years	—	Smoking not associated with progression of nephropathy
Cohort Klein et al. Wisconsin, USA 1999[55]	Wisconsin Epidemiology Study of Diabetic Retinopathy 891 individuals with diabetes onset <30 years and taking insulin followed 10 years	Smoking not related to change in creatinine clearance or incidence of renal insufficiency	—
Klein, Klein and Moss Wisconsin, USA 1993[41]	Wisconsin Epidemiology Study of Diabetic Retinopathy 839 individuals with diabetes onset ≥30 years mean follow-up = 4.1 years	Smoking associated with proteinuria incidence, increased risk with increasing pack-years OR = 3.47, CI 1.95–6.1 (per 45 pack-years, multivariate)	—
Microalbuminuria Collaborative Study England 1993[56]	Microalbuminuria Collaborative Study 137 patients with type 1 diabetes and normoalbuminuria from 9 clinics followed 4 years	Smoking associated with microalbuminuria incidence p <0.05 (ever smoking, multivariate)	—

'–' indicates not reported; OR = odds ratio; CI = 95% confidence interval; ns = not significant.

Table 19.3. Risk of development of neuropathy in diabetic smokers versus nonsmokers.

Study	Participants	Neuropathy Development	Progression
Patient series Mitchell et al. Michigan, USA 1990[57]	160 patients with type 1 diabetes and 166 patients with type 2 diabetes mean age = 34 years (type 1) mean age = 58 years (type 2)	Smoking associated with neuropathy prevalence in type 1 (but not in type 2) patients $OR = 3.32$, $p = 0.026$ ($\geq$ versus <30 pack-years, multivariate)	—
Cross-sectional Tesfaye et al. Europe 1996[58]	EURODIAB IDDM Complications Study 3250 individuals with type 1 diabetes from 31 centers in 16 countries mean age = 33 years	Smoking associated with neuropathy prevalence $OR = 2.4$, $p = 0.02$ (current smoking, multivariate)	—
Maser et al. Pennsylvania, USA 1989[59]	Epidemiology of Diabetes Complications Study 400 individuals with type 1 diabetes from Pittsburgh IDDM Registry mean age = 28 years	Smoking associated with neuropathy prevalence $OR = 2.2$, $p < 0.01$ (ever smoking, multivariate)	—
Trial participants Christen et al. United States 1999[22]	Sorbinil Retinopathy Trial 407 participants with type 1 diabetes aged 18–56 years median follow-up = 3.3 years	Smoking associated with definite distal symmetric polyneuropathy incidence $HR = 1.87$, $p = 0.023$ (ever smoking, multivariate)	—

Table 19.3. contd.

Reichard *et al.* Stockholm, Sweden 1991[54]	Stockholm Diabetes Intervention Study 96 participants with type 1 diabetes and non-proliferative retinopathy mean age = 30 years followed 5 years	—	Smoking not associated with progression of neuropathy
DCCT Research Group United States 1988[60]	Diabetes Control and Complications Trial (DCCT) 278 participants with type 1 diabetes, but no hypertension, renal impairment or severe neuropathy, aged 13–39 years baseline data	Smoking not associated with mild neuropathy prevalence	—
Cohort Forrest *et al.* Pennsylvania, USA 1997[61]	Epidemiology of Diabetic Complications Study 453 individuals with type 1 diabetes from Pittsburgh IDDM Registry mean age = 25 years mean follow-up = 5.3 years	Smoking associated with distal symmetrical polyneuropathy incidence HR = 1.73, p = 0.03 (ever smoking, multivariate)	—
Sands *et al.* Colorado, USA 1997[62]	San Luis Valley Diabetes Study 231 individuals with type 2 diabetes aged 20–74 years, 71% Hispanic mean follow-up = 4.7 years	Smoking associated with distal symmetric sensory neuropathy incidence OR = 2.2, p = 0.05 (current smoking, multivariate)	—

'–' indicates not reported; OR = odds ratio; HR = hazards ratio; CI = 95% confidence interval; ns = not significant.

RETINOPATHY

Evidence of an association between smoking and retinopathy in individuals with diabetes is inconsistent[28,49,50,53,54,63–70] (see Table 19.4). Given the great number of cross-sectional studies of patients, only multinational studies are presented. Neither of the WHO reports found evidence of an association between smoking and the prevalence of retinopathy or small vessel eye disease, using data on 6695 and 3583 individuals from 14 centers[28,63]. In contrast, the EURODIAB IDDM Complications Study based on 3250 individuals from 31 centers found a significant association between current smoking and retinopathy prevalence, but only among men[50].

Among prospective studies examining retinopathy incidence, five found no association with smoking[66–70]. The United Kingdom Prospective Diabetes Study[64] found a significant reduction in the incidence of retinopathy among individuals with type 2 diabetes who smoked, RR = 0.63 (95% confidence interval 0.48–0.82). One study reported a weak positive association in individuals with type 1 diabetes[53].

Among six cohort studies examining retinopathy progression, three found no association with smoking[49,65,68]. The United Kingdom Prospective Diabetes Study[64] found a significant reduction in risk among individuals with type 2 diabetes, RR = 0.50 (95% confidence interval 0.36–0.71), while two studies of individuals with type 1 diabetes found significantly increased risk[53,54].

In summary, the majority of studies of smoking and retinopathy have found no significant association. Of those that found an association, one study found a reduced risk[64] and three found an increased risk[50,53,54], one of which found the association only in men[50]. This inconsistency across gender, ethnic groups, countries and study designs, argues against an association between smoking and retinopathy.

HEART DISEASE MORBIDITY AND MORTALITY

Smoking is an established risk factor for heart disease in persons without diabetes. As shown in Table 19.5, most studies have also identified smoking as a risk factor for heart disease in persons with diabetes[31,34,35,38,39,71–74]. In these studies, representing three different countries, smoking increased the risk of fatal heart disease in individuals with both type 1 and type 2 diabetes about two-fold. In addition, data from the Multiple Risk Factor Intervention Trial (MRFIT) identified a significant dose-response; risk of cardiovascular mortality increased with increasing numbers of cigarettes smoked for 5163 men with diabetes as well as 342 815 men without diabetes[73]. Only the Whitehall Study in England[37] failed to identify smoking as a risk factor for coronary heart disease mortality in individuals with diabetes; however, only 40 diabetic men (24%) reported never having smoked. While the majority of the studies of

Table 19.4. Risk of development and progression of retinopathy in diabetic smokers versus nonsmokers.

Study	Participants	Retinopathy	
		Development	Progression
Cross-sectional			
Chaturvedi et al. Europe 1995[50]	EURODIAB IDDM Complications Study 3250 individuals with type 1 diabetes from 31 centers in 16 countries aged 15–60 years	Smoking associated with retinopathy prevalence in men only (multivariate) OR = 1.71, p <0.01 (current) OR = 1.82, p <0.05 (past)	—
WHO Diabetes Drafting Group Multinational 1985[28]	WHO Multinational Study of Vascular Disease in Diabetics 6695 individuals with diabetes from 14 centers, 13 populations aged 35–54 years	Smoking not associated with small vessel eye disease	—
West et al. Multinational 1982[63]	WHO Multinational Study of Vascular Disease in Diabetics 3583 individuals with diabetes from 9 populations aged 34–56 years	Smoking not associated with retinopathy prevalence	—
Trial participants			
Stratton et al. England 2001[64]	United Kingdom Prospective Diabetes Study (UKPDS) 1919 individuals with type 2 diabetes mean age = 52 years followed for 6 years	Smoking associated with reduced retinopathy incidence RR = 0.63, p = 0.0043 (current smoking, multivariate)	Smoking associated with reduced retinopathy progression RR = 0.50, p = 0.0045 (current smoking, multivariate)
Cohen et al. United States 1999[65]	Sorbinil Retinopathy Trial 485 participants with type 1 diabetes in RCT of aldose reductase inhibition aged 18–56 years median follow-up = 3.4 years	—	Smoking not associated with progression of retinopathy RR = 0.8, ns (current smoking, multivariate)
Mühlhauser et al. Germany 1995[53]	Trial of intensive insulin therapy 613 participants with type 1 diabetes mean age = 27 years followed 6 years	Smoking weakly associated with retinopathy incidence OR = 1.17, p = 0.2	Smoking associated with progression of retinopathy OR = 1.44, p = 0.0075 (per 10 pack-years, multivariate)

Table 19.4. contd.

Reichard et al. Stockholm, Sweden 1991[54]	Stockholm Diabetes Intervention Study. 96 participants with type 1 diabetes and non-proliferative retinopathy in RCT of intense versus regular treatment mean age = 30 years followed 5 years	—	Smoking associated with progression of retinopathy OR = 3.0, p <0.05 (multivariate)
Cohort			
Chaturvedi et al. Europe 2001[66]	EURODIAB Prospective Complications Study. 764 individuals with type 1 diabetes followed for 7.3 years	Current smoking not associated with retinopathy incidence	—
Tudor et al. Colorado, USA 1998[67]	San Luis Valley Diabetes Study. 244 individuals with type 2 diabetes (65% Hispanic) median follow-up = 4.8 years	Smoking not associated with retinopathy incidence OR = 1.23, p = 0.63 (ever smoking, multivariate)	—
Moss, Klein and Klein Wisconsin, USA 1996[68]	Wisconsin Epidemiologic Study of Diabetic Retinopathy. Incidence: 130 younger-onset and 447 older-onset Progression: 529 younger-onset and 904 older-onset followed 10 years	Smoking not associated with retinopathy incidence (current, past, pack-years, multivariate)	Smoking not associated with retinopathy progression (current, past, pack-years, multivariate)
Chase et al. Colorado, USA 1991[49]	359 patients with type 1 diabetes mean age ≈ 20 years mean follow-up = 2.4 years	—	Smoking not associated with retinopathy progression
Ballard et al. Rochester, MN, USA 1986[69]	1135 individuals with type 2 diabetes followed 13–37 years	Smoking not associated with retinopathy incidence p = 0.96 (smoking at time of diagnosis, multivariate)	—
Yanko et al. Israel 1983[70]	Israel Ischaemic Heart Disease Project. 178 men with diabetes aged 40–65 years followed approximately 15 years	Smoking not associated with retinopathy incidence	—

* indicates not reported; OR = odds ratio; RR = relative risk; CI = 95% confidence interval; ns = not significant.

Table 19.5. Risk of heart disease morbidity and mortality in diabetic and nondiabetic smokers versus nonsmokers.

Study	Participants	Heart disease morbidity and mortality	
		Diabetes	No diabetes
Case Control Schumacher and Smith Utah, USA 1988[31]	1986 telephone survey 255 individuals with type 2 diabetes and 622 matched controls aged 20–79 years	Ever smoking associated with CHD morbidity POR = 2.63, CI 1.41–4.91 (Age-, sex- and county matched)	Ever smoking associated with CHD morbidity POR = 1.43, CI 0.84–2.45 (Age-, sex- and county matched)
DeStefano *et al.* 35 states, USA 1993[71]	1986 National Mortality Followback Survey and 1988 Behavioral Risk Factor Surveillance System (BRFSS) Survey Younger men 25–44, women 25–54 years: 867 cases and 27 749 controls Older men ≥ 45 women ≥ 55 years: 2589 cases and 19 568 controls	Current smoking associated with CHD mortality Younger OR = 1.5, CI 0.9–2.5 Older OR = 1.8, CI 1.3–2.6 Past smoking not associated with CHD mortality Younger OR = 1.0, CI 0.6–1.8 Older OR = 1.1, CI 0.8–1.4 (multivariate)	Current smoking associated with CHD mortality Younger OR = 4.8, CI 3.8–6.1 Older OR = 2.2, CI 1.8–2.5 Past smoking not associated with CHD mortality Younger OR = 1.4, CI 1.0–1.8 Older OR = 1.0, CI 0.8–1.1 (multivariate)
Trial participants Alderberth *et al.* Sweden 1998[72]	Multifactorial Primary Prevention Trial 249 men with diabetes and 6851 men without diabetes aged 51–59 years followed 16 years	Smoking predicted CHD mortality HR = 1.74, CI 1.09–2.77 (current smoking, multivariate)	Smoking predicted CHD mortality HR = 1.95, CI 1.66–2.28 (current smoking, multivariate)

Stamler *et al.*
USA
1993[73]
	Multiple Risk Factor Intervention Trial (MRFIT)
	5163 men with diabetes and 342 815 men without diabetes free of myocardial infarction at baseline aged 35–57 years mean follow-up = 12 years
		Increasing # cigarettes associated with increasing risk of CVD mortality
		p = 0.0024 (multivariate)
			Increasing # cigarettes associated with increasing risk of CVD mortality
			p = 0.0006 (multivariate)

Cohort Morrish *et al.* London, England 1991[39]	London cohort of the WHO Multinational Study of Vascular Disease in Diabetics 243 patients with type 1 diabetes and 254 patients with type 2 diabetes mean age ≈ 46 years mean follow-up = 8.3 years	Smoking associated with ECG abnormality (type 2), myocardial infarction and ischaemic heart disease (types 1 and 2), p <0.05 (multivariate)	—

Table 19.5. contd.

Study	Population		
Ford and DeStefano, United States 1991[34]	NHANES I Epidemiologic Follow-Up Study. 602 individuals with diabetes and 12562 without diabetes aged 25–74 years followed 10 years	Smoking predicted CHD mortality HR = 2.49, CI 0.94–6.59 (current smoking, multivariate)	Smoking predicted CHD mortality HR = 1.71, CI 1.19–2.47 (current smoking, multivariate)
Manson et al., 11 states, USA 1991[35]	Nurses Health Study. 1483 female nurses with type 2 diabetes and 114694 without diabetes aged 30–55 years followed 8 years	Smoking predicted CHD morbidity and mortality RR current = 2.6 RR past = 1.6 (age-adjusted)	Smoking predicted CHD morbidity and mortality RR current = 4.6 RR past = 1.4 (age-adjusted)
Moy et al., Pennsylvania, USA 1990[74]	IDDM Morbidity and Mortality Study. 548 patients with type 1 diabetes from Pittsburgh IDDM Registry aged ≥18 years followed 6 years	Smoking predicted CHD mortality in women HR = 5.16, CI 1.29–20.57 but not men HR = 0.78, CI 0.21–2.86 (heavy smoking, multivariate)	–
Jarrett and Shipley, London, England 1985[37]	Whitehall Study. 168 male civil servants with diabetes and 18229 without diabetes aged 40–64 years followed 10 years	Smoking did not predict CHD mortality current smoking, ns past smoking, ns #cigarettes/day, ns (multivariate)	Smoking predicted CHD mortality current smoking, p<0.001 past smoking, ns #cigarettes/day, p <0.05 (multivariate)
Suarez, Barrett-Connor Rancho Bernardo, CA USA 1984[38]	Rancho Bernardo Study. 229 individuals with type 2 diabetes and 2391 without diabetes aged 60–79 years followed 9 years	Smoking predicted CVD mortality men RR = 2.6, p = 0.05 women RR = 2.4, ns (current smoking, age-adjusted) 65% CVD deaths attributed to interaction of diabetes and smoking	Smoking did not predict CVD mortality men RR = 1.1, ns women RR = 1.4, ns (current smoking, age-adjusted)

'–indicates not reported; OR = odds ratio; RR = relative risk; HR = hazards ratio; POR = prevalence risk ratio; CHD = coronary heart disease; CVD = cardiovascular disease; CI = 95% confidence interval; ns = not significant.

smoking and heart disease among individuals with diabetes report only fatal heart disease, a study from England[39] found that smoking significantly predicted ECG abnormalities, myocardial infarction, and ischemic heart disease incidence, and a survey in Utah[31] identified an association with the prevalence of heart disease.

Table 19.5 also indicates that the relative risk of smoking and heart disease is generally of a similar magnitude among individuals with and without diabetes (approximately two-fold). Only among younger individuals, in the cross-sectional study by DeStefano and colleagues[71], was the relative risk for fatal coronary heart disease substantially lower among those with diabetes compared to those without diabetes (1.5 versus 4.8). In contrast, data from the National Health and Nutrition Examination Survey[34] and the Rancho Bernardo Study[38] suggest that smoking may be a stronger risk factor for fatal heart disease among those with diabetes compared to those without (relative risk ≈ 2.5 and 1.5, respectively). Suarez and Barrett-Connor[38] estimated that 65% of cardiovascular disease deaths could be attributed to the interaction between diabetes and smoking. In addition, Stamler and colleagues[73] note that, based on data from the Multiple Risk Factor Intervention Trial (MRFIT), the absolute excess risk of cardiovascular death was greater for diabetic heavy smokers compared to diabetic nonsmokers (89.64 versus 56.28/10 000 person-years).

ALL CAUSE MORTALITY

As can be seen in Table 19.6, smoking is almost universally associated with an increased overall mortality among individuals with diabetes.[34,72,74–77,79] Only the Whitehall Study in England[37] and a community study from Maryland in the USA[78] failed to identify smoking as a risk factor for overall mortality among those with diabetes.

For the two studies that allow a direct comparison, the relative risk of overall mortality associated with smoking was nearly identical among those with and without diabetes[34,72]. In the study from Sweden[72], the relative risks were 1.95 and 1.96 respectively for those with and without diabetes. In the study from USA[34], based on data from the National Health and Nutrition Examination Study, the relative risks were 1.79 and 1.60 respectively for those with and without diabetes.

CLINICAL TRIALS OF SMOKING CESSATION AMONG INDIVIDUALS WITH DIABETES

There is overwhelming evidence that smoking cessation decreases the risk of coronary heart disease, cancer, stroke and lung disease[1]. While no clinical trials have randomized individuals with diabetes to smoking cessation versus no intervention and then monitored individuals for incidence or progression

Table 19.6. Risk of all-cause mortality in diabetic and nondiabetic smokers versus nonsmokers.

Study	Participants	All-cause mortality Diabetes	All-cause mortality No diabetes
Trial participants			
Mühlhauser et al. Germany 2000[75]	Trial of Intensive Insulin Therapy 3570 participants with type 1 diabetes mean age = 27 years mean follow-up = 10.3 years	Smoking predicted mortality HR = 1.92, p = 0.0001 (current smoking, multivariate)	—
Alderberth et al. Sweden 1998[72]	Multifactorial Primary Prevention Trial 249 men with diabetes and 6851 men without diabetes aged 51–59 years mean follow-up = 16 years	Smoking predicted mortality RR = 1.95; CI 1.41–2.70 (current smoking, multivariate)	Smoking predicted mortality RR = 1.96; CI 1.79–2.15 (current smoking, multivariate)
Cohort			
Chaturvedi et al. Multinational 1997[76]	WHO Multinational Study of Vascular Disease in Diabetes 4427 patients with type 1 and 2 diabetes from 10 centers aged 35–55 years followed 11 years	Smoking predicted mortality; risk increased with duration and quantity, and decreased with time since quit RR = 1.45, p = 0.001 (current smoking, age-adjusted) RR = 1.53, p = 0.001 (quit 1–9 years, age-adjusted) RR = 1.25, p = 0.02 (quit ≥10 years, age-adjusted)	—
Ford and DeStefano United States 1991[34]	NHANES I 602 individuals with diabetes and 12 562 without diabetes aged 25–74 years followed 10 years	Smoking predicted mortality HR = 1.79, CI 1.10–2.91 (current smoking, multivariate)	Smoking predicted mortality HR = 1.60, CI 1.34–1.90 (current smoking, multivariate)

Table 19.6. contd.

Reference	Study		
Moy et al. Pennsylvania, USA 1990[74]	IDDM Morbidity and Mortality Study 548 patients with type 1 diabetes from Pittsburgh IDDM Registry aged ≥18 years followed 6 years	Smoking predicted mortality Women HR = 2.57, CI 1.04–6.36 Men HR = 1.21, CI 0.57–2.55 (heavy smoking, multivariate)	–
Klein et al. Wisconsin, USA 1989[77]	Wisconsin Epidemiologic Study of Diabetic Retinopathy 2366 individuals with onset either before or after 30 years followed 6 years	Smoking predicted mortality Younger onset HR = 2.36, p = 0.05 Older onset HR = 1.58, p = 0.0001 (current smoking, multivariate)	–
Jarrett and Shipley London, England 1985[37]	Whitehall Study 168 male civil servants with diabetes and 18229 without diabetes aged 40–64 years followed 10 years	Smoking did not predict mortality ns (current/past, multivariate)	Smoking predicted all-cause mortality p <0.001 (current/past, multivariate)
Dupree and Meyer Maryland, USA 1980[78]	371 individuals with types 1 and 2 diabetes and 742 age, race and sex-matched controls without diabetes from a community-wide survey aged 20–75 years followed 39 months	Smoking did not predict mortality RR = 1.1, ns (ever smoking)	Smoking did not predict mortality RR = 1.3, ns (ever smoking)
Intervention study Yudkin USA 1993[79]	Multiple Risk Factor Intervention Trial (MRFIT) 5163 men with diabetes and 342815 men without diabetes free of myocardial infarction at baseline aged 35–57 years followed 10 years (Intervention estimates from meta-analysis of MRFIT data)	Smoking cessation would prolong life by a mean of 3 years in a 45-year-old man with diabetes	Smoking cessation would prolong life by a mean of 4 years in a 45-year-old man without diabetes

'–' indicates not reported; RR = relative risk; HR = hazard ratio; CI = 95% confidence interval; ns = not significant.

of complications, Yudkin[79] estimated the benefits of smoking cessation for persons with and without diabetes, using data from the Multiple Risk Factor Intervention Trial (MRFIT)[80]. He estimated that smoking cessation would prolong the life of a 45-year-old man with diabetes by a mean of three years, compared to four years in a 45-year-old man without diabetes[79]. This estimate is based on a multifactorial intervention in primarily white men. Cessation benefits among those with diabetes may vary by ethnicity, gender and the presence of other complications.

Current intervention techniques have low success in diabetic populations[56,81–84] and may not be as effective for individuals with diabetes compared to those without diabetes[56,81,84]. Factors potentially inhibiting success include fear of weight gain, depression, and the use of smoking to suppress stress and anxiety related to diabetes management[81–84]. Some of these beliefs were specifically assessed in a survey of 64 patients with type 1 diabetes (mean age 41 years)[81]. Approximately 50% agreed with the statement that they were reluctant to quit smoking because they might gain weight, 46% that smoking helped them not eat sweets, 38% that when they were worried about diabetes, smoking helped calm them down, and 42% that diabetes makes them give up so many things that they like that they don't also want to give up cigarettes. These attitudes may influence a diabetic smoker's desire to quit and confidence to succeed.

Data from the US National Health Interview Surveys indicate that between 1974 and 1990 the prevalence of smoking declined in individuals with diabetes (from 36% to 26%), similar to those without diabetes (from 37% to 26%)[85]. While a greater proportion of smokers with diabetes compared to those without reported that they had been advised by a physician to quit or cut down on smoking in 1990 (58% versus 46%), more than 40% of smokers with diabetes reported never having received advice from a physician to quit smoking[85].

SUMMARY

In addition to the known benefits of smoking cessation for decreasing the risk of coronary heart disease, cancer, stroke, and lung disease[1], individuals with diabetes may also be able to reduce their risk of some diabetic complications by quitting smoking. As reviewed in this chapter and summarized in Table 19.7, there is substantial evidence from patient series, case-control and cohort studies that smoking is associated with both the development and progression of heart disease and nephropathy, and with the development of neuropathy. (Evidence of an association with retinopathy, however, is inconsistent.) In addition, smoking increases the risk of overall mortality in individuals with diabetes.

There are no randomized controlled trials of smoking cessation among those with diabetes, but evidence from studies of nondiabetic individuals suggests that smoking cessation will be associated with a significant reduction

Table 19.7. Summary of evidence: Benefits of not smoking or quitting smoking in type 1 or type 2 diabetes.

Benefit	Level of evidence	Strength of recommendation
Reduction in development of		
Nephropathy	II-2	B
Neuropathy	II-2	B
Retinopathy	II-2	D
Reduction in progression of		
Nephropathy	II-2	B
Neuropathy	none	–
Retinopathy	II-2	C
Reduction in morbidity or mortality from		
Heart disease	II-2	A
Reduction in mortality from		
All-causes	I*	A

I   at least one randomized controlled trial
II-1 controlled trial without randomization
II-2 cohort or case-control studies
II-3 timed series or uncontrolled experiment
III clinical expertise or expert committee

A   good evidence supporting quitting smoking or not smoking
B   fair evidence in support of quitting smoking or not smoking
C   insufficient evidence
D   fair evidence in support of no association
E   good evidence in support of no association
*   intervention estimates from meta-analysis of MRFIT data[79]

in risk of cardiovascular disease and death. Given that individuals with diabetes are already at increased risk of cardiovascular disease and diabetes complication, even a small decrease in their risk would be clinically meaningful. Unfortunately individuals with diabetes appear to be smoking at the same rate as nondiabetic individuals (or even higher among black males). Development of group-specific approaches to smoking cessation and trials of the effectiveness of such programs among diabetic adults are critically needed.

ACKNOWLEDGMENT

This work was partially supported by grant DK31801 from the National Institute of Diabetes, Digestive and Kidney Disease, Bethesda, MD.

REFERENCES

1. US Department of Health and Human Services (1990) The Health Benefits of Smoking Cessation: A Report of the Surgeon General. Atlanta, GA, US Department of Health and Human Services, Public Health Service, Centers for Disease Control and Prevention, National Center for Chronic Disease Prevention and Health Promotion, Office on Smoking and Health.

2. Mühlhauser I (1990) Smoking and diabetes. *Diabetic Medicine* **7**: 10–15.
3. Mühlhauser I (1994) Cigarette smoking and diabetes: an update. *Diabetic Medicine* **11**: 336–343.
4. Dierkx RIJ, van de Hoek W, Hoekstra JBL, Erkelens DW (1996) Smoking and diabetes mellitus (Review). *The Netherlands Journal of Medicine* **48**: 150–162.
5. Haire-Joshu D, Glasgow RE, Tibbs TL (1999) Smoking and diabetes (technical review). *Diabetes Care* **22**: 1887–1898.
6. Ritz E, Ogata H, Orth SR (2000) Smoking: A factor promoting onset and progression of diabetic nephropathy. *Diabetes and Metabolism* **26**: 54–63.
7. American Diabetes Association (2000) Smoking and diabetes (Position Statement). *Diabetes Care* **23**: 93–94.
8. Bott U, Jorgens V, Grusser M, Bender R, Mühlhauser I, Berger M (1994) Predictors of glycaemic control in type 1 diabetic patients after participation in an intensified treatment and teaching programme. *Diabetic Medicine* **11**: 362–371.
9. Lundman BM, Asplund K, Norberg A (1990) Smoking and metabolic control in patients with insulin-dependent diabetes mellitus. *Journal of Internal Medicine* **227**: 101–106.
10. Modan M, Meytes D, Rozeman P, Yosef SB, Sehayek E, Yosef NB (1988) Significance of high HbA1 levels in normal glucose tolerance. *Diabetes Care* **11**: 422–428.
11. Cryer PE, Haymond MW, Santiago JV, Shah SD (1976) Norepinephrine and epinephrine release and adrenergic mediation of smoking-associated hemdynamic and metabolic events. *New England Journal of Medicine* **295**: 573–577.
12. Baer L, Radichevich I (1985) Cigarette smoking in hypertensive patients – blood pressure and endocrine responses. *American Journal of Medicine* **78**: 564–568.
13. Chiodera P, Volpi R, Capretti L (1997) Abnormal effect of cigarette smoking on pituitary hormone secretions in insulin-dependent diabetes mellitus. *Clinical Endocrinology* **46**: 351–357.
14. Targher G, Alberiche M, Zenere M, Bonadonna R, Muggeo M, Bonora E (1997) Cigarette smoking and insulin resistance in patients with non-insulin-dependent diabetes mellitus. *Journal of Clinical Endocrinology and Metabolism* **82**: 3619–3624.
15. Hleve E, Yki-Jarvinen H, Koivisto VA (1986) Smoking and insulin sensitivity in type 1 diabetic patients. *Metabolism* **35**: 874–877.
16. Ganda OMP (1980) Pathogenesis of macrovascular disease in the human diabetic. *Diabetes* **29**: 931–942.
17. Craig WY, Palomaki GE, Haddow JE (1989) Cigarette smoking and serum lipid and lipoprotein concentrations: an analysis of published data. *British Medical Journal* **298**: 784–788.
18. The DCCT Research Group (1992) Lipid and lipoprotein levels in patients with IDDM. *Diabetes Care* **15**: 886–894.
19. Oliver MF (1989) Cigarette smoking, polyunsaturated fats, linoleic acid, and coronary heart disease. *Lancet* **I**: 1241–1243.
20. Groppelli A, Giorgi DMA, Omboni S, Parati G, Mancia G (1992) Persistent blood pressure increase induced by heavy smoking. *Journal of Hypertension* **10**: 495–499.
21. Morgando P, Chen H, Patel V, Herbert L, Kohner E (1994) The acute effect of smoking on retinal blood flow in subjects with and without diabetes. *Ophthalmology* **101**: 1220–1224.
22. Christen WG, Manson JE, Bubes V, Glynn RJ (1999) Risk factors for progression of distal symmetric polyneuropathy in type 1 diabetes mellitus. *American Journal of Epidemiology* **150**: 1142–1151.
23. Ford ES, Malarcher AM, Herman WH, Aubert RE (1994) Diabetes mellitus and cigarette smoking: Findings from the 1989 National Health Interview Survey. *Diabetes Care* **17**: 688–692.

24. Ford ES, Newman J (1991) Smoking and diabetes mellitus: Findings from 1988 Behavioral Risk Factor Surveillance System. Diabetes Care **14**: 871–874.
25. Barrett-Connor E, Khaw KT (1989) Cigarette smoking and increased central adiposity. *Annals of Internal Medicine* **111**: 783–787.
26. Troisi RJ, Heinold JW, Vokonas PS, Weiss ST (1991) Cigarette smoking, dietary intake, and physical activity: effects on body fat distribution – the Normative Aging Study. *American Journal of Clinical Nutrition* **53**: 1104–1111.
27. Randrianjohany A, Balkau B, Cubeau J, Ducimetiere P, Warnet JM, Eschwege E (1993) The relationship between behavioral pattern, overall and central adiposity in a population of healthy French men. *International Journal of Obesity and Related Metabolic Disorders* **17**: 651–655.
28. WHO Diabetes Drafting Group (1985) Prevalence of small vessel and large vessel disease in diabetic patients from 14 centres. The World Health Organization Multinational Study of Vascular Disease in Diabetics. *Diabetologia* **28**: 615–640.
29. Gay EC, Cai Y, Gale SM, Baron A, Cruickshanks, Kostraba JN, Hamman RF (1992) Smokers with IDDM experience excess morbidity: The Colorado IDDM Registry. *Diabetes Care* **15**: 947–952.
30. Songer TJ (1988) What impact does insulin-dependent diabetes mellitus (IDDM) have upon health behaviors? *Diabetes* **37**(Suppl. 1): 124A.
31. Schumacher MC, Smith KR (1988) Diabetes in Utah among adults: Interaction between diabetes and other risk factors for microvascular and macrovascular complications. *American Journal of Public Health* **78**: 1195–1201.
32. Kesson CM, Slater SD (1979) Smoking in diabetics. *Lancet* **I**(814): 504–505.
33. Czyzyk A, Krolewski AS (1976) Is cigarette smoking more frequent among insulin-treated diabetics. *Diabetes* **25**: 717–718
34. Ford ES, DeStefano F (1991) Risk factors for mortality from all causes and from coronary heart disease among persons with diabetes. Findings from the National Health and Nutrition Examination Survey. I. Epidemiologic Follow-Up Study. *American Journal of Epidemiology* **133**: 1220–1230.
35. Manson JE, Colditz GA, Stampfer MJ, Willett WC, Krolewski AS, Rosner B, Arky RA, Speizer FE, Hennekens CH (1991) A prospective study of maturity-onset diabetes mellitus and risk of coronary heart disease and stroke in women. *Archives of Internal Medicine* **151**: 1141–1147.
36. Brand FN, Abbott RD, Kannel WB (1989) Diabetes, intermittent claudication and risk of cardiovascular events. The Framingham Study. *Diabetes* **38**: 504–509.
37. Jarrett RJ, Shipley MJ (1985) Mortality and associated risk factors in diabetics. *Acta Endocrinologica* **110 (Suppl 272)**: 21–26.
38. Suarez L, Barrett-Connor E (1984) Interaction between cigarette smoking and diabetes mellitus in the prediction of death attributed to cardiovascular disease. *American Journal of Epidemiology* **120**: 670–675.
39. Morrish NJ, Stevens LK, Fuller JH, Jarrett RJ, Keen H (1991) Risk factors for macrovascular disease in diabetes mellitus: the London follow-up to the WHO Multinational Study of Vascular Disease in Diabetics. *Diabetologia* **34**: 590–594.
40. Lundman B, Engstrom L (1998) Diabetes and its complications in a Swedish country. *Diabetes Research and Clinical Practice* **39**: 157–164.
41. Klein R, Klein BE, Moss SE (1993) Incidence of gross proteinuria in older-onset diabetes: a population-based perspective. *Diabetes* **42**: 381–389.
42. Pijls LTJ, de Vries H, Kriegsman DMW, Donker AbJM, van Eijk JThM (2001) Determinants of albuminuria in people with type 2 diabetes mellitus. *Diabetes Research and Clinical Practice* **52**: 133–143.

43. Forsblom CM, Groop PH, Ekstrand A, Totterman KJ, Sane T, Saloranta C, Groop L (1998) Predictors of progression from normoalbuminuria to microalbuminuria in NIDDM. *Diabetes Care* **21**: 1932–1938.
44. Biesenbach G, Grafinger P, Janko O, Zazgornik J (1997) Influence of cigarette smoking on the progression of clinical diabetic nephropathy in type 2 diabetic patients. *Clinical Nephrology* **48**: 146–150.
45. Gall MA, Hougaard P, Johnsen KB, Parving HH (1997) Risk factors for development of incipient and overt diabetic nephropathy in patients with non-insulin-dependent diabetes mellitus: prospective, observational study. *British Medical Journal* **314**: 783–799.
46. Ikeda Y, Suehiro T, Takamatsu K, Yamashita H, Tamura T, Hashimoto K (1997) Effect of smoking on the prevalence of albuminuria in Japanese men with non-insulin-dependent diabetes mellitus. *Diabetes Research Clinical Practice* **36**: 57–61.
47. Sawicki PT, Didjurgeit U, Mühlhauser I, Bender R, Heinemann L, Berger M (1994) Smoking is associated with progression of diabetic nephropathy. *Diabetes Care* **17**: 126–131.
48. Couper JJ, Staples AJ, Cocciolone R, Nairn J, Badcock N, Henning P (1994) Relationship of smoking and albuminuria in children with insulin-dependent diabetes. *Diabetes Medicine* **11**: 666–669.
49. Chase HP, Garg SK, Marshall G, Berg CL, Harris S, Jackson WE, Hamman RE (1991) Cigarette smoking increases the risk of albuminuria among subjects with type 1 diabetes. *JAMA* **265**: 614–617.
50. Chaturvedi N, Stephenson JM, Fuller JH (1995) The relationship between smoking and microvascular complications in the EURODIAB IDDM Complications Study. *Diabetes Care* **18**: 785–792.
51. Haffner SM, Morales A, Gruber MK, Hazuda HP, Stern MP (1993) Cardiovascular risk factors in non-insulin-dependent diabetic subjects with microalbuminuria. *Arteriosclerosis and Thrombosis* **13**: 205–210.
52. Mehler PS, Jeffers BW, Biggerstaff SL, Schrier RW (1998) Smoking as a risk factor for nephropathy in non-insulin-dependent diabetics. Journal of General and Internal Medicine **13**: 842–845.
53. Mühlhauser I, Bender R, Bott U, Jorgens V, Grusser M, Wagener W, Overmann H, Berger M (1995) Cigarette smoking and progression of retinopathy and nephropathy in type 1 diabetes. *Diabetic Medicine* **13**: 536–543.
54. Reichard P, Berglund B, Britz A, Nilsson BY, Rosenqvist U (1991) Intensified conventional insulin treatment retards the microvascular complications of insulin-dependent diabetes mellitus (IDDM): the Stockholm Diabetes Intervention Study (SDIS) after five years. *Journal of Internal Medicine* **230**: 101–108.
55. Klein R, Klein BEK, Moss SE, Cruickshanks KJ, Brazy PC (1999) The 10-year incidence of renal insufficiency in people with type 1 diabetes. *Diabetes Care* **22**: 743–751.
56. Microalbuminuria Collaborative Study Group, United Kingdom (1993) Risk factors for development of microalbuminuria in insulin dependent diabetic patients: a cohort study. *British Medical Journal* **306**: 1235–1239.
57. Mitchell BD, Hawthorne VM, Vinik AI (1990) Cigarette smoking and neuropathy in diabetic patients. *Diabetes Care* **13**: 434–437.
58. Tesfaye S, Stephenson JM, Fuller JH, Plater M, Ionescu-Tirgoviste C, Nuber A, Pozza G, Ward JD, EURODIAB IDDM Study Group (1996) Prevalence of diabetic peripheral neuropathy and its relation to glycaemic control and potential risk factors: the EURODIAB IDDM Complications Study. *Diabetologia* **39**: 1377–1384.

59. Maser RE, Steenkiste AR, Dorman JS, Nielsen VK, Bass EB, Manjoo Q, Drash AL, Becker DJ, Kuller LH, Greene DA, Orchard TJ (1989). Epidemiological correlates of diabetic neuropathy: Report from Pittsburgh Epidemiology of Diabetes Complications Study. *Diabetes* **38**: 1456–1461.
60. The DCCT Research Group (1988) Factors in development of diabetic neuropathy. Baseline analysis of neuropathy in feasibility phase of Diabetes Control and Complications Trial (DCCT). *Diabetes* **37**: 476–481.
61. Forrest KY-Z, Maser RE, Pambianco G, Becker DJ, Orchard TJ (1997) Hypertension as a risk factor for diabetic neuropathy. A prospective study. *Diabetes* **46**: 665–670.
62. Sands ML, Shetterly SM, Franklin GM, Hamman RF (1997) Incidence of distal symmetric (sensory) neuropathy in NIDDM. *Diabetes Care* **20**: 322–329
63. West KM, Ahuja MMS, Bennett PH, Grab B, Grabauskas V, Mateo-de-Acosta O, Fuller JH, Jarrett RJ, Keen H, Kosaka K, Krolewski AS, Miki E, Schliack V, Teuscher A (1982) Interrelationships of microangiopathy, plasma glucose and other risk factors in 3583 diabetic patients: a multinational study. *Diabetologia* **22**: 412–420.
64. Stratton IM, Kohner EM, Aldington SJ, Turner RC, Holman RR, Manley SE, Matthews DR (2001) UKPDS 50: Risk factors for incidence and progression of retinopathy in type II diabetes over 6 years from diagnosis. *Diabetologia* **44**: 156–163.
65. Cohen RA, Hennekens CH, Christen WG, Krolewski A, Nathan DM, Peterson MJ, LaMotte F, Manson JE (1999) Determinants of retinopathy progression in type 1 diabetes mellitus. *American Journal of Medicine* **107**: 45–51.
66. Chaturvedi N, Sjoelie A-K, Porta M, Aldington SJ, Fuller JH, Songini M, Kohner EM (2001) Markers of insulin resistance are strong risk factors for retinopathy incidence in type 1 diabetes. The EURODIAB Prospective Complications Study. *Diabetes Care* **24**: 284–289.
67. Tudor SM, Hamman RF, Baron A, Johnson DW, Shetterly SM (1998) Incidence and progression of diabetic retinopathy in Hispanics and Non-Hispanic whites with type 2 diabetes. San Luis Valley Diabetes Study, Colorado. *Diabetes Care* **21**: 53–61.
68. Moss SE, Klein R, Klein BE (1996) Cigarette smoking and ten-year progression of diabetic retinopathy. *Ophthalmology* **103**: 1438–1442.
69. Ballard DJ, Melton LJ, Dwyer MS, Trautmann JC, Chue CP, O'Fallon WM, Palumbo PJ (1986) Risk factors for diabetic retinopathy: a population-based study in Rochester, Minnesota. *Diabetes Care* **9**: 334–342.
70. Yanko B, Goldbourt U, Michaelson IC, Shapiro A, Yaari S (1983) Prevalence and 15-year incidence of retinopathy and associated characteristics in middle-aged and elderly diabetic men. *British Journal of Ophthalmology* **67**: 759–765.
71. DeStefano F, Ford ES, Newman J, Stevenson JM, Wetterhall SF, Anda RF, Vinicor F (1993) Risk factors for coronary heart disease mortality among persons with diabetes. *Annals of Epidemiology* **3**: 27–34.
72. Alderberth AM, Rosengren A, Wilhelmsen L (1998) Diabetes and long-term risk of mortality from coronary and other causes in middle-aged Swedish men. A general population study. *Diabetes Care* **21**: 539–545.
73. Stamler J, Vaccaro O, Neaton JD, Wentworth D, the Multiple Risk Factor Intervention Trial Research Group (1993) Diabetes, other risk factors and 12-year cardiovascular mortality for men screened in the Multiple Risk Factor Intervention Trial. *Diabetes Care* **16**: 434–444.

74. Moy CS, LaPorte RE, Dorman JS, Songer TJ, Orchard TJ, Kuller LH, Becker DJ, Drash AL (1990) Insulin-dependent diabetes mellitus mortality. *Circulation* **82**: 37–43.
75. Mühlhauser I, Overmann H, Bender R, Jorgens V, Berger M (2000) Predictors of mortality and end-stage diabetic complications in patients with type 1 diabetes mellitus on intensified insulin therapy. *Diabetic Medicine* **17**: 727–734.
76. Chaturvedi N, Stevens L, Fuller JH, the World Health Organization Multinational Study Group (1997) Which features of smoking determine mortality risk in former cigarette smokers with diabetes? *Diabetes Care* **20**: 1266–1272.
77. Klein R, Moss SE, Klein BEK, DeMets DL (1989) Relation of ocular and systemic factors to survival in diabetes. *Archives of Internal Medicine* **149**: 266–272.
78. Dupree EA, Meyer MB (1980) Role of risk factors in complications of diabetes mellitus. *American Journal of Epidemiology* **112**: 100–112.
79. Yudkin JS (1993) How can we best prolong life? Benefits of coronary risk factor reduction in non-diabetic and diabetic subjects. *British Medical Journal* **306**: 1313–1318.
80. Ockene JK, Kuller LH, Svendsen KH, Meilahn E (1990) The relationship of smoking cessation to coronary heart disease and lung cancer in the Multiple Risk Factor Intervention Trial. *Journal of Public Health* **80**: 954–958.
81. Haire-Joshu D, Heady S, Thomas L, Schechtman K, Fisher EB (1994) Beliefs about smoking and diabetes care. *Diabetes Educator* **20**: 410–415.
82. Kirkman MS, Weinberger M, Landsman PB, Samsa GP, Shortliffe EA, Simel DL, Feussner JR (1994) A telephone-delivered intervention for patients with NIDDM. Effect on coronary risk factors. *Diabetes Care* **17**: 840–846.
83. Sawicki PT, Didjurgeit U, Mühlhauser I, Berger M (1993) Behavioral therapy versus doctor's anti-smoking advice in diabetic patients. *Journal of Internal Medicine* **234**: 407–409.
84. Fowler PM, Hoskins PL, McGill M, Dutton SP, Yue DK, Turtle JR (1989) Anti-smoking programme for diabetic patients: The agony and the ecstasy. *Diabetic Medicine* **6**: 698–702.
85. Malarcher AM, Ford ES, Nelson DE, Chrismon JH, Mowery P, Merritt RK, Herman WH (1995) Trends in cigarette smoking and physicians' advice to quit smoking among people with diabetes in the US. *Diabetes Care* **18**: 694–697.

20

Prevention of Complications: A Commentary

DAVID SIMMONS

University of Melbourne, Victoria, Australia

The reviews of the benefits to those with diabetes of glycaemic control, and, of smoking cessation, physical activity participation, dietary interventions, weight, blood pressure and lipid control in Chapters 12–15, and from interventions for diabetes-related complications in Chapter 16 cover evidence for the prevention of associated complications and reduction in their severity, following diagnosis of diabetes. This chapter collates and further describes the evidence provided in relation to risk factors (other than glycaemia), highlights the positive and negative synergies between the risk factors and comments on the integrated implementation of the strategies. Implementation of strategies is covered further in Chapters 21 and 22 which review evidence for how care should be delivered to individuals and over whole populations and communities respectively.

It needs to be emphasised that while there is evidence for the efficacy of a range of pharmacological and non-pharmacological interventions, there is not universal access to those with the greatest effect. For example, ACE-inhibitors and statins are expensive medications, which are not always available in some countries[1]. Chapter 19 has therefore been helpful in describing the evidence for the benefits of some of the older, less expensive pharmaceutical products in, for example, hypertension, even if the newer agents are unavailable. There is considerable scope for comparative studies in phamaco-economics, which have yet to be developed in those without diabetes. For example, in hypertension, the balance is yet to be calculated between direct costs of newer and older treatments and comparative costs of managing side-effects, including days off work, set against effectiveness or actual impact on health achieved (e.g. through differential adherence to different medication types, as well as

The Evidence Base for Diabetes Care. Edited by R. Williams, W. Herman, A.-L. Kinmonth and N. J. Wareham.
© 2002 John Wiley & Sons, Ltd

efficacy)[2]. The outcome from such analyses will vary according to the direct and indirect costs in different health systems.

OVERVIEW OF THE EVIDENCE REGARDING THE ASSOCIATION BETWEEN INDIVIDUAL RISK FACTORS AND DIABETES-RELATED COMPLICATIONS

Smoking cessation, physical activity participation, dietary factors, weight, blood pressure and lipids have been generally treated as independent risk factors for cardiovascular disease (heart disease, cerebrovascular disease and other peripheral vascular disease including amputation), nephropathy, retinopathy and neuropathy. In general, reviewers have addressed the following range of questions:

Question 1
What is the evidence that a chronic diabetes-related complication is associated with having the risk factor? i.e. evidence from cross-sectional studies.

Question 2
What is the evidence that having a risk factor is associated with developing the chronic diabetes related complication? i.e. evidence from prospective studies.

Question 3
What is the evidence that risk/severity of a chronic diabetes-related complication is improved by 'improving' the risk factor concerned? i.e. evidence from intervention studies and specifically randomised control trials.

Table 20.1 summarises the evidence for the five risk factors for each of these three questions.

Areas to note are:

1. The lack of studies demonstrating a direct relationship between weight, physical activity and weight control on the one hand and macrovascular or microvascular complications on another (except through extrapolation from an impact on glycaemia).

2. The lack of studies demonstrating or refuting a relationship between these key non-glycaemic risk factors and peripheral vascular disease (and perhaps amputation) in diabetic patients.

3. The shortage of studies demonstrating that an improvement in the diabetes-related risk factor leads to a reduction in risk or severity of a complication independent of any impact on blood pressure or glycaemia.

4. The apparent contradiction between the evidence required to state 'there is good evidence to support an intervention' by the authors and the evidence required to state 'improving the risk factor is associated with improving the

complication' in Table 20.1. The best example of this is where Wingard recommends quitting smoking or not smoking to reduce progression of nephropathy and morbidity/mortality from heart disease (B and A level respectively), but the evidence comes from case-control and cohort studies, not randomised controlled trials (C and B in Table 20.1 respectively).

Table 20.1 assumes a homogenous association between risk factor and diabetes complication and between management of risk factor and improvement in a given complication. However, this is not necessarily the case. Table 20.2 takes the studies with a likely implication of a risk factor for a given complication and summarises patient participation in studies with significant relationships known to be across ages, genders and type of diabetes (type 1 or 2).

As can be seen, unlike many of the early studies into heart disease which focused on relatively restricted study populations, most studies of diabetic patients have included a range of ages and both sexes and there has been little evidence of substantial differences between genders and by age. Intervention studies for the impact of elevated blood pressure and dyslipidaemia on macrovascular disease in type 1 diabetes are lacking. Generally, if studies exist, and if significant risk factors and interventions are found, they are important in both type 1 and type 2 diabetes. Few studies have differentiated between pre- and postmenopausal women. While in studies of Europid women with type 2 diabetes, this may be understandable, further studies are needed, particularly in the ethnic groups at high risk of type 2 diabetes where age at onset is often younger. Similarly, whether the extent of the benefit gained by intervention differs, beyond that due to the initial absolute risk of a given complication in a given age group, gender or by type of diabetes, requires further work

The impact of ethnic differences in risk and natural history of type 2 diabetes on the efficacy of interventions remains unclear. Most intervention studies have been undertaken among people of European ancestry with various degrees of admixture between European ethnic groups. Tables 20.1 and 20.2 often cannot be created for non-European groups. While many cross-sectional studies have been undertaken of the prevalence of diabetes, detailed studies of relationships between non-glycaemic risk factors and complications are less common, prospective studies are uncommon and intervention studies are rare[3]. Where prospective studies have been undertaken, generally, blood pressure remains a predictor of both macro- and microvascular disease across ethnic groups.

Publications of intervention studies in non-European groups are uncommon, although the UKPDS included a sizable proportion of Afro-Caribbeans and South Asians[4]. At the commencement of the study, South Asians had the lowest mean body mass index and systolic blood pressure and Afro-Caribbeans the lowest triglyceride and highest HDL concentrations. Along with Afro-Caribbeans, South Asians experienced the lowest weight

Table 20.1. Overall answers to the three questions among diabetic patients.

Risk factor	Question 1 The risk factor is associated with having the complication					Question 2 The risk factor is associated with developing the complication					Question 3 Improving the risk factor is associated with improving the complication				
	BP	L	S	Weight	PA	BP	L	S	Weight	PA	BP	L	S	W	PA
HD	A	A	A	C	C	A	A	A	C	C	A	A	B	C	C
CD	A	C	C	C	C	A	C	C	C	C	A	C	C	C	C
PVD	C	C	C	C	C	C	C	C	C	C	C	C	C	C	C
Neph.	A	A	A	C	C	A	C	B	C	C	A	C	C	C	C
Retin.	A	A	E	C	C	A	C	E	C	C	A	C	C	C	C
Neuro.	C	B	A	C	C	C	E	A	C	C	C	C	C	C	C

Levels of evidence: A = Yes. B = Probably, but either conflicting data or inadequate data. C = Insufficient evidence. D = Probably not, but either conflicting data or inadequate data. E = No.

Table 20.2. Answers to the three questions according to age, sex and type of diabetes where impact is known

	The risk factor is associated with having the complication					Improving the risk factor is associated with improving the complication				
Risk factor	BP	L	S	Weight	PA	BP	L	S	Weight	PA
HD	TAG	TAG	TAG			T2AG	T2AG	TAG		
CD	TAG					T2AG				
PVD										
Neph.	TAG	TAG	TAG			TAG				
Retin.	TAG	TAG				TAG				
Neuro.	T1AG	T1AG	TAG							

BP = Blood pressure; L = Lipids (any abnormality); S = smoking; W = weight control; PA = physical activity; HD = heart disease; CD = cerebrovascular disease; PVD = peripheral vascular disease; Neph = nephropathy; Retin = retinopathy; Neuro = neuropathy; A = known to be across all ages; G = known to be in both genders; M = male only; F = female only; T1 = known to be affected in type 1 diabetes; T2 = affected in type 2 diabetes; T = both type 1 and type 2 diabetes in at least one study.

gain over the nine years. Afro-Caribbeans experienced the greatest increase in HDL cholesterol and South Asians the least decrease in diastolic blood pressure. By the end of the study, Afro-Caribbeans had experienced a greater rise in systolic blood pressure than Europids. No ethnic differences in efficacy of individual antihypertensive agents were reported, although the randomised trial of beta-blocker versus ACE-inhibitor may have included too few people from these ethnic groups for confident interpretation. Most reports suggest that African-Americans respond less well to monotherapy with ACE-inhibitor and beta-blocker than Caucasians, but equally well to diuretics, central alpha agonists and calcium channel blockers (CCBs)[5]. Among those without diabetes, adding a diuretic is reported to bring the antihypertensive potency among African-Americans up to that of other groups[14].

Although microvascular complications are generally pathognomonic for diabetes, macrovascular disease affects those with and without diabetes. The question therefore arises whether those with diabetes have a comparable benefit from interventions for cardiovascular disease when compared with those without diabetes. In general, the potency of the interventions are similar, although Wareham points out that there is some suggestion that people with diabetes find it harder to lose weight (page?) and Wingard *et al.* suggest that smoking cessation programmes may be less effective among diabetic patients (Chapter 19). Overall, the data in this chapter suggest that the relative reductions in cardiovascular end-points are generally similar or greater among diabetic patients than the general population studied. Furthermore, with their higher absolute risk, the absolute benefits are greater among those with diabetes.

OTHER RISK FACTORS AND ASSOCIATIONS

While smoking, traditional lipid measurements (LDL, HDL, cholesterol triglycerides), weight control, physical activity and blood pressure are the conventional non-glycaemic risk factors for diabetes complications, there are others.

ALCOHOL

Wareham has described the impact of vitamin and mineral supplementation, altering fat and carbohydrate content of the diet and alcohol on metabolic measures. There have also been studies investigating the association between alcohol consumption and diabetes-related complications. The Wisconsin Epidemiologic Study of Diabetic Retinopathy followed up 983 patients with 'older onset diabetes' for up to 12.3 years. Alcohol consumption was inversely associated with risk of coronary heart disease mortality, with those drinking 14 or more g/day alcohol (1 or more drinks per day) having a relative risk of 0.21 (0.09–0.48) when compared with teetotallers[6]. A similar finding was shown in the 2790 men in the Physicians Health Study[7]. The relative benefits were similar to those found in men without diabetes. Similarly, although not analysed separately, the protective effects of moderate alcohol consumption (up to two drinks per day) against stroke persisted after adjusting for diabetes in a case control study in a multiethnic population in New York[8]. No data are available for risk of peripheral vascular disease. Although in painful diabetic neuropathy, it is recommended on clinical grounds that alcohol be avoided[9], overall there is no epidemiological evidence to suggest alcohol is a risk factor for the more common distal symmetric sensory neuropathy[10]. No substantive studies have investigated the relationship between alcohol consumption and either retinopathy or nephropathy among those with diabetes.

HOMOCYSTEINE

In cross-sectional studies among patients with both types of diabetes, hyper-homocysteinaemia is associated with coronary artery disease and nephropathy, possibly peripheral and carotid atherosclerotic disease and retinopathy but not neuropathy[11–13,15,16]. Relationships with retinopathy and microalbuminuria are not consistent however, in type 1 diabetes[17,18]. Such cross-sectional studies are difficult to interpret due to the usual inability to determine cause and effect. For example, total homocysteine concentration (tHcy) is increased according to degree of nephropathy[19].

Hyperhomocysteinaemia is associated with an increased prevalence of cardiovascular disease[20,21] in type 2 diabetes. Hyperhomocysteinaemia is also associated with an increase in all cause mortality in type 2 diabetes[22] and in types 1 and 2 diabetes when combined[23]. Prospective studies in relation to microvascular disease have not yet been reported.

Work in those without diabetes suggest that lowering tHcy by 5 μmol/l may reduce the risk of cardiovascular death by almost 10% in men and 6% in women[24]. Folic acid supplementation reduces the risk factor in plausible ways[24] but folate intervention studies to achieve this have not yet been reported.

CIGAR AND PIPE SMOKING

The data presented by Wingard and colleagues in Chapter 19 comprehensively shows the relationship between tobacco consumption and diabetes-related complications. The review only includes cigarette smoking and no data exist for either pipe or cigar smoking. In the British Regional Heart Study[25],of 7124 men without diabetes, tobacco consumption was associated with an increased risk of diabetes and this was equal among those who switched from cigarettes to pipe or cigars. A link between smoking and insulin resistance has been suggested and, if this is the case, then the relationship with at least macrovascular disease might be expected to be the same between different modalities of tobacco consumption[26]. However, further studies are required.

LIPOPROTEIN (A)

Orchard (Chapter 18) focused on the lipoprotein fractions in standard clinical practice, and a review of the evidence that measuring other lipoproteins may be important in the future is not possible here. Lipoprotein (a) was commented upon, and at one time was thought to have potential as a risk factor for macrovascular disease, but the contribution is now considered relatively small in comparison with the other lipoproteins (such as HDL cholesterol)[27]. Lp (a) is not elevated in type 2 diabetes and slightly (if at all) in type 1 diabetes[28]. Just as there have been mixed findings for Lp (a) in nephropathy and neuropathy (as commented upon by Orchard), the relationship between Lp (a) concentrations and diabetic retinopathy is unclear . Some studies report little relationship[29,30], and others a significant relationship[31,32]. The positive studies have been in type 2 diabetes in Asians rather than Europids, and further work is required to clarify these findings. Similarly, findings in macrovascular disease are mixed. Lp (a) is not related to atherosclerosis or cardiovascular disease in type 1 diabetes[29,33–36], but there are relationships in type 2 diabetes in some[37–40] but not all studies[33–35]. Peripheral atherosclerosis is associated with Lp (a) in both type 1 and type 2 diabetes[41].

TYPE OF BP MEASUREMENT

The evidence presented by Fuller in Chapter 17 focuses principally on the relationship between diabetes-related complications and systolic and/or diastolic blood pressure. There is debate as to which Korotkof sound is more predictive of complications (i.e. I, IV or V) and the importance of derived measures such as mean blood pressure and pulse pressure. The variation associated with clinic-based blood pressure measures, including those related to 'white coat' hypertension, have led to the introduction of both ambulatory blood pressure monitoring (ABPM) and home blood pressure monitoring (HBPM). As the earliest prospective studies did not have the required technology (or the technology was unreliable), prospective and intervention studies using ABPM remain limited.

In cross-sectional studies in patients with type 1 diabetes, retinopathy, microalbuminuria and nephropathy are associated with a higher night/day ratio of diastolic blood pressure ('non-dippers') and blunted circadian blood pressure variation[42–44]. The additional precision of exposure measurement derived from ABPM was shown with retinopathy, where previous doubt regarding the importance of elevated blood pressure as a risk factor was dispelled using ABPM. The loss of diurnal variation is associated with autonomic neuropathy, which may in turn increase the risk of microvascular disease[45,46]. Studies using ABPM are more limited in type 2 diabetes, although higher night-time systolic blood pressure and night/day systolic blood pressure ratios are associated with the presence of microalbuminuria and proteinuria[47–49]. Cross-sectional studies of ABPM in macrovascular disease remain limited in both type 1 and type 2 diabetes.

In a small (n = 75), five-year, clinic-based follow-up study among British patients with either type 1 or type 2 diabetes, non-dippers were found to have a higher mortality (26% versus 8%) and higher cardiovascular event rate than dippers[50]. A similar finding among Japanese patients with type 2 diabetes included increased renal events[51]. In this four-year follow-up study of 288 patients, those with a reversed circadian blood pressure rhythm were also more likely to have retinopathy, nephropathy and both somatic and autonomic neuropathy at baseline. Increments in ABPM are associated with progression of microalbuminuria in type 2 diabetes[52].

ABPM is able to detect differences in blood pressure indices undetected by clinical BP measurements. In a randomised trial of 58 type 1 patients with early microalbuminuria, ABPM was able to detect differences in night recordings with lisinopril which were undetectable with clinical BP measurements and associated with improvements in urinary albumin excretion[53].

Home blood pressure monitoring has been the subject of few studies and, while unable to detect 'non-dippers', there is better comparability with 24-hour ABPM than clinic blood pressure measurement[54].

WAIST CIRCUMFERENCE

Wareham has focused on weight and body mass index as risk factors for diabetes-related complications. Visceral or abdominal adiposity (central fat distribution) often measured as waist circumference (or waist:hip ratio) has emerged as a further risk factor in this area, with predictive value additional to that provided by other overall measures of adiposity. Although part of the effect is possibly through other risk factors[55], residual effects remain after adjustment for other metabolic measures. Among diabetic patients, abdominal fat distribution has been found to be associated with increased frequency of peripheral vascular disease, coronary heart disease, proliferative retinopathy, neuropathy and nephropathy[55–57]. In the EURODIAB study among type 1 diabetic patients, development of retinopathy was also associated with increased measures of central fat distribution[58].

MICROALBUMINURIA

Although microalbuminuria is a risk factor for diabetic nephropathy in type 1 and type 2 diabetes (see Chapter 22), it is also an independent predictor of mortality and atherosclerotic vascular disease[59–61]. Management of microalbuminuria is covered in Chapter 22, but it is important to appreciate here the current evidence for the additional predictive value of microalbuminuria for cardiovascular disease and mortality among diabetic patients, over and above that mediated through nephropathy.

INTERDEPENDENCE OF RISK FACTORS

Chapters 12 and 19 have been divided to review the major risk factors for diabetes complications individually. This has allowed a depth of interrogation of the data to systematically answer the question of whether intervening to address a given risk factor provides benefit. However, although the risk factors have an independent effect, the overall impact on risk is often at least additive and at times risk factors combine to become permissive for harm or create harm greater than that expected by simple addition. One of the points made by Orchard is that the failure to intervene for one risk factor (dyslipidaemia) to investigate its impact on one adverse outcome (nephropathy) may be unethical because of the increased risk of other outcomes (cardiovascular) without treatment. Tables 20.1 and 20.2 clearly show the gaps in our knowledge and the resulting need to use impact on surrogate end-points and 'clinical judgement' to balance risk and benefit. As evidence grows for a given intervention, gaining further evidence of efficacy in demographic and clinical sub-groups may also become difficult. The question clearly becomes, at what stage is evidence for a given intervention sufficient to warrant implementation? Table 20.1 does not need to be completed if there is sufficient evidence to justify action to manage one complication and no adverse impact has been shown in other areas.

CAUSE, EFFECT AND EPIPHENOMENON

Metabolic Syndrome: Dyslipidaemia, hyperglycaemia, insulin resistance, obesity, visceral obesity, hypertension and increased risk of cardiovascular disease are the key components included in the Metabolic Syndrome (MS)[62,63]. There is marked heterogeneity of the MS both between and within populations, and relationships between components are inconsistent. However, given this clustering of phenomena it is possible that the relationship between a given risk factor (e.g. low HDL) and a complication (e.g. cardiovascular disease) is due not to the risk factor itself but to other causal factors related through proximal genetic and environmental interactions. In such a case, prospective studies will still show an apparent relationship, but attempts at modulation may not result in a reduction in complication risk or severity unless they unwittingly affect the true causal path. Similarly the measurement of a given risk factor may serve in part as a surrogate for another metabolic measure: disentangling the influence of such related parameters in studies in humans using multivariate analysis is fraught with difficulties.

Smoking: Clustering is not just confined to the Metabolic Syndrome. For example, in a study of 60 patients with type 1 diabetes, tHcy levels were higher in smokers than in non-smokers in a dose-dependent fashion[64]. If this is the case, and given difficulties with patients stopping smoking, it may be appropriate to provide folate to patients who smoke. This is an area for further research. The association between stopping smoking and weight gain is another example of the confounding which can occur with a single risk factor approach, and this is further elaborated by Wingard *et al*.

Glycaemia and dyslipidaemia: Dyslipidaemia, even with dietary intervention, can be improved to reach the criteria set by the various guidelines for lipid lowering pharmaceutical intervention (see Table 18.1 on page 000), but may be better managed by introducing a pharmaceutical intervention to reduce hyperglycaemia[65, 66].

HDL cholesterol and triglyerides are especially sensitive to improvements in blood glucose, although LDL cholesterol is less likely to be influenced by improvements in glucose control. However, this then begs the question of whether and for how long we should wait to treat those who are hyperglycaemic with lipid lowering agents. With such dyslipidaemia, atheroma formation is likely to be progressing and cumulative and the coronary arteries 'do not forget'. This is an issue which has bearing on the absolute risk approaches discussed below.

Weight control and lipids/blood pressure: Wareham has presented the evidence that in some studies weight control and physical activity can improve glycaemia. Weight and waist circumference are associated with both dyslipidaemia and blood pressure and these in turn are related to cardiovascular disease. Weight loss and waist circumference reduction can be associated with improvements in lipid profile and blood pressure among patients with type 2 diabetes[67–69].

Once patients with diabetes have developed dyslipidaemia and/or hypertension warranting intervention, it needs to be considered whether and for how long it is appropriate to reinforce 'lifestyle' advice that may have been offered repeatedly since diagnosis before pharmaceutical intervention, as is recommended.

CALCULATING ABSOLUTE RISK

The clustering of risk factors and interrelationship between different risk factors makes it difficult to calculate the combined risk of an event on a risk factor by risk factor basis. The continuous nature of the distributions of variables and their biological and measurement variation make the calculations yet more difficult. There have been a number of attempts to create tables to guide the clinician in calculating the risk of cardiovascular disease in a given individual, which can be applied to those with diabetes[70–74,75].

These 'absolute risk' tables have been designed to allow the absolute risk and therefore absolute benefit of a given intervention to be tailored to the patient. None of the charts includes measures of central fat distribution. The data have been based on Europid population based cohorts (Framingham, PROCAM (Germany) and the United Kingdom Heart Disease Prevention Project) and most recently the UKPDS study population. The impact of secular change (e.g. as shown with the observed association between birth weight and MS[76] are not considered).

Only one table has included HDL as a continuous variable (albeit as the cholesterol/HDL ratio) and microalbuminuria, and that is the Yudkin-Chaturvedi risk stratification chart[73]. This is shown in Figure 20.1. The risks of coronary heart disease predicted in these tables have been compared with the predictions in the Dundee and PROCAM tables. Substantial differences have been shown. This table recognises some of the additional risk factors by suggesting that for South Asians, people with cardiovascular disease, a family history of coronary heart disease at an early age, central obesity or left ventricular hypertrophy, the risk level is increased by about one category. The UKPDS risk engine remains under development and includes the largest diabetes cohort with which to project cardiac outcomes[75]. Using a study rather than a population-based sample could be problematic. The model includes the Total cholesterol/HDL ratio and will allow the risk for Afro-Caribbeans to be viewed separately. South Asians have been grouped with Europids as they were not a significant entrant into the model ($p > 0.5$). Triglycerides were also not a significant entrant into the final model. Interestingly, the model includes the HbA_{1c} as a risk factor for coronary heart disease, even though a causal relationship between glycaemia and coronary heart disease susceptible to

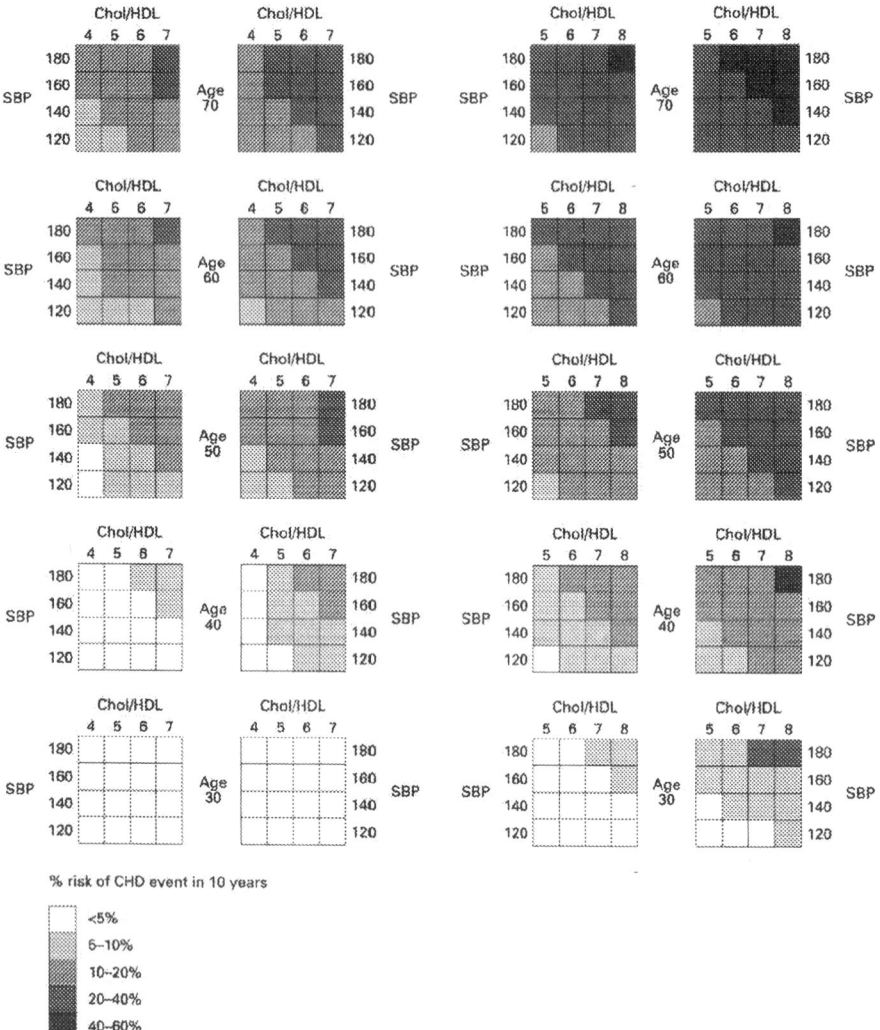

Figure 20.1a. Ten-year risk of coronary heart disease event in nondiabetic men and women. An event is defined as coronary heart disease death, myocardial infarction or angina pectoris. In order to read a person's risk, identify the chart relating to the person's gender, age and smoking status. Within the chart, find the cell nearest to the person's level of total:high density lipoprotein cholesterol ratio and systolic blood pressure. Compare the cell tone with the key and read the risk level. For south Asian subjects, people with symptomatic or asymptomatic cardiovascular disease, a family history of coronary disease at an early age, central obesity, or left ventricular hypertrophy, the risk level will be greater than that indicated in the chart by around one category. The risk will be higher at lower levels, or if concentrations of triglyceride exceed 2.2 mmol/l. Chol/HDL, total cholesterol:high density lipoprotein cholesterol ratio; SBP, systolic blood pressure in mmHg. Reproduced with permission from Blackwell Science Ltd[73].

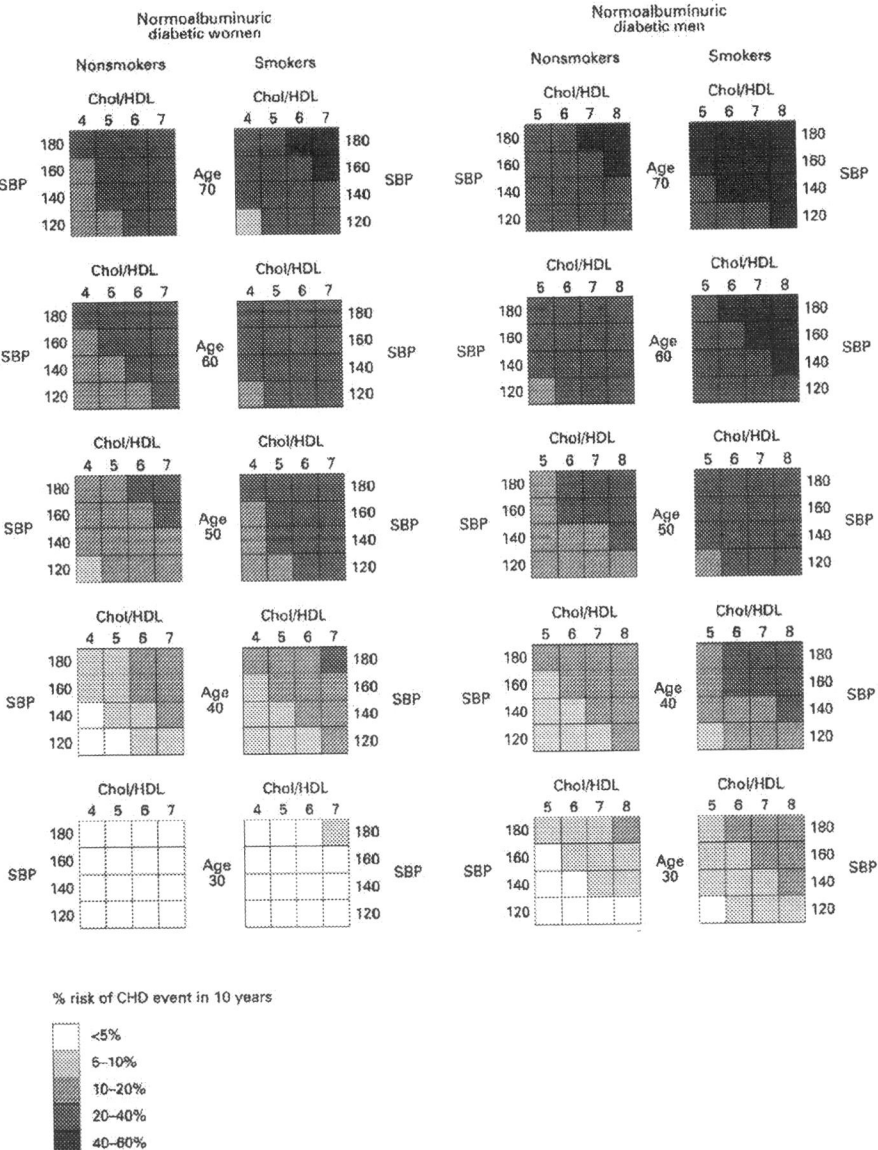

Figure 20.1b. Ten-year risk of coronary heart disease event in diabetic men and women without microalbuminuria (see legend to Figure 20.1a).

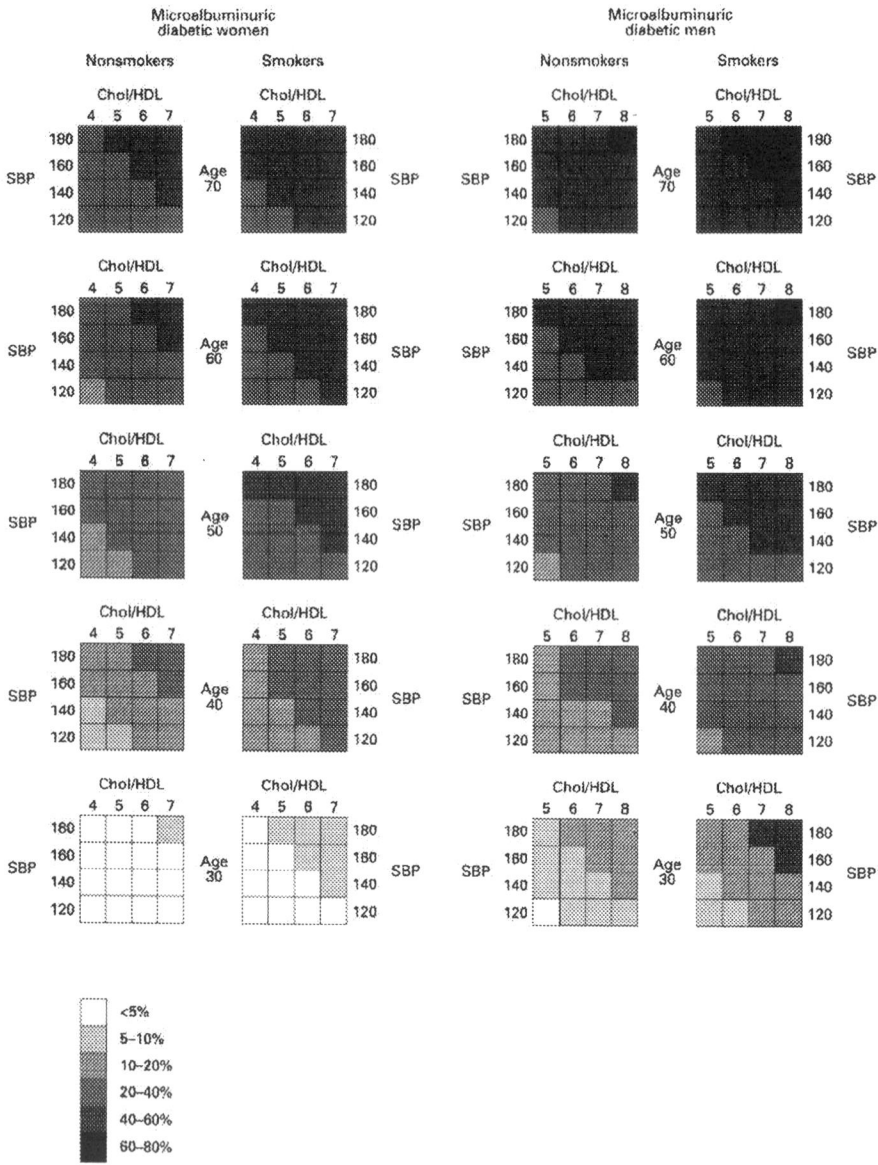

Figure 20.1c. Ten-year risk of coronary heart disease event in diabetic men and women with microalbuminuria (see legend to Figure 20.1a).

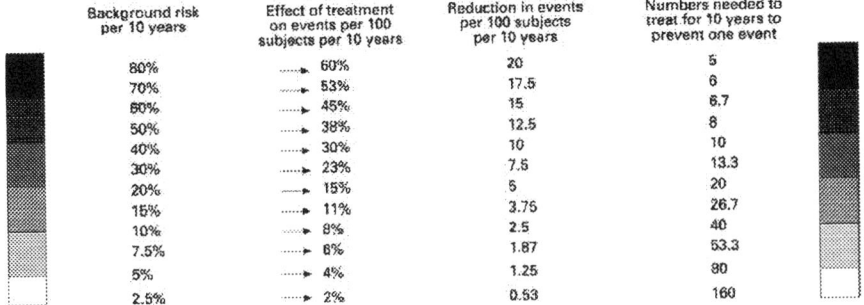

Background risk per 10 years	Effect of treatment on events per 100 subjects per 10 years	Reduction in events per 100 subjects per 10 years	Numbers needed to treat for 10 years to prevent one event
80%	60%	20	5
70%	53%	17.5	6
60%	45%	15	6.7
50%	38%	12.5	8
40%	30%	10	10
30%	23%	7.5	13.3
20%	15%	5	20
15%	11%	3.75	26.7
10%	8%	2.5	40
7.5%	6%	1.87	53.3
5%	4%	1.25	80
2.5%	2%	0.53	160

Figure 20.1d. Numbers needed to treat for 10 years to prevent one coronary heart disease event. The tonal codes are those employed in Figures 20.1a–c. The calculations assume that the intervention reduces the risk of a coronary heart disease event by 25% (see text).

intervention remains unproven. However, microalbuminuria has not been considered as a risk factor in the UKPDS risk engine. While the model created predicts the event rate seen retrospectively, it is hoped the model will also predict events in the post-study period and in other cohorts.

There are other caveats to these early tables. First, there are other new risk factors such as hyperhomocysteinaemia which have not been included. Second, the tables only include coronary heart disease (myocardial infarction, CHD death and angina pectoris) as outcomes for treatment when other cardiovascular outcomes such as congestive cardiac failure, cerebrovascular disease and possibly peripheral vascular disease are significant. Furthermore, when considering antihypertensive medication, the additional benefits on preventing renal and retinal outcomes should be included. In some ethnic groups (e.g. New Zealand Maori and Australian Aborigines)[77-78], these are major causes of death and disability even in those with type 2 diabetes. Thresholds for treatment might be lowered significantly if these outcomes were included.

TARGETS

In spite of these caveats, the absolute risk tables should benefit those who would not be treated on single risk factor assessment and yet are at increased risk because of slightly raised levels of risk across several areas. Having said this, many studies have attempted to identify the risk level at which it is 'worthwhile' epidemiologicaly intervening for a single risk factor. The HOT study and UKPDS have demonstrated that the lower blood pressure targets are of value on their own[79,80]. But there is still debate over what the lower limit for blood pressure lowering should be to provide optimal benefit to patients. Absolute risk tables can certainly help with probabilistic answers choosing an 'agreed' long-term cardiovascular risk. The introduction of ABPM and its interpretation now generates a new area for discussion. Work is still underway to understand the comparability between 24-hour blood pressure targets and clinic blood pressure targets[81]. Similar discussions regarding targets are underway for lipids, weight control and physical activity.

WHICH IS THE BEST INTERVENTION?

Having demonstrated that managing a risk factor is associated with a reduction in risk of a given complication, the next question is, 'What is the best intervention?' Fuller and Orchard and Fried have provided the evidence regarding the use of the major classes of antihypertensive and antidyslipidaemia agents. However, evidence supporting use of individual agents and interchangeability within a class is limited. Differences in side-effect profiles are often taken into account among clinicians and patients in deciding on which agent to use within and between classes, but these are difficult to include in pharmaco-economic discussions in countries deciding on which drugs to subsidise and the extent of the subsidy. The recent withdrawal of cerivostatin as a result of its side-effects and the debate over the impact of the dihydropyridine calcium channel blockers provide examples of how, within a class, there may be clear differences between agents which do not emerge until significant time has passed. Head to head studies of agents within and sometimes between classes are not common, and it is often difficult to know which agent is 'the best' for a given patient. Even where head to head studies have been undertaken, results can be conflicting, with some showing superiority of one agent over another and others failing to show such a difference, or the converse. The comparison between ACE-inhibitors and beta blockers, and ACE inhibitors and CCBs are good examples of this and are well debated by Fuller in Chapter 17.

The issue of 'which agent' has become even more complicated with the realisation that a large number of patients may require more than one agent to treat a given risk factor. Hypertension often requires three or more agents[80]. Confounding may occur in a long-lasting randomised trial where over the years the 'other drug' may be prescribed for other indications (e.g. ACE-inhibitors for heart failure, beta-blockers for angina). Furthermore, as the number and frequency of medications increase, the adherence to the pharmaceutical regimen declines[82–83]. This can be helped partly with the use of, for example, blister calender packs[84].

The issue of the best intervention does not only apply among pharmaceutical agents. Lifestyle interventions to increase physical activity, reduce calorie intake, control weight, stop smoking and enhance dietary intake are fraught with queries over 'the best' intervention. Wareham has already pointed out the difficulties in determining how much and what kind of physical activity is to be recommended from an evidence-based perspective (e.g. differences between people with and without manual occupations, low versus high intensity activity, resistance training or not). The need to tailor such interventions to 'stage of change' needs to be shown conclusively, but is likely to be one confounder that is relatively easily ameliorated. The dearth of data in relation to how to achieve lifestyle change remains a clear area of need, in spite of the costs and difficulties involved, and is considered further in Chapters 30 and 31.

DO WE KNOW ALL THE RISKS?

The absolute risk tables lay down in concrete terms the average risks for groups of individuals according to the data available to date. The Yudkin–Chaturvedi tables are a major advance on earlier tables which did not include microalbuminuria and adjustments for HDL, rather than assuming the same HDL for all. The UKPDS risk engine is also likely to be helpful with its inclusion of HbA_{1c}[75]. Similarly, the advent of other risk factors makes the multidimensional matrix required yet more complicated. On the whole, their omission will have resulted in an underestimate of absolute risk. On the other hand, the risks and benefits associated with particular drugs should also be introduced into the absolute risk tables, and an attempt made to demonstrate the expected impact on risks of particular lifestyle choice, such as amounts of physical activity taken.

The medications currently used have been introduced with monitoring of the known complications, over a limited period of time. Drugs such as cerivostatin have recently been withdrawn because of unexpected side-effects, which do not seem to be class effects and have appeared as usage has increased. Such events will continue and contribute to the absolute risk associated with a given condition (albeit a potential iatrogenic component). Many of the agents currently used (such as ACE-inhibitors and statins) can affect key components of the cellular architecture or key cellular activities. The long lead time for some side-effects such as malignancy and dementia means that their discovery depends upon population-based disease surveillance systems which remain poorly developed in most cases. Thus it may be many years before such sequelae emerge (in the unlikely event that they do).

IMPROVING IMPLEMENTATION OF INTERVENTIONS

It is interesting on looking at Table 20.1 that we appear to know so much about the relationship between risk factors for diabetes complications and the complications themselves, yet so little about what actually works (outside of hypertension) to reduce them. Wareham points out a range of barriers to undertaking trials of lifestyle interventions and Wingard calls for trials in smoking cessation. However, the observations by Fuller and Wingard of the systematic failure to implement existing knowledge, i.e. to translate knowledge into action, is a major concern. There is a great deal of evidence regarding personal and system barriers to implementation of care, and these will be covered in Chapters 30 and 32 .

CONCLUSION

The growth in knowledge quantifying the risk factors for diabetes-associated complications and developing strategies to address them has grown exponentially over the last five or 10 years. The evidence that we can make a difference is beyond doubt in some areas and intervening early rather than awaiting for the 'risk' to materialise into harm needs to be systematically embedded within every system for diabetes care, particularly in relation to blood pressure, blood lipids and blood glucose itself. Risk factors that deserve early attention for introduction into clinical care include waist circumference, ABPM and homocysteine. Absolute risk tables appear useful, but their precision and validity in the clinical setting require further definition. Beyond translation of current knowledge into action (e.g. using absolute risk tables), pharmacological developments will continue to progress. The reviews have shown a range of gaps, particularly in areas where interest by pharmaceutical companies is limited and randomised trial study designs are difficult (e.g. lifestyle approaches). Many of the questions requiring answers identified here need targeted funding: it is time to debate how this is to be achieved.

REFERENCES

1. Mafi G, Simmons D, Harry T, Patel A, Wellingham J., Cutfield R. Diabetes in general practice: Tongans in Tonga and South Auckland. *J. Quality in Clinical Practice* 2001; **21**: 17–20.
2. Giles TD. Pharmacoeconomic issues in antihypertensive therapy. *Am. J. Cardiol.* 1999; **84 (Supp 1)**: 25–28.
3. Keen H, Fuller JH (eds). WHO multinational study of vascular disease in diabetes: follow-up. *Diabetologia* 2001; 4(supp 2): S1–S88.
4. Davis TM, Cull CA, Holman RR, The UK Prospective Diabetes Study (UKPDS) Group (2001). Relationship between ethnicity and glycemic control, lipid profiles and blood pressure during the first 9 years of type 2 diabetes: UK Prospective Diabetes Study (UKPDS 55). *Diabetes Care* 24(7):1167–74.
5. Kaplan N. Ethnic aspects of hypertension. *Lancet* 1994; **344**: 450–452.
6. Valmadrid CT, Klein R, Moss SE, Klein B, Cruickshanks KJ. Alcohol intake and the risk of coronary heart disease mortality in persons with older onset diabetes mellitus. *JAMA* 1999; **282**: 239–246.
7. Ajani UA, Gaziano JM, Lotufo PA, Liu S, Hennekens CH, Buring JE, Manson JE. Alcohol consumption and risk of coronary heart disease by diabetes status. *Circulation* 2000; **102**: 500–505.

8. Sacco RL, Elkind M, Boden-Albala B, Lin IF, Kargman DE, Hauser WA, Shea S, Paik M. The protective effect of moderate alcohol consumption on ischaemic stroke. *JAMA* 1999; **28**: 53–60.

9. Riddle MC. Diabetic neuropathies in the elderly: management update. *Geriatrics* 1990; **45**: 32–6.

10. Sands ML, Shetterly SM, Franklin GM, Hamman RF. Incidence of distal symmetric (sensory) neuropathy in NIDDM: The San Luis Valley Diabetes Study. *Diabetes Care* 1997; **20**: 322–329.

11. Buysschaert M, Dramias A, Wallemacq PE, Hermans MP. Hyperhomocysteinemia in type 2 diabetes: relationship to macroangiopathy, nephropathy and insulin resistance. *Diabetes Care* 2000; **23**: 1816–1822.

12. Chico A, Perez A, Cordoba A, Arcelus R, Carreras G, de Leiva A, Gonzalez-Sastre F, Blanco-Vaca F. Plasma homocysteine is related to albumin excretion rate in patients with diabetes mellitus: a new link between diabetic nephropathy and cardiovascular disease? *Diabetologia* 1998; **41**: 684–693.

13. Chiarelli F, Pomilio M, Mohn A, Tumini S, Vanelli M, Morgese G, Spagnoli A, Verrotti A. Homocysteine levels during fasting and after methionine in adolescents with diabetic retinopathy and nephropathy. *J. Pediatr.* 2000; **137**: 386–392.

14. Cruickshank JK. Diabetes: contrasts between peoples of black (west African), Indian and white European origin. In: Cruickshank JK, Beevers DG (eds) *Ethnic Factors in Health and Disease*. Butterworth Heinemann: London **1994**: 289–304.

15. Vaccaro O, Ingrosso D, Rivellese A, Greco G, Riccardi G. Moderate hyperhomocysteinaemia and retinopathy in insulin dependent diabetes. *Lancet* 1997; **349**: 1102–1103.

16. Lanfredini M, Fiorina P, Peca MG, Veronelli A, Mello A, Astorri E, Dallagio P, Craveri A. Fasting and post-methionine load homocyst(e)ine values are correlated with microalbuminuria and could contribute to worsening vascular damage in non-insulin dependent diabetes mellitus patients. *Metabolism* 1998; **47**: 915–921.

17. Agardh CD, Agardh E, Andersson A, Hultberg B. lack of association between plasma homocysteine levels and microangiopathy in type 1 diabetes mellitus. *Scand. J. Clin. Lab. Invest.* 1994; **54**: 637–644.

18. Cronin CC, McPartlin JM, Barry DG, Ferriss JB, Scott JM, Weir DG. Plasma homocysteine concentrations in patients with type 1 diabetes. *Diabetes Care* 1998; **21**: 1843–1847.

19. Emoto M, Kanda H, Shoji T, Kawagishi T, Komatsu M, Mori K, Tahara H, Ishimura E, Inaba M, Okuno Y, Nishizawa Y. Impact of insulin resistance and nephropathy on homocysteine in type 2 diabetes. *Diabetes Care* 2001; **24**: 533–538.

20. Hoogeveen EK, Kostense PJ, Beks PJ. Hyperhomocysteinemia is associated with an increased risk of cardiovascular disease, especially in non-insulin dependent diabetes mellitus: a population based study. *Arterioscler. Thromb. Vasc. Biol.* 1998; **18**: 133–138.

21. Okada E, Oida K, Tada H, Asazuma K, Eguchi K, Tohda G, Kosaka S, Takahashi S, Miyamori I. Hyperhomocysteinemia is a risk factor for coronary arteriosclerosis in Japanese patients with type 2 diabetes. *Diabetes Care* 1999; **22**: 484–490.

22. Hoogeveen EK, Kostense P, Jakobs C, Dekker J, Nijpels G, Heine R, Bouter L, Stehouwer CDA. Hyperhomocysteinemia increases risk of death, especially in type 2 diabetes: five year follow-up of the Hoorn study. *Circulation* 2000; **101**: 1506–1511.

23. Kark JD, Selhub J, Adler B, Rosenberg IH. Plasma homocysteine and all cause mortality in diabetes. *Lancet* 1999; **353**: 1936–1937.

494 *The Evidence Base for Diabetes Care*

24. Boushey CJ, Beresford SAA, Omenn GS, Motulsky AG. A quantitative assessment of plasma homocysteine as a risk factor for vascular disease. *JAMA* 1995; **274**: 1049–1057.
25. Wannamethee SG, Shaper AG, Perry IJ. Smoking as a modifiable risk factor for type 2 diabetes in middle aged men. *Diabetes Care* 2001; **24**: 1590-1595.
26. Facchini FS, Hollenbeck CB, Jeppesen J, Chen YD, Reaven GM. Insulin resistance and cigarette smoking. *Lancet* 1992; 1128–1130.
27. Ridker PM, Stampfer MJ, Hennekens CH. Plasma concentration of lipoprotein(a) and the risk of future stroke. *JAMA* 1995; **273**: 1269–1273.
28. Kronenberg F, Steinmetz A, Kostner GM, Dieplinger H. Lipoprotein(a) in health and disease. *Critl. Rev. Clin. Lab. Sci.* 1996; **33**(6): 495–543.
29. Maser RE, Usher D, Becker DJ, Drash AL, Kuller LH, Orchard TJ. Lipoprotein (a) concentration shows little relationship to IDDM complications in the Pittsburgh Epidemiology of Diabetes Complications Study cohort. *Diabetes Care* 1993; **16**: 755–758.
30. Massimo B, Cristina S, Amadio L, Fumelli P, James RW. Lipoprotein (a) and retinopathy in IDDM and NIDDM patients. *Diabetes Care* 1997; **20**: 115.
31. Kim C-H, Park H-J, Park J-Y, Hong S-K, Yoon Y-H. High serum lipoprotein (a) levels in Korean type 2 diabetic patients with proliferative diabetic retinopathy. *Diabetes Care* 1998; **21**: 2149–2151.
32. Morisaki N, Yokote K, Tashiro J, Inadera H, Kobayashi J, Kanzaki T, Saito Y, Yoshida S. Lipoprotein (a) is a risk factor for diabetic retinopathy in the elderly. *J. Am. Geriatr. Soc.* 1994; **42**: 965–967.
33. Heller FR, Jamart J, Honore P, Derue G, Novik V, Galanti L, Parfonry A, Hondekijn JC, Buysschaert M. Serum lipoprotein(a) in patients with diabetes mellitus. *Diabetes Care* 1993; **16**: 819–823.
34. Ritter MM, Loscar M, Richter WO, Schwandt P: Lipoprotein (a) in diabetes mellitus. *Clin. Chim. Acta* 1993; **214**: 45–54.
35. Haffner SM, Moss SE, Klein BE, Klein R. Lack of association between lipoprotein (a) concentrations and coronary heart disease mortality in diabetes: the Wisconsin Epidemiological Study of Diabetes Retinopathy. *Metabolism* 1992; **41**: 194–197.
36. Winocour PH, Durrington PN, Bhatnagar D, MBewu AD, Ishola M, Mackness M, Arrol S. A cross-sectional evaluation of cardiovascular risk factors in coronary heart disease associated with type 1 (insulin-dependent) diabetes mellitus. *Diabetes Res. Clin. Pract.* 1992; **18**: 173–184.
37. Velho G, Erlich D, Turpin E, Neel D, Cohen D, Froguel P, Passa P. Lipoprotein(a) in diabetic patients and normoglycemic relatives in familial NIDDM. *Diabetes Care* 1993; **16**: 742–747.
38. James RW, Boemi M, Sirolla C, Amadio L, Fumelli P, Pometta D. Lipoprotein (a) and vascular disease in diabetic patients. *Diabetologia* 1995; 38: 711–714.
39. Ruiz J, Thillet J, Huby T, James RW, Erlich D, Flandre P, Froguel P, Passa P. Association of elevated lipoprotein (a) levels and coronary heart disease in NIDDM patients: relationship with apolipoprotein (a) phenotypes. *Diabetologia* 1994; **37**: 585–591.
40. Hiraga T, Kobayashi T, Okubo M, Nakanishi K, Sugimoto T, Ohashi Y, Murase T: Prospective study of lipoprotein(a) as a risk factor for atherosclerotic cardiovascular disease in patients with diabetes. *Diabetes Care* 1995; **18**: 241–244.
41. Wollesen F, Dahlen G, Berglund L, Berne C. Peripheral atherosclerosis and serum lipoprotein (a) in diabetes. *Diabetes Care* 1999; **22**: 93–98.
42. Hansen KW, Christensen CK, Andersen PH, Pedersen MM, Christiansen JS, Mogensen CE. Ambulatory blood pressure in microalbuminuric type 1 diabetic patients. *Kidney Int.* 1992; **41**: 847–854.

43. Hansen KW, Pedersen MM, Marshall SM, Christiansen JS, Mogensen CE. Circadian variation of blood pressure in patients with diabetic nephropathy. *Diabetologia* 1992; **35**: 1074–1079.

44. Poulsen PL, Bek T, Ebbehoj E, Hansen KW, Mogensen CE. 24 h ambulatory blood pressure and retinopathy in normoalbuminuric IDDM patients. *Diabetologia* 1998; **41**: 105–110.

45. Poulsen PL, Ebbehoj E, Hansen KW, Mogensen CE. 24 h blood pressure and autonomic function is related to albumin excretion within the normoalbuminuric range in IDDM patients. *Diabetologia* 1997; **40**: 718–725.

46. Lafferty AR, Werther G, Clarke CF. Ambulatory blood pressure, micro-albuminuria and autonomic neuropathy in adolescents with type 1 diabetes. *Diabetes Care* 2000; **23**: 533–538.

47. Mitchell TH, Nolan B, Henry M, Cronin C, Baker H, Greely G. Microalbuminuria in patients with non-insulin dependent diabetes mellitus relates to nocturnal systolic blood pressure. *Am. J. Med.* 1997; **102**: 531–535.

48. Rutter MK, McComb JM, Forster J, Brady S, Marshall SM. Increased left ventricular mass and nocturnal systolic blood pressure in patients with type 2 diabetes mellitus and microalbuminuria. *Diabetic Med.* 2000; **17**: 321–325.

49. Equiliz-Bruck S, Schnack C, Kopp HP, Schernthaner G. Nondipping of nocturnal blood pressure is related to urinary albumin excretion rate in patients with type 2 diabetes. *Am. J. Hypertens.* 1996; **9**: 1139–1143.

50. Sturrock ND, George E, Pound N, Stevenson J, Peck GM, Sowter H. Nondipping circadian blood pressure and renal impairment are associated with increased mortality in diabetes mellitus. *Diabetic Med.* 2000; **17**: 360–364.

51. Nakano S, Fukuda M, Horta F, Ito T, Ishii T, Kitazawa M, Nishizawa M. Kigoshi T, Uchida K. Reversed circadian blood pressure rhythm is associated with occurrences of both fatal and non-fatal vascular events in NIDDM. *Diabetes* 1998; **47**: 1501–1506.

52. Nielsen S, Schmitz A, Poulsen PL, Hansen KW, Mogensen CE. Albuminuria and 24-h ambulatory blood pressure in normoalbuminuric and microalbuminuric NIDDM patients. A longitudinal study. *Diabetes Care* 1995; **18**: 1434–1441.

53. Poulsen PL, Ebbehoj E, Nosadini R, Fioretto P, Defarri G, Crepaldi G, Mogensen CE. Early ACE-I intervention in microalbuminuric patients with type 1 diabetes: effects on albumin excretion, 24 h ambulatory blood pressure and renal function. *Diabetes Metab.* 2001; **27**: 123–128.

54. Masding MG, Jones JR, Bartley E, Sandeman DD. Assessment of blood pressure in patients with type 2 diabetes: comparison between home blood pressure monitoring, clinic blood pressure measurement and 24 hour blood pressure monitoring. *Diabetic Med.* 2001; **18**: 431–437.

55. Stuhldreher WL, Becker DJ, Drash AL, Allis D, Kuller LH, Wolfson SK, Orchard TJ. The association of waist/hip ratio with diabetes complications in an adult IDDM population. *J. Clin. Epi.* 1994; **47**: 447–456.

56. Van Gaal L, Rillaerts E, Creten W, De Leeuw L. Relationship of body fat distribution pattern to atherogenic risk factors in NIDDM. Preliminary results. *Diabetes Care* 1988; **11**: 103–106.

57. Simmons D, Shaw LS, Kenealy T, Scott DJ, Scragg RK. Ethnic differences in diabetic nephropathy and microalbuminuria: the South Auckland Diabetes Survey. *Diabetes Care* 1994; **17**: 1405–1409.

58. Chaturvedi N, Sjoelie AK, Porta M, Aldington SJ, Fuller JH, Songini M, Kohner EM, The EURODIAB Prospective Complications Study Group. Markers of insulin resistance are strong risk factors for retinopathy incidence in type 1

diabetes: The EURODIAB prospective complications study. *Diabetes Care* 2001; **24**: 284–289.

59. Beilin J, Stanton KG, McCann VJ, Knuiman MW, Divitini ML. Microalbuminuria in type 2 diabetes: an independent predictor of cardiovascular mortality. *Aust. NZ J. Med.* 1996; **26**: 519–525.

60. Jarrett RJ, Viberti GC, Argyropoulis A, Hill RD, Mahmud U, Murrells TJ. Microalbuminuria predicts mortality in non insulin dependent diabetes. *Diabetic Med.* 1984; **1**: 17–19.

61. Deckert T, Yokoyama H, Mathiesen E, Ronn B, Jensen T, Feldt–Rasmussen B, Borch-Johnsen K, Jensen JS. Cohort study of predictive value of urinary albumin excretion for atherosclerotic vascular disease in patients with insulin dependent diabetes. *BMJ* 1996; **312**: 871–874.

62. Reaven GM. Role of insulin resistance and disease. Diabetes 1988; 37: 1595–1607.

63. Alberti KGMM, Zimmet PZ, for the WHO Consultation: Definition, diagnosis and classification of diabetes mellitus and its complications. Part 1: diagnosis and classification of diabetes mellitus, provisional report of a WHO consultation. *Diabetic Med* 1998; **15**: 539–553.

64. Giovanni T, Bertolini L, Zenari L, Cacciatori V, Muggeo M, Faccini G, Zoppini G. Cigarette smoking and plasma total homocysteine levels in young adults with type 1 diabetes. *Diabetes Care* 2000; **23**: 524–528.

65. Haffner SM. Management of dyslipidemia in adults with diabetes. *Diabetes Care* 1998; **21**: 160–178.

66. Johnston PS, Feig PU, Coniff RF, Krol A, Kelley DE, Mooradian A. Chronic treatment of African-American type 2 diabetic patients with alpha glucosidase inhibition. *Diabetes Care* 1998; **21**: 416–422.

67. Markovic T, Campbell LV, Balasubramanian S, Jenkins A, Fleury AC, Simons LA, Chisholm DJ. Beneficial effect on average lipid levels from energy restriction and fat loss in obese individuals with or without type 2 diabetes. *Diabetes Care* 1998; **21**: 695–700.

68. Heilbronn LK, Noakes M, Clifton PM. Effect of energy restriction, weight loss and diet composition on plasma lipids and glucose in patients with type 2 diabetes. *Diabetes Care* 1999; **22**: 889–895.

69. Halle M, Berg A, Garwers U, Grathwohl D, Knisel W, Keul J. Concurrent reductions of serum leptin and lipids during weight loss in obese men with type 2 diabetes. *Am. J. Physiol.* 1999; **277**: E277–E282.

70. Tunstall-Pedoe H. The Dundee coronary risk disk for management of change in risk factors. *BMJ* 1991; **303**: 744–747.

71. Haq IU, Jackson PR, Yeo WW, Ramsey LE. Sheffield risk and treatment table for cholesterol lowering for primary prevention of coronary heart disease. *Lancet* 1995; **346**: 1467–1471.

72. Wood D, de Backer G, Faergeman O, Graham I, Mancia G, Pyorala K, together with members of the taskforce. Prevention of coronary heart disease in clinical practice. Recommendations of the Second Joint Task-Force of European and other Societies on Coronary Prevention. *Eur. Heart J.* 1998; **19**: 1434–1503.

73. Yudkin JS, Chaturvedi N. Developing risk stratification charts for diabetic and nondiabetic subjects. *Diabetic Med.* 1999; **16**: 219–227.

74. McLeod AJ, Armitage M. Use of statins but New Zealand tables are better. *BMJ* 1998; **317**: 474.

75. Stevens RJ, Kothari V, Adler AI, Stratton IM, Holman RR. The UKPDS risk engine: a model for the risk of coronary heart disease in Type II diabetes (UKPDS 56). *Clin. Sci.* 2001; **101**: 671–679.

76. Hales CN, Barker DJP. Type 2 (non-insulin-dependent) diabetes mellitus: the thrifty phenotype hypothesis. *Diabetologia* 1992; **35**: 595–601.
77. Simmons D, Schaumkel J, Cecil A, Scott J, Kenealy T. High impact of nephropathy on 5-year mortality rates among patients with type 2 diabetes mellitus from a multi-ethnic population in New Zealand. *Diab. Med. J.* 1999; **16**: 926–931.
78. De Courten M, Hodge A, Dowse G, King I, Vickery J, Zimmet P. Review of the epidemiology, aetiology, pathogenesis and preventability of diabetes in Aboriginal and Torres Strait Islander populations. Office for Aboriginal and Torres Strait Islander Health Services, Canberra, Australia, 1998.
79. Hansson L, Zanchetti A, Carruthers SG, Dahlof B, Elmfeldt D, Julius S, Menard J, Rahn KH, Wedel H, Westerling S. Effects of intensive blood pressure lowering and low-dose aspirin in patients with hypertension: principal results of the Hypertension Optimal Treatment (HOT) randomized trial. *Lancet* 1998; **351**: 1755–1762.
80. UK Prospective Diabetes Study Group. Tight blood pressure control and risk of macrovascular and microvascular complications in type 2 diabetes: UKPDS 38. *BMJ* 1998; **317**: 703–713.
81. Hansen KW, Poulsen PL, Abbehoj E, Mogensen CE. What is hypertension in diabetes? Ambulatory blood pressure in 137 normotensive and normoalbuminuric type 1 diabetic patients. *Diabetic Med* 2001; **18**: 370–373 .
82. Wright EC. Non-compliance or how many aunts has Matilda? *Lancet* 1993; **342**: 909–913 .
83. Paes AHP, Bakker A, Soe-Agnie CJ. Impact of dosage frequency on patient compliance. *Diab. Care* 1997; **20**: 1512–1517.
84. Simmons D, Upjohn M, Gamble G. Can medication packaging improve glycaemic control and blood pressure in type 2 diabetes? Results from a randomised controlled trial. *Diabetes Care* 2000; 153–156.

Part VII

TREATMENT OF ESTABLISHED COMPLICATIONS

21

Treatment of Retinopathy

T. MARK JOHNSON and RON M. KURTZ

National Retina Institute, MD 21204, USA and
University of California, Irvine, CA 92697–4375, USA

DIABETIC RETINOPATHY

Diabetic retinopathy was one of the first conditions extensively studied using clinical trials, beginning in the 1970s and continuing until now (Table 21.1). Together, these studies have defined indications, safety and efficacy of various therapeutic interventions, while also detailing the natural history and epidemiology of the disease. In this chapter, we summarize the findings of the major diabetic retinopathy studies, concluding with evidence-based management recommendations. While the role of glycemic control in delaying the onset and/or decreasing the severity of diabetic retinopathy is discussed in Chapters 6 and 7, the implications of these findings are incorporated in these guidelines.

CLASSIFICATION

Diabetic retinopathy classification schemes recognize two distinct, visually significant clinical entities: proliferative diabetic retinopathy (PDR) and diabetic macular edema (DME). Progressive retinal changes in each entity may be graded in a manner that is predictive of increasing risk for significant visual loss[1]. In PDR, untreated retinal ischemia from small vessel closure can produce neovascularization, vitreous hemorrhage and retinal detachment, any of which may lead to severe visual loss. In diabetic macular edema, decreased vascular competence and microaneurysm formation produce exudation and swelling in the central retina that also can significantly decrease visual acuity. DME can occur with any level of retinal ischemia, with clinically significant levels predicting a high risk for visual loss[2] (Table 21.2).

The Evidence Base for Diabetes Care. Edited by R. Williams, W. Herman, A.-L. Kinmonth and N. J. Wareham.

Table 21.1. Major diabetic retinopathy studies.

Study name	Abbreviation
Diabetic Retinopathy Study	DRS
Early Treatment Diabetic Retinopathy Study	ETDRS
Diabetic Retinopathy Vitrectomy Study	DRVS
Wisconsin Epidemiologic Study of Diabetic Retinopathy	WESDR
Diabetes Control and Complications Trial	DCCT
United Kingdom Prospective Diabetes Study	UKPDS

Table 21.2: Diabetic retinopathy classification criteria.

Category	Abbreviation	Findings
Ischemic changes		
Mild non-proliferative diabetic retinopathy	NPDR	Microaneurysms only
Moderate non-proliferative diabetic retinopathy	NPDR	Extensive microaneurysms with or without cotton wool spots, intraretinal microvascular abnormalities (IRMA), venous beading
Severe non-proliferative diabetic retinopathy	NPDR	Extensive microaneurysms, hemorrhages, cotton wool spots, venous beading or IRMA
Early proliferative diabetic retinopathy	PDR	Mild neovascularization of disc or retina, without vitreous hemorrhage
High risk proliferative diabetic retinopathy	HR-PDR	Moderate neovascularization of disc or retina, often with vitreous hemorrhage
Vascular competence changes		
Non-clinically significant macular edema	NCS-DME	Retinal thickening/hard exudates within 1 disc diameter of the center of macula
Clinically significant macular edema	CSDME	Retinal thickening/hard exudates less than 500 μm from center of fovea or an area greater than 1 disc diameter within 1 disc diameter of center of fovea

MODIFIED NATURAL HISTORY DATA AS A BASIS FOR RETINAL EXAMINATION GUIDELINES

PRIMARY PATIENT CHARACTERISTICS

An individual's risk of developing vision-threatening PDR or CSDME is dependent mainly on their duration and type of diabetes, existing level of retinopathy

Table 21.3. Approximate 10-year incidence of any retinopathy, proliferative retinopathy and clinically significant macular edema in type 1 and type 2 diabetes.*

	10-year incidence of any retinopathy %	10-year incidence of proliferative retinopathy (for patients with some retinopathy at baseline) %	10-year incidence of clinically significant macular edema (for patients with some retinopathy at baseline) %
Type 1 diabetics, traditional glucose control	90	24	27
Type 1 diabetics, intensive glucose control	70	8	15
Type 2 diabetics, traditional glucose control	80	25 (insulin controlled) 10 (non-insulin controlled)	25 (insulin controlled) 14 (non-insulin controlled)
Type 2 diabetics, intensive glucose control	50	~12.5 (insulin controlled) ~5 (non-insulin controlled)	~12.5 (insulin controlled) ~7 (non-insulin controlled)

* Adapted from DCCT, WESDR and ETDRS results

and glycemic control[3-7]. As seen in Table 21.3, even with excellent glycemic control, most diabetics eventually develop retinopathy[7]. A significant percentage of both type 1 and 2 diabetics go on to develop sight- threatening PDR and/or CSDME, again even with excellent glycemic control[7].

While diabetic retinopathy appears to satisfy criteria generally required to justify routine examinations, no randomized trial has ever demonstrated that a particular screening protocol reduces the rate of visual loss in diabetics. Since withholding routine examination in a randomized trial would be ethically untenable, referral guidelines are based on natural history findings from several clinical trials.

For example, current recommendations for type 1 diabetics call for an initial examination five years after diagnosis, with follow-up thereafter annually if no disease is present, or more frequently based on the level of retinopathy found[8]. This recommendation is based on the following observations:

- Over 30% of type 1 diabetics, with traditional glucose control and no pre-existing diabetic retinopathy, will develop some level of disease after four years[7].
- It is rare for type 1 patients with no baseline retinopathy to develop sight-threatening PDR (less than 1% risk within four years)[7].

- In patients with known diabetic retinopathy, approximately 40% with mild baseline retinopathy (NPDR) will show significant progression within a four-year period, with approximately 10–15% developing sight-threatening PDR or CSDME. Intensive insulin control reduces, but does not eliminate, this risk, with about 20% still progressing to more severe diabetic retinopathy levels[7]
- Type 1 diabetics with severe NPDR baseline retinopathy have a much higher risk of progression, with an 80% chance of going on to PDR and a 20% risk of HR-PDR[5,6]

Recommendation for immediate retinal examination upon diagnosis of type 2 diabetes is based on the delay in diagnosis that commonly occurs with this disease. Annual follow-up examination has also traditionally been recommended for all type 2 diabetics without retinopathy at the time of diagnosis[9]. However, recently some have advocated less stringent examination schedules for this group, especially when glucose control is good[10]. More frequent follow-up may be indicated, based on the level of retinopathy. These recommendations are based on the following observations:

- For insulin-dependant, type 2 diabetics under traditional insulin control and followed for four years, there is a 50% risk of developing some diabetic retinopathy, a 35% risk of progression to a more severe level of diabetic retinopathy, and an 8% risk of PDR[6]
- CSDME develops in approximately 8.4% of such patients over four years[3].
- The incidence of both PDR and CSDME is significantly lower in diet-controlled diabetics, 2% and 8% respectively over four years[3,6].

OTHER RISK FACTORS: PREGNANCY, PUBERTY, NEPHROPATHY, RACE

The development and progression of diabetic retinopathy during pregnancy is well documented[11]. Recommendations for retinal examination early in the first trimester, with follow-up based on the level of retinopathy found, are based on the following observations:

- In patients with no background retinopathy at the onset of pregnancy, 10% will develop NPDR and 0.2% will develop PDR. Of these, 60% will demonstrate regression post-partum[11].
- In patients with some retinopathy at pregnancy onset, 50% will show progression, with 5% progressing to PDR[11].
- Finally, in patients with PDR at onset of pregnancy, 60% not treated with laser will progress, while 25% will progress even after laser treatment[11].

Although puberty and nephropathy have also been shown to influence the progression of diabetic retinopathy, no specific additional recommendations have been developed. The four-year incidence of retinopathy in patients that are post-menarche at baseline is significantly greater compared to those who are pre-menarche[12], possibly due to elevated pre-puberty levels of insulin like growth factor I[13]. Although renal dysfunction is closely correlated with the development of retinopathy, hypertension does not appear to be an independent risk factor when its association with nephropathy is calculated[14].

Although most epidemiological studies on diabetic retinopathy have been performed in predominately white populations, studies in non-white populations have not identified consistent differences in incidence or prevalence, when other variables are controlled[15,16]. High rates of blindness in Afro-Americans from diabetic retinopathy may indicate less access to appropriate medical care, or poorer glycemic control[15]. Studies in Native Americans and Hispanic populations have had mixed results, with some showing higher prevalence rates[17,18] and other the same rate as whites[19,20].

ALTERNATIVE SCREENING PROTOCOLS

Alternative screening procedures have been tested against standard techniques of ophthalmic examination and photography to try to improve compliance with current guidelines, which now hover at around 50%[21]. The current accepted gold standard for retinopathy screening is a series of seven high-quality fundus photographs graded by an experienced observer[1]. High sensitivity and specificity rates have been found when screening is performed by experienced clinicians in patients with a widely dilated pupil[22]. Significantly lower rates have been seen with non-ophthalmologist examination or photography through an undilated pupil[23]. The usefulness of current non mydriatic cameras is limited by a high rate of poor quality photographs[23,24]. Improvements in photographic technology may increase the sensitivity and specificity rates, making remote diagnosis of diabetic retinopathy more practical[24].

MANAGEMENT

PROLIFERATIVE DIABETIC RETINOPATHY: PAN-RETINAL PHOTOCOAGULATION

The management of PDR is based on several large, randomized clinical trials that have established a generally accepted progression from laser to surgical treatment based on the severity of disease. In both techniques, laser photocoagulation of the peripheral retina (pan-retinal photocoagulation, PRP) reduces production of vasoproliferative factors induced by retinal ischemic, thereby leading to regression of retinal neovascularization[25,26].

In PRP, approximately 1500 to 2000 laser burns are applied to the retinal periphery leading to destruction of approximately 15% of the retinal surface area[26]. PRP can be applied with topical or retrobulbar anesthesia in one to four outpatient sessions, though single-session treatments have been associated with a greater risk of transient choroidal effusions and secondary angle closure glaucoma[27]. Postoperatively, most patients report some loss of night vision and mild constriction of visual field. Approximately 10% of patients experience a mild decrease in central visual acuity following PRP[26]. Even with optimal laser therapy, at least 5% of eyes eventually go on to require surgical intervention due to complications of progressive retinopathy[25].

Current recommendations specify that patients be followed until development of HR-PDR, prior to initiating PRP. PRP may be considered at earlier stages in patients with poor outcomes in the fellow eye, or patients in whom follow-up may be difficult or inconsistent. These recommendations are based on the following findings:

- PRP reduces the rate of severe visual loss (visual acuity less than 5/200 at two years) in patients with HR-PDR[26].
- In patients with less severe PDR, PRP also reduces progression to HR-PDR and the rate of severe visual loss. However the rate of severe visual loss in non HR-PDR patients is low, even without treatment[25] (Table 21.4).

PROLIFERATIVE DIABETIC RETINOPATHY: PARS PLANA VITRECTOMY

Surgical intervention with pars plana vitrectomy (PPV) has been supported in several randomized trials for specific indications (Table 21.5)[28-30]. In type 1 diabetics, PPV performed within four months of onset of vitreous hemorrhage significantly increases the likelihood of better final visual acuity, when compared to observation[28]. Though no significant difference in final visual acuity was found in type 2 diabetics with vitreous hemorrhage, surgery speeds the rate of visual recovery in severe hemorrhages of greater than three-month duration[28]. Overall about 60% of patients will recover better than 20/200 visual acuity with vitrectomy for severe vitreous hemorrhage[28].

PPV for tractional retinal detachment involving the fovea is also supported, although visual outcomes are significantly poorer than in patients with vitreous hemorrhage alone[29,30]. Early PPV has also been found to improve chances for

Table 21.4. High-risk PDR: indications for PRP.*

Neovascularization of the disc greater than half the disc area
Neovascularization of the disc greater than half the disc area with vitreous hemorrhage
Neovascularization of the disc less than half the disc area with vitreous hemorrhage
Neovascularization of the retina greater than half the disc area with vitreous hemorrhage

* Generally, three of four criteria must be present to support PRP.

Table 21.5. Indications for pars plan vitrectomy

High-risk proliferative diabetic retinopathy
Non-clearing vitreous hemorrhage
Traction retinal detachment

better visual acuity in type 1 patients with severe, progressive PDR (even without PRP), although final visual outcomes are frequently limited[29]. Improvements in surgical instrumentation and technique may broaden indications for vitrectomy in clinical practice, especially in patients with poor vision in the fellow eye[29,30].

DIABETIC MACULAR EDEMA: FOCAL LASER THERAPY

Laser photocoagulation in the central macula reduces exudation and swelling, stabilizing visual acuity[31]. Focal laser applications are applied to leaking microaneurysms within two disc diameters of the center of the macula. In areas of diffuse leakage due to capillary non-perfusion, a 'grid' pattern of laser spots one burn width apart is applied[32]. Laser is not used within 500 microns of the center of the fovea unless the visual acuity drops below 20/40, since patients with better visual acuity are more likely to notice side-effects related to treatment[33]. Focal laser therapy is guided by pre-operative fluorescein angiography to identify areas of significant leakage, and may need to be repeated several times to produce significant improvement[32].

Focal laser therapy is only recommended in patients with CSDME (Table 21.6)[31]. In eyes with clinically insignificant DME, the risk of visual loss is low, so laser therapy is deferred until these criteria are met[31]. These guidelines are based on the following study results:

- Focal laser therapy reduces the rate of visual loss in eyes with so-called clinically significant diabetic macular edema by approximately 50%[31].
- At three years follow-up, the incidence of moderate visual loss was reduced to 15% in treated eyes with CSDME compared with 32% in untreated eyes. However, significant visual improvement is rare with laser, with less than 3% of treated patients regaining more than 3 lines of visual acuity[31]. Although patients with 20/20 visual acuity and macular edema involving the center of the macula benefit from laser, such treatment remains controversial[33].

Table 21.6. Indications for focal laser therapy in CSDME.

Retinal thickening/hard exudates less than 500μm from center of fovea
Area of retinal thickening greater than one disc diameter within one disc diameter of center of fovea

DIABETIC MACULAR EDEMA: PARS PLANA VITRECTOMY

The role for pars plana vitrectomy in the treatment of CSDME is unclear. A few case series have suggested that patients with macular edema may benefit from removal of the posterior hyaloid (the back surface of the vitreous gel) that can exert traction on the macula and contribute to vascular leakage[34–37]. In one series, 50% of patients with macular edema unresponsive to standard laser photocoagulation had a modest improvement in visual acuity following PPV[37]. Since surgery can be associated with severe complications, including retinal detachment, cataract and vitreous hemorrhage, larger trials may be beneficial in assessing its utility for this condition.

COEXISTING DIABETIC RETINOPATHY AND CATARACT

Cataract is common in diabetic patients, with approximately 10% of type 1 and 25% of type 2 diabetics undergoing cataract surgery over a 10-year period[38]. Results of cataract surgery in diabetic patients without active retinopathy is excellent, with 85% experiencing visual improvement of two or more lines and 70% achieving 20/40 visual acuity or better[39]. Although progression of retinopathy after cataract surgery has been proposed, the evidence for this association is weak. In one study of 65 eyes undergoing monocular cataract extraction, progression of retinopathy in the operative eye correlated well with progression in the fellow, non-operative eye[40]. Similarly, in the deferred photocoagulation arm of the ETDRS trial, patients undergoing lens extraction did not experience significant progression of retinopathy[41]. In contrast, existing macular edema not treated prior to cataract surgery may limit visual prognosis, with only 25% of such patients attaining vision better than 20/40, compared to 46% of patients receiving early photocoagulation[42].

Table 21.7 shows evidence-based recommendations for various conditions and their treatment.

REFERENCES

1. Early Treatment of Diabetic Retinopathy Study Group (1991) Grading diabetic retinopathy from stereoscopic color fundus photographs – an extension of the modified Airlie House classification. ETDRS Report No. 10. *Ophth.* **98**: 786–806.
2. ETDRS Group (1985) Photocoagulation for diabetic macular edema: ETDRS Report number 1. *Arch Ophth.* **103**: 1796–1806.
3. Klein R, Moss SE, Klein BEK *et al.* (1989) The Wisconsin Epidemiologic Study of Diabetic Retinopathy XI. The incidence of macular edema. *Ophth.* **96**: 1501–1510.
4. Klein R, Moss SE, Klein BEK *et al.* (1995) The Wisconsin Epidemiologic Study of Diabetic Retinopathy XV. The long-term incidence of macular edema. *Ophth.* **102**: 7–16.

Table 21.7. Evidence-based recommendations.

Condition	Intervention	Evidence	Reference
Type 1 diabetes	Retinal examination at 5 years from diagnosis, with follow-up annually if no retinopathy, or more frequently based on level of retinopathy	II-1 A	5
Type 2 diabetes	Retinal examination at time of diagnosis, with follow-up annually if no retinopathy, or more frequently based on level of retinopathy	II-1 A	6
Pregnancy and pre-existing type 1 or 2 diabetes	Retinal examination early in first trimester, follow-up based on level of retinopathy	II-1A	11
Non proliferative retinopathy	Observation: PRP reduces rate of moderate visual loss, but may not outweigh risks. May be beneficial in selected patients	I/A III / C	25
Non high risk proliferative retinopathy (PDR)	Observation: PRP reduces risk of severe visual loss, but overall risk is low, so careful observation for progression to HR-PDR	I/A	26
High risk proliferative retinopathy (HR-PDR)	Panretinal photocoagulation reduces risk of severe visual loss	I/A	26
Clinically significant macular edema	Focal/grid laser improves visual outcome at 6 months versus observation in selected patients with acuity < 20/40.	I/A	31
Non-clearing vitreous hemorrhage	Pars plana vitrectomy improves visual outcome in type 1 diabetics and speeds recovery of vision in type 2 patients	I/A	28
Tractional retinal detachment (TRD)	Pars plana vitrectomy improves visual outcome when TRD involves fovea	I/A	30
Progressive retinopathy	Pars plana vitrectomy improves visual outcome in type 1 diabetics with progressive PDR unresponsive to PRP or with certain very high-risk characteristics	II/A	29
Cataract and diabetes	Cataract extraction improves visual acuity, as long as pre-existing macular edema is treated pre-operatively	II-2/B	41

5. Klein R, Klein BEK, Moss SE *et al.* (1989) The Wisconsin Epidemiologic Study of Diabetic Retinopathy IX. Four-year incidence and progression of diabetic retinopathy when age at diagnosis is less than 30 years. *Arch. Ophth.* **107**: 237–243.
6. Klein R, Klein BEK, Moss SE *et al.* (1989) The Wisconsin Epidemiologic Study of Diabetic Retinopathy X. Four-year incidence and progression of diabetic retinopathy when age at diagnosis is 30 years or more. *Arch Ophth.* **107**: 244–49.
7. The Diabetes Complications and Control Trial Research Group (1993) The effect of intensive treatment of diabetes on the development and progression of long

term complications in insulin dependent diabetes mellitus. *New Engl. J. Med.* **329**: 977–986.

8. Javitt JC, Aiello LP, Chiang Y *et al.* (1994) Preventitive eye care in people with diabetes is cost-saving to the federal government: implications for health care reform. *Diab. Care* **17**: 909–917.

9. Klein R, Klein BEK, Moss SE *et al.* (1984) The Wisconsin Epidemiologic Study of Diabetic Retinopathy III. Prevalence and risk of diabetic retinopathy when age at diagnosis is 30 or more years. *Arch Ophth.* **102**: 527–532.

10. Vijan S, Hofer TP, Hayward RA (2000) Cost utility analysis of screening intervals for diabetic retinopathy in patients with type 2 diabetes mellitus. *JAMA* **283**: 889–896.

11. Klein BEK, Moss SE, Klein R (1990) Effect of pregnancy on progression of diabetic retinopathy. *Diab. Care* **13**: 34–40.

12. Klein BEK, Moss SE, Klein R (1990) Is menarche associated with diabetic retinopathy? *Diab. Care* **13**: 1034–1038.

13. Haffner SM, Klein R, Moss SE *et al.* (1993) Sex hormones and the incidence of severe retinopathy in male subjects with type I diabetes. *Ophth.* **100**: 1782–1786.

14. Knuiman MW, Welborn TA, McCann VJ *et al.* (1986) Prevalence of diabetic complications in relation to risk factors. *Diabetes* **35**: 1332–1339.

15. Rabb MF, Gaglianio DA, Sweeny NE (1990) Diabetic retinopathy in blacks. *Diab. Care* **31**: 1202–1206.

16. Cruickshank JK, Alleyne SA, (1987) Black West Indian and matched white diabetics in Britain compared with diabetics in Jamaica: body mass, blood pressure and vascular disease. *Diab. Care.* **10**: 170–179.

17. Haffner SM, Fong D, Stern MP *et al.* (1988) Diabetic retinopathy in Mexican Americans and non Hispanic whites. *Diabetes* **37**: 878–884.

18. Nelson RG, Wolder JA, Horton MB *et al.* (1989) Proliferative retinopathy in NIDDM : incidence and risk factors in Pima Indians. *Diabetes* **38**: 435–440.

19. Hamman RF, Franklin GA, Mayer EJ *et al.* (1991) Microvascular complications of NIDDM in Hispanic and non Hispanic whites. San Luis Valley Diabetes Study. *Diab. Care* **14**(Suppl.): 655–664.

20. Lee ET, Lee VS, Kingsley RM *et al.* (1992) Diabetic retinopathy in Oklahoma Indians with NIDDM. *Diab. Care* **15**: 1620–1627.

21. Wyllie-Rosett J, Basch C, Walker EA *et al.* (1995) Ophthalmic referral rates for patients with diabetes in primary care clinics located in disadvantaged urban communities. *J. Diabetes Compl.* **9**: 49–54.

22. Williams R, Nussey S, Humphry R *et al.* (1986) Assessment of non-mydriatic fundus photography in detection of diabetic retinopathy. Br. Med. J. 1986:293: 1140–1142.

23. Buxton MJ, Sculpher MJ, Ferguson BA *et al.* A relative cost effectiveness analysis of different methods of screening for diabetic retinopathy. *Diabetic Med.* **8**: 644–650.

24. Taylor R, Lovelock L, Turnbridge WMG *et al.* (1990) Comparison of non-mydriatic retinal photography with ophthalmoscopy in 2159 patients: mobile retinal camera study. *Br. Med. J.* **301**: 1243–1247.

25. ETDRS Group (1991) Early photocoagulation for diabetic retinopathy. ETDRS Report No. 9. *Ophth.* **98 (Suppl)**: 766–785.

26. DRS Group (1978) Photocoagulation treatment of proliferative diabetic retinopathy. *Ophth.* **85**: 82–105.

27. Doft BH *et al.* (1982) Single versus multiple sessions of argon laser panretinal photocoagulation for proliferative diabetic retinopathy. *Ophth.* **89**: 772–779.

28. Diabetic Retinopathy Vitrectomy Research Group (1990) Early vitrectomy for severe vitreous hemorrhage in diabetic retinopathy. Four-year results of a randomized trial. The Diabetic Retinopathy Vitrectomy Study Report No. 5. *Arch. Ophth.* **108**: 958–964.

29. Diabetic Retinopathy Vitrectomy Research Group (1985) Two-year course of visual acuity in severe proliferative diabetic retinopathy with conventional management. Diabetic Retinopathy Vitrectomy Study Report No. 1. *Ophth.* **92**: 492–502.

30. Diabetic Retinopathy Vitrectomy Research Group (1988) Early vitrectomy for severe proliferative diabetic retinopathy in eyes with useful vision: Results of a randomized trial. Diabetic Retinopathy Vitrectomy Study Report No. 3. *Ophth.* **95**: 1307–1320.

31. ETDRS Group (1987) Photocoagulation for diabetic macular edema: ETDRS Report No. 4. *Int. Ophth. Clin.* **27**: 265–272.

32. ETDRS Group (1987) Treatment techniques and clinical guidelines for photo-coagulation of diabetic macular edema. ETDRS Report No. 2. *Ophth.* **94**: 761–774.

33. Ferris FL, Davis MD (1999) Treating 20/20 eyes with diabetic macular edema. *Arch. Ophth.* **117**: 675–676.

34. Nasrallah FP, Jalkh AE, Van Coppenolle F *et al.* (1988) The role of the vitreous in diabetic macular edema. *Ophth.* **95**: 1335–1339.

35. Harbour JW, Smiddy WE, Flynn HW *et al.* (1996) Vitrectomy for diabetic macular edema associated with a thickened and taut posterior hyaloid membrane. *Am. J. Ophth.* **121**: 405–413.

36. Lewis H, Abrams GW, Blumenkranz MS *et al.* (1992) Vitrectomy for diabetic macular traction and edema associated with posterior hyaloidal traction. *Ophth.* **99**: 753–759.

37. Tachi N, Ogino N (1996) Vitrectomy for diffuse macular edema in cases of diabetic retinopathy. *Am. J. Ophth.* **122**: 258–260.

38. Klein BEK, Klein R, Moss SE (1995) Incidence of cataract surgery in the Wisconsin Epidemiologic Study of Diabetic Retinopathy. *Am. J. Ophth.* **119**: 295–300.

39. Tsujikawa A. *et al.* (1997) Long-term prognosis of extracapsular cataract extraction and intraocular lens implantation in diabetic patients. *Jpn. J. Ophth.* **41**: 319–323.

40. Chew EY, Benson WE, Remaley NA *et al.* (1999) Results after lens extraction in patients with diabetic retinopathy. ETDRS Report No. 25. *Arch. Ophth.* **117**: 1600–1606.

41. Early Treatment Diabetic Retinopathy Study Group (1999) Results after lens extraction in patients with diabetic retinopathy. ETDRS Report No. 25. *Arch. Ophth.* **117**: 1600–1606.

42. Cunliffe IA *et al.* (1991) Extracapsular cataract surgery with lens implantation in diabetics with and without proliferative retinopathy. *Br. J. Ophth.* **75**: 547–551.

22

Treatment of Nephropathy

AKINLOLU OJO

University of Michigan Health System, MI 4809-0364, USA

INTRODUCTION

Diabetic nephropathy is the single most important cause of end-stage renal failure. Twenty-five percent of patients entering chronic dialysis programs and 35–40% of renal transplant recipients have diabetic nephropathy as the primary cause of end-stage renal disease (ESRD). A brief discuss of the pathogenesis is essential for full comprehension of the efficacious therapy for different stages of the wide spectrum of diabetic renal disease. The pathogenesis of diabetic nephropathy results from several abnormalities of the diabetic milieu. Glomerular hyperfiltration due to hyperglycemia-induced alteration in renal hemodynamics is the first pathogenic abnormality observed in diabetic nephropathy. There is increased plasma flow and sustained increase in renal perfusion and glomerular capillary pressure. Subsequently, chronic hyperglycemia provides conditions for excess glucose to combine with free amino acids on cells and tissue proteins to form irreversible advanced glycosylation end products (AGES) via an Amadori rearrangement. AGES promote abnormal crosslinkage of collagen, which is then trapped with albumin and IgG in the extracellular matrix. The tissue accumulation of AGES ultimately participates in vasculopathy of the microcirculation of the kidneys and other target organs affected by diabetes mellitus. Experimental studies point to increased mesangial glucose concentration as a potent stimulus for mesangial cell matrix formation and increased expression of transforming growth factor beta (TGF-β) in the glomeruli which then contributes to the cellular hypertrophy and collagen synthesis. These processes lead to the development of nodular glomerulosclerosis, tubulointerstitial scarring, proteinuria, hypertension and progressive decline in glomerular filtration rate (GFR). ESRD supervenes unless the process is arrested by efficacious therapeutic interventions.

The Evidence Base for Diabetes Care. Edited by R. Williams, W. Herman, A.-L. Kinmonth and N. J. Wareham.
© 2002 John Wiley & Sons, Ltd

CLINICAL STAGES OF DIABETIC NEPHROPATHY

To serve as a guide to disease management, the natural course of diabetic nephropathy can be conventionally divided into four stages (Table 22.1). Each of these stages have distinct, albeit overlapping, pathogenetic correlates and calls for specific therapeutic interventions. Stage 1 (initial nephropathy) is detectable within two to four weeks after the onset of glucose intolerance and is characterized by hemodynamic alterations. The principal abnormality during stage 1 diabetic nephropathy is a 25–50% increase in glomerular filtration rate. Stage 2 (quiescent stage) is usually well established by five years after onset of diabetes mellitus, and is typified by thickening of the glomerular basement membrane, mesangial expansion and nephromegaly. Stage 3 (incipient nephropathy) is generally diagnosed 10–15 years after duration of hyperglycemia and is marked by onset of microalbuminuria (30 mg/24hrs or 20 µg/min), progressive increase in systemic blood pressure and further mesangial expansion. Stage 4 (overt nephropathy) is characterized by increasing proteinuria, established hypertension and progressive decline in glomerular filtration rate. Pathognomonic nodular glomerulosclerotic lesion (Kimmelstiel–Wilson lesion) and tubulointerstitial scarring may be detected as early as the incipient nephropathy stage but may be uniformly present during the overt nephropathy stage, which is often accompanied by nephrotic syndrome. In time, end-stage renal disease (stage 5) invariably supervenes after overt nephropathy. The rate

Table 22.1. Clinical stages, pathologic features and treatment of diabetic nephropathy.

Stage	Clinical marker	Pathological features	Time (years)	Treatment
1: Initial	Onset of diabetes mellitus	GFR, kidney size, reversible albuminuria	0	Glycemic control, ACE-inhibitor/ARB
2: Incipient	Microalbuminuria	GBM thickening, mesangial expansion, rising BP	2–5	ACEI/ARB
3: Overt	Overt proteinuria	Nodular glomerulo-sclerosis, hypertension	11–23	Protein restriction (0.8 g/Kg/d)
4: Chronic renal failure	Rising serum creatinine		13–25	Blood pressure control 125/70–80 mmHg
5: End-stage renal disease (ESRD)	Uremic syndrome	GFR <20 cc/min, persistent nephromegaly	15–27	Kidney and pancreas transplantation and dialysis

of progression from overt nephropathy to ESRD is variable, lasting from seven to 10 years, but an average patient loses 1 cc/min of GFR per month.

THE RISK FACTORS FOR MANANGEMENT OF DIABETIC NEPHROPATHY

The intensity with which preventative therapeutic measures are implemented should be guided by the fact that not all diabetic patients develop nephropathy. Although nephropathy is a major complication of both type 1 and type 2 diabetes mellitus (DM), epidemiological studies indicate that the cumulative incidence of clinical significant nephropathy is 25–45% in patients with type 1 and 15–30% in patients with type 2 DM. Because the incidence ratio of type 2 to type 1 DM is 10:1, the number of type 2 patients with nephropathy far exceeds type 1 patients. A number of risk factors are associated with increased risk of diabetic nephropathy (Table 22.2). The presence of these risk factors should be taken into account when implementing a treatment program for individual patients. Several studies have shown genetic susceptibility to nephropathy. The likelihood of developing diabetic nephropathy is markedly increased if a diabetic sibling or parent has diabetic nephropathy. Noncaucasian race groups (Mexican Americans, Pima Indians and Blacks) are also at markedly increased risk of diabetic nephropathy. In one epidemiological study of Pima Indians, the risk of overt proteinuria was 14% if neither parent had proteinuria, 23% if one parent had proteinuria, and 46% if both parents had proteinuria. In Western Europe and North America, the excess risk of diabetic nephropathy in disadvantaged socioeconomic groups suggests an interaction between genetic susceptibility and socioeconomic factors. Evidence indicates that genetic susceptibility to diabetic nephropathy is likely to be of polygenic origin. Genes that have been implicated include those encoding two enzymes – angiotensin converting enzyme (ACE) and aldose reductase. Another independent risk factor for diabetic nephropathy is the degree of initial glomerular hyperfiltration. Glomerular hyperfiltration greater than 125 cc/min in type 1 diabetics in whom duration of hyperglycemia was less than five years is associated with increased risk of proteinuria compared to lower levels of GFR. The relationship between hyperfiltration nephropathy in type 2 diabetes mellitus is less clear because patients are older at the onset of disease and are more likely to have lower degrees of hyperfiltration due to a greater likelihood of concomitant arteriosclerotic vascular disease, which limits increases in glomerular filtration and nephromegaly. The degree of glycemic control, hypertension, plasma prorenin activity and abnormalities of the sodium-lithium and sodium-hydrogen countertransport mechanisms have been implicated as risk factors for the development of diabetic nephropathy.

Table 22.2. Risk factors for diabetic nephropathy.

Duration of diabetes
Systemic blood pressure
Glomerular hyperfiltration
Glycemic control
Genetic predisposition
Renal hypertrophy
Race

EVALUATION FOR DIABETIC NEPHROPAHY

The first step towards an effective treatment program is staging of the disease with appropriate diagnostic testing. Urinary protein excretion and renal function should be quantified in all patients with diabetes mellitus[1]. Serum creatinine measurement or endogenous creatinine clearance is sufficient to evaluate renal function in most cases. However, more precise methods such as isotopic glomerular filtration rates measurement, which is more cumbersome, may be indicated if other factors which may introduce unacceptable error to simpler methods are in attendance (e.g. diminished muscle mass), particularly if significant renal dysfunction is suspected. There is no specific guideline for the frequency of renal function testing, as this is best determined by individual clinical scenarios. Because of its importance as a determinant of disease treatment and outcome, all patients should be evaluated for microalbuminuria/proteinuria. Microalbuminuria is defined as an albumin excretion rate of greater than 300 mg/24 hrs. Microalbuminuria or total protein excretion greater than 300 mg/24 hrs is considered to be overt proteinuria. The routine urinalysis is positive for albuminuria only when the concentration exceeds 30 mg/dL and therefore should not be used to evaluate microalbuminuria. Quantitative albumin determination in a timed urine specimen is most appropriate but the testing can be simplified by analyzing a first void, clean-catch (spot) urine specimen for its albumin (mg) to creatinine (g) ratio. The albumin/creatinine ratio value is approximately equal to the 24 hr albumin excretion divided by 100, so that a P:C ratio greater than 0.3 is considered abnormal. The recommended guidelines for evaluation of microalbuminuria are shown in Table 22.3.

TREATMENT OF DIABETIC NEPHROPATHY

Achievable therapeutic goals should be established for each stage of the disease. It is important to educate the patient about the intended goals and secure participation. Coexisting risk factors and other systemic illness may call for modification of the specific treatment goals in individual patients. In

Table 22.3 Evaluation of microalbuminuria.

1. Test type 1 patients of greater than five years duration. If negative, repeat every two years. Test type 2 patients at diagnosis. If negative, repeat once a year or at each periodic health examination.
2. Rule out causes of transient microalbuminuria: urinary tract infection, essential hypertension, physical exercise, congestive heart failure, water loading.
3. If albumin excretion is elevated, repeat twice over three months to verify microalbuminuria.

general, treatment should be directed at preservation of renal function and prevention and reduction of microalbuminuria and overt proteinuria. More specific treatment goals are summarized in Table 22.1. The primary aim of therapy during stage 1 is to prevent the development of microalbuminuria. In stage 2, treatment should aim to achieve remission/reduction of micro-albuminuria. In addition, nonpharmacological and pharmacological anti-hypertensive measures should be taken to prevent elevation of blood pressure to supranormal levels (<120/70 mmHg). With onset of overt proteinuria (stage 3), the focus of treatment is to reduce proteinuria and to control blood pressure to a normal level (<125/75 mmHg). An integrated program of renal replacement therapy, including various forms of dialysis and renal trans-plantation best accomplishes treatment of ESRD. Evidence-based treatment recommendations are presented in detail below. Most of the evidence support-ing the beneficial role of individual therapeutic modalities have been obtained from studies of type 1 patients. There is enough evidence to indicate that similar benefits applies to type 2 patients. Given the greater prevalence of type 2 and the presence of other risk factors for renal disease in this population, it is no longer appropriate to treat type 2 patients less aggressively than type 1 to prevent diabetic nephropathy, since type 2 patients constitute the over-whelming majority of patients at risk of end-stage nephropathy.

BLOCKADE OF THE RENIN-ANGIOTENSIN ALDOSTERONE (RAA) SYSTEM

Glomerular hemodynamic aberrations attendant to diabetic renal disease are mediated in part by increased tonicity of the RAA system. Angiotensin II plays a central role both in hemodynamic perturbation and the ensuing mesangial expansion, matrix accumulation and glomerulosclerosis. Consequently, thera-peutic manipulation of the RAA system with Angiotensin Converting Enzyme (ACE) inhibitors (ACEI) and/or Angiotensin Receptor Blockers (ARBs) have been shown to beneficial effect in all stages of diabetic nephropathy[2,3,4]. A number of studies have evaluated the effect of ACEI in both type 1 and 2 DM patients with nephropathy. The overwhelming evidence indicates that ACEI preserve GFR and decrease microalbuminuria. In a meta-analysis of 77 experimental groups, ACEI decreased microalbuminuria and proteinuria in addition to preserving renal function. This beneficial effect was also demonstrable in normotensive patients in whom ACEI decreased both albumin excretion and progression to diabetic nephropathy at two years compared to placebo-treated patients. In the European Diabetes (EURODIAB) Controlled Trial of Lisinopril in Insulin Dependent Diabetes (EUCLID) which enrolled over 500 patients[5], ACEI significantly reduced the albumin excretion rate (AER) in both normoalbuminuric and microalbuminuric patients, with the greatest treatment benefit observed in patients with baseline AER $\geq$20 μg/min.

In the European Microalbuminuria Captopril Study group[6], captopril impeded progression to overt proteinuria and prevented increase in AER in normotensive type 1 patients with stage 2 (incipient) nephropathy. The North American Microalbuminuria Study Group also found that after 24 months of ACEI, only 6% of captopril-treated patients progressed to overt proteinuria compared to 18% in the placebo group. Creatinine clearance remained stable in the captopril group (-0.9 mL/min per 1.73 m^2 per year) but declined by 4.9 ml/min per 1.73 m^2 per year in the placebo group. The Collaborative Study Group of Angiotensin Converting Enzyme Inhibition in Diabetic Nephropathy provided the best evidence of the antiproteinuric and renoprotective effect of ACEI in patients with diabetic nephropathy[2]. In this study, 409 type 1 diabetics with overt proteinuria and plasma creatinine concentration $\leq$2.5mg/dL were randomized to receive captopril or placebo with addition of further antihypertensive drugs (except ACEI and calcium channel blockers) as needed. After four years of equivalent blood pressure control, both hypertensive and normotensive patients who received captopril had a slower rate of progression to ESRD or death. The rate of rise in plasma serum creatinine was reduced by over 50% in patients in the captopril group who had an initial serum creatinine greater than 1.4 mg/dL. The rate of progression in patients with plasma creatinine less than 1.4 mg/dl was too small for this study to detect a difference between captopril and placebo in this subset of 'slow progressors'. In another prospective controlled study of normotensive patients with type 2 DM, ACEI treatment for five years was associated with stabilization of proteinuria and renal function decline, whereas the placebo group had a 2.5-fold increase in proteinuria and a 13% rise in plasma creatinine concentration.

A large number of studies have shown reduction in AER and proteinuria with ARBS. The antiprotienuric effect of ARB appears to be similar to that of ACEI. Long-term studies of preservation of GFR with this newer class of RAA system antagonist are in progress[7].

PROTEIN RESTRICTION

Dietary protein restriction in the range of 0.6–0.8 g/Kg per day has been shown to slow the progressive decline in GFR in diabetic nephropathy. Low-protein diet reduces intraglomerular pressure and preserves kidney function. Type 1 patients with stage 1 and stage 2 diabetic renal disease showed a reduction in glomerular hyperfiltration and urinary albumin excretion on low-protein diets[8]. In one report of 35 type 1 patients with a mean follow-up of 37 months, the rate of decline in GFR was 1.01 mL/min/month in the patients on a high-protein diet compared to 0.26 mL/min/month for those on a low-protein diet. In separate controlled trials, protein and phosphate restriction (0.6 g/Kg per day) slowed the rate of decline in GFR from 12 mL/min per year to 3 mL/min per year. In another study of 22 type 1 patients with diabetic nephropathy, moderate protein restriction (0.8 g/Kg per day) resulted in a marked decrease in proteinuria of 1.13–21.15 g/day and stabilization of GFR, whereas in the controlled group who were allowed an unrestricted protein diet (>1.6 g/Kg per day), GFR declined by 1.3 mL/min per month with no change in proteinuria[9]. In a meta-analysis of five experimental groups (total = 108 patients)[10], dietary protein restriction ranging from 0.50 to 0.85 g/Kg/per day reduced the risk of decline in GFR or increase in AER (relative risk 0.56 [CI, 04.0–0.77]; P < 0.001).

Dietary protein restriction is problematic and difficult to achieve. Difficulty may ensue due to concurrent fat and simple carbohydrate restriction. Even in experimental settings, drop-out rates for this treatment modality may exceed 40%. Moreover, patients with DM are at increased risk for protein malnutrition because the reduction in protein intake may enhance protein catabolism induced by insulin deficiency. Indeed, substantial protein restriction was barely feasible in 121 type patients studied for six months. However, a small reduction of 0.10 g/Kg per day was associated with an 11.1% reduction in albuminuria. Therefore, whenever feasible, a modest restriction of protein intake should be encouraged in patients with diabetic nephropathy. In the advanced uremic state, drastic reduction in protein intake is no longer beneficial and may lead to malnutrition and poorer patient outcomes on renal replacement therapy.

PENTOXIFYLLINE

Hyperviscosity syndrome in renal microcirculation has been implicated in the microcirculatory derangement of diabetes mellitus. During the glomerular filtration process, an increase in peritubular hemoconcentration occurs, which worsens hyperviscosity and hyperfiltration, causing glomerular injury. Poor glycemic control and dehydration enhance this derangement. Furthermore, diabetics have decreased erythrocyte deformability, high platelet adhesivity and increased release of von Willebrand's factor and tissue plasminogen activator. These conditions reduce microcirculatory blood flow and promote the development of systemic and renal macroangiopathy. Pentoxifylline (PTF) is a methylxanthine derivative with hemorrheological properties that has been used in the management microcirculatory abnormalities. PTF has been shown to reduce proteinuria in diabetic patients with normal renal function because of its rheological and renal hemodynamic actions. It has been demonstrated that PTF increases erythrocyte deformability and thus reduces blood viscosity in the peripheral and central circulation. Therefore, its use to improve micro-circulatory derangement in diabetes is theoretically attractive. In a study of 41 type 1 and 2 patients, treated with PTF 1200 mg/day for four months, AER declined from 63 $\pm$ 19 μg/min to zero and overt proteinuria declined from 752 $\pm$ 214 to 103 $\pm$ 63 μg/min to zero in type 1 patients. An equally marked reduction in AER and proteinuria were noted in type 2 patients. PTF has also been shown to reduce proteinuria in diabetic patients with advanced renal failure (CrCl <35 min/min). PTF was administered in a dose of 400 mg/day for six months from 2.7 to 1.1 gram/day. Although these results are encouraging, there are currently no large-scale long-term trials of PTF in diabetic nephropathy. Furthermore, its effect on renal function is unclear. At the present time, the use of PTF is limited to experimental protocols and carefully selected and closely monitored patients who have not responded adequately to ACEI/ARB and moderate protein restriction.

AMINOGLYCOSANS

Initial experimental evidence suggests that sulfated glycosaminoglycans may have therapeutic potential in diabetic nephropathy. The theoretic basis of this therapeutic approach derives from the fact that decreased expression of heparan sulfate is a consistent structural abnormality in the glomerular basement membrane of patients with overt diabetic nephropathy. Administration of low molecular weight heparan and other highly sulfated glycosaminoglycans has been shown to decrease UAE in patients with incipient and overt diabetic nephropathy[11]. Due to the small number of patients included in clinical trials and the potential adverse effects including hematological problems associated with sulfated glycosaminoglycans, these agents cannot be recommended for use in diabetic nephropathy at the present time.

DIALYSIS, KIDNEY AND PANCREAS TRANSPLANTATION

Patients with diabetic end-stage nephropathy can be treated with maintenance dialysis and kidney transplantation. Type 1 patients with end-stage nephropathy can also be treated with combinations of kidney and pancreas transplantation. Hemodialysis and peritoneal dialysis are equally effective in diabetic patients. The choice of dialytic modality should be guided by the same factors operative in patients with ESRD from nondiabetic causes. However, special considerations should be entertained for the following reasons. First, diabetic patients experience uremic manifestations at a higher level of residual renal function than nondiabetic ESRD patients. Thus, early initiation of renal replacement therapy is in order. Timely institution of renal replacement therapy requires vigilance for uremic signs and symptoms when renal function is still well above the range at which dialysis is required in other ESRD populations (GFR $\approx$ 20–25cc/min). Second, the excess prevalence of advanced systemic atherosclerotic disease in diabetic ESRD patients often causes problems with hemodialysis vascular access in terms of poor maturity of native arteriovenous fistula and diminished patency and longevity of the vascular access. Third, cardiovascular autonomic dysfunction associated with diabetic neuropathy may make hemodialysis sessions more arduous with repeated hypotensive episodes during hemofiltration. This may limit the ability to deliver adequate dialysis therapy. In this respect, peritoneal dialysis is often more tolerable because of less abrupt fluid shifts between the vascular and the interstitial compartments. However, diabetic patients on peritoneal dialysis are at greater risk of infectious peritonitis and excessive caloric gain from the peritoneal dialysis dextrose. Because of diminished muscle mass, monitoring of dialysis adequacy should rely more on careful measurement of delivered therapy and systemic manifestation of uremia. Despite adequate dialysis treatment, patients with diabetic end-stage nephropathy have significantly higher morbidity and mortality than patients with ESRD from nondiabetic causes.

Renal transplantation improves the quality of life and longevity of patients with end-stage diabetic nephropathy. Allograft survival is now similar between patients with diabetic ESRD and other renal transplant recipient groups. The improved patient survival associated with renal transplantation is proportionally greater for patients with end-stage diabetic nephropathy than other renal transplant recipient groups. However, overall mortality and the risk of death with a functioning renal allograft still exceed the average in transplant recipients with diabetic nephropathy. Whole-organ, cadaveric donor pancreatic transplantation is widely accepted as the treatment of choice for type 1 diabetics with ESRD. Pancreatic transplantation may be performed simultaneously with same-donor cadaveric kidney transplantation or after kidney transplantation. Simultaneous pancreas-kidney transplantation (SPK) accounts for 85–90% of pancreatic transplantation in diabetics with ESRD and pancreas-after-kidney transplantation (PAK) accounts for the remainder. Currently, segmental living-donor pancreas and islet cell transplantation are done in humans on an experimental basis. Recipients of SPK or PAK transplantation report a substantial improvement in their quality of life compared to their counterparts who received solitary renal transplantation. Other documented benefits of pancreas transplantation include prevention of recurrent diabetic nephropathy in the renal allograft, freedom from insulin therapy, dietary restrictions and frequent glucose monitoring, and stabilization or improvement of neuropathy and retinopathy. It is unclear whether pancreas transplantation improves the survival of patients with end-stage nephropathy when compared to solitary renal transplantation. Pancreas transplantation is not recommended for patients with type 2 diabetes mellitus.

The treatments described here should be integrated with other interventions that have been shown to be beneficial in preventing diabetic complications. These include glycemic control and anithypertensive therapy, which are discussed elsewhere in this book.

REFERENCES

1. Bakris GL, Williams M, Dworkin L, Elliot WJ, Epstein M, Toto R, Tuttle K, Douglas J, Hsueh W, Sowers J (2000) for the National Kidney Foundation Hypertension and Diabetes Working Group. Preserving renal function in adults with hypertension and diabetes: a consensus approach. *Am J Kidney Dis* **36**: 646–661.
2. Lewis EJ, Hunsicker LG, Bain RP, Rohde RD (1993) for the Collaborative Study Group. The effect of angiotensin-converting-enzyme inhibition on diabetic nephropathy. *N Engl J Med* **329**: 1456–1462.
3. Parving HH, Rossing P, Hommel E, Smidt UM (1995) Angiotensin-converting enzyme inhibition in diabetic nephropathy: ten years' experience. *Am J Kidney Dis* **126**: 99–107.
4. Heart Outcomes Prevention Evaluation (HOPE) Study Investigators (2000) Effects of ramipril on cardiovascular and microvascular outcomes in people with diabetes mellitus: results of the HOPE study and MICRO-HOPE substudy. *Lancet* **355**: 253–2599.
5. The EUCLID study group (1997) Randomised placebo-controlled trial of lisinopril in normotensive patients with insulin-dependent diabetes and Normoalbuminuria. *Lancet* **349**: 1787–1792.
6. Viberti G, Mogensen CE, Groop LC, Pauls JF (1994) Effect of captopril on progression to clinical proteinuria in patients with insulin-dependent diabetes mellitus and microalbuminuria. European Microalbuminuria Captopril Study Group. *JAMA* **271**: 275–279.
7. Brenner BM, Cooper ME, de Zeeuw D, Keane WF, Mitch WE, Parving HH, Remuzzi G, Snapinn SM, Zhang Z, Shahinfar S (2001) for the RENAAL Study Investigators. Effects of losartan on renal and cardiovascular outcomes in patients with type 2 diabetes and nephropathy. *N Engl J Med* **345**: 861–869.
8. Zeller K, Whittaker E, Sullivan L, Raskin P, Jacobson HR (1991) Effect of restricting dietary protein on the progression of renal failure in patients with insulin-dependent diabetes mellitus. *N Engl J Med* **324**: 78–84.
9. Pijls LTJ, de Vries H, Donker AJM, van Eijk JTM (1999) The effect of protein restriction on albuminuria in patients with type 2 diabetic mellitus: a randomized trial. *Nephrol Dial Transplant* **14**: 1445–1453.
10. Pedrini MT, Levey AS, Lau J, Chalmers TC, Wang PH (1996) The effect of dietary protein restriction on the progression of diabetic and nondiabetic renal diseases: a meta-analysis. *Ann Intern Med* **124**: 627–632.
11. Gambaro G, Van der Woude FJ (2000) Glycosaminoglycans: use in treatment of diabetic nephropathy. *J Am Soc Nephrol* **11**: 359–368.

23

Treatment of Periodontal Disease

GEORGE W. TAYLOR and SARA G. GROSSI

The University of Michigan School of Dentistry
State University of New York at Buffalo

INTRODUCTION

Clinicians have long assumed that diabetes and periodontal diseases are biologically linked. However, it is only recently that there has been sufficient cumulative evidence from cross-sectional and longitudinal studies to provide strong support for this association being a causal relationship. An increased susceptibility of people with diabetes to many types of infection is a widely held view regarding the presumed link between diabetes mellitus and periodontitis, though this concept has been questioned[1,2]. Some people have suggested that diabetes adversely affects host resistance to certain infections which influence the endocrinologic-metabolic status of the patient. Gram-negative anaerobes, several of which have been recognized as periodontal pathogens, have been implicated in this latter set of infections, with *Bacteroides* species being among the organisms identified[3-5].

Periodontal disease is a chronic, potentially progressive bacterial infection resulting in inflammation and destruction of tooth-supporting tissues. Gingivitis and periodontitis are the most common periodontal diseases. Gingivitis is an inflammatory condition of the gingiva, in which the junctional epithelium is altered by the disease but remains attached to the tooth at its original level[6]. The most common form of gingivitis (often occurring in otherwise healthy individuals) is caused by supragingival bacterial plaque and, if untreated, may be observed to progress to more destructive periodontitis[7]. The most common form of destructive periodontal disease is adult periodontitis, a bacterially

The Evidence Base for Diabetes Care. Edited by R. Williams, W. Herman, A.-L. Kinmonth and N. J. Wareham.
© 2002 John Wiley & Sons, Ltd

induced, chronic inflammatory disease in which gram-negative anaerobes, including *Porphyromonas gingivalis* and *Prevotella intermedia* (classified in the genus Bacteroides until 1988 and 1990 respectively[8,9]), spirochetes, and occasionally the microaerophilic organism *Actinobacillus actinomycetemcomitans*, are prominent micro-organisms of the flora in subgingival bacterial plaque. These organisms are considered putative periodontopathogens[10–17]. Destructive periodontitis is characterized by destruction of periodontal tissues (gingiva, periodontal ligament, alveolar bone and cementum) and loss of connective tissue attachment[6].

Typically, adult periodontitis begins in adolescence[18] and, in its most common presentation, is thought to have a cyclic pattern of progression followed by periods of remission[19]. If untreated, it is thought to progress over time, typically from the initial lesions confined to interdental areas of the posterior teeth to a general pattern involving the entire dentition[20]. Severe periodontitis can lead to oral pain and tooth loss, and may affect dietary intake and overall quality of life.

While gingivitis is common, with approximately 50% of the US population in all age groups exhibiting reversible gingival inflammation[21], moderate or severe periodontitis with destruction of periodontal attachment tissues is much less common, affecting approximately 13% of the entire US population[22].

DIABETES MELLITUS AND ITS EFFECTS ON PERIODONTAL DISEASE

Current evidence supporting the link between diabetes mellitus and periodontal diseases comes from a review of English language literature published since 1960. This review was conducted using a Medline search as well as reviewing reference lists of relevant papers obtained from a search to identify primary research reports on investigations of relationships between diabetes and peridontal diseases. The reports included in the review were restricted to those that compared periodontal health in subjects with and without diabetes.

To summarize the evidence on the relationship between diabetes and periodontal disease, studies were broadly classified by age group and type of diabetes (Table 23.1). Using this classification scheme, 10 reports focused principally on children and adolescents with type 1 diabetes[23–32]; all except one[23] reported greater prevalence, extent or severity of at least one measure of periodontal disease. Another set of studies of subjects aged 15–35 with type 1 diabetes all reported greater prevalence, extent or severity of at least one measure or index of periodontal disease[33–38]. A third set of studies with type 1 diabetes (or with subjects reported as being insulin dependent without diabetes type being specified), included adults aged 20–70[39–43]. All five of these studies also reported greater prevalence, extent or severity of at least one measure or index of periodontal disease.

Table 23.1. Summary of studies of the association between diabetes and periodontal diseases, classified by strength of evidence, diabetes type and age group.

Author	Country	Study design	Diabetes Type[2]	No. of subjects a. Diabetic b. Control	Ages[3] a. Diabetic b. Control	Perio. measure: Diabetes effect[4]	Other diabetes-related variables considered in the study	Evidence level[1]
Firatli 1997	Turkey	Prospective	1	a. 44 b. 20	a. 12.2 (mean) b. 12.3 (mean)	Ging: 0s Ppd: 0s Lpa: 1s	Glycemic control Duration of diabetes	II-2
Cohen et al. 1970	USA	Prospective	1*	a. 21 b. 18	a. 18, 35 b. 18, 35	Ging: 1s Lpa: 1r, 1s	None	II-2
Tervonen and Karjalainen 1997	Finland	Prospective	1	a. 36 b. 10	a. 24, 36 b. 24, 36	Ging: 0e Ppd: 1r Lpa: 1e	Glycemic control Duration of diabetes Diabetes complications	II-2
Novaes, Jr. et al. 1996	Brazil	Prospective	2	a. 30 b. 30	a. 30, 77 b. 30, 67	Ppd: 1s, 1r Lpa. 1s, 1r	Glycemic control	II-2
Nelson et al. 1990	USA	Prospective	2	a. 720 b. 1553	a. 15, 55+ b. 15, 55+	XRBL: 1i, 1p	None	II-2
Taylor et al. 1998	USA	Prospective	2	a. 24 b. 338	a. 15, 57 b. 15, 57	XRBL: 1i, 1r	None	II-2
Taylor et al. 1998	USA	Prospective	2	a. 21 b. 338	a. 15, 49 b. 15, 49	XRBL: 1i, 1r	Glycemic control	II-2
Goteiner et al. 1986	USA	Cross-sectional	1	a. 169 b. 80	a. school ages b. 5, 18	Ging: 0s Lpa: 0p, 0s PDI: 0s	None	III
Harrison and Bowen 1987	USA	Cross-sectional	1	a. 30 b. 30	a. 4, 19 b. 4, 19	Ging: 1s Lpa: 1p	Glycemic control	III
Novaes AB et al. 1991	Brazil	Cross-sectional	1	a. 30 b. 30	a. 5, 18 b. 5, 18	Ging: 1s Ppd: 0s XRBL: 1s	None	III

Table 23.1. contd.

Study	Country	Type		Sample	Age	Measurements	Confounders	Grade
Cianciola et al. 1982	USA	Cross-sectional	1	a. 263 b. 208	a. <10, >19 b. <10, >19	Ging: 1p Lpa: 1p XRBL: 1p, 1s JPS: 1p,1s	Duration of diabetes	III
de Pommereau et al. 1992	France	Cross-sectional	1	a. 85 b. 38	a. 12, 18 b. 12, 18	Ging: 1e Lpa: 0e, 0p, 0s XRBL: 0e, 0p, 0s	Glycemic control Duration of diabetes	III
Ringleberg et al. 1977	USA	Cross-sectional	1	a. 56 b. 41	a. 10, 16 b. 10, 12	Ging: 1s MGI: 1s	None	III
Firatli et al. 1996	Turkey	Cross-sectional	1	a. 77 b. 77	a. 12.5 (mean) b. 12.6 (mean)	Ging: 0s Ppd: 1s Lpa: 1s	Duration of diabetes	III
Pinson et al. 1995	USA	Cross-sectional	1	a. 26 b. 24	a. 7–18 b. 7–18	Ging: 1s Ppd: 0s Lpa: 0s	Glycemic control Duration of diabetes	III
Faulconbridge et al. 1981	England	Cross-sectional	1	a. 94 b. 94	a. 5, 17 b. 5, 17	Ging: 1s	Duration of diabetes	III
Kjellman et al. 1970	Sweden	Cross-sectional	1*	a. 105 b. 52	a. 15, 24 b. 15, 24	Ging: 1e Ppd: 0s XRBL: 0s	Glycemic control Diabetes complications	III
Guven et al. 1996	Turkey	Cross-sectional	1	a. 10 b. 52	a. 18, 27 b. 19, 22	Ging: 1e	None	III
Rylander et al. 1987	Sweden	Cross-sectional	1	a. 46 b. 41	a. 18, 26 b. 19, 25	Ging: 1e, 1p Ppd: 0e Lpa: 1e, 1p XRBL: 0p	Diabetes complications	III
Sznajder et al. 1978	Argentina	Cross-sectional	1*	a. 20 b. 26	a. 9, 29 b. 9, 29	Ging: 1s Lpa: 0s	None	III
Galea et al. 1986	Malta	Cross-sectional	1*	a. 82 b. unknown	a. 5, 29 b. 5, 29	Ging: 1s Ppd: 1p	Glycemic control Duration of diabetes Diabetes complications	III

Table 23.1. contd.

Study	Country	Study type	Group	Sample	Age	Measures	Confounders	Quality
Hugoson et al. 1989	Sweden	Cross-sectional	1	a. 154 b. 77	a. 20, 70 b. 20, 70	Ging: 1e; Ppd: 1e, 1p, 1s; XRBL: 1s	Duration of diabetes	III
Glavind et al. 1968	Denmark	Cross-sectional	1*	a. 51 b. 51	a. 20, 40 b. 20, 40	Ging: 0s; Ppd: 0s; Lpa: 1s; XRBL: 1s	Duration of diabetes; Diabetes complications	III
Thorstennsson and Hugoson 1993	Sweden	Cross-sectional	1	a. 117 b. 99	a. 40, 70 b. 40, 70	Ging: 0e; Ppd: 1e, 1s; XRBL: 1s	Duration of diabetes; Onset age	III
Tervonen et al. 2000	Finland	Cross-sectional	1	a. 35 b. 10	a. 29,7 (mean) b. 29,0 (mean)	XRBL: 1e	Glycemic control; Duration of diabetes; Diabetes severity based on presence of complications	III
Morton et al. 1995	Mauritius	Cross-sectional	2	a. 24 b. 24	a. 26, 76 b. 25, 73	Ging: 1p; Ppd: 1s; Lpq: 1s	None	III
Shlossman et al. 1990	USA	Cross-sectional	2	a. 736 b. 2483	a. 5, 45+ b. 5, 45+	Lpa: 1p; XRBL: 1p	None	III
Emirich et al. 1990	USA	Cross-sectional	2	a. 254 b. 1088	a. 15, 55+ b. 15, 55+	Lpa: 1p, 1s; XRBL: 1p, 1s	None	III
Sandberg et al. 2000	Sweden	Cross-sectional	2	a. 102 b. 102	a. 64.8 (mean) b. 64.9 (mean)	Ging: 1e; Ppd: 1e; XRBL: 1p	Glycemic control; Duration of diabetes	III
Wolf, 1977	Finland	Cross-sectional	1,2	a. 186 b. 156	a. 16, 60 b. 16, 60	Ging: 1s; Lpa: 1s; XRBL: 1s	Glycemic control; Duration of diabetes; Diabetes complications	III
Benveniste et al. 1967	USA	Cross-sectional	1,2*	a. 53 b. 71	a. 5, 72 b. 5, 72	Ging: 0s; Ppd: 0p, 0s	None	III
Finestone and Boorujy 1967	USA	Cross-sectional	1,2*	a. 189 b. 64	a. 20, 79 b. 20, 79	PI: 1s	Glycemic control; Duration of diabetes; Diabetes complications	III

Table 23.1. contd.

Study	Country	Design	Code	Sample	Age	Outcome	Adjustment	Quality
Belting et al. 1964	USA	Cross-sectional	1, 2*	a. 78 b. 79	a. 20, 79 b. 20, 79	PI: 1s	Diabetes severity	III
Oliver and Tervonen 1993	USA	Cross-sectional	1, 2	a. 114 b. 15132	a. 20, 64 b. 20, 64	Ppd: 1e, 1p Lpa: 1e, 0p, 0s	None	III
Yavuzyilmaz et al. 1996	Turkey	Cross-sectional	1, 2	a. 17 b. 17	a. 25, 74 b. 19, 29	Ppd: 1s	None	III
Bridges et al. 1996	USA	Cross-sectional	1, 2	a. 118 b. 115	a. 24, 78 b. 24, 78	Ging: 0s Ppd: 0s Lpa: 1s	Glycemic control Duration of diabetes	III
Sandler and Stahl 1960	USA	Cross-sectional	1, 2*	a. 100 b. 3894	a. 20, 69 b. 20, 69	PDR: 1e	None	III
Bacic et al. 1988	Yugoslavia	Cross-sectional	1, 2	a. 222 b. 189	a. <20, 60+ b. <20, 60+	Ppd: 1e, 1p, 1s	Glycemic control Duration of diabetes Diabetes complications	III
Hove and Stallard 1970	USA	Cross-sectional	1, 2*	a. 28 b. 16	a. 20, 40+ b. 20, 40+	Ging: 0s Ppd: 0s XRBL: 0s	Duration of diabetes Diabetes severity	III
Mackenzie and Millard 1963	USA	Cross-sectional	9	a. 124 b. 92	a. 32, 78 b. 32, 78	XRBL: 0s	None	III
Sznajder et al. 1978	Argentina	Cross-sectional	9	a. 63 b. 39	a. 30, 49 b. 30, 50	Ging: 1s Lpa: 1s	None	III
Dolan et al. 1997	USA	Cross-sectional	9	Wt'd a. 107 b. 554	a. 45, 75+ b. 45, 75+	Lpa: 1e, 1p, 1s	None	III
Grossi et al. 1994	USA	Cross-sectional	9	a. 1426 b. 69	All: 25, 74; unknown for diabetes	Lpa: 1s, 1p	None	III
Tervonen and Knuuttila 1986	Finland	Cross-sectional	9	a. 50 b. 53	a. <30, 40+ b. <30, 40+	Ging: 1e Ppd: 1e, 1p XRBL: 0s	Glycemic control	III

Table 23.1. contd.

Campbell 1972	Australia	Cross-sectional	9	a. 70 b. 102	a. 17, 39 b. 17, 39	PI: 1p, 1s	None	III
Albrecht et al. 1988	Hungary	Cross-sectional	9	a. 1360 b. 625	a. 15, 65+ 15, 65+	Ging: 1s PI: 0s	None	III
Szpunar et al. 1989 (NHANES I)	USA	Cross-sectional	9	a. 474 b. 15174	a. 6, 65+ b. 6, 65+	PI: 1s	None	III
Szpunar 1989 (HHANES)	USA	Cross-sectional	9	a. 322 b. 8040	a. 15, 65+ b. 12, 65+	PI: 1s	None	III

1. Hierarchy of evidence based on classification scheme used by US Preventive Services Task Force, where I = evidence obtained from at least one properly randomized controlled trial; II-1 = evidence obtained from well-designed controlled trial without randomization; II-2 = evidence obtained from well-designed cohort or case-control analytic studies, preferably from more than one center or research group; II-3 = evidence obtained from multiple time series with or without intervention. Dramatic results in uncontrolled experiments (such as the results of the introduction of penicillin treatment in the 1940s) could also be regarded as this type of evidence; III = opinions of respected authorities, based on clinical experience; descriptive studies and case reports; or reports of expert committees.

2. Diabetes type: 1 – type 1 diabetes mellitus; 2 – type 2 diabetes mellitus; 1,2 – subjects with both type 1 and type 2 diabetes mellitus included; 9 – diabetes type not specified and not clearly ascertainable from other information in the report; * – diabetes type not specified but ascertained by reviewer from other information in the report.

3. Ages: subjects' ages presented as minimum, maximum reported for those with diabetes and controls unless otherwise specified.

4. Measure of periodontal disease status. Measures used include Ging – gingivitis or gingival bleeding, Ppd – probing pocket depth, Lpa – loss of periodontal attachment, XRBL – radiographic bone loss, JPS – juvenile periodontal score, MGI – modified gingival index, PI – Russell's Periodontal Index, PDR – periodontal disease rate (proportion of teeth affected by periodontal disease). The number following the measure corresponds to greater disease in those with diabetes (1) or no difference between those with diabetes and controls (0). The letters following the number correspond to the parameter(s) assessed in the study: e – extent, i – incidence, p – prevalence, s – severity, r – progression.

There are a smaller number of studies on the relationship between type 2 diabetes and periodontitis. The review identified eight reports limited to subjects with type 2 diabetes. Three of these reports[44–46] included only adults. The remaining five reports are from an epidemiological study of the Pima Indians of the Gila River Indian Community, Arizona, USA and include subjects aged 5 and older[47] or 15 and older[48–51]. These eight studies all reported significantly poorer periodontal health in subjects with diabetes. A subset of these reports provided additional epidemiologic parameter estimates of association and risk. Emirich *et al.*[49] reported that the odds were approximately three times greater for people with diabetes to have destructive periodontal disease after controlling for other important factors; Nelson *et al.*[48] found a 2.6-fold greater risk of advanced periodontal disease incidence, and Taylor *et al.*[50] reported that subjects with type 2 diabetes had a four-fold greater risk for more severe alveolar bone loss progression.

Several reports consist of analyses where subjects with type 1 and type 2 diabetes were not distinguished. All of the studies in this subset were cross-sectional and included adult subjects, although two studies in this group also included children or adolescents as well[52,53]. Eight of these 10 studies reported greater prevalence, extent or severity of periodontal disease for at least one measure or index of periodontal disease[52,54–60]. Hove and Stallard[61] and Benveniste *et al.*[53] did not find significant differences in periodontal disease between subjects with and without diabetes.

Finally, there is a set of cross-sectional studies in which the type of diabetes was not specified and which was not easily determined from other information provided. Five of the eight reports in this set included adults only[37,62–65]. The other three reports included subjects with ages ranging from childhood to older adulthood[66–68]. All of these studies found subjects with diabetes to have increased prevalence, extent, or severity of periodontal disease. Two of the population-based surveys, Grossi *et al.*[64] and Dolan *et al.*[63] provide epidemiologic estimates of association for diabetes and attachment loss severity, with individuals having diabetes being approximately twice as likely to have more severe attachment loss than those without diabetes, after controlling for other variables.

As with other complications of diabetes, current evidence also supports poorer glycemic control contributing to poorer periodontal health. Primary research reports in the literature investigating relationships between glycemic control level and periodontal disease have predominantly been studies where subjects either had type 1 diabetes, a combination of both type 1 and type 2 diabetes, or where the diabetes type was not specified (Table 23.2). There have only been five reports published on the association between glycemic control and periodontal disease specifically in type 2 diabetes[44,46,50,69,70]. Each of these studies found poorer glycemic control to be a significant factor associated with poorer periodontal health. Among the studies providing information on differ-

Table 23.2. Summary of reports with information on effects of glycemic control on periodontal status, sorted by strength of evidence, diabetes type and age groups.

Authors	Country	Study design	Diabetes type[2]	Age group	Effect[3]	Non-DM comparison group[4]	Evidence level[1]
Seppala et al. 1993	Finland	Prospective	1	adults	1	N	II-2
Tervonen and Karjalainen 1997	Finland	Prospective	1	adults	1	Y	II-2
Karjalainen and Knuuttila 1996	Finland	Prospective	1	children	1	N	II-2
Firatli et al. 1997	Turkey	Prospective	1	children	1	Y	II-2
Seppala and Ainamo 1994	Finland	Prospective	1, 2	adults	1	N	II-2
Wolf, 1977	Finland	Prospective	1, 2	mixed ages	0	Y	II-2
Novaes et al. 1996	Brazil	Prospective	2	adults	1	Y	II-2
Taylor et al. 1998	USA	Prospective	2	mixed ages	1	Y	II-2
Sastrowijoto et al. 1989	Netherlands	Cross-sectional	1	adults	0	N	III
Moore et al. 1999	USA	Cross-sectional	1	adults	0	N	III
Tervonen et al. 2000	Finland	Cross-sectional	1	adults	1	Y	III
Gusberti et al. 1983	USA	Cross-sectional	1	children	1	N	III
Barnett et al. 1984	USA	Cross-sectional	1	children	0	N	III
Harrison and Bowen, 1987	USA	Cross-sectional	1	children	1	Y	III
Sandholm et al. 1989	Finland	Cross-sectional	1	children	0	Y	III
de Pommereau et al. 1992	France	Cross-sectional	1	children	0	Y	III
Pinson et al. 1995	USA	Cross-sectional	1	children	0	Y	III
Galea et al. 1986	Malta	Cross-sectional	1	children and young adults	1	Y	III
Kjellman et al. 1970	Sweden	Cross-sectional	1	children and young adults	1	Y	III
Rylander et al. 1987	Sweden	Cross-sectional	1	mixed ages	0	Y	III
Safkan-Seppala and Ainamo 1992	Finland	Cross-sectional	1	mixed ages	1	N	III
Finestone and BooruJy 1967	USA	Cross-sectional	1, 2	adults	1	Y	III
Bacic et al. 1988	Yugoslavia	Cross-sectional	1, 2	adults	0	Y	III

Table 23.2. contd.

Study	Country	Design	Diabetes type[2]	Age	Effect[3]	Non-DM comparison[4]	Evidence[1]
Oliver et al. 1993	USA	Cross-sectional	1, 2	adults	1	N	III
Tervonen and Oliver 1993	USA	Cross-sectional	1, 2	adults	1	N	III
Bridges et al. 1996	USA	Cross-sectional	1, 2	adults	0	Y	III
Ainamo et al. 1990	Finland	Prospective (case report)	2	adults (n = 2)	1	N	III
Unal et al. 1993	Turkey	Cross-sectional	2	adults	1	Y	III
Sandberg et al. 2000	Sweden	Cross-sectional	2	adults	0	Y	III
Hove and Stallard 1970	USA	Cross-sectional	9	adults	0	Y	III
Nichols et al. 1978	USA	Cross-sectional	9	adults	0	N	III
Tervonen and Knuuttila 1986	Finland	Cross-sectional	9	adults	1	Y	III
Albrecht et al. 1988	Hungary	Cross-sectional	9	mixed ages	0	Y	III
Hayden and Buckley 1989	Ireland	Cross-sectional	9	mixed ages	0	N	III

[1] Hierarchy of evidence based on classification scheme used by US Preventive Services Task Force, where I = evidence obtained from at least one properly randomized controlled trial; II-1 = evidence obtained from well-designed controlled trial without randomization; II-2 = evidence obtained from well-designed cohort or case-control analytic studies, preferably from more than one center or research group; II-3 = evidence obtained from multiple time series with or without intervention. Dramatic results in uncontrolled experiments (such as the results of the introduction of penicillin treatment in the 1940s) could also be regarded as this type of evidence; III = opinions of respected authorities, based on clinical experience; descriptive studies and case reports; or reports of expert committees.

[2] Diabetes type: 1 – type 1 diabetes mellitus; 2 – type 2 diabetes mellitus; 1, 2 – subjects with both type 1 and type 2 diabetes mellitus included; 9 – diabetes type not specified and not clearly ascertainable from other information in the report; * – diabetes type not specified but ascertained by reviewer from other information in the report.

[3] Effect: 1 – Subjects with poorer glycemic control had poorer health than the comparison group(s); 0 – no difference in the periodontal health status between subjects with poorer glycemic control and comparison group(s).

[4] Non-DM comparison group: Y – the report included subjects without diabetes as well as subjects classified by glycemic control status.

ences in periodontal health classified by glycemic control status, most have been cross sectional, with 19 out of 34 reporting more frequent or severe periodontal disease in those with poorer glycemic control[24,30,34,38,42–44,51,54,56,65,69–76] and 15 reporting no differences[27,31,46,52,56,58,60,61,67,77–82]. Among the follow-up studies in this body of literature, 8 out of 9 reported poorer periodontal health in subjects with poorer glycemic control[30,42,44,51,70,73,74,76]. Additionally, among reports published before 1990, 6 out of 16 reported more frequent or severe periodontal disease in subjects with poorer glycemic control[24,34,38,54,65,71], whereas 13 out of 18 papers published since 1990 reported results supporting poorer glycemic control associated with or contributing to more severe or frequent periodontal disease[30,42–44,51,56,69–76].

Although the preponderance of studies included in this review of the adverse effects of diabetes on periodontal health are cross-sectional and describe findings of convenience samples, principally from outpatients in hospitals and clinics, the smaller subset of longitudinal and population-based studies also strongly supports the association between diabetes and increased occurrence and severity of periodontal diseases. While limitations on causal inference must be considered, the literature provides consistent evidence of greater prevalence, severity or extent of at least one manifestation of periodontal disease in the large majority of studies. Additionally, there are no studies reported in the literature with superior design features to refute this assessment. The studies were conducted in distinctly different settings with subjects from different ethnic populations, different age mixes and with a variety of measures of periodontal status (i.e. gingival inflammation, pathologic probing pocket depth, loss of periodontal attachment or radiographic evidence of alveolar bone loss). The studies also used various parameters to summarize periodontal disease occurrence (prevalence, incidence, extent, severity or progression). Hence this inevitable variation in methodology and study populations limits the possibility that the same biases or confounding factors apply in all the studies, and provides support for concluding that diabetes is a risk factor for periodontal disease incidence, progression and severity. Further, there is substantial evidence to support a 'dose-response'; i.e. as glycemic control worsens, the adverse effects of diabetes on periodontal health become greater.

BIOLOGIC MECHANISMS: CELLULAR AND MOLECULAR DYNAMICS

Moving from the review of clinical and epidemiolgical evidence, this section reviews the biological mechanisms currently considered in explaining the increased risk for destructive periodontal disease observed in people with diabetes.

As with other complications of diabetes, biological mechanisms important in diabetes-associated periodontitis are probably multifactoral, consisting of complex, iterative interrelated cellular and molecular interactions resulting from the metabolic abnormalities that characterize diabetes mellitus. Micro-angiopathy, alterations in the composition of gingival crevicular fluid, alterations in collagen metabolism and impaired wound healing, altered host immunoinflammatory response, altered subgingival microflora and hereditary predisposition have all been proposed to contribute to increased periodontal inflammation and alveolar bone loss in diabetes[83-89]. Hence, a biological explanation for more frequent and more severe periodontal infection in dia-betes involves synthesis of observations from several lines of inquiry.

In the stable periodontal environment where there is effective oral hygiene and a systemically healthy host, there is a series of protective cellular and molecular interactions occurring in response to the bacterial challenge asso-ciated with dental plaque biofilm. In this 'normal' situation, neutrophils, which are principal host defense cells responding to this microbial challenge, accu-mulate at the surface of the dental plaque biofilm and limit its lateral and apical extension[90].

For individuals who are not otherwise susceptible to development of periodontitis, normal host defenses, accompanied by effective daily oral hygiene practices, prevent the extension of bacterial proliferation into the gingival sulcus and the subsequent initiation of chronic inflammation and periodontal pocket formation[90]. In this uncompromised state, the immunoinflammatory response is tightly regulated to act in concert with normal tissue turnover, regeneration and repair.

The colonizing bacteria in the dental plaque biofilm and their metabolic processes the gingiva a tissue continuously subject to repetitive pathological injury, and hence it is in a constant state of repair. This continual healing process is necessary to maintain structural integrity. When tissue healing cannot keep pace with tissue injury, progressive gingivitis develops, and may eventually lead to destructive periodontitis.

In susceptable individuals where bacterial plaque is not effectively removed, bacteria colonize the teeth, forming an adherent plaque that progressively becomes more gram-negative, anaerobic and virulent in composition as it matures. Substances released from the surface of the dental plaque, such as bacterial lipopolysaccharides (LPS), activate a destructive inflammatory response comprised of periodontal epithelial cell proliferation, increased inflammatory cell infiltration and heightened secretion of inflammatory mediators and matrix metalloproteinases. This net catabolic response results in the degradation of collagen and the components of the connective tissue extracellular matrix and destruction of the collagen fibers attached to the root surface, followed by lateral and apical extension of the sulcular epithelium[90]. This process results in deepening of the periodontal pockets, gingival recession, clinical attachment loss, increased tooth mobility and, in severe cases, tooth loss.

Impaired neutrophil function has been observed in diabetes. The impaired chemotaxis[91–95], adherence[96,97], phagocytosis and bacteriocidal activity[98–100] could result in increased propensity for colonization and proliferation of periodontal pathogens in the dental plaque biofilm.

Recent evidence has provided additional insights into potential metabolic and genetic factors that could contribute to the increased risk and severity of periodontal tissue destruction found in diabetes. In the metabolic dysregulation of diabetes, persisting hyperglycemia causes nonenzymatic glycation and oxidation of proteins and lipids, and the subsequent formation of advanced glycation end-products (AGEs), which accumulate in the plasma and tissues[101]. Hyperglycemia and resultant AGE formation are considered to be a major causal factor in the pathogenesis of diabetes complications[101,102]. In subjects with diabetes who also have periodontitis, AGEs with accompanying markers for increased oxidant stress have been demonstrated in human gingiva[103]. Cell surface binding sites or receptors for AGE (RAGE) have been identified on the cell surfaces of mononuclear phagocytes and endothelial cells[104]. The underlying postulate associated with these findings is that enhanced oxidant stress in the gingival tissues could contribute to more frequent and more severe periodontal tissue destruction in individuals with diabetes. It has been hypothesized that the AGE–RAGE interaction induces an oxidant stress that may contribute to chronic monocytic upregulation, activation of NF-κB, and subsequent expression of mRNA and secretion of proinflammatory cytokines (such as TNFα, IL-1β, and IL-6) by monocytic phagocytes involved in periodontal tissue inflammation and destruction[103,105–111]. These mediators are recognized as effectors in periodontal tissue inflammation and destruction[112]. Additionally, AGE interaction with endothelial cell RAGE has been shown to enhance endothelial cell vascular hyperpermeability and expression of vascular cell adhesion molecule-1, an adherence molecule capable of attracting mononuclear cells to the vascular wall[113–115]. Hence, AGE–RAGE interaction has been proposed to result in pertubation of cellular properties, exaggerated and sustained inflammatory response, impaired wound healing and more severe diabetes-associated periodontal disease[116].

Iacopino[89], in an extensive review, provides an additional perspective on metabolic dysregulation in diabetes and the effects of hyperlipidemia on monocyte/macrophage function in wound signaling. The monocyte/ macrophage is considered the major mediator of the inflammatory phase in wound healing, having primary roles in wound signal transduction and in the initiation of the transition of healing from the inflammatory to the granulation phase[89,117–123]. One hypothesized effect of hyperlipidemia occurs through fatty acid interaction with the monocyte cell membrane, causing impaired function of membrane-bound receptors and enzyme systems[89,124,125]. This leads to impaired amplification and transduction of the wound signal. Another postulated pathway leading to impaired monocyte function in diabetes and wound signaling is via the nonenzymatic glycosylation of lipids and triglycerides[89,126–128] in addition to proteins. These AGEs are thought to affect normal differentiation and maturation of specific monocyte phenotypes throughout the different stages of wound healing[89]. The net result of both these pathways is exacerbated host-mediated inflammatory tissue destruction. In impairing monocyte function, diabetes-associated lipid dysregulation, leading to high levels of low density lipoproteins (LDL) and triglycerides (TRG), may be a major factor in the incidence and severity of periodontal disease where the periodontal tissues experience chronic, pathological wounding and tissue destruction[89,129,130].

Other recent studies of periodontal disease in diabetes provide evidence that a significant subset of individuals with type 1 diabetes have a monocytic hyperresponsive phenotype that predisposes them to an exaggerated response to gram-negative bacterial infections[131–134]. It has been suggested that this hyperresponsive monocytic phenotype is genetically determined, possibly regulated by genes in the HLA-DR3/4 and HLA-DQ regions[112,132,134–138]. Several important putative periodontal pathogens are gram-negative anerobes. Salvi *et al.*[83,131] have reported elevated gingival crevicular fluid levels (i.e. PGE2, IL-1β and possibly TNFα) and enhanced peripheral blood monocytic response to LPS challenge, as evidenced by increased secretion of PGE2, IL-1β and TNFα in individuals with type 1 diabetes and periodontal disease when compared to controls without diabetes. The reported enhanced inflammatory mediator response is functionally consistent with the type and levels of mediators required to induce alveolar bone resorption and other periodontal connective tissue destruction. In addition to the increased monocytic secretory response in type 1 diabetes patients in general, they found significantly greater levels of these inflammatory mediators in subjects with both type 1 diabetes and severe periodontitis. This evidence suggests that the enhanced PGE2, IL-1β and TNFα secretory responsiveness of peripheral blood monocytes in individuals with type 1 diabetes may contribute to explaining the increased risk for severe periodontal disease found in diabetes.

PERIODONTAL DISEASE: ITS EFFECTS ON GLYCEMIC CONTROL IN DIABETES MELLITUS

While there is substantial evidence to support considering diabetes as a risk factor for poor periodontal health, there is also evidence for periodontal infection adversely affecting glycemic control in diabetes, although this has been less extensively studied. Indirect evidence comes from investigations of the relationship between insulin resistance and active inflammatory connective tissue diseases[139,140], other clinical diseases[139–142] and acute infection[143,144].

Due to the high vascularity of the inflamed periodontium, this inflamed tissue may serve as an endocrine-like source for TNFα and other inflammatory mediators[145,146]. Because of the predominance of gram-negative anaerobic bacteria in periodontal infection, the ulcerated pocket epithelium could constitute a chronic source of systemic challenge for bacterial products and locally produced inflammatory mediators. TNFα, IL6 and IL1, all mediators important in periodontal inflammation, have been shown to have important effects on glucose and lipid metabolism, particularly following an acute infectious challenge or trauma[88,14,3,148]. TNFα has been reported to interfere with lipid metabolism and to be an insulin antagonist[149,150]. IL6 and IL1 have also been reported to antagonize insulin action[148,151,152]. To date, all reports on an infection-related alteration of the endocrinologic-metabolic status of the host have been with acute infections. There is a compelling need to evaluate these relationships in the chronic infection context applicable to periodontal infection.

More direct evidence regarding the effects of periodontal infection on glycemic control diabetes comes from treatment studies[52,73,74,153–159] and observational studies[160–162] (Table 23.3). There is evidence to support periodontal infection/severe periodontitis having an adverse, yet modifiable, effect on glycemic control[52,73,153–156]. However, not all investigations report an improvement in glycemic control after periodontal treatment[74,157–159,162]. There are major variations in the design, conduct and results of these studies, as described in recent detailed reviews[88,163]. Perhaps most notable is the identification of only three published controlled clinical trials, with one trial specifically designed for periodontal treatment in patients with type 2 diabetes[153,154] and potential limitations in length of follow-up time to assess changes in glycated hemoglobin in studies reporting no improvement of glycemic control.

Despite the variation in the literature, there is a distinction in the effect of periodontal treatment on glycemic control related to the mode of therapy[88]. Studies involving mechanical periodontal treatment alone[74,157,158,162] reported an improvement in periodontal status only (i.e. no change in glycemic control), while studies including systemic antibiotics accompanying mechanical therapy reported both an improvement in periodontal status and an improvement in glycemic control[153–156]. It has been hypothesized that these differential results due to antibiotic use (especially doxycycline) may involve several mechanisms, including an antimicrobial effect, a modulation of host response and, possibly, inhibition of the nonenzymatic glycosylation process.

Additional evidence to support the effect of severe periodontitis on increased risk for poorer glycemic control comes from two longitudinal observational studies. In a longitudinal epidemiological study of the Pima Indians in Arizona, USA, Taylor *et al.*[160] found that subjects with type 2 diabetes in good to moderate control and with severe periodontitis at baseline were approximately six times more likely to have poor glycemic control at approximately

Table 23.3. Effects of periodontal disease and its treatment on glycemic control: clinical and epidemiological evidence

Reference	Study design	Diabetes	No. of Subjects a. Treatment (ages) b. Control (ages)	Follow-up time	Periodontal treatment	Metabolic control outcome measure	Effects on metabolic control	Evidence level[1]
Aldridge *et al.* Study 1, 1995	RCT	Type 1	a. 16 (16–40) b. 15 (16–40)	2 months	Exp. group: oral hygiene instruction, scaling, adjustment of restoration margins and reinforcement after one month. Control group: no treatment	Glycated hemoglobin, fructosamine	Periodontal treatment had no effect on change in glycated hemoglobin	I
Aldridge *et al.* Study 2, 1995	RCT	Type 1	a. 12 (20–60) b. 10 (20–60)	2 months	Exp. group: oral hygiene instruction, scaling and root planing, extractions, root canal therapy. Control group: no treatment	Glycated hemoglobin	Periodontal treatment had no effect on change in glycated hemoglobin	I
Grossi *et al.* 1996, 1997	RCT	Type 2	a. 89 (25–65) b. 24 (25–65)	12 months	Exp. groups received either systemic doxycycline or placebo and ultrasonic bactericidal curettage with irrigation using either H$_2$O, chlorhexidine or povidone-iodine. Control groups received ultrasonic bacterial curettage with H2O irrigation and placebo	Glycated hemoglobin	The three groups receiving doxycycline and ultrasonic bacterial curettage showed significant reductions (p ≤0.04) in mean glycated hemoglobin at 3 months	I

Table 23.3. contd.

Study	Study type	Diabetes type	Subjects	Duration	Treatment	Outcome measure	Results	Quality
Smith et al. 1996	Treatment study, non-RCT	Type 1	a. 18 (26–57) b. 0	2 months	Scaling and root planing with ultrasonic and curetes; oral hygiene instruction	Glycated hemoglobin	Found no statistically or clinically significant change in glycated hemoglobin	II-1
Westfelt et al. 1996	Treatment* study, non-RCT	Types 1 and 2	a. 20 (45–65) b. 20 (45–65)	5 years	Baseline oral hygiene instruction, scaling and root planing followed by periodic prophys, OHI, localized subgingival plaque removal, and surgery at sites with bleeding on probing and PPD >5 mm	Glycated hemoglobin	The mean value of HbA_{1c} between BL-24 months was not signif different from that between 24-60 months.	II-1
Christgau et al. 1998	Treatment study, non-RCT	Types 1 and 2	a. 20 (30–66) b. 20 (30–66)	2 months	Scaling/root planing, subgingival irrigation with chlorhexidine, OHI and extractions	Glycated hemoglobin	No effect on glycated hemoglobin	II-1
Taylor et al. 1996	Historical prospective cohort	Type 2	a, b: no tx or control subjects, all type 2 DM 49 (severe periodis.) 56 (less severe periodis.)	2–4 years	Not applicable	Glycated hemoglobin	Those with severe periodontitis were ~6 times more likely to have poor glycemic control at follow-up	II-2
Collin et. al. 1998	Retrospective cohort	Type 2	a, b: no subjects received treatment 25 with diabetes (ages 58–76) 40 without diabetes (ages 59–77)	2-3 years	Not applicable	Glycated hemoglobin	Among subjects with type 2 diabetes the HbA_{1c} level significantly increased in those with advanced periodontitis, but not in those without advanced periodontitis	II-2

Table 23.3. contd.

Williams and Mahan 1960	Descriptive clinical study	Not specified	a. 9 (20–32) b. 0	3–7 months	Extractions, scaling and curettage, gingivectomy, systemic antibiotics	Insulin requirement, diabetes control (not operationally defined)	7/9 subjects had 'significant' reduction in insulin requirements	III
Wolf 1977	Treatment study, non-RCT	Types 1 and 2	a. 117 (16–60) b. 0	8–12 months	Scaling and home care instructions; periodontal surgery, extractions, endodontic treatment, restorations, denture replacement or repair	Blood glucose, 24-h urinary glucose, insulin dose	Compared 23 subjects with improved oral infection with 23 who had no improvement after tx for inflammation. The subject with improved oral inflam. and infect. tended to demonstrate diabetic control improvement ($p < 0.1$). However, Wolf states in discussion, 'tx of periodontal inflammation and periapical lesions ... does little to improve the control of diabetes'.	III
Miller et al. 1992	Treatment study, non-RCT	Type 1	a. 10 (not given) b. 0	8 weeks	Scaling and root planing, systemic doxycycline	Glycated hemoglobin, glycated albumin	Found decrease in glycated hemoglobin and glycated albumin in patients with improvement in gingival	III

Table 23.3. contd.

| Seppala *et al.* 1993, 1994 | Treatment study, non-RCT | Type 1 | a. 38-1y; 22-2y² 26 PIDD-1y (48 ± 6) 12 CIDD-1y (43 ± 5) 16 PIDD-2y 6 CIDD-2y b. 0 | 2 years | Scaling and root planing, periodontal surgery and extractions | Medical history for baseline control status; glycosylated hemoglobin A1 and blood glucose for assessing response to treatment | inflammation (p <0.01). Patients with no improvement in gingival inflammation had either no change or an increase in glycated hemoglobin post-treatment Reported an improvement of HBA1 levels in PIDD and CIDD subjects (p <0.068, t-test) | III |

¹ Hierarchy of evidence based on classification scheme used by US Preventive Services Task Force, where I = evidence obtained from at least one properly randomized controlled trial; II-1 = evidence obtained from well-designed controlled trial without randomization; II-2 = evidence obtained from well-designed cohort or case-control analytic studies, preferably from more than one center or research group; II-3 = evidence obtained from multiple time series with or without intervention. Dramatic results in uncontrolled experiments (such as the results of the introduction of penicillin treatment in the 1940s) could also be regarded as this type of evidence; III = opinions of respected authorities, based on clinical experience; descriptive studies and case reports; or reports of expert committees.
² 38 subjects were followed for 1 year and 22 for 2 years. PIDD – poorly controlled insulin-dependent diabetes; CIDD – controlled insulin-dependent diabetes.

two-years follow-up than those without severe periodontitis at baseline. In another observational study of 25 adults with type 2 diabetes, aged 58–77, Collin *et al.*[161] also reported an association between advanced periodontal disease and impaired metabolic control.

The clinical and epidemiological evidence reviewed provides support for the concept that periodontal infection contributes to poorer glycemic control in people with diabetes. However, further rigorous, controlled trials in diverse populations are necessary to establish that treating periodontal infections can be influential in contributing to glycemic control management and possibly to the reduction of the burden of complications of diabetes mellitus.

TREATMENT OF PERIODONTAL DISEASE IN PATIENTS WITH DIABETES MELLITUS

Treatment of periodontal disease in patients with diabetes should be guided toward arresting the periodontal infection and control of the inflammatory destructive process. Controlled studies have demonstrated that the short-term clinical response of patients with diabetes to nonsurgical and surgical periodontal therapy is similar to responses in those without diabetes. A study by Ternoven *et al.*[164] compared the short-term (three or four month) response to nonsurgical periodontal therapy in patients with diabetes and controls. There was a comparable percentage reduction in both groups in pockets 4–5 mm (moderate depth) and >6 mm (severe depth). Similar reductions in moderate and deep pockets in both patients with and without diabetes were reported following mechanical periodontal treatment combined with subgingival irrigation with 0.2% chlorhexidine and local application of 1% chlorhexidine gel[162]. Subgingival bacteria were reduced in both groups following this antimicrobial treatment. *P. gingvalis*, however, persisted in 60% of patients with diabetes compared to 40% of those who did not have diabetes. The long-term response to nonsurgical periodontal therapy was compared in patients with diabetes and controls by Ternoven and Karjalainen[42]. Patients with diabetes were divided according to their degree of metabolic control into good, moderate and poor control. Again, the short-term response to periodontal therapy was no different between groups. However, significant differences were seen between the groups in the long-term response (12 months) to periodontal therapy. Patients with poorly-controlled diabetes exhibited a three-fold greater number of pockets >4 mm and more subgingival calculus at 12 months after periodontal therapy than the other groups with diabetes. These results suggest that risk for periodontal disease recurrence may be greater in patients with poorly-controlled diabetes than in those who are well or moderately controlled. Periodontal disease recurrence may be reduced, however, in patients with moderately-controlled diabetes, provided dental plaque is carefully controlled with a rigorous periodontal maintenance program[159]. Studies by Seppala and Ainamo[74] and Aldridge *et al.*[157] also examined the effect of mechanical periodontal therapy in type 1 diabetes patients and reported improved periodontal condition, as measured by changes in pocket depth. Smith *et al.*[158] evaluated the effect of nonsurgical periodontal therapy, including ultrasonic debridement, in 18 patients with type 1 diabetes with moderate to severe periodontitis and included measures for the presence of periodontal pathogens. Significant reduction in pocket depth and gain in attachment level were seen two months after therapy. In spite of a favorable short-term clinical outcome, patients continued to harbor *P. gingivalis* and *B. forsythus* in subgingival plaque. Smith *et al.*[158] posited that elimination of pathogenic periodontal bacteria in at least some patients with diabetes may not be achieved by mechanical treatment alone. A conclusion from this set of reviewed studies is that mechanical periodontal therapy is effective in reducing periodontal inflammation in patients with diabetes, but in certain subgroups of individuals with diabetes (e.g. those who are poorly controlled or have advanced periodontal disease) adjunct therapy with antibiotics may be required to aid in control of periodontal infection. Failure to completely resolve the periodontal infection may, in turn, explain the lack of effect of periodontal therapy on glycemic control in several of the studies reviewed.

In contrast, three studies incorporating systemic antibiotics with conventional mechanical periodontal therapy reported both improved clinical outcome in periodontal status as well as an improvement in diabetes metabolic control[154–156]. In one of these studies, Grossi *et al.*[154] demonstrated that periodontal treatment incorporating ultrasonic debridement, topical antimicrobial and systemic doxycycline (100 mg/day for 14 days) resulted in elimination of *P. gingvalis* infection, significant gain in attachment level and a 1% reduction in levels of HbA_{1c} at three months after treatment. This reduction represents approximately 10% of the initial HbA_{1c} concentration and was independent of the effect of diet, oral hypoglicemics and insulin, conventional methods for lowering glycemia and controlling diabetes. Although no assessment of subgingival infection was conducted in the other two studies that included systemic antibiotics as part of periodontal treatment, they both reported either a reduction in insulin requirements[155] or a reduction in levels of HbA_{1c}[156]. Therefore, it appears that elimination of periodontal infection in certain patients with diabetes may not be achieved by mechanical modes of treatment alone; systemic antibiotic therapy may be indicated in order to effectively eliminate the chronic infection associated with periodontal disease. When this is achieved, individuals with diabetes may also exhibit an improvement in glycemia and diabetes control, as measured by glycated hemoglobin. One may conclude from these studies that the effect of periodontal treatment on diabetes metabolic control is dependent on the mode of therapy, mechanical versus mechanical combined with systemic antibiotic. When mechanical periodontal treatment alone is provided, the treatment outcome may be strictly improvement in periodontal status or a *local effect* only. On the contrary, when systemic antibiotics are incorporated with mechanical therapy, a *systemic effect* may be seen as well, i.e. an improvement in diabetes control measured as a reduction in glycated hemoglobin or a reduction in insulin requirements.

SUMMARY AND CONCLUSION

The evidence reviewed in this chapter supports viewing the relationship between diabetes and periodontal diseases as bidirectional. That is, diabetes is associated with increased occurrence and progression of periodontitis, and periodontal infection is associated with poorer glycemic control in people with diabetes. While treating periodontal infection in people with diabetes is clearly an important component in maintaining oral health, it may also have an important role in establishing and maintaining glycemic control. Further rigorous, systematic study in diverse populations is necessary to support existing evidence that treating periodontal infections can be influential in contributing to glycemic control management and possibly to the reduction of the burden of complications of diabetes mellitus.

ACKNOWLEDGEMENTS

Portions of this text and the tables have been adapted, from the Surgeon General's Report on Oral Health[165] and papers published in the *Journal of Public Health Dentistry*[166] and *Annals of Periodontology*[167].

REFERENCES

1. Kaslow RA (1985). Infections in diabetics. In: Harris MI (ed) *Diabetes in America.* NIH Publication No. 85–1468. Washington DC: Government Printing Office, XIX-1–XIX-18.
2. Wilson RM (1991). Infection and diabetes mellitus. In: Pickup JC and Williams W (eds) *Textbook of Diabetes*. London: Blackwell Scientific Publications, pp. 813–818.
3. Rayfield EJ, Ault MJ, Keusch GT, Brothers MJ, Nechemias C, Smith H (1982). Infection and diabetes: the case for glucose control. *American Journal of Medicine* **72**: 439–450.
4. Wheat JL (1980). Infection in diabetes melllitus. *Diabetes Care* **3**: 187–197.
5. Lewis RP, Sutter VL, Finegold SM (1978). Bone infections involving anaerobic bacteria. *Medicine* **57**: 279–305.
6. Genco RJ (1990). Classification and clinical and radiographic features of periodontal disease. In: Genco RJ, Goldman HM, Cohen DW (eds) *Contempory periodontics*. St. Louis: Mosby, pp. 63–81.

7. Page RC (1986). Gingivitis. J Clin Perio **13**: 345–355.
8. Shah HN, Collins DM (1988). Proposal for reclassification of *Bacteroides asaccharolyticus*, *Bacteroides gingivalis*, and *Bacteroides endodontalis* in a new genus, Porphyromonas. *International Journal of Systematic Bacteriology* **38**: 128–131.
9. Shah HN, Collins DM (1990). *Prevotella*, a new genus to include Bacteroides melaninogenicus and related species formerly classified in the genus *Bacteroides*. *International Journal of Systematic Bacteriology* **40**: 205–208.
10. Dzink JL, Socransky SS, Haffajee AD (1988). The predominant cultivable microbiota of active and inactive lesions of destructive periodontal diseases. *Journal of Clinical Periodontology* **15**: 316–323.
11. Loesche WJ, Syed SA, Schmidt E, Morrison EC (1985). Bacterial profiles of subgingival plaques in periodontitis. *J Periodontol* **56**: 447–456.
12. Slots J, Genco RJ (1984). Black-pigmented Bacteroides species, Capnocytophaga species, and *Actinobacillus actinomycetemcomitans* in human periodontal disease: Virulence factors in colonization, survival and tissue destruction. *J Dent Res* **63**: 412–421.
13. Moore WEC (1987). Microbiology of periodontal disease. *Journal of Periodontolal Research* 1987; **22**: 335–341.
14. Zambon JJ (1985). *Actinobacillus actinomycetemcomitans* in human periodontal disease. *Journal of Clinical Periodontology* **12**: 1–20.
15. Kornman KS, Robertson PB (1985). Clinical and microbiological evaluation of therapy for juvenile periodontitis. *Journal of Periodontic Research* **56**: 443–446.
16. Slots J, Hafstrom C, Rosling B, Dahlen G (1985). Detection of *Actinobacillus actinomycetemcomitans* and Bacteroides gingivalis in subgingival smears by the indirect fluorescent-antibody technique. *Journal of Periodontolal Research* **20**: 613–620.
17. Genco RJ, Zambon JJ, Christersson LA (1988). The origin of periodontal infections. *Advances in Dental Research* **2**: 245–259.
18. Loe H, Morrison E (1986). Periodontal health and disease in young people: screening for priority care. *International Dental Journal* **36**: 162–167.
19. Socransky SS, Haffajee AD, Goodson JM, Lindhe J (1984). New concepts of destructive periodontal disease. *Journal of Clinical Periodontology* **11**: 21–32.
21. Albandar JM, Kingman A (1999). Gingival recession, gingival bleeding, and dental calculus in adults 30 years of age and older in the United States, 1988–1994. *Journal of Periodontology* **70**: 30–43.
22. Albandar JM, Brunelle JA, Kingman A (1999). Destructive periodontal disease in adults 30 years of age and older in the United States, 1988–1994 [published erratum appears in *Journal of Periodontology* **70**: 351]. *Journal of Periodontology* 1999; **70**(1): 13–29.
23. Goteiner D, Vogel R, Deasy M, Goteiner C (1986). Periodontal and caries experience in children with insulin-dependent diabetes mellitus. *Journal of the American Dental Association* **113**: 277–279.
24. Harrison R, Bowen WH (1987). Periodontal health, dental caries, and metabolic control in insulin-dependent diabetic children and adolescents. *Pediatric Dentistry* **9**: 283–286.
25. Novaes Jr. AB, Pereira, ALA, de Moraes N, Novaes AB (1991). Manifestations of insulin-dependent diabetes mellitus in the periodontium of young brazilian patients. *Journal of Periodontology* **62**: 116–122.
26. Cianciola LA, Park BH, Bruck E, Mosovich L, Genco RJ (1982). Prevalence of periodontal disease in insulin-dependent diabetes mellitus (juvenile diabetes). *Journal of American Dental Association* **104**: 653–660.

27. de Pommereau V, Dargent-Pare C, Robert JJ, Brion M (1992). Periodontal status in insulin-dependent diabetic adolescents. *Journal of Clinical Periodontology* **19**: 628–632.

28. Ringelberg ML, Dixon DO, Francis AO, Plummer RW (1977). Comparison of gingival health and gingival crevicular fluid flow in children with and without diabetes. *Journal of Dental Research* **56**: 108–111.

29. Firatli E, Yilmaz O, Onan U (1996). The relationship between clinical attachment loss and the duration of insulin-dependent diabetes mellitus (IDDM) in children and adolescents. J*ournal of Clinical Periodontology* **23**: 362–366.

30. Firatli E (1997). The relationship between clinical periodontal status and insulin-dependent diabetes mellitus. Results after five years. *Journal of Periodontology* **68**: 136–140.

31. Pinson M, Hoffman WH, Garnick JJ, Litaker MS (1995). Periodontal disease and type I diabetes mellitus in children and adolescents. *Journal of Clinical Periodontology* **22**: 118–23.

32. Faulconbridge AR, Bradshaw WC, Jenkins PA, Baum JD (1981). The dental status of a group of diabetic children. *British Dental Journal* **151**: 253–255.

33. Cohen DW, Friedman LA, Shapiro J, Kyle GC, Franklin S (1970). Diabetes mellitus and periodontal disease: two-year longitudinal observations. I. *Journal of Periodontology* **41**: 709–712.

34. Kjellman O, Henriksson CO, Berghagen N, Andersson B (1970). Oral conditions in 105 subjects with insulin-treated diabetes mellitus. *Svensk Tandlakaretidskrift* **63**: 99–110.

35. Guven Y, Satman I, Dinccag N, Alptekin S (1996). Salivary peroxidase activity in whole saliva of patients with insulin-dependent (type 1) diabetes mellitus. *Journal of Clinical Periodontology* **23**: 879–881.

36. Rylander H, Ramberg P, Blohme G, Lindhe J (1987). Prevalence of periodontal disease in young diabetics. *Journal of Clinical Periodontology* **14**: 38–43.

37. Sznajder N, Carraro JJ, Rugna S, Sereday M (1978). Periodontal findings in diabetic and nondiabetic patients. *Journal of Periodontology* **49**: 445–448.

38. Galea H, Aganovic I, Aganovic M (1986). The dental caries and periodontal disease experience of patients with early onset insulin dependent diabetes. *International Dental Journal* **36**: 219–224.

39. Hugoson A, Thorstensson H, Falk H, Kuylenstierna J (1989). Periodontal conditions in insulin-dependent diabetics. *Journal of Clinical Periodontology* **16**: 215–223.

40. Glavind L, Lund B, Loe H (1968). The relationship between periodontal state and diabetes duration, insulin dosage and retinal changes. *Journal of Periodontology* **39**: 341–347.

41. Thorstensson H, Hugoson A (1993). Periodontal disease experience in adult long-duration insulin-dependent diabetics. *Journal of Clinical Periodontology* **20**: 352–358.

42. Tervonen T, Karjalainen K (1997). Periodontal disease related to diabetic status. A pilot study of the response to periodontal therapy in type 1 diabetes. *Journal of Clinical Periodontology* **24**: 505–510.

43. Tervonen T, Karjalainen K, Knuuttila M, Humonen S (2000). Alveolar bone loss in type 1 diabetic subjects. *Journal of Clinical Periodontology* **27**: 567–571.

44. Novaes Jr. AB, Gutierrez FG, Novaes AB (1996). Periodontal disease progression in type II non-insulin-dependent diabetes mellitus patients (NIDDM). Part I–Probing pocket depth and clinical attachment. *Brazilian Dental Journal* **7**: 65–73.

45. Morton AA, Williams RW, Watts TLP (1995). Initial study of periodontal status in non-insulin-dependent diabetics in Mauritius. *Journal of Dentistry* **23**: 343–345.

46. Sandberg GE, Sundberg HE, Fjellstrom CA, Wikblad KF (2000). Type 2 diabetes and oral health: A comparison between diabetic and non-diabetic subjects. *Diabetes Research and Clinical Practice* **50**: 27–34.

47. Shlossman M, Knowler WC, Pettitt DJ, Genco RJ (1990). Type 2 diabetes mellitus and periodontal disease. *Journal of the American Dental Association* **121**: 532–536.

48. Nelson RG, Shlossman M, Budding LM, Pettitt DJ, Saad MF, Genco RJ Knowler WC (1990). Periodontal disease and NIDDM in Pima Indians. *Diabetes Care* **13**: 836–840.

49. Emirich LJ, Shlossman M, Genco RJ (1991). Periodontal disease in non-insulin-dependent diabetes mellitus. *Journal of Periodontology* Feb; **62**: 123–130.

50. Taylor G.W, Burt BA, Becker MP, Genco RJ, Shlossman M, Knowle, WC, Pettitt DJ (1998). Non-insulin dependent diabetes mellitus and alveolar bone loss progression over two years. *Journal of Periodontology* **69**: 76–83.

51. Taylor GW, Bur, BA, Becker MP, Genco RJ, Shlossman M (1998). Glycemic control and alveolar bone loss progression in Type II diabetes. *Annals of Periodontology* **3**: 30–39.

52. Wolf J (1977). Dental and periodontal conditions in diabetes mellitus. A clinical and radiographic study. *Proceedings of the Finnish Dental Society* **73 (4–6 Suppl VI)**: 1–56.

53. Benveniste R, Bixler D, Conneally PM (1967). Periodontal disease in diabetics. *Journal of Periodontology* **38**: 271–279.

54. Finestone AJ, Boorujy SR (1967). Diabetes mellitus and periodontal disease. *Diabetes* **16**: 336–340.

55. Belting CM, Hiniker JJ, Dummett CO (1964). Influence of diabetes mellitus on the severity of periodontal disease. *Journal of Periodontology* **35**: 476–480.

56. Oliver RC, Tervonen T (1993). Periodontitis and tooth loss: comparing diabetics with the general population. *Journal of the American Dental Association* **124**: 71–76.

57. Yavuzyilmaz E, Yumak O, Akdoganli T, Yamalik N, Ozer N, Ersoy F (1996). The alterations of whole saliva constituents in patients with diabetes mellitus. *Australian Dental Journal* **41**: 193–197.

58. Bridges RB, Anderson JW, Saxe SR, Gregory K, Bridges SR (1996). Periodontal status of diabetic and non-diabetic men: effects of smoking, glycemic control, and socioeconomic factors. *Journal of Periodontology* **67**: 1185–1192.

59. Sandler HC, Stahl SS (1960). Prevalence of periodontal disease in a hospitalized population. *Journal of Dental Research* **39**: 439–449.

60. Bacic M, Plancak D, Granic M (1988). CPITN assessment of periodontal disease in diabetic patients. *Journal of Periodontology* **59**: 816–822.

61. Hove KA, Stallard RE (1970). Diabetes and the periodontal patient. *Journal of Periodontology* **41**: 713–718.

62. Mackenzie RS, Millard HD (1963). Interrelated effects of diabetes, arteriosclerosis and calculus on alveolar bone loss. *The Journal of the American Dental Association* **66**: 191–198.

63. Dolan TA, Gilbert GH, Ringelberg ML, Legler DW, Antonson DE, Foerster U, Heft MW (1997). Behavioral risk indicators of attachment loss in adult floridians. *Journal of Clinical Periodontology* **24**: 223–232.

64. Grossi SG, Sambon JJ, Ho AW, Koch G, Dunford RG, Machtei EE, Norderyd OM, Genco RJ (1994). Assessment of risk for periodontal disease. I. Risk indicators for attachment loss. *Journal of Periodontology* **65**: 260–267.

548   *The Evidence Base for Diabetes Care*

65. Tervonen T, Knuuttila M (1986). Relation of diabetes control to periodontal pocketing and alveolar bone level. *Oral Surgery, Oral Medicine, Oral Pathology* **61**: 346–349.
66. Campbell MJ (1972). Epidemiology of periodontal disease in the diabetic and the non-diabetic. *Australian Dental Journal* **17**: 274–278.
67. Albrecht M, Banoczy J, Tamas G, Jr. (1988) Dental and oral symptoms of diabetes mellitus. *Community Dentistry & Oral Epidemiology* **16**: 378–80.
68. Szpunar SM, Ismail AI, Eklund SA (1989). Diabetes and periodontal disease: analyses of NHANES I and HHANES [Abstr #1605]. *Journal of Dental Research* **68 (Special Issue)**: 383.
69. Unal T, Firatli E, Sivas A, Meric H, Oz H (1993). Fructosamine as a possible monitoring parameter in non-insulin dependent diabetes mellitus patients with periodontal disease. *Journal of Periodontology* **64**: 191–194.
70. Ainamo J, Lahtinen A, Uitto VJ (1990). Rapid periodontal destruction in adult humans with poorly controlled diabetes. A report of two cases. *Journal of Clinical Periodontology* **17**: 22–28.
71. Gusberti FA, Syed SA, Bacon G, Grossman N, Loesche WJ (1983). Puberty gingivitis in insulin-dependent diabetic children. I. Cross-sectional observations. *Journal of Periodontology* **54**: 714–720.
72. Safkan-Seppala B, Ainamo J (1992). Periodontal conditions in insulin-dependent diabetes mellitus. *Journal of Clinical Periodontology* **19**: 24–29.
73. Seppala B, Seppala M, Ainamo J. A (1993). longitudinal study on insulin-dependent diabetes mellitus and periodontal disease. *Journal of Clinical Periodontology* **20**: 161–165.
74. Seppala B, Ainamo J (1994). A site-by-site follow-up study on the effect of controlled versus poorly controlled insulin-dependent diabetes mellitus. *Journal of Clinical Periodontology* **21**: 161–165.
75. Tervonen T, Oliver RC (1993). Long-term control of diabetes mellitus and periodontitis. *Journal of Clinical Periodontology* **20**: 431–435.
76. Karjalainen KM, Knuuttila ML (1996). The onset of diabetes and poor metabolic control increases gingival bleeding in children and adolescents with insulin-dependent diabetes mellitus. *Journal of Clinical Periodontology* **23**: 1060–7.
77. Nichols C, Laster LL, Bodak-Gyovai LZ (1978). Diabetes mellitus and periodontal disease. *Journal of Periodontology* **49**: 85–88.
78. Barnett ML, Baker RL, Yancey JM, MacMillan DR, Kotoyan M (1984). Absence of periodontitis in a population of insulin-dependent diabetes mellitus (IDDM) patients. *Journal of Periodontology* 402–405.
79. Hayden P, Buckley LA (1989). Diabetes mellitus and periodontal disease in an Irish population. *Journal of Periodontal Research* **24**: 298–302.
80. Sandholm L, Swanljung O, Rytomaa I, Kaprio EA, Maenpaa J (1989). Morphotypes of the subgingival microflora in diabetic adolescents in Finland. *Journal of Periodontology* **60**: 526–528.
81. Sastrowijoto SH, Hillemans P, van Steenbergen TJ, Abraham-Inpijn L, de Graaff J (1989). Periodontal condition and microbiology of healthy and diseased periodontal pockets in type 1 diabetes mellitus patients. *Journal of Clinical Periodontology* **16**: 316–322.
82. Moore PA, Weyant RJ, Mongelluzzo MB, Myers DE, Rossie K, Guggenheimer J, Block HM, Huber H, Orchard T (1999). Type 1 diabetes mellitus and oral health assessment of periodontal disease. *Journal of Periodontolal Research* **70**: 409–417.

83. Salvi GE, Collins JG, Yalda B, Arnold RR, Lang NP, Offenbacher S (1997). Monocytic TNFα secretion patterns in IDDM patients with periodontal diseases. *Journal of Clinical Periodontology* **24**: 8–16.
84. Wilton JM, Griffiths GS, Curtis MA, Maiden MF, Gillett IR, Wilson DT, Sterne JA, Johnson NW (1988). Detection of high-risk groups and individuals for periodontal diseases. Systemic predisposition and markers of general health. *Journal of Clinical Periodontology* **15**: 339–346.
85. Murrah VA (1985). Diabetes mellitus and associated oral manifestations: a review. *Journal of Oral Pathology* **14**: 271–281.
86. Manouchehr-Pour M, Bissada NF (1983). The *Journal of the American Dental Association* **107**: 766–770.
87. Oliver RC, Tervonen T (1994). Diabetes – a risk factor for periodontitis in adults? *Journal of Periodontolal Research* **65 (5 Suppl)**: 530–538.
88. Grossi SG, Genco RJ (1998). Periodontal disease and diabetes mellitus: a two-way relationship. *Annals of Periodontology* **3**: 51–61.
89. Iacopino, A (1995). Diabetic periodontitis: possible lipid-induced defect in tissue repair through alteration of macrophage phenotype and function. *Oral Diseases* **1**: 214–229.
90. Page R (1998). The pathobiology of periodontal diseases may affect systemic diseases: inversion of a paradigm. *Annals of Periodontology* **3**: 108–120.
91. Brayton RG, Stokes PE, Schwartz MS, Louria DB (1970). Effect of alcohol and various diseases on leukocyte mobilization, phagocytosis and intracellular bacterial killing. *N Engl J Med* **282**: 123–128.
92. Hill HR, Sauls HS, Dettloff JL, Quie PG (1974). Impaired leukotactic responsiveness in patients with juvenile diabetes mellitus. *Clinical Immunology and Immunopathology* **2**: 395.
93. Mowat AG, Baum J (1971). Chemotaxis of polymophonuclear leukocytes from patients with diabetes mellitus. *N Engl J Med* **284**: 621.
94. Miller M, Baker L (1974). Leukocytes function and juvenile diabetes mellitus: humoral and cellular aspects. *J Pediatr* **81**: 979.
95. Molenaar DM, Palumbo PJ, Wilson WR, Ritts RE (1976). Leukocyte chemotaxis in diabetic patients and their nondiabetic first-degree relatives. *Diabetes* **25**: 880–883.
96. Bagdade JD, Stewart M, Walters E (1978). Impaired granulocyte adherence. A reversible defect in host defense in patients with poorly controlled diabetes. *Diabetes* **27**: 677–681
97. Bagdade JD, Walters E (1980). Impaired granulocyte adherence in mildly diabetic patients: effects of tolazamide treatment. *Diabetes* **29**: 309–311.
98. Bagdade JD, Nielson KL, Bulger RJ (1972). Reversible abnormalities in phagocytic function in poorly controlled diabetic patients. *The American Journal of the Medical Sciences* **263**: 451–456.
99. Bagdade JD, Root RK, Bulger RJ (1974). Impaired leukocyte function in patients with poorly controlled diabetes. *Diabetes* **23**: 9–15.
100. Walters MI, Lessler MA, Stevenson TD (1971). Oxidative metabolism of leukocytes from nondiabetic and diabetic patients. *Journal of Laboratory and Clinical Medicine* **78**: 158–166.
101. Brownlee M (1994). Lilly Lecture 1993: Glycation and diabetic complications. *Diabetes* **43**: 836–841.
102. Vlassara H (1994). Recent progress on the biological and clinical significance of advanced glycosylation end products. *Journal of Laboratory and Clinical Medicine* **124**: 19–30.

103. Schmidt AM, Weidman E, Lalla E, Yan SD, Hori O, Cao R, Brett JG, Lamster IB (1996). Advanced glycation endproducts (AGEs) induce oxidant stress in the gingiva: a potential mechanism underlying accelerated periodontal disease associated with diabetes. *Journal of Periodontal Research* **31**: 508–515.
104. Brett J, Schmidt AM, Yan SD, Zou YS, Weidman E, Pinsky D, Nowygrod R, Neeper M, Przysiecki C, Shaw A (1993). Survey of the distribution of a newly characterized receptor for advanced glycation end products in tissues. *American Journal of Pathology* **143**: 1699–1712.
105. Yan SD, Schmidt AM, Anderson GM, Zhang J, Brett J, Zou YS, Pinsky D, Stern D (1994). Enhanced cellular oxidant stress by the interaction of advanced glycation end products with their receptors/binding proteins. *Journal of Biological Chemistry* **269**: 9889–9897.
106. Schmidt AM, Hasu M, Popov D, Zhang JH, Chen J, Yan SD, Brett J, Cao R, Kuwabara K, Costache G (1994). Receptor for advanced glycation end products (AGEs) has a central role in vessel wall interactions and gene activation in response to circulating AGE proteins. *Proceedings of the National Academy of Sciences of the United States of America* **91**: 8807–8811.
107. Moughal N, Adonogianaki E, Rthornhill M, Kinane D (1992). Endothelial cell leukocyte adhesion molecule-I and intercellular adhesion molecule-I expression in gingival tissue during health and experimentally-induced gingivitis. *Journal of Periodontal Research* **27**: 623–630.
108. Baeuerle P (1991). The inducible transcription activator NF-kappa B: regulation by distinct protein subunits. *Biochimica et Biophysica Acta* **1072**: 63–80.
109. Collins T (1993). Endothelial nuclear factor-kappa B and the initiation of the atherosclerotic lesion. *Laboratory Investigation* **68**: 499–508.
110. Schreck R, Rieber P, Baeuerle PA (1991). Reactive oxygen intermediates as apparently widely used messengers in the activation of the NF-kappa B transcription factor and HIV-1. *EMBO Journal* **10**: 2247–2258.
111. Takahasi K, Takashiba S, Nagai A, Miyamoto M, Kurihara H, Murayama Y (1994). Assessment of IL-6 in the pathogenesis of periodontal disease. *Journal of Periodontology* **65**: 147–153.
112. Salvi GE, Beck JD, Offenbacher S (1998). PGE2, IL-1 beta, and TNF-alpha responses in diabetics as modifiers of periodontal disease expression. *Annals of Periodontology* **3**: 40–50.
113. Lalla E, Lamster IB, Schmidt AM (1998). Enhanced interaction of advanced glycation end products with their cellular receptor RAGE: implications for the pathogenesis of accelerated periodontal disease in diabetes. *Annals of Periodontology* **3**: 13–19.
114. Wautier JL, Zoukourian C, Chappey O, Wautier MP, Guillausseau PJ, Cao R, Hori O, Stern D, Schmidt, AM (1996). Receptor-mediated endothelial cell dysfunction in diabetic vasculopathy. Soluble receptor for advanced glycation end products blocks hyperpermeability in diabetic rats. *Journal of Clinical Investigation* **97**: 238–243.
115. Schmidt AM, Hori O, Chen JX, Li JF, Crandall J, Zhang J, Cao R, Yan SD, Brett J, Stern D (1995). Advanced glycation endproducts interacting with their endothelial receptor induce expression of vascular cell adhesion molecule-1 (VCAM-1) in cultured human endothelial cells and in mice. A potential mechanism for the accelerated vasculopathy of diabetes. *Journal of Clinical Investigation* **96**: 1395–1403.
116. Lalla E, Lamster IB, Feit M, Huang L, Schmidt AM (1998). A murine model of accelerated periodontal disease in diabetes. *Journal of Periodontolal Research* **33**: 387–399.

117. Clark RAF, Henson PM (1988). *The Molecular and Cellular Biology of Wound Repair*. New York: Plenum Press.
118. Andreesen R, Kreutz M, Lohr GW (1990). Surface phenotype analysis of human monocyte to macrophage maturation. *Journal of Leukocyte Biology* **47**: 490–497.
119. Messadi DV, Bertolami CN (1991). General principles of healing pertinent to the periodontal problem. *Dental Clinics of North America* **35**: 443–457.
120. Kreutz M, Krause SW, Rehm A, Andreesen R (1992). Macrophage heterogeneity and differentiation. *Research into Immunology* **143**: 107–115.
121. Martin P, Hopkinson-Woolley J, McCluskey J (1992). Growth factors and cutaneous wound repair. *Progress in Growth Factor Research* **4**: 25–44.
122. Wikesjo UME, Nilveus RE, Selvig KA (1992). Significance of early healing events on periodontal repair: a review. *Journal of. Periodontology* **63**: 158–165.
123. Kiritsy CP, Lynch SE (1993). Role of growth factors in cutaneous wound healing: a review. *Critical Reviews in Oral Biology and Medicine* **4**: 729–760.
124. Sullivan DR, Conney G, Caterson I, Turtle JR, Hensley WJ (1990). The effects of dietary fatty acid in animal models of type 1 and type 2 diabetes. *Diabetes Research and Clinical Practice* **9**: 225–230.
125. Clarke SD, Jump DB (1993). Regulation of gene expression by polyunsaturated fatty acids. *Progress in Lipid Research* **32**: 139–149.
126. Hicks M, Delbridge L, Yue D, Reeve TS (1988). Catalysis of lipid peroxidation by glucose and glycosylated proteins. *Biochemical and Biophysical Research* **151**: 649–655.
127. Hunt J, Smith C, Wolff S (1990). Autooxidative glycosylation and possible involvement of peroxides and free radicals in LDL modification by glucose. *Diabetes* **30**: 1420–1424.
128. Bucala R, Makita Z, Koschinsky T, Cerami A, Vlassara H (1993). Lipid advanced glycosylation: pathway for lipid oxidation in vivo. *Proceedings of the National Academy of Sciences* **90**: 6434–6438.
129. Salbach PB, Specht E, von Hodenberg E, Kossmann J, Janssen-Timmen U, Schneider WJ, Hugger P, King WC, Glomset JA, Habenicht AJ (1992). Differential low-density lipoprotein receptor-dependent formation of eicosanoid in human blood-derived monocytes. *Proceedings of the National Academy of Sciences* **89**: 2439–2443.
130. Jambou D, Dejour N, Bayer P, Poiree JC, Fredenrich A, Issa-Sayegh M, Adjovi-Desouza M, Lapalus P, Harter M (1993). Effect of human native low-density and high-density lipoproteins on prostaglandin production by mouse macrophage cell line P388D1: Possible implications in pathogenesis of atherosclerosis. *Biochimica et Biophysica Acta* **1168**: 115–121.
131. Salvi GE, Yalda B, Collins JG, Jones BH, Smith FW, Arnold RR, Offenbacher S (1997). Inflammatory mediator response as a potential risk marker for periodontal diseases in insulin-dependent diabetes mellitus patients. *Journal of Clinical Periodontology* **68**: 127–135.
132. Santamaria P, Gehrz RC, Bryan MK, J.J. B (1989). Involvement of class II MHC molecules in the LPS-induction of IL-1/TNF secretions by human monocytes. *Journal of Immunology* **143**: 913–922.
133. Pociot F, Molvig J, Wogensen L, Worsaae H, Dalboge H, Baek L, Nerup J (1991). A tumour necrosis factor beta gene polymorphism in relation to monokine secretion and insulin-dependent diabetes mellitus. *Scandinavian Journal of Immunology* **33**: 37–49.
134. Pociot F, Wilson AG, Nerup J, Duff GW (1993). No independent association between a tumor necrosis factor-α promotor region polymorphism and insulin-dependent diabetes mellitus. *European Journal of Immunology* **23**: 3043–3049.

135. Salvi GE, Lawrence HP, Offenbacher S, Beck JD (2000). Influence of risk factors on the pathogenesis of periodontitis. *Periodontology* **14**: 173–201.
136. Leslie RDG, Lazarus NR, Vergani D (1989). Etiology of insulin dependent diabetes mellitus. *Br Med Bull* **45**: 58–72.
137. Reinhardt RA, Maze CS, Seagren-Alley CD, Dubois LM (1991). HLA-D types associated with type 1 diabetes and periodontitis. *Journal of Dental Research* 70.
138. Todd JA (1990). Genetic control of autoimmunity in type 1 diabetes. *Immunol Today* **11**: 122–129.
139. Svenson KL, Lundqvist G, Wide L, Hallgren R (1987). Impaired glucose handling in active rheumatoid arthritis: relationship to the secretion of insulin and counter-regulatory hormones. *Metabolism: Clinical and Experimental* **36**: 940–3.
140. Hallgren R, Lundquist G (1983). Elevated serum levels of pancreatic polypeptide are related to impaired glucose handling in inflammatory states. *Scandinavian Journal of Gastroenterology* **18**: 561–564.
141. Beck-Nielsen H (1992). Clinical disorders of insulin resistance. In: Alberti KGMM, Defronzo RA, Keen H, Zimmet P (eds) *International Textbook of Diabetes Mellitus*. New York: Wiley; p. 531–568.
142. Beisel WR (1975). Metabolic response to infection. *Annual Review of Medicine* **26**: 9–20.
143. Drobny EC, Abramson EC, Baumann G (1984). Insulin receptors in acute infection: a study of factors conferring insulin resistance. *Journal of Clinical Endocrinology and Metabolism* **58**: 710–716.
144. Sammalkorpi K (1989). Glucose intolerance in acute infections. *Journal of Internal Medicine* **225**: 15–19.
145. Offenbacher S, Katz V, Fertik G, Collins J, Boyd D, Maynor G, McKaig R, Beck J (1996). Periodontal infection as a possible risk factor for preterm low birth weight. *Journal of Periodontolal Research* **67**: 1103–1113.
146. Grossi SG, Genco RJ (1998). Periodontal disease and diabetes mellitus: a two-way relationship. *Ann Peridontal* **3**(1): 51–61.
147. Feingold KR, Soued M, Serio MK, Moser AH, Dinarello CA, Grunfeld C (1989). Multiple cytokines stimulate hepatic lipid synthesis in vivo. *Endocrinology* **125**: 267–274.
148. Ling PR, Istfan NW, Colon E, Bistrian BR (1995). Differential effects of interleukin-1 receptor antagonist in cytokine- and endotoxin-treated rats. *American Journal of Physiology* **268**(2 Pt. 1): E255–E261.
149. Feingold KR, Grunfeld C (1992). Role of cytokines in inducing hyperlipidemia. *Diabetes* **41 (Suppl 2)**: 97–101.
150. Grunfeld C, Soued M, Adi S, Moser AH, Dinarello CA, Feingold KR (1990). Evidence for two classes of cytokines that stimulate hepatic lipogenesis: relationships among tumor necrosis factor, interleukin-1 and interferon-alpha. *Endocrinology* **127**: 46–54.
151. Pickup JC, Mattock MB, Chusney GD, Burt D (1997). NIDDM as a disease of the innate immune system: association of acute-phase reactants and interleukin-6 with metabolic syndrome X. *Diabetologia* **40**: 1286–1292.
152. Michie HR (1996). Metabolism of sepsis and multiple organ failure. *World Journal of Surgery* **10**: 460–464.
153. Grossi SG, Skrepcinski FB, DeCaro T, Zambon JJ, Cummins D, Genco RJ (1996). Response to periodontal therapy in diabetics and smokers. *Journal of Periodontology* **67 (10 Suppl)**: 1094–1102.
154. Grossi SG, Skrepcinski FB, DeCaro T, Robertson D, Ho AW, Dunford R, Genco RJ (1997). Treatment of periodontal disease in diabetics reduces glycated hemoglobin. *Journal of Periodontology* **68**: 713–719.

155. Williams R, Mahan C (1960). Periodontal disease and diabetes in young adults. *JAMA* **172**: 776–778.
156. Miller LS, Manwell MA, Newbold D, Reding ME, Rasheed A, Blodgett J, Kornman KS (1992). The relationship between reduction in periodontal inflammation and diabetes control: A report of 9 cases. *Journal of Periodontolal Research* **63**: 843–848.
157. Aldridge JP, Lester V, Watts TLP, Collins A, Viberti G, Wilson RF (1995). Single-blind studies of the effects of improved periodontal health on metabolic control in type 1 diabetes mellitus. *Journal of Clinical Periodontology* **22**: 271–275.
158. Smith GT, Greenbaum CJ, Johnson BD, Persson GR (1996). Short-term responses to periodontal therapy in insulin-dependent diabetic patients. *Journal of Periodontal Research* **67**: 794–802.
159. Westfeld E, Rylander H, Blohme G, Jonasson P, Lindhe J (1996). The effect of periodontal therapy in diabetics: results after five years. *Journal of Clinical Periodontology* **23**: 92–100.
160. Taylor GW, Burt BA, Becker MP, Genco RJ, Shlossman M, Knowler WC, Pettitt DJ (1996). Severe periodontitis and risk for poor glycemic control in patients with non-insulin-dependent diabetes mellitus. *Journal of Periodontology* **67(10 Suppl.)**: 1085–1093.
161. Collin HL, Uusitupa M, Niskanen L, Kontturi-Narhi V, Markkanen H, Koivisto AM, Meurman JH (1998). Periodontal findings in elderly patients with non-insulin dependent diabetes mellitus. *Journal of Periodontology* **69**: 962–966.
162. Christgau M, Palitzsch K-D, Schmalz G, Kreiner U, Frenzel S (1998). Healing response to non-surgical periodontal therapy in patients with diabetes mellitus: clinical, microbiological and immunological results. *Journal of Clinical Periodontology* **25**: 112–124.
163. Taylor GW (1999). Periodontal treatment and its effects on glycemic control: a review of the evidence. Oral Surgery, Oral Medicine, *Oral Pathology, Oral Radiology and Endodontics* **87**: 311–316.
164. Tervonen T, Knuutila M, Pohjamo L, Nurkkala H (1991). Immediate response to non-surgical periodontal treatment in subjects with diabetes mellitus. *Journal of Clinical Periodontology* **18**: 65–68.
165. U.S. Department of Health and Human Services (2000). Oral Health in America: A Report of the Surgeon General. Rockville, MD: US Department of Health and Human Services, National Institute of Dental and Craniofacial Research, National Institutes of Health.
166. Taylor GW, Loesche WJ, Terpenning MS (2000). Impact of oral diseases on systemic health in the elderly: diabetes mellitus and aspiration pneumonia. *Journal of Public Health Dentistry* **60**: 313–320.
167. Taylor GW (2001). Bidirectional interrelationships between diabetes and periodontal diseases: an epidemiologic perspective. *Annals of Periodontology* **6**: 99–112.

24

Treatment of Diabetic Neuropathy

ZACHARY SIMMONS, [1] and EVA L. FELDMAN[2]

[1]Pennsylvania State University, Hershey, Pennsylvania, USA
[2]University of Michigan, Ann Arbor, Michigan, USA

PREVALENCE OF DIABETIC NEUROPATHY

Diabetes is the most common cause of neuropathy in the Western world. Neuropathy may occur in both type 1 and type 2 diabetes. A large cross-sectional study of 6487 diabetic patients in the UK found the prevalence of diabetic neuropathy to be 28.5%[1]. However, prevalence varies greatly among various series, from a low of less than 5% to a high of 100%[2]. Differences in prevalence arise partially from differences in age, but primarily from differences in the definition of diabetic neuropathy, and whether this is based on symptoms only, signs and symptoms, nerve conduction abnormalities or composite definitions. Using a definition based on symptoms, signs, nerve conduction studies, quantitative sensory testing and autonomic testing[3], neuropathy was present in 66% of all diabetic patients in one series[4]. The most common neuropathy was polyneuropathy, with a prevalence of 54% in patients with type 1 diabetes, and 45% in patients with type 2 diabetes. The neuropathy was subclinical in most of these. Neuropathy appears to be less common in children, with a prevalence of 2% or less[2]. The prevalence of diabetic neuropathy increases with the known duration of diabetes, as illustrated in Table 24.1.

CLASSIFICATION OF DIABETIC NEUROPATHY

Diabetic neuropathy is very heterogeneous[2]. One classification scheme is presented in Table 24.2.

The Evidence Base for Diabetes Care. Edited by R. Williams, W. Herman, A.-L. Kinmonth and N. J. Wareham.
© 2002 John Wiley & Sons, Ltd

Table 24.1. Changes in the prevalence of diabetic neuropathy over time.

Reference	Initial prevalence (%)	Time of initial prevalence	Later prevalence (%)	Time of later Prevalence
134	7.5	At diagnosis	50	25 years after diagnosis
135	4	Within five years of diagnosis	15	20 years after diagnosis
	20.8	Less than five years duration	36.8	Greater than 10 years duration
136	8.3	At diagnosis	41.9	10 years after diagnosis

Table 24.2. Classification of diabetic neuropathies

Symmetric polyneuropathies
- Sensory or sensorimotor polyneuropathy
- Selective small-fiber polyneuropathy
- Autonomic neuropathy

Focal and multifocal neuropathies
- Cranial neuropathy
- Limb mononeuropathy

    - Compression and entrapment neuropathies
    - Nerve infarction

- Trunk mononeuropathy
- Mononeuropathy multiplex
- Asymmetric lower limb motor neuropathy (amyotrophy)

Mixed forms

DISTAL SENSORY AND SENSORIMOTOR POLYNEUROPATHY

Symptoms and signs. A distal sensory neuropathy with an insidious onset is the most common neuropathy in patients with diabetes[2]. This is a length-dependent process, with the most distal portions of the longest nerves affected earliest. Thus, the earliest symptoms typically involve the toes, and then ascend. Upper extremity involvement is later, less severe and less common, also proceeding distally to proximally. A 'stocking–glove' pattern of sensory loss results. If severe, the midline abdomen may be involved. The most common symptoms are numbness, tingling and pain. The pain is particularly troubling to most patients, and it is common for such patients to present primarily because of pain in the feet. This neuropathic pain may be described as sharp, stabbing, burning or aching. It is often worst at night, disturbing sleep, and the patient may have to sleep with his or her feet out from under the covers. Despite the pain, there is numbness. Gait ataxia may be reported. Weakness is typically minor and occurs later. Examination generally demonstrates distal sensory loss, with reduced or absent ankle jerks. Distal weakness is less common and typically mild.

Diagnostic studies. Electrodiagnostically, this neuropathy is usually classified as having features of both axon loss and demyelination[5].On nerve conduction studies, the lower extremity nerves are affected first and most severely. The earliest and most sensitive findings are changes in sensory nerve conduction studies, which demonstrate a reduction in conduction velocity and a decrease in amplitude. With more severe neuropathy, sensory responses may disappear. Motor nerve studies demonstrate some slowing even when patients have no symptoms or signs of neuropathy, with a greater slowing in symptomatic patients. A decrease in motor amplitudes may be seen in more advanced cases. Needle electromyography may be normal in mild or neurologically asymptomatic subjects, but demonstrate denervation in more severe cases, most prominent distally[2,6]. On sural nerve biopsy, there is loss of both myelinated and unmyelinated axons. Demyelination is also seen on teased fiber studies. There is thickening of the walls of small neural blood vessels, particularly endoneurial capillaries, due to reduplication of the basal lamina[2].

Pathogenesis. Both metabolic and vascular factors appear to be involved in the pathogenesis of diabetic polyneuropathy. It now appears that hyperglycemia results in increased activity of the enzyme aldose reductase, with changes in the polyol pathway. This eventually leads to oxidative stress, mitochondrial dysfunction, and ischemic nerve damage[7].

Treatment of the neuropathy. Treatment of diabetic polyneuropathy has traditionally focused on control of hyperglycemia as a means of slowing progression or delaying the appearance of neuropathy. The Diabetes Control and Complications Trial found that intensive therapy of type 1 diabetes reduced the frequency of appearance of neuropathy by 60% over a five-year period in patients who did not have neuropathy at the onset of the study[8]. Pancreatic transplantation appears to halt the progression of diabetic neuropathy, but does not clearly reverse existing neuropathy[9,10].

Aldose reductase inhibitors (ARIs) have been studied as a means of preventing or improving diabetic polyneuropathy. They act by reducing the flux of glucose through the polyol pathway. There have been many human clinical trials of ARIs since 1981, with mixed results[11]. A recent meta-analysis of 13 randomized, controlled trials of ARIs found that the effects on motor nerve conduction velocity were inconsistent on different nerves within studies and were also inconsistent between studies, leading the authors to state that no clear conclusions can be drawn regarding the benefits of ARIs in the treatment of diabetic neuropathy[12]. An analysis of 32 trials of ARIs on patients with distal symmetrical diabetic polyneuropathy found that ARIs showed promise for possibly slowing the progression of diabetic neuropathy, but that many of these trials were flawed, being of insufficient duration and size[11]. A recent double-blind, placebo-controlled trial of the ARI zenarestat demonstrated that doses producing >80% suppression of nerve sorbitol content were required to demonstrate efficacy, so that even low residual levels of aldose reductase activity might be neurotoxic[13]. Thus, the issue of whether ARIs are effective in the treatment of diabetic polyneuropathy has not yet been settled.

Nerve growth factor (NGF) may be useful. Recombinant human NGF was found to be well tolerated in an open-label, phase I clinical trial[14]. A randomized, double-blind, placebo-controlled phase II study of NGF in the treatment of diabetic polyneuropathy was recently completed[15]. Improvement was noted compared to placebo on the sensory component of the neurological exam, on quantitative sensory testing and in the impression of the subjects. The results of two phase III trials will soon be available.

Diabetic foot care. Twenty-five per cent of patients with diabetes develop foot complications at some point[16], and patients with diabetes account for approximately half of all nontraumatic lower extremity amputations performed in the USA each year[17]. Plantar ulceration often precedes amputation[18]. Patients with diabetic neuropathy develop foot problems for several reasons[19-22]: (1) They have a loss of protective sensation on their feet, which may result in painless injuries; (2) Atrophy of the intrinsic foot muscles can lead to foot deformities and an abnormal distribution of weight when walking, producing increased plantar pressures; (3) There is often autonomic neuropathy, causing dry skin which can crack and cause arteriovenous shunting, leading to altered skin and bone perfusion. These factors may lead to foot deformities (a Charcot foot) with disruption of the normal bony architecture and with plantar ulcers.

Good preventative foot care has been emphasized, including such practical measures as careful inspection, proper trimming of nails and proper footwear. The evidence base for such preventative care in patients with diabetes has recently been reviewed[19]. There have not been randomized, controlled trials of treatment of the Charcot foot. However, in patients with diabetic neuropathy and plantar ulcers, a total contact cast often leads to healing of the ulcers[23,24].

Control of pain. In managing diabetic neuropathy, a major goal of most patients and their physicians is control of pain. A large number of agents have been studied in both uncontrolled and controlled clinical trials. A placebo-controlled, single-blind, crossover study demonstrated both ibuprofen 600 mg qid and sulindac 200 mg bid to be more effective than placebo in relieving the pain of diabetic neuropathy. The response to sulindac was significantly better than the response to ibuprofen[25]. Caution must be exercised when using nonsteroidal anti-inflammatory medications in patients with diabetes, due to the risk of nephrotoxicity, although none was noted in the study above.

Tricyclic antidepressants have been studied extensively. They act by blocking neuronal reuptake of norepinephrine and serotonin, thereby potentiating the inhibitory effect of these neurotransmitters in nociceptive pathways[26]. Amitriptyline, imipramine and desipramine were all found to relieve pain in patients with diabetic neuropathy better than placebo in double-blind, placebo-controlled trials. These compounds were effective in both depressed and nondepressed patients, and the efficacy appeared to be independent of any antidepressant effect[27–31]. Additional support for the efficacy of tricyclic antidepressants was provided by a meta-analysis of 21 different clinical trials[32]. Although nortriptyline as monotherapy would also be expected to be effective in treatment of painful diabetic neuropathy, and is often used in this manner, there is no study to support this. When used in combination with fluphenazine, it has been shown to be more effective than placebo and as effective as carbamazepine in double-blind, crossover studies[33,34]. The use of neuroleptics may produce extrapyramidal symptoms, and therefore we do not recommend their use in the routine treatment of diabetic neuropathy pain.

All of the tricyclic antidepressants may produce sedation, confusion and anticholinergic side-effects such as constipation, dry mouth, blurred vision, urinary hesitancy and orthostatic dizziness. These agents are contraindicated in patients with a variety of heart diseases, and must be used with great caution in patients with orthostatic hypotension or angle-closure glaucoma. Arranged in order from most to least potent anticholinergic effects, the most commonly used agents are amitriptyline, imipramine, nortriptyline and desipramine[35]. Thus, for patients who do not tolerate amitriptyline, other tricyclic antidepressants, particularly despiramine, may represent useful alternatives. The usual dosage schedule is 10–25 mg at bedtime initially, increasing as tolerated up to 100 or 150 mg as a single bedtime dose.

Serotonin reuptake inhibitors (SRIs) are another category of antidepressants which may have some efficacy, but the evidence for this is less convincing than that for tricyclic antidepressants. In a randomized, double-blind, crossover study, paroxetine 40 mg per day reduced symptoms significantly more than placebo, although it was somewhat less effective than imipramine[36]. Fluoxetine at a mean daily dose of 40 mg was shown to be no more effective than placebo except in patients who were depressed, in a double-blind, placebo-controlled study[30]. Open-label sertraline up to 150 mg/day was shown to lead to a reduction in pain from diabetic neuropathy in a small study of eight patients, but a placebo-controlled study has not yet been carried out[37]. Trazodone is often used empirically. Open-label use raises the possibility that it may have some efficacy in treating painful diabetic neuropathy, but there are no controlled studies[38].

Another group of medications with utility in pain control is the anticonvulsants. Gabapentin has been shown to be more effective than placebo when used in doses ranging from 900–3600 mg per day[39]. The lower end of this dosage range may be relatively ineffective; another placebo-controlled study did not demonstrate efficacy at a dose of 900 mg per day[40]. The main side-effects of gabapentin are dizziness, somnolence, headache, diarrhea, confusion and nausea. The dose is typically started at 300 mg per day or less, and increased very gradually, up to a maximum of 2400–3600 mg per day if tolerated and as needed for control of pain. Carbamazepine 200 mg tid was more effective than placebo in a double-blind crossover trial[41]. An open-label trial[42] also appeared to demonstrate efficacy. Side-effects are somnolence, dizziness, unsteadiness, nausea and vomiting. We suggest beginning at 100 mg bid or tid, increasing gradually to 200 qid as tolerated and if needed for pain control. Because aplastic anemia and agranulocytosis may occur on rare occasions, patients should undergo hematologic monitoring at baseline and regularly while being treated. Double-blind studies have not demonstrated efficacy of phenytoin in patients with diabetic neuropathy[43,44].

Randomized, double-blind, placebo-controlled trials of the antiarrhythmic agent mexiletine have demonstrated efficacy in the treatment of painful diabetic neuropathy[45–47], although one small, double-blind study did not demonstrate efficacy[48]. The most common side-effects are gastrointestinal distress (nausea, vomiting, heartburn), dizziness/lightheadedness, tremor, nervousness and uncoordination. We recommend an initial dose of 150 mg per day, increasing gradually until there is relief of pain, up to a maximum dose of 600–800 mg per day in three or four divided doses. Obtain a baseline ECG to make sure there are no cardiac contraindications, and consult a cardiologist if there are any concerns. The response to oral mexiletine can be predicted by an infusion of intravenous lidocaine[49].

Several other oral agents have been used. Tramadol acts via low-affinity binding to micro-opioid receptors and weak inhibition of norepinephrine and serotonin reuptake[50]. It was recently found to be effective in treatment of pain in diabetic neuropathy in a double-blind, placebo-controlled, randomized trial[51]. It is often good treatment for breakthrough or refractory pain, and can be given as 50–100 mg every four to six hours, up to 400 mg per day. Levodopa at a dosage of 100 mg three times a day was used in conjunction with a dopa decarboxylase inhibitor in a four-week placebo-controlled trial, and was found to be more effective than placebo from the second week onward[52]. The proof of efficacy of clonidine is questionable. Two double-blind, placebo-controlled trials have not shown a significant effect[53,54]. However, one trial in which the positive responders to clonidine were entered into a second double-blind, placebo-controlled phase demonstrated some benefit, suggesting that clonidine may be effective in a subset of patients[55].

Some rather unconventional systemic agents have been tried. Based on the impaired conversion of linoleic acid to gamma-linolenic acid in patients with diabetes, gamma-linolenic acid 360 mg per day was found to be superior to placebo for control of pain in a small, six-month, randomized, placebo-controlled double-blind trial[56]. Intravenous infusion of alpha-lipoic acid, an antioxidant, was shown to reduce pain in a large multicenter randomized, double-blind, placebo-controlled trial[57]. Dextromethorphan was superior to placebo in a randomized, double-blind crossover trial of pain control in diabetic neuropathy. The initial dose of 30 mg qid was increased gradually to 240 mg qid. Side-effects were sedation, dizziness, lightheadedness, ataxia and confusion[58].

Not all agents for pain control must be administered systemically. Topical capsaicin cream stimulates the release and subsequent depletion of substance P from sensory fibers. A placebo-controlled study[59,60] demonstrated the superiority of capsaicin cream 0.075% to placebo in control of pain and improvement of daily activities, while another double-blind study found it to be overall as effective as amitriptyline[61].In contrast, a double-blind, placebo-controlled study of capsaicin cream in patients with chronic distal painful neuropathy of various causes demonstrated no benefit over placebo[62]. Overall, capsaicin cream appears to be effective. A meta-analysis of four randomized, double-blind, placebo-controlled trials of capsaicin in diabetic neuropathy found capsaicin to be more effective overall than placebo[63]. Poor compliance is common, due to the need for frequent applications, an initial exacerbation of symptoms, and frequent burning and redness at the application site. Other nonsystemic treatments which have been studied include transcutaneous electrical nerve stimulation (TENS) units and acupuncture. In a controlled study, TENS was more effective than sham treatment in reducing pain in patients with diabetic neuropathy[64]. Uncontrolled studies of TENS and of acupuncture have been reported to decrease pain in over 75% of patients with diabetic neuropathy[65,66]. However, the powerful effect of placebo treatment in diabetic neuropathy, documented in multiple studies, raises questions about the reliability of such uncontrolled trials.

Narcotic analgesics are often used for severe, refractory pain, but are controversial for treatment of this chronic condition, due to the habituation which typically occurs. Some experts use it at night for sleep, but patients must be cautioned not to escalate the dose.

A summary of treatments used for painful diabetic polyneuropathy is provided in Table 24.3.

SMALL-FIBER POLYNEUROPATHY

Some patients have a selective small-fiber polyneuropathy, or small-fiber sensory neuropathy (SFSN)[67–72]. The patient with SFSN typically presents with pain as a chief complaint, most commonly in the distal limb, which he or she describes in a variety of terms, including tingling, prickling, burning, coldness,

Table 24.3. Summary of treatments for painful diabetic polyneuropathy.

Treatment	Double-blind, controlled	Open-label	Other (see text)
Nonsteroidal antiinflammatory agents			
Ibuprofen			X
Sulindac			X
Tricyclic antidepressants			
Amitriptyline	X		
Imipramine	X		
Desipramine	X		
Nortriptyline			X
Serotonin reuptake inhibitors			
Paroxetine	X		
Sertraline		X	
Anticonvulsants			
Gabapentin	X		
Carbamazepine	X	X	
Antiarrhythmics			
Mexiletine	X		
Other oral agents			
Tramadol	X		
Levodopa	X		
Clonidine			X
Gamma-linolenic acid	X		
Dextromethorphan	X		
Phenothiazines			X
Narcotics			X
Intravenous agent			
Alpha-lipoic acid	X		
Non-systemic treatment			
Capsaicin cream	X		
Nonpharmacological treatments			
TENS unit		X	X
Acupuncture		X	

deep aching, jabbing or shooting. Autonomic dysfunction is frequently present. The examination demonstrates distal sensory loss affecting pain and temperature, with relative preservation of large-fiber-mediated modalities (vibration and proprioception). Reflexes are generally preserved (although ankle jerks may be decreased or absent), and strength is normal. Nerve conduction studies are normal or minimally abnormal, since such tests assess primarily the largest, fastest-conducting fibers. Quantitative sensory testing (QST) is abnormal in 60–100% of patients tested. Autonomic testing may be abnormal. Biopsies of the sural nerve show predominantly small fiber loss, but may rarely be normal. Skin biopsies demonstrate abnormalities of intra-epidermal nerves. Treatment is directed toward control of pain, using the agents discussed above.

AUTONOMIC NEUROPATHY

Visceral autonomic neuropathy was present in 7% of patients with type 1 diabetes and 5% of those with type 2 diabetes in one series[24]. The clinical features of diabetic autonomic neuropathy are varied[2], and are presented in Table 24.4. Treatment of some of the major clinical manifestations is discussed here.

Treatment of orthostatic hypotension: This involves the use of nonpharmacological as well as pharmacological measures. Many of the nonpharmacological treatments are based on commonly-accepted clinical practices, rather than controlled studies[2,73–77]. Such measures include the following: (1) Avoidance of sudden changes in body posture to the head-up position, particularly in warm weather, and after taking a warm bath, both of which produce cutaneous vasodilation; (2) Avoiding medications that aggravate hypotension, such as tricyclic antidepressants and phenothiazines; (3) Taking small, frequent meals to avoid the postprandial hypotension which may occur after a large carbohydrate-containing meal; (4) Avoiding activities that involve straining, since increased intra-abdominal and intrathoracic pressure decrease venous return. In contrast, the efficacy of some nonpharmacological treatments has been demonstrated in case reports or small uncontrolled studies: (1) Elevation of the head of the bed 18 inches at night improved symptoms in a small series of patients with orthostatic hypotension from various causes[78]; (2) The efficacy of a compressive garment over the legs and abdomen has been demonstrated

Table 24.4. Clinical features of diabetic autonomic neuropathy.

Pupillary dysfunction

Cardiovascular disturbances
- Abnormalities of heart rate
- Orthostatic hypotension

Gastrointestinal disturbances
- Esophageal, gastric, duodenal and colonic atony
- Diarrhea
- Gall bladder atony
- Anal sphincter weakness

Genito-urinary disturbances
- Bladder dysfunction
- Retrograde ejaculation
- Impotence
- Female sexual dysfunction

Unawareness of hypoglycemia

Abnormalities of sweating

in multiple case reports[79–82]; (3) An inflatable abdominal band was shown to be effective in a small study of six patients with orthostatic hypotension[83]; (4) A low portable chair used by patients as needed for symptoms was found to be effective in one study[84].

Some pharmacological means are part of commonly accepted clinical practice, but without studies to document efficacy. Plasma expansion by increased salt intake or by the use of prostaglandin inhibitors such as ibuprofen or indomethacin are commonly recommended[73]. One of the first effective pharmacological treatments which was studied was plasma expansion with 9-alpha-fluorohydrocortisone, a compound that has potent mineralocorticoid activity. The earliest report described a single patient[85]. Other case reports followed[86]. A small, open-label study of 14 patients demonstrated symptomatic as well as objective improvement[87]. The effects are not immediate, but occur over a one- to two-week period. Supine hypertension, hypokalemia and hypomagnesemia may occur. Caution must be used, particularly in patients with congestive heart failure, to avoid fluid overload[88,89]. We recommend beginning at 50 μg at bedtime, and titrating upward gradually to a maximum of 200 μg daily. The dose can ultimately be titrated up to 400 μg, but at these higher doses there is more of a tendency to develop hypokalemia and excessive fluid retention with resulting hypertension and congestive heart failure.

Sympathomimetic drugs can be helpful. Ephedrine is often used empirically at a dosage of 15–45 mg three times a day. It is best given upon awakening, at lunch and at dinner. Side effects which may limit its use are tremulousness, irritability, insomnia, hypertension, tachycardia, reduction in appetite and, in males, urinary retention (Mathias 1998). An alternative is midodrine, an alpha agonist which activates alpha-1 receptors on arterioles and veins to increase total peripheral resistance[90,91]. Because it does not cross the blood–brain barrier, it has fewer central side-effects than ephedrine. Several double-blind, placebo-controlled studies have documented its efficacy in the treatment of orthostatic hypotension[92–94]. The main adverse effects are piloerection, pruritis, paresthesias, urinary retention and supine hypertension. Of course, all sympathomimetic drugs must be used with caution in patients with ischemic heart disease, cardiac arrhythmias and peripheral vascular disease. The usual dose of midodrine is 2.5–10 mg three times a day.

Dihydroergotamine, in combination with caffeine, indomethacin and the alpha-2 adrenergic antagonist yohimbine has been used in refractory patients[76,77]. In an experimental animal model of orthostatic hypotension, yohimbine has been found to delay the fall in blood pressure (BP) elicited by head-up tilting, but not to modify its magnitude[95].

Beta-blockers have shown efficacy in some open-label studies of patients with orthostatic hypotension due to varying etiologies[96–98], but a double-blind, placebo-controlled crossover study of eight patients with diabetic autonomic neuropathy and orthostatic hypotension failed to demonstrate efficacy[99].

Treatment of diabetic gastroparesis. Some treatments are based simply on commonly accepted clinical practices. These include the use of multiple small feedings and changes in diet such as a decrease in dietary fat and fiber[74,76,77,100]. The principal pharmacological means of treatment has been the use of a pro-kinetic agent such as metoclopramide, cisapride, erythromycin or domperidone.

Metoclopramide has antiemetic properties, stimulates acetylcholine release in the myenteric plexus, and is a dopamine antagonist[100]. There have been one open trial, two single-blind trials, and five double-blind trials. The single-blind and double-blind trials demonstrated improvement in gastric emptying, while the open trial demonstrated no improvement[101]. Extrapyramidal symptoms such as acute dystonic reactions, drug-induced parkinsonism, akathisia and tardive dyskinesia may be side-effects. Galactorrhea, amenorrhea, gyneco-mastia and hyperprolactinemia are potential side-effects as well. The usual dose is 10 mg given 30 minutes before meals and at bedtime.

Cisapride increases gut motility by increasing the release of acetylcholine from postganglionic myenteric neurons[100]. There have been 10 open trials and seven double-blind trials which demonstrated improvement in gastric empty-ing[101]. It appears to maintain efficacy in long-term use[102]. It does not have the dopaminergic activity of metoclopramide, and so avoids the extrapyramidal and other side-effects noted above. It is contraindicated in some patients with heart disease or abnormal electrocardiograms. The usual dose is 10–20 mg given 15–30 minutes before meals and at bedtime.

Erythromycin is effective in accelerating gastric emptying. It is believed to act by stimulating motilin receptors in the gut[103]. It may be used orally or intravenously[104,105]. There have been five open trials involving 71 patients, with a mean improvement in gastric emptying of over 40%[101]. One single-blind trial also demonstrated an improvement in gastric emptying of 50%[101].

Domperidone has also demonstrated efficacy, although only small numbers of patients have been studied. There have been two open trials involving 18 patients and two double-blind trials involving 28 patients, all of which demon-strated improvement in gastric emptying[101]. A double-blind, randomized trial has demonstrated that domperidone and metoclopramide are equally effect-ive[106].

An analysis of 36 studies of prokinetic agents found all four of these agents appear to have efficacy in improving gastric emptying times and symptoms[101]. When compared with one another, improvement in gastric emptying time was greatest with erythromycin, followed by domperidone, cisapride then meto-clopramide. Improvement in symptoms was greatest with erythromycin, then domperidone, then metoclopramide then cisapride. The choice of an agent will usually be determined by availability, cost and side-effects.

Persistent vomiting may require a surgical approach: placement of a feeding jejunostomy to bypass an atonic stomach has been advocated, based on clinical practice[100]. Radical surgery, consisting of resection of a large portion of the stomach, with performance of a Roux-en-Y loop, has been reported to be successful in a small series of patients[107]. A recent, novel approach is gastric pacing. In one series of nine patients with gastroparesis, five of whom had diabetes, gastric pacing accelerated gastric emptying and improved symptoms[108].

Treatment of diabetic diarrhea: Diarrhea in diabetics is often due to bacterial overgrowth, which can be diagnosed via a hydrogen breath test. An early double-blind study involving a single patient demonstrated that the diarrhea subsided when the patient was treated with an oral antibiotic preparation (a combination of tetracycline, amphotericin B and potassium metaphosphate), then recurred when placebo was substituted[109]. Broad-spectrum antibiotics are commonly used to treat diabetic diarrhea, either when the breath test is positive, or as an empiric trial. Several different regimens have been advocated: (1) Ampicillin or tetracycline 250 mg every eight hours[76,77]; (2) Amoxicillin 875 mg and clavulanate potassium twice daily for 14 days[100]. (3) Metronidazole 500 mg every six hours or 750 mg every eight hours for three weeks[76,77]; caution must be used since long-term use of metronidazole can lead to neuropathy.

Other treatments have been based largely on accepted clinical practice patterns[76,77]. Cholestyramine can be used in an attempt to chelate bile salts if the hydrogen breath test is normal, or if patients fail an empiric trial of broad-spectrum antibiotics. Diphenoxylate with atropine or loperamide can also be used.

Octreotide (a somatostatin analog) 50–75 ug subcutaneously twice a day was effective in a case report of a single patient with diabetic diarrhea[110]. A recent study demonstrated that octreotide was effective in accelerating gastric emptying, inhibiting small bowel transit, reducing ileocolonic bolus transfers, inhibiting post-prandial colonic tonic response and increasing colonic phasic pressure activity in healthy volunteers, and thus should be of value in the treatment of diarrheal states[111].

Treatment of the neurogenic bladder. Dysfunction of the lower urinary tract occurs in 26–87% of patients with diabetes[112]. These patients experience a decrease in the ability to sense a distended bladder, due to loss of afferent autonomic innervation. As a result, they urinate less frequently, and develop a hypocontractile bladder and urinary retention[112–114]. This leads to recurrent urinary tract infections, overflow incontinence, dribbling and poor stream. Recommendations from a number of sources are similar, and are based largely on commonly-accepted clinical practices[74,76,77]. The patient should be scheduled for an evaluation by a urologist with a cystometrogram. If abnormal, scheduled voiding is recommended, often coupled with Crede's maneuver: manual squeezing of the bladder to initiate urination. Bethanechol, a parasympathomimetic agent, 10–30 mg three times a day may be helpful. Some patients may require intermittent catheterization. Transurethral surgery of the bladder neck may be needed in selected cases, and occasionally patients may require an indwelling catheter. Based on an animal model, some patients may benefit from surgery to reduce bladder size[115].

Treatment of impotence. The prevalence of erectile dysfunction in men with diabetes is high, varying from 35–75%[116–119]. The treatment of choice is now sildenafil which was shown to be significantly more effective than placebo in a randomized, double-blind, placebo-controlled study of 268 men with diabetes and erectile dysfunction[120]. The main side effects were headache, dyspepsia and respiratory tract disorder. The dose is 25–100 mg taken one hour before sexual activity.

Traditionally, a number of other treatments have been used, based on clinicians' experience and case reports, including vacuum devices, rigid penile implants and inflatable prostheses[121,122]. Direct injections into the corpus cavernosum of either papaverine or alprostadil represent another option. The success rate of intracavernosal injections is high, with nearly 90% of patients achieving erection[122,123]. Yohimbine, an alpha-2 adrenergic antagonist, is occasionally used. A meta-analysis of seven randomized clinical trials found it to be more effective than placebo[124].

CRANIAL NEUROPATHIES

Cranial neuropathies affecting extraocular movements occur more frequently in diabetic than nondiabetic patients. Patients are usually over 50 years of age. The onset is typically abrupt, and may be painless or associated with a headache. A lesion of oculomotor nerve (CN III) is the most common single cranial neuropathy in diabetes, often sparing the pupil. Dysfunction of the trochlear nerve (CN IV) is less common. The abducens nerve (CN VI) is rarely involved by itself, but may be involved with other cranial nerves. While facial palsy (CN VII) and other cranial neuropathies occur in patients with diabetes, their relationship to the diabetes is uncertain[2,125]. There is no specific treatment, although gradual recovery typically occurs.

LIMB MONONEUROPATHIES

Compression and entrapment neuropathies are common in patients both with and without diabetes, and it not uncertain whether these are causally related to diabetes. The most commonly involved nerve is the median nerve at the wrist (carpal tunnel syndrome). Symptomatic carpal tunnel syndrome occurs in 11% of patients with type 1 diabetes, and 6% of patients with type 2 diabetes.

Asymptomatic carpal tunnel syndrome is much more common[4]. Ulnar neuropathy at the elbow also occurs commonly. Typically such neuropathies are slowly-developing lesions characterized by variable amounts of pain and weakness. Treatment has been empiric, and may be conservative or surgical. The presence of a superimposed generalized polyneuropathy does not preclude surgical intervention in such patients, but the degree of polyneuropathy which is contributing to the patient's symptoms must be taken into account when making decisions regarding surgery[126].

Dysfunction of some nerves may be abrupt and painful, likely secondary to nerve infarctions. Common examples include the radial nerve (wrist drop), peroneal nerve (foot drop), femoral nerve (quadriceps weakness) and lateral femoral cutaneous nerve ('meralgia paresthetica'). Electrodiagnostic tests reveal axon loss. Recovery typically occurs over months or years, and depends on the extent of axon loss and the site (proximal versus distal) of the lesion. Distal muscle strength is often recovered incompletely. If multiple nerve are affected in this way, a mononeuropathy multiplex will result. There is no specific treatment for these abrupt limb neuropathies, though some have advocated immunomodulating therapy when there is multinerve involvement, similar to that used by some for treatment of diabetic amyotrophy (see below).

DIABETIC TRUNCAL MONONEUROPATHY

This is typically characterized by pain around the abdomen or lower chest. Cutaneous hyperesthesia may occur, as may abdominal wall weakness. Some cases appear to be a restricted form of diabetic radiculopathy, and demonstrate paraspinal muscle denervation on needle electromyography[2]. Once structural abnormalities have been ruled out, treatment consists of pain management. Gradual improvement generally occurs.

ASYMMETRIC LOWER LIMB MOTOR NEUROPATHY (DIABETIC AMYOTROPHY)

There are many names for this syndrome, including proximal diabetic neuropathy, diabetic polyradiculopathy, diabetic femoral neuropathy, diabetic lumbar plexopathy and diabetic lumbosacral plexus neuropathy. Affected individuals have type 2 diabetes mellitus, and are usually males aged over 50. The initial symptom is pain in most patients, usually in the territory of the lower thoracic and upper lumbar nerve roots. The pain typically is worst at onset, and gradually subsides. Paresthesia and hyperesthesia are common. Weakness, generally in the upper legs, commonly follows the pain. Weight loss is common. On examination, weakness is most common in the L2–L4 distribution.

Thus, the weakness primarily affects the iliopsoas, quadriceps and adductor muscles, usually sparing hip extensors and hamstrings. The weakness may be unilateral or bilateral, and when bilateral it is frequently asymmetric. Sensory loss is mild and mainly distal in most patients, consistent with a coexisting distal sensory or sensorimotor polyneuropathy. Knee and/or ankle jerks are lost in most patients[127].

Progression of symptoms and signs occurs over a very variable period of time; as short as one or two weeks, and as long as a year or more. Most patients experience improvement or resolution of pain or dysesthesia. Recovery of motor function is often incomplete and usually slower, proceeding for up to 18 months. Nerve conduction studies often reveal evidence of a sensory or sensorimotor polyneuropathy. The needle examination typically reveals fibrillation potentials and positive sharp waves in lower extremity muscles and in thoracic and/or lumbar paraspinal muscles. Most commonly affected are the L2–L4 levels, although low thoracic and L5–S1 levels are abnormal in some patients. The etiology appears to be microscopic vasculitis producing nerve ischemia, with multifocal involvement of lumbosacral roots, plexus and peripheral nerves. This has led to the recent use of the term 'diabetic lumbosacral radiculoplexus neuropathy' to characterize this type of neuropathy[128,129].

Typically, no treatment is given other than controlling the diabetes. However, the inflammatory changes on biopsy have raised the issue of whether immunomodulating agents might be useful for treatment of this type of diabetic neuropathy. In patients with particularly severe cases, prednisone, intravenous immunoglobulin (IVIg) and plasmapheresis have shown some promise in open-label, uncontrolled studies. Patients appeared to stop worsening and to begin to improve after beginning these treatments. However, since untreated patients also gradually improve, the efficacy of these treatments is unproven at this time[130–133].

ACKNOWLEDGMENTS:

This work was supported by National Institutes of Health grants NIH NS36778 and NIH NS38849, and grants from the Juvenile Diabetes Foundation and American Diabetes Association (ELF).

REFERENCES

1. Young MJ, Boulton AJM, Macleod AF, Williams DRR and Sonksen PH (1993) A multicentre study of the prevalence of diabetic peripheral neuropathy in the United Kingdom hospital clinic population. *Diabetologia* **36**: 150–154.
2. Thomas PK and Tomlinson DR (1993) Diabetic and hypoglycemic neuropathy. In *Peripheral Neuropathy*, 3rd ed (eds Dyck PJ, Thomas PK, Griffin JW, Low PA, and Poduslo JF), WB Saunders: Philadelphia, pp. 1219–1250.

3. Dyck PJ, Karnes JL, O'Brien PC, Litchy WJ, Low PA and Melton LJ (1992) The Rochester diabetic neuropathy study: reassessment of tests and criteria for diagnosis and staged severity. *Neurology* **42**: 1164–1170.
4. Dyck PJ, Kratz KM, Karnes JL, Litchy WJ, Klein R, Pach JM, Wilson DM, O'Brien PC and Melton LJ (1993) The prevalence by staged severity of various types of diabetic neuropathy, retinopathy and nephropathy in a population-based cohort: the Rochester diabetic neuropathy study. *Neurology* **43**: 817–824.
5. Donofrio PD and Albers JW (1990) AAEM minimonograph #34: polyneuropathy: classification by nerve conduction studies and electromyography. *Muscle Nerve*, **13**: 889–903.
6. Dumitru D (1995) *Electrodiagnostic Medicine*. Hanley & Belfus: Philadelphia, pp. 821–824.
7. Feldman EL, Russell JW, Sullivan KA and Golovoy D (1999) New insights into the pathogenesis of diabetic neuropathy. *Curr. Opin. Neurol.* **12**: 553–563.
8. Diabetes Control and Complications Trial Research Group (1993) The effect of intensive treatment of diabetes on the development and progression of long-term complications in insulin-dependent diabetes mellitus. *N. Engl. J. Med* **329**: 977–986.
9. Kennedy WR, Navarro X, Goetz FC, Sutherland DE and Najarian JS (1990) Effects of pancreatic transplantation on diabetic neuropathy. *N. Engl. J. Med* **322**: 1031–1037.
10. Navarro X, Sutherland DER and Kennedy WR (1997) Long-term effects of pancreatic transplantation on diabetic neuropathy. *Ann. Neurol.* **42**: 727–736.
11. Pfeifer MA, Schumer MP and Gelber DA (1997) Aldose reductase inhibitors: the end of an era or the need for different trial designs? *Diabetes* **46**(suppl. 2), S82–S89.
12. Nicolucci A, Carinci F, Cavaliere D, Scorpiglione N, Belfiglio M, Labbrozzi D, Mari E, Massi Bendetti M, Tognoni G and Liberati A (1996) A meta-analysis of trials on aldose reductase inhibitors in diabetic peripheral neuropathy. *Diabetic Med.* **13**: 1017–1026.
13. Green DA, Arezzo JC, Brown MB and the Zenarestat Study Group (1999) Effect of aldose reductase inhibition on nerve conduction and morphometry in diabetic neuropathy. *Neurology* **53**: 580–591.
14. Petty BG, Cornblath DR, Adornato BT, Chaudhry V, Flexner C, Wachsman M, Sinicropi D, Burton LE and Peroutka SJ (1994) The effect of systemically administered recombinant human nerve growth factor in healthy human subjects. *Ann. Neurol.* **36**: 244–246.
15. Apfel SC, Kessler JA, Adornato BT, Litchy WJ, Sanders C, Rask CA and the NGF Study Group (1998) Recombinant human nerve growth factor in the treatment of diabetic polyneuropathy. *Neurology* **51**: 695–702.
16. Most RS and Sinnock P (1983) The epidemiology of lower-extremity amputations in diabetic individuals. *Diabetes Care* **6**: 87–91.
17. Bild DE, Selby JV, Sinnock P, Browner WS, Braveman P, and Showstack JA (1989) Lower-extremity amputation in people with diabetes. *Diabetes Care* **12**: 24–31.
18. Pecoraro RE, Ahroni JH, Boyko EJ and Stensel VL (1991) Chronology and determinants of tissue repair in diabetic lower-extremity ulcers. *Diabetes* **40**: 1305–1313.
19. Mayfield JA, Janisse D, Reiber GE, Pogach LM and Sanders LJ (1998) Preventive foot care in people with diabetes. *Diabetes Care* **21**: 2161–2177.
20. Cavanagh PR, Ulbrecht JS and Caputo GM (1996) Biomechanical aspects of diabetic foot disease: aetology, treatment, and prevention. *Diabetic Medicine*, **13**(suppl. 1), S17–S22.

21. Stevens MJ, Edmonds ME, Foster AV and Watkins PJ (1992) Selective neuropathy and preserved vascular responses in the diabetic Charcot foot. *Diabetologia* **35**: 148–154.
22. Boulton AJM (1990) The diabetic foot: neuropathic in aetiology? *Diab. Med.* **7**: 852–858.
23. Caputo GM, Ulbrecht JS and Cavanagh PR (1997) The total contact cast: a method for treating neuropathic diabetic ulcers. *Am. Fam. Physician* **55**: 425–426.
24. Caputo GM, Ulbrecht J and Cavanagh PR (1998) The Charcot foot in diabetes: six key points. *Am. Fam. Physician* **57**: 2705–2710.
25. Cohen KL and Harris S (1987) Efficacy and safety of nonsteroidal anti-inflammatory drugs in the therapy of diabetic neuropathy. *Arch. Intern. Med.* **147**: 1442–1444.
26. Joss JD (1999) Tricyclic antidepressant use in diabetic neuropathy. Ann. Pharmacother. **33**: 996–1000.
27. Kvinesdal B, Molin J, Froland A and Gram LF (1984) Imipramine treatment of painful diabetic neuropathy. *JAMA* **251**: 1727–1730.
28. Max MB, Culnane M, Schafer SC, Gracely RH, Walther DJ, Smoller B and Dubner R (1987) Amitriptyline relieves diabetic neuropathy pain in patients with normal or depressed mood. *Neurology* **37**: 589–596.
29. Max MB, Kishore-Kumar R, Schafer SC, Meister B, Gracely RH, Smoller B and Dubner R (1991) Efficacy of desipramine in painful diabetic neuropathy: a placebo-controlled trial. *Pain* **45**: 3–9.
30. Max MB Lynch SA, Muir J, Shoaf SE, Smoller B and Dubner R (1992) Effects of desipramine, amitriptyline, and fluoxetine on pain in diabetic neuropathy. *N. Engl. J. Med* **326**: 1250–1256.
31. Sindrup SH, Ejlertsen B, Froland A, Sindrup EH, Brosen K and Gram LF (1989) Imipramine treatment in diabetic neuropathy: relief of subjective symptoms without changes in peripheral and autonomic nerve function. *Eur. J. Clin. Pharmacol.* **37**: 151–153.
32. McQuay HJ, Tramer M, Nye BA, Carroll D, Wiffen PJ and Moore RA (1996) A systematic review of antidepressants in neuropathic pain. *Pain* **68**: 217–227.
33. Gomez-Perez FJ, Rull JA, Dies H, Rodriguez-Rivera JG, Gonzalez-Barranco J and Lozano-Castaneda O (1985) Nortriptyline and fluphenazine in the symptomatic treatment of diabetic neuropathy. A double-blind crossover study. *Pain* **23**: 395–400.
34. Gomez-Perez FJ, Choza R, Rios JM, Reza A, Huerta E, Aguilar CA and Rull JA (1996) Nortriptyline-fluphenazine vs. carbamazepine in the symptomatic treatment of diabetic neuropathy. *Arch. Med. Res.* **27**: 525–529.
35. Richelson E (1994) Pharmacology of antidepressants – characteristics of the ideal drug. *Mayo. Clin. Proc.* **69**: 1069–1081.
36. Sindrup SH, Gram LF, Brosen K, Eshoj O and Morgensen EF (1990) The selective serotonin reuptake inhibitor paroxetine is effective in the treatment of diabetic neuropathy symptoms. *Pain* **42**: 135–144.
37. Goodnick PJ, Jimenez I and Kumar A (1997) Sertraline in diabetic neuropathy: preliminary results. *Ann. Clin. Psychiatry* **9**: 255–257.
38. Khurana RC (1983) Treatment of painful diabetic neuropathy with trazodone. *JAMA* **250**: 1392.
39. Backonja M, Beydoun A, Edwaards KR, Schwartz SL, Fonseca V, Hes M, LaMoreaux L and Garofalo E (1998) Gabapentin for the symptomatic treatment of painful neuropathy in patients with diabetes mellitus: a randomized controlled trial. *JAMA* **280**: 1831–1836.

40. Gorson KC, Schott C, Herman R, Ropper AH and Rand WM (1999) Gabapentin in the treatment of painful diabetic neuropathy: a placebo-controlled, double blind crossover trial. *J. Neurol. Neurosurg. Psychiatry* **66**: 251–252.
41. Rull JA, Quibrera R, Gonzalez-Millan H and Lozano Castaneda O (1969) Symptomatic treatment of peripheral diabetic neuropathy with carbamazepine (Tegretol): double-blind crossover trial. *Diabetologia* **5**: 565–568.
42. Chakrabarti AK and Samantaray SK (1976) Diabetic peripheral neuropathy: nerve conduction studies before, during and after carbamazepine therapy. *Aust. NZ J. Med.* **6**: 565–568.
43. Ellenberg M (1968) Treatment of diabetic neuropathy with diphenylhydantoin. *NY State J. Med.* **68**: 2653–2655.
44. Saudek C, Werns S and Reidenberg M (1977) Phenytoin in the treatment of diabetic symmetrical polyneuropathy. *Clin. Pharmacol. Ther.* **22**: 196–199.
45. Dejgard A, Petersen P and Kastrup J (1988) Mexiletine for treatment of chronic painful diabetic neuropathy. *Lancet,* **2**: 9–11.
46. Stracke H, Meyer UE, Schumacher HE and Federlin K (1992) Mexiletine in the treatment of diabetic neuropathy. *Diabetes Care* **15**: 1550–1555.
47. Oskarsson P, Ljunggren J-G, Lins P-E and the Mexiletine Study Group (1997) Efficacy and safety of mexiletine in the treatment of painful diabetic neuropathy. *Diabetes Care* **20**: 1594–1597.
48. Wright JM, Oki JC and Graves L (1997) Mexiletine in the symptomatic treatment of diabetic peripheral neuropathy. *Ann. Pharmacother.* **31**: 29–34.
49. Galer BS, Harle J and Rowbotham MC (1996) Response to intravenous lidocaine infusion predicts subsequent response to oral mexiletine: a prospective study. *J. Pain Symptom Manage.* **12**: 161–167.
50. Raffa RB, Friderichs E, Reimann W, Shank RP, Codd EE and Vaught JL (1998) Opioid and nonopioid components independently contribute to the mechanism of action of tramadol, an 'atypical' opioid analgesic. J. Pharmacol. Exp. Ther. **260**: 275–285.
51. Harati Y, Gooch C, Swenson M, Edelman S, Greene D, Raskin P, Donofrio P, Cornblath D, Sachdeo R, Siu CO and Kamin M (1998) Double-blind randomized trial of tramadol for the treatment of the pain of diabetic neuropathy. *Neurology* **50**: 1842–1846.
52. Ertas M, Sagduyu A, Arac N, Uludag B and Ertekin C (1998) Use of levodopa to relieve pain from painful symmetrical diabetic polyneuropathy. *Pain* **75**: 257–259.
53. Ziegler D, Lynch SA, Muir J, Benjamin J and Max MB (1992) Transdermal clonidine versus placebo in painful diabetic neuropathy. *Pain* **48**: 403–408.
54. Cohen KL, Lucibello FE and Chomiak MA (1990) Lack of effect of clonidine and pentoxifylline in short-term therapy of diabetic peripheral neuropathy. *Diabetes Care* **13**: 1074–1077.
55. Byas-Smith MG, Max MB, Muir J and Kingman A (1995) Transdermal clonidine compared to placebo in painful diabetic neuropathy using a two-stage 'enriched enrollment' design. *Pain* **60**: 267–274.
56. Jamal GA and Carmichael H (1990) The effect of gamma-linolenic acid on human diabetic peripheral neuropathy: a double-blind placebo-controlled trial. *Diabetic Med.* **7**: 319–323.
57. Ziegler D, Hanefeld M, Ruhnau KJ, Meissner HP, Lobisch M, Schutte K, Gries FA and the ALADIN Study Group (1995) Treatment of symptomatic diabetic peripheral neuropathy with the antioxidant alpha-lipoic acid. *Diabetologia* **38**: 1425–1433.

58. Nelson KA, Park KM, Robinovitz E, Tsigos C and Max MB (1997) High-dose oral dextromethorphan versus placebo in painful diabetic neuropathy and postherpetic neuralgia. *Neurology* **48**: 1212–1218.

59. Capsaicin Study Group (1991) Treatment of painful diabetic neuropathy with topical capsaicin. A multicenter, double-blind, vehicle-controlled study. *Arch. Intern. Med.* **151**: 2225–2229.

60. Capsaicin Study Group (1992) Effect of treatment with capsaicin on daily activities of patients with painful diabetic neuropathy. *Diabetes Care* **15**: 159–165.

61. Biesbroek R, Bril V, Hollander P, Kabadi U, Schwartz S, Singh SP, Ward WK and Bernstein JE (1995) A double–blind comparison of topical capsaicin and oral amitriptyline in painful diabetic neuropathy. Adv. Therapy **12**: 111–120.

62. Low PA, Opfer-Gehrking TL, Dyck PJ, Litchy WJ and O'Brien PC (1995) Double-blind, placebo-controlled study of the application of capsaicin cream in chronic distal painful polyneuropathy. *Pain* **62**: 163–168.

63. Zhang WY and Po ALW (1994) The effectiveness of topically applied capsaicin: a meta-analysis. *Eur. J. Clin. Pharmacol.* **46**: 517–522.

64. Kumar D and Marshall HJ (1997) Diabetic peripheral neuropathy: amelioration of pain with transcutaneous electrostimulation. *Diabetes Care* **20**: 1702–1705.

65. Julka IS, Alvaro M and Kumar D (1998) Beneficial effects of electrical stimulation on neuropathic symptoms in diabetes patients. *J. Foot Ankle Surg.* **37**: 191–194.

66. Abuaisha BB, Costanzi JB and Boulton AJ (1998) Acupuncture for the treatment of chronic painful peripheral diabetic neuropathy: a long-term study. *Diabetes Res. Clin. Prac.* **39**, 115–121.

67. Brown MJ, Martin JR and Asbury AK (1976) Painful diabetic neuropathy: a morphometric study. *Arch. Neurol.* **33**: 164–171.

68. Said G, Slama G and Selva J (1983) Progressive centripetal degeneration of axons in small fibre type diabetic polyneuropathy. A clinical and pathological study. *Brain* **106**: 791–807.

69. Kennedy WR and Wendelschafer-Crabb G (1996) Utility of skin biopsy in diabetic neuropathy. *Sem. Neurol.* **16**: 163–171.

70. Kennedy WR, Wendelschafer-Crabb G and Johnson T (1996) Quantitation of epidermal nerves in diabetic neuropathy. *Neurology* **47**: 1042–1048.

71. Holland NR, Crawford TO, Hauer P, Cornblath DR, Griffith JW and McArthur JC (1998) Small-fiber sensory neuropathies: clinical course and neuropathology of idiopathic cases. *Ann. Neurol.* **44**: 47–59.

72. Herrmann DN, Griffin JW, Hauer P, Cornblath DR and McArthur JC (1999) Epidermal nerve fiber density and sural nerve morphometry in peripheral neuropathies. *Neurology* **53**: 1634–1640.

73. Onrot J, Goldberg MR, Hollister AS, Biaggioni I, Robertson RM and Robertson D (1986) Management of chronic orthostatic hypotension. *Am. J. Med.* **80**: 454–464.

74. Hilsted J and Low PA (1997) Diabetic autonomic neuropathy. In *Clinical Autonomic Disorders: Evaluation and Management*, 2nd edn (ed. Low PA), Lippincott-Raven: Philadelphia, pp. 487–507.

75. Mathias CJ and Kimber JR (1998) Treatment of postural hypotension. *J. Neurol. Neurosurg. Psychiatry* **65**: 285–289.

76. Vinik AI (1999) Diabetic neuropathy: pathogenesis and therapy. *Am. J. Med.* **107**(2B), 17S–26S.

77. Vinik AI (1999) Diagnosis and management of diabetic neuropathy. *Clin. Ger. Med.* **15**: 293–320.

78. MacLean AR and Allen BV (1940) Orthostatic hypotension and orthostatic tachycardia. Treatment with 'head-up' bed. *JAMA* **115**: 2162–2167.

79. Schatz IJ, Podolsky S and Frame B (1963) Idiopathic orthostatic hypotension: diagnosis and treatment. *JAMA* **186**: 537–540.
80. Levin JM, Ravenna P and Weiss M (1964) Idiopathic orthostatic hypotension: treatment with a commercially available counterpressure suit. *Arch. Int. Med.* **114**: 145–148.
81. Lewis HD Jr. and Dunn M (1967) Orthostatic hypotension syndrome: a case report. *Am. Heart. J.* **74**: 396–401.
82. Sheps SG (1976) Use of an elastic garment in the treatment of orthostatic hypotension. *Cardiology* **61**(suppl. 1), 271–279.
83. Tanaka H, Yamaguchi H and Tamai H (1997) Treatment of orthostatic intolerance with inflatable abdominal band. *Lancet* **349**: 175.
84. Smit AAJ, Hardjowkjono MA and Wieling W (1997) Are portable folding chairs useful to combat orthostatic hypotension? *Ann. Neurol.* **42**: 975–978.
85. Hickler RB, Thompson GR, Fox LM and Hamlin JT (1959) Successful treatment of orthostatic hypotension with 9-alpha-fluorohydrocortisone. *N. Engl. J. Med*, **261**: 788–791.
86. Bannister R, Ardell L and Fenten P (1969) An assessment of various methods of treatment of idiopathic orthostatic hypotension. *Q.J. Med.* **38**: 377–395.
87. Campbell IW, Ewing DJ and Clarke BF (1976) Therapeutic experience with fludrocortisone in diabetic postural hypotension. *Br. Med. J.* **1**: 872–874.
88. Chobanian AV, Volicer L, Tifft CP, Gavras H, Liang C and Faxon D (1979) Mineralocorticoid-induced hypertension in patients with orthostatic hypotension. *N. Engl. J. Med* **301**: 68–73.
89. Robertson D and Davis TL (1995) Recent advances in the treatment of orthostatic hypotension. *Neurology* **45**(suppl. 5), S26–S32.
90. Zachariah PK, Bloedow DC, Moyer TP, Sheps SG, Schirger A and Fealey RD (1986) Pharmacodynamics of midodrine, an antihypotensive agent. *Clin. Pharmacol. Ther.* **39**: 586–591.
91. McTavish D and Goa KL (1989) Midodrine: a review of its pharmacological properties and therapeutic use in orthostatic hypotension and secondary hypotensive disorders. *Drugs* **38**: 757–777.
92. Low PA, Gilden JL, Freeman R, Sheng K-N and McElligott MA (1997) Efficacy of midodrine vs. placebo in neurogenic orthostatic hypotension: a randomized, double-blind multicenter study. *JAMA* **277**: 1046–1051.
93. Kaufman H, Brannan T, Krakoff L, Yahr MD and Mandeli J (1988) Treatment of orthostatic hypotension due to autonomic failure with a peripheral alpha-adrenergic agonist (midodrine) *Neurology* **38**: 951–956.
94. Wright RA, Kaufmann HC, Perera R, Opfer-Gehrking TL, McElligott MA, Sheng KN and Low PA (1998) A double-blind, dose–response study of midodrine in neurogenic orthostatic hypotension. *Neurology* **51**: 120–124.
95. Verwaerde P, Tran MA, Montastruc JL, Senard JM and Portolan G (1997) Effects of yohimbine, an alpha 2-adrenoceptor antagonist, on experimental neurogenic orthostatic hypotension. *Fund. Clin. Pharmacol.* **11**: 567–575.
96. Chobanian AV, Volicer L, Liang CS, Kershaw G and Tifft C (1977) Use of propranolol in the treatment of idiopathic orthostatic hypotension. *Trans. Assoc. Am. Physicians* **90**: 324–334.
97. Brevetti G, Chiariello M, Giudice P, DeMichele G, Mansi D and Campanella G (1981) Effective treatment of orthostatic hypotension by propranolol in the Shy–Drager syndrome. *Am. Heart J.* **102**: 938–941.
98. Man in't Veld AJ and Schalekamp MA (1981) Pindolol acts as beta-adrenoceptor agonist in orthostatic hypotension: therapeutic implications. *Br. Med. J.* **282**: 929–931.

99. Dejgaard A and Hilsted J (1988) No effect of pindolol on postural hypotension in type 1 (insulin-dependent) diabetic patients with autonomic neuropathy. A randomised double-blind controlled study. *Diabetologia* **31**: 281–284.
100. Verne GN and Sninsky CA (1998) Diabetes and the gastrointestinal tract. *Gastroenterology Clin.* **27**: 861–874.
101. Sturm A, Holtman G, Goebell H and Gerken G (1999) Prokinetics in patients with gastroparesis: a systematic analysis. *Digestion* **60**: 422–427.
102. Kendall BJ, Kendall ET, Soykan I and McCallum RW (1997) Cisapride in the long-term treatment of chronic gastroparesis: a two-year open-label study. *J. Int. Medical Res.* **25**: 182–189.
103. Peeters T, Matthijs G, Depoortere I, Cachet T, Hoogmartens J and Vantrappen G (1989) Erythromycin is a motilin receptor agonist. Am J Physiol, 257: G470–474.
104. Richards RD, Davenport K and McCallum RW (1993) The treatment of idiopathic and diabetic gastroparesis with acute intravenous and chronic oral erythromycin. *Am. J. Gastroenterol.* **88**: 203–207.
105. DiBaise JK and Quigley EMM (1999) Efficacy of prolonged administration of intravenous erythromycin in an ambulatory setting as treatment of severe gastroparesis: one center's experience. *J. Clin. Gastroenterol.* **28**: 131–134.
106. Patterson D, Abell T, Rothstein R, Koch K and Barnett J (1999) A double-blind multicenter comparison of domperidone and metoclopramide in the treatment of diabetic patients with symptoms of gastroparesis. *Am. J. Gastroenterol.* **94**: 1230–1234.
107. Ejskjaer NT, Bradley JL, Boxton-Thomas MS, Edmonds ME, Howard ER, Purewal T, Thomas PK and Watkins PJ (1999) Novel surgical treatment and gastric pathology in diabetic gastroparesis. *Diabetic Medicine* **16**: 488–495.
108. Green PA, Berge KG and Sprague RG (1968) Control of diabetic diarrhea with antibiotic therapy. *Diabetes*, **17**: 385.
108. McCallum RW, Chen J de Z, Lin Z, Schirmer BD, Williams RD and Ross RA (1998) Gastric pacing improves emptying and symptoms in patients with gastroparesis. *Gastroenterology* **114**: 456–461.
110. Tsai ST, Vinik AI and Brunner JF (1986) Diabetic diarrhea and somatostatin. *Ann. Intern. Med.* **104**: 894.
111. Von der Ohe M, Camilleri M, Thomforde GM and Klee GG (1995) Differential regional effects of octreotide on human gastrointestinal motor function. *Gut* **36**: 743–748.
112. Frimodt-Moller C (1980) Diabetic cystopathy: epidemiology and related disorders. *Ann. Intern. Med.* **92**: 318–321.
113. Buck AC, Reed PL, Siddiq YK, Chisholm GD and Fraster TR (1976) Bladder dysfunction and neuropathy in diabetes. *Diabetologia* **12**: 251–258.
114. Menendez V. Cofan F, Talbot-Wright R, Ricart MJ, Gutierrez R and Carretero P (1996) Urodynamic evaluation in simultaneous insulin-dependent diabetes mellitus and end-stage renal disease. *J. Urol.* **155**: 2001–2004.
115. Watanabe T and Miyagawa I (1999) The effect of partial cystectomy on the residual urine of a large bladder demonstrated in diabetic rats. *J. Urol.* **161**: 1010–1014.
116. Rundles RW (1945) Diabetic neuropathy. *Medicine (Baltimore)* **24**: 111–159.
117. Rubin A and Babbott D (1958) Impotence in diabetes mellitus. *JAMA* **168**: 498–500.
118. McCulloch DK, Campbell IW, Wu FC, Prescott RJ and Clarke BF (1980) The prevalence of diabetic impotence. *Diabetologia* **18**: 279–283.
119. Zemel P (1988) Sexual dysfunction in the diabetic patient with hypertension. Am. J. Cardiol. **61**: 27H–33H.

120. Rendell MS, Rajfer J, Wicker P, Smith MD and the Sildenafil Diabetes Study Group (1999) Sildenafil for treatment of erectile dysfunction in men with diabetes: a randomized controlled study. *JAMA* **281**: 421–426.
121. Saulie BA and Campbell RK (1997) Treating erectile dysfunction in diabetes patients. *Diabetes Educator* **23**: 29–38.
122. Spollett GR (1999) Assessment and management of erectile dysfunction in men with diabetes. *Diabetes Educator* **25**: 65–73.
123. Virag R, Frydman D, Legman M and Virag H (1984) Intracavernous injection of papaverine as a diagnostic and therapeutic method in erectile failure. *Angiology* **35**: 79–87.
124. Ernst E and Pitter MH (1998) Yohimbine for erectile dysfunction: a systematic review and meta-analysis of randomized clinical trials. J. Urol. **159**: 433–436.
125. Asbury AK (1987) Focal and multifocal neuropathies of diabetes. In *Diabetic Neuropathy* (eds Dyck PJ, Thomas PK, Asbury AK, Winegrad AI and Porte D) WB Saunders: Philadelphia, pp. 45–55.
126. al-Quattan MM, Manktelow RT and Bowen CV (1994) Outcome of carpal tunnel release in diabetic patients. *J. Hand Surg. (Br.)* **19**: 626–629.
127. Bastron JA and Thomas JE (1981) Diabetic polyradiculopathy: clinical and electromyographic findings in 105 patients. *Mayo Clin. Proc.* **56**: 725–732.
128. Dyck PJB, Norell JE and Dyck PJ (1999) Microvasculitis and ischemia in diabetic lumbosacral radiculoplexus neuropathy. *Neurology* **53**: 2113–2121.
129. Llewelyn JG, Thomas PK and King RH (1988) Epineurial microvasculitis in proximal diabetic neuropathy. *J. Neurol.* **245**: 159–165.
130. Krendel DA, Costigan DA and Hopkins LC (1995) Successful treatment of neuropathies in patients with diabetes mellitus. *Arch. Neurol.* **52**: 1053–1061.
131. Krendel DA, Zacharias A and Younger DS (1997) Autoimmune diabetic neuropathy. *Neurol. Clin.* **15**: 959–971.
132. Pascoe MK, Low PA, Windebank AJ and Litchy WJ (1997) Subacute diabetic proximal neuropathy. *Mayo Clin. Proc.* **72**: 1123–1132.
133. Jaradeh SS, Prieto TE and Lobeck LJ (1999) Progressive polyradiculoneuropathy in diabetes: correlation of variables and clinical outcome after immunotherapy. *J. Neurol. Neurosurg. Psychiatry* **67**: 607–612.
134. Pirart J (1978) Diabetes mellitus and its degenerative complications: a prospective study of 4400 patients observed between 1947 and 1973. *Diabetes Care* **1**: 168–188.
135. Palumbo PJ, Elveback LR and Whisnant JP (1978) Neurologic complications of diabetes mellitus: transient ischemic attack, stroke and peripheral neuropathy. *Adv. Neurol.* **19**: 593–601.
136. Partanen J, Niskanen L, Lehtinen J, Mervaala E, Shtonen O and Uusitupa M (1995) Natural history of peripheral neuropathy in patients with non-insulin-dependent diabetes mellitus. *N. Engl. J. Med.* **333**: 89–94.

25

Cardiac Complications and Management

AMAN CHUGH[1], KIM A. EAGLE[2] and
RAJENDRA H. MEHTA[3]

[1] Division of Cardiology, MI 48109, USA
[2] University Hospital, MI 48109-0366, USA
[3] Veterans Hospital, MI 48105, USA

INTRODUCTION

Evidence from a variety of epidemiological studies indicate that patients with type 1 and type 2 diabetes are at a high risk for cardiac disorders: coronary artery disease, cardiomyopathy and congestive heart failure[1–4]. Cardiovascular complications account for the majority of morbidity and mortality associated in diabetic patients. Thus, more than 75% of hospitalizations and about 80% of mortality among diabetics are attributable to cardiovascular diseases (30% related to acute myocardial infarction)[4–6]. Cardiovascular mortality is increased two-fold in men and four-fold in women[1]. Similarly, diabetic men succumb to sudden death 50% more often and diabetic women 300% more often then do their counterparts[7]. Diabetics who develop cardiovascular disease have a worse prognosis than those patients with cardiovascular disease without diabetes[8,9].

The overall prevalence of coronary artery disease, as assessed by various diagnostic methods, is as high as 55% among adult patients with diabetes compared with 2%–4% for the general population[10]. Coronary artery disease is not only more prevalent, but also more extensive, in diabetics than in nondiabetic patients[11]. Patients with diabetes have a higher incidence of double and triple vessel disease and a lower incidence of single vessel disease than those seen in their nondiabetic counterparts at coronary angiography or

The Evidence Base for Diabetes Care. Edited by R. Williams, W. Herman, A.-L. Kinmonth and N. J. Wareham.
© 2002 John Wiley & Sons, Ltd

autopsy[10,12]. The incidence of severe left main coronary disease is also significantly higher in diabetics[13]. While some evidence supports the fact that coronary atherosclerosis is more diffuse, other studies have argued that this is merely expressed as a greater number of discrete stenosis[13,14]. The left ventricular ejection fraction is often disproportionately lower in diabetics in relation to the degree of their epicardial coronary artery stenosis[15].

The burden on health care delivery posed by cardiovascular disease in diabetics is enormous and increasing. This is related to several factors: first, the number of older patients in the USA is increasing and the incidence of type 2 diabetes increases with aging[16]. Second, improved medical care has led to more screening of susceptible individuals and thus to greater detection of type 2 diabetes. Third, better treatment of diabetes leads to increased survival of these patients and their cardiovascular risk increases with each additional year of survival. Fourth, there is a growing population of susceptible individuals: African-Americans, Native Americans, Hispanics, Pacific Islanders, and Asians (especially South Asians), which increases the prevalence of patients with diabetes[17]. Fifth, an estimated 97 million Americans are overweight or obese and three-quarters of the US population take part in daily exercise[18]. The increasing significance of diabetes as the leading cause of cardiovascular disease has led to its designation as a major risk factor for cardiovascular disease along with cigarette smoking, hypertension and elevated cholesterol by the American Heart Association[19].

FACTORS FAVORING CARDIOVASCULAR DISEASE IN DIABETICS

ASSOCIATED CARDIOVASCULAR RISK FACTORS

Several risk factors for the development of coronary artery disease exist simultaneously with diabetes, and are responsible for the development of atherosclerotic heart disease in diabetics. These factors include hereditary, advanced age, sex, obesity and lack of physical exercise. While the interaction of these factors with diabetes in causing atherosclerosis is complex, they often exacerbate and accelerate the effect of diabetes and other major risk factors such as hypertension, smoking and hyperlipidemia.

Hypertension has long been recognized as a major risk factor for cardiovascular disease, with increased risk of coronary artery disease, congestive heart failure and stroke[3]. It has been known to be associated with an increased tendency for plaque fissuring and rupture a major precursor to acute myocardial infarction[20]. Hypertension is more common in diabetics than in nondiabetics, and is found in >50% of diabetics over the age of 45 years, with an

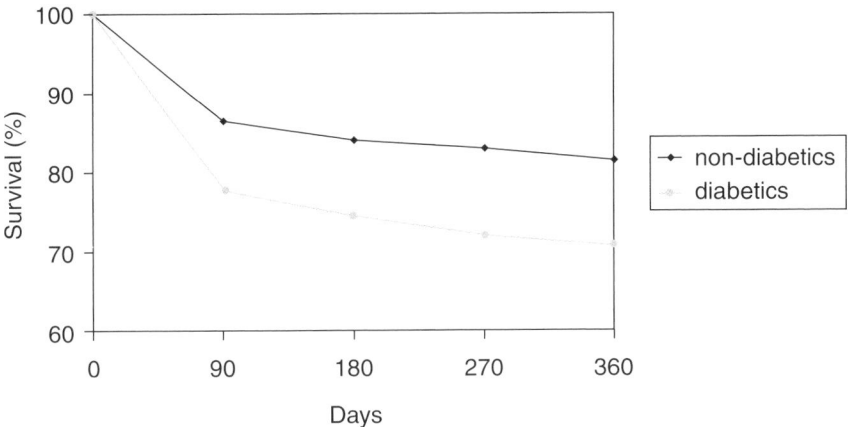

Figure 25.1. One-year survival rates following acute myocardial infarction. Reproduced from Duell[189].

especially high prevalence among women[21]. Hypertension, also, is an associated component of the 'metabolic syndrome' that is associated with type 2 diabetes and accounts for a two-fold increase in the risk of diabetic nephropathy[22,23].

Abnormalities of lipid metabolism exist in most diabetics and promote vascular damage and atherosclerosis. Pathological studies of coronary arteries in patients with myocardial infarction suggests that lipid-rich plaques are more likely to rupture than fibrous plaques[24]. Compared with persons without diabetes, patients with hypertension, diabetes or both, appear to have a higher propensity of such fissured plaques[20]. An increased serum LDL cholesterol is a major risk factor for coronary artery disease[25]. In the absence of elevated serum LDL cholesterol, coronary artery disease is relatively uncommon even when other major risk factors such as hypertension, diabetes or smoking are present[26]. Similarly, elevated LDL cholesterol leads to accelerated atherosclerosis even with no other known risk factors[27].

Diabetics often have lipoprotein abnormality characterized by an elevated low density lipoprotein (LDL), low high-density lipoprotein (HDL) and small LDL cholesterol particles, a combination that often exists with insulin resistance[28–31]. This atherogenic lipoprotein abnormality leads to premature coronary artery disease, even in the absence of elevated LDL cholesterol[28,32]. Often, an elevated serum apolipoprotein B level is associated with this atherogenic dyslipidemia[33].

Despite a preponderance of lipid abnormalities in patients with diabetes, the independent contribution of total cholesterol to coronary artery disease is the same as that in patients without diabetes[21]. The average total cholesterol level in the Framingham study was similar in patients with or without diabetes[34]. While the atherogenic lipoprotein abnormality described above was more common in diabetics, serum LDL cholesterol levels were similar in diabetics and nondiabetics[35].

Hyperinsulinemia is particularly common in type 2 diabetics with insulin resistance, and appears to be a risk factor for atherogenesis[36]. Factors commonly associated with insulin resistance include abdominal obesity, atherogenic dyslipidemia, impaired glucose tolerance, hypertension and a prothrombotic state[36]. While genetic factors play an important role in insulin resistance, obesity, physical inactivity and advanced age contribute to the development of this abnormality[37–39]. Hyperinsulinemia may play a role in promoting atherosclerosis by causing smooth muscle cell proliferation and cholesterol synthesis, and by increasing the level of growth hormone[40].

Cigarette smoking is an independent risk factor for cardiovascular disease. In diabetics, smoking is an independent predictor of mortality, especially in women, since it increases their cardiac mortality more than two-fold[41]. For patient, who continue to smoke despite having diabetes, the benefits of modification of other major risk factors is mitigated.

Microalbuminuria is the first clinical sign of diabetic nephropathy and is associated with increased risk of cardiovascular disease[42–44]. The risk of developing coronary artery disease is eight or more times higher in patients with microalbuminuria[23,45]. Similarly, the risk of cardiovascular mortality is increased up to four-fold (in type 2) and 37 times (in type 1) in diabetic patients as compared with the general population [44,46]. Most type 1 diabetics over the age of 45 have over 50% stenosis of one or more of their epicardial

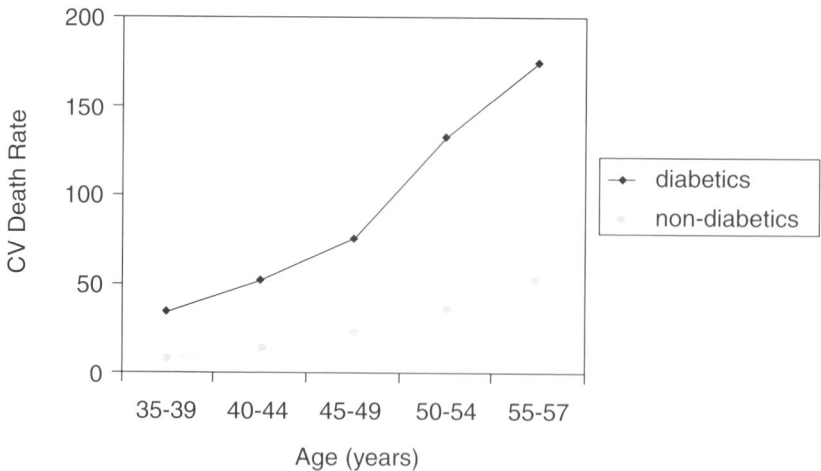

Figure 25.2. Cardiovascular mortality in diabetics. Reproduced from Duell[189].

coronary arteries[47]. Thus, microalbuminuria or persistent protenuria is not only a marker of diabetic nephropathy, but also a potent indicator of coronary artery disease.

HEMO-RHEOLOGICAL ABNORMALITIES IN DIABETIC PATIENTS

Patients with diabetes have elevated whole plasma and blood viscosity due to high levels of plasma proteins, increased red cell aggregation and decreased red cell deformity[48,49], particularly during periods of metabolic derangement such as diabetic ketoacidosis. The tendency for plaque rupture is enhanced due to increased viscosity. This rheological abnormality probably contributes to the extension of infarction by impeding the collateral blood flow, especially in areas of low blood flow at baseline.

Spontaneous as well as induced platelet aggregation has been shown to be higher in diabetics than in nondiabetics, and this has been shown to correlate with an increase in cardiovascular events[50–52]. Thomboxane A_2 synthesis is abnormally high in the platelets of diabetic patients, particularly in those with poor glycemic control or vascular complications, and may lead to increased platelet aggregation and vasospasm[52–55]. Platelet consumption is higher in diabetic patients and two platelet-specific proteins, beta-thromboglobulin and platelet factor 4, thought to reflect in vivo platelet activation, may be elevated in these patients[49,52]. Platelet reactivity in diabetic patients has been shown to be elevated consistently throughout the day, unlike in the general population, in whom the period of greatest platelet aggregability occurs in the early morning[56,57]. Thus, unlike in the general population, which exhibits an early morning peak in the onset of their acute myocardial infarction coinciding with their period of greatest platelet aggregability[57], among diabetic patients myocardial infarction occurs more evenly throughout the day[58].

Plasma fibrinogen levels are elevated in patients with diabetes and have been shown to be associated with myocardial infarction and sudden death in diabetic men[50,52]. High fibrinogen levels in diabetics have been shown to predict vascular complications[59]. Factor VIII and the von Willebrand factor are elevated in diabetic patients as well[50,52,60]. The Atherosclerosis Risk In Communities (ARIC) Study documented a strong association between plasma von Willebrand factor and several components of insulin resistance syndrome[61]. Endothelial dysfunction or damage precedes both macrovascular and microvascular complications in diabetic patients, and results in deficient production of prostacyclin and elevated levels of procoagulant von Willebrand factor[49,50,52,61]. Endogenous fibrinolysis has also been shown to be deficient in these patients from elevated levels of plasminogen activator inhibitor-1, the principal physiological inhibitor of endogenous tissue plasminogen activator[52,62].

SPECIFIC CARDIAC DISEASES IN DIABETIC PATIENTS

CORONARY ARTERY DISEASE AND ACUTE CORONARY SYNDROMES

Both type 1 and type 2 diabetes are independent risk factors for coronary heart disease[1,2]. Further myocardial ischemia occurs without any symptoms in patients with diabetes[63]. This is due to blunted appreciation of ischemic pain by diabetic patients. Unrecognized infarctions tend to be more frequent in diabetic patients, occurring in 39% of their infarctions as opposed to 22% in those without diabetes[64,65]. These data parallel the observation that myocardial scars in the absence of a pre-mortem history of myocardial infarction is found three times more often in autopsies in a diabetic patients[66]. Furthermore, the incidence of painless ST segment depression during exercise stress tests is almost double that seen in patients without diabetes (69% versus 35%)[67]. Furthermore, diabetic patients who experience angina become aware of their symptoms later in the course of ischemia than do nondiabetic patients[68]. The delay in time from onset of ST segment depression to angina may be twice as long in diabetics as in nondiabetics, and correlates with the extent of autonomic nervous dysfunction[68]. Histological damage to cardiac afferent nerve fibers as well as physiologic abnormalities in afferent and efferent nerve fibers have been shown in diabetic patients, suggesting the existence of neuropathy involving these fibers that may play a role in altered pain perception in patients with diabetes[69–70]. As a result, accurate diagnosis of infarction based on historical grounds may be difficult. Atypical symptoms such as confusion, dyspnoea, fatigue or nausea and vomiting (mimicking those from hypo- or hyperglycemia) may be a presenting complaint in 32–42% of diabetic patients with myocardial infarction, compared with 6–15% of non-diabetic patients[71]. These atypical presentations may lower the clinician's suspicion of infarction, leading to less than optimal care with up to one-third of diabetic patients with acute myocardial infarction admitted initially to general hospital wards rather than to coronary care units[72]. This may also lead to underutilization, as well as delays in the institution of appropriate treatment in diabetic patients with myocardial infarction[73]. Atypical symptoms may alter patients' perception of the nature of their illness and interfere with their decision to seek medical attention. More than one-third of patients with diabetes without chest pain during their infarction wait 24 or more hours to seek medical care[74]. Nonpainful myocardial infarction has been shown to be associated with increased morbidity and mortality[74]. It is likely that the delay in seeking and receiving appropriate medical care may contribute to the observed increase in morbidity and mortality[73,74].

Mortality is especially high in diabetic patients with unstable angina or with acute myocardial infarction. A recent prospective study indicated a three-

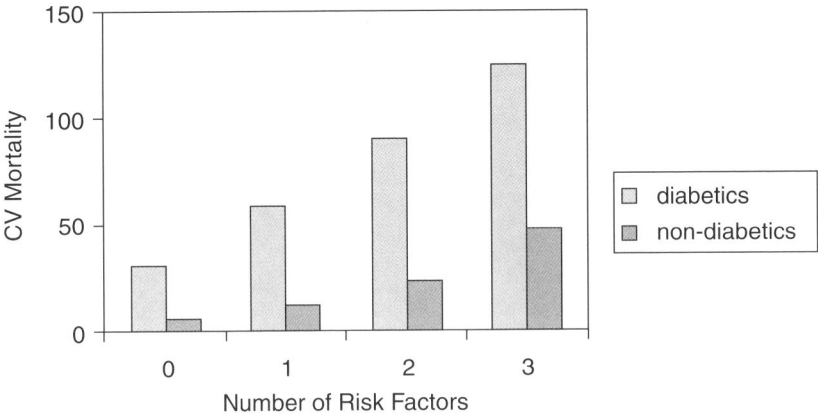

Figure 25.3. Cardiovascular mortality in diabetics with additional risk factors. Reproduced from Jensen[23].

month mortality of 8.6% and one-year mortality of 16.7% in diabetics versus 2.5% and 8.6%, respectively, in nondiabetic patients with unstable angina[75]. The one-year mortality in diabetic patients is reported to be as high as 25% after acute myocardial infarction, and is twice as high in patients with than without a history of prior infarction[76]. Diabetic women with acute myocardial infarction have a poorer prognosis than do diabetic men and nearly twice the in-hospital mortality, attributed to high incidence of severe congestive heart failure and cardiogenic shock[76,77]. Even in younger diabetic patients with acute myocardial infarction, mortality rates are significantly greater than in younger nondiabetic patients, who generally seem to tolerate infarction better than the elderly[78].

Several factors contribute to this increased in-hospital and long-term mortality. The size of infarct tends to be greater, and anterior infarcts are more common in diabetic than in nondiabetic patients[8,78-81]. Congestive heart failure and cardiogenic shock are more common and more severe than can be predicted from the size of infarct in patients with diabetes than in those without diabetes, with a reduction in global as well as regional ejection fractions[76,77,82-84]. Reinfarction, recurrent or persistent ischemia, myocardial rupture and atrioventricular and intraventricular conduction abnormalities are more common in diabetics than in nondiabetic patients[8,80-82].

DIABETIC CARDIOMYOPATHY

Patients with diabetes are unusually prone to enhanced myocardial dysfunction leading to accelerated heart failure[85-89]. In epidemiological studies, the frequency of congestive heart failure was two times and five times in diabetic

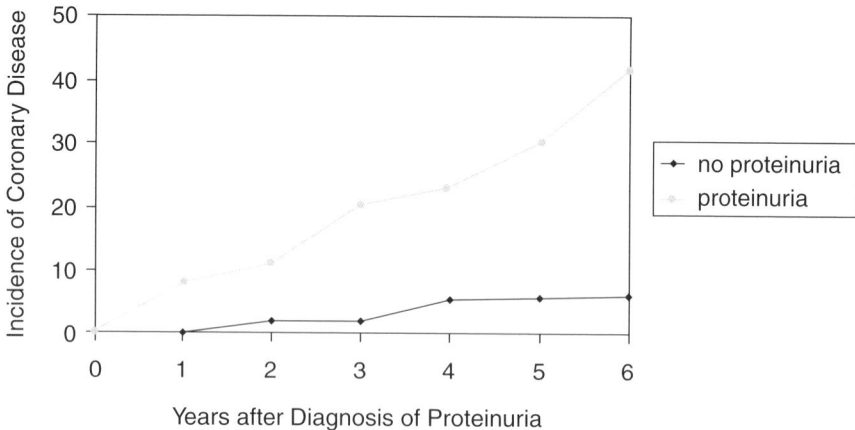

Figure 25.4. Proteinuria and the incidence of coronary disease in type 1 diabetics. Reproduced from Krolewski[45].

men and women, respectively, that in their cohorts without diabetes[88]. Several factors underlie the development of diabetic cardiomyopathy: severe diffuse coronary artery disease, chronic hyperglycemia, prolong high blood pressure, microvascular disease, glycosylation of myocardial proteins and autonomic neuropathy[85-87]. Pathological findings in diabetic cardiomyopathy include myocardial enlargement, hyopertrophy and fibrosis as well as an increase in basement membrane thickening with periodic acid-Schiff positive deposits in the interstitium and microaneurysm formation[86,90-93]. These pathological abnormalities are reflected in a wide spectrum of abnormalities of left ventricular function ranging from asymptomatic diastolic dysfunction to overt decreased systolic function[83,84]. While diastolic abnormalities are greater in hypertensive diabetic patients, they are frequently demonstrated in diabetics without high blood pressure[86]. Left ventricular hypertrophy, particularly in women, has been shown to occur in diabetic patients even in the absence of hypertension[94]. Further, decreased contractile reserve, as reflected by lower augmentation of left ventricular ejection fraction with exercise, has been shown in diabetic patients[95,96]. Frank systolic dysfunction occurs late in long-standing diabetes with microvascular and macrovascular complications[97].

AUTONOMIC NEUROPATHY IN DIABETIC PATIENTS

Cardiac autonomic neuropathy has been shown to evolve very early in the course of diabetes[98,99]. Cardiac parasympathetic nerve fibers are affected before sympathetic fibers, leading to a relative excess of sympathetic tone that initially manifests as tachycardia, reduced heart rate variability at rest and attenuation of heart rate and blood pressure response to exercise[29-101]. An absent parasympathetic tone may also be responsible for exaggerated or inappropriate coronary vasoconstriction, which may produce or worsen ischemia[100,101]. Sympathetic nervous system dysfunction is evident in five years from the onset of parasympathetic abnormalities, and manifests as orthostatic hypotension[102]. Autonomic dysfunction is responsible for the lack of pain perception during ischemia or exercise testing and for the higher incidence of silent ischemia, as discussed above. In addition, autonomic neuropathy may be responsible for sudden death in diabetic patients[103–106]. Although arrhythmias precipitated by silent ischemia may predispose to sudden death, autopsy studies have demonstrated a surprising absence of significant coronary artery disease in some diabetic patients who suffer sudden cardiac death[103,107]. A relationship has been noted between diabetic cardiac autonomic neuropathy and prolonged QT interval on electrocardiogram, which may predispose to life-threatening ventricular arrhythmia and sudden death[104–106].

ASSESSMENT OF CORONARY RISK FACTORS IN DIABETIC PATIENTS

Risk assessment in diabetics like that for any patient at risk of coronary artery disease, should begin with assessing the presence of major risk factors such as hypertension, cigarette smoking, hyperlipidemia and family history of premature coronary artery disease. In addition, factors that contribute to the risk (excess body weight, abdominal obesity, lack of physical activity) should also be sought. The value of a detailed history, physical examination and appro-

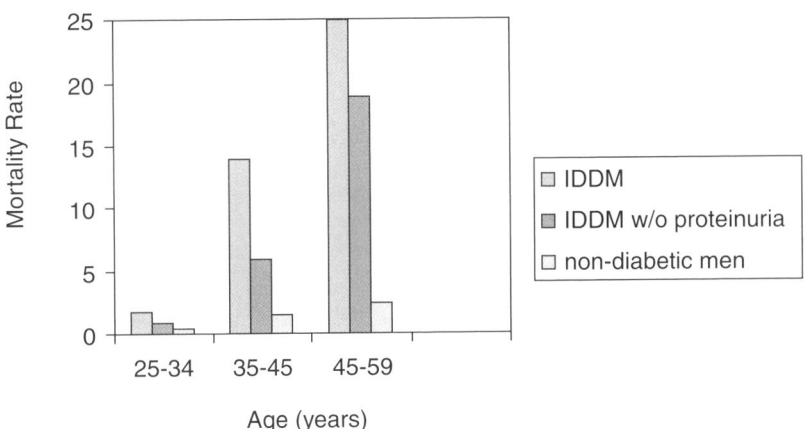

Figure 25.5. Proteinuria in patients with IDDM and mortality rates. Reproduced from Kjekshus[123].

priate laboratory tests for the identification of these risk factors cannot be overemphasized. Specialized testing such as 24-hour monitoring of ambulatory blood pressure through automated techniques may help to detect hypertension. Lipoprotein analysis should be a routine part of screening for all diabetic patients. The effectiveness of glycemic control could be best determined by periodic measurement of hemoglobin A_{1c} levels. Similarly, an assessment of micro- or macroalbuminuria should be considered for all diabetic patients, not only because it predicts the development of diabetic nephropathy, but as suggested earlier, it is also associated with greater risk of developing coronary artery disease. A careful assessment of the status of the predisposing risk factors can set the stage for therapeutic modifications known to reduce the risk of coronary artery disease.

DETECTION OF CLINICAL AND SUBCLINICAL CORONARY ARTERY DISEASE

Early diagnosis of coronary artery disease is imperative in patients with diabetes for effective treatment and to decrease the high morbidity and mortality associated with diabetes. A careful history should include the presence of angina, dypnoea, cerebrovascular events or claudications. The lack of typical symptoms in many patients makes early diagnosis of coronary artery difficult, and requires a high index of suspicion on part of physicians for detection of coronary atherosclerotic disease. Physical examination should, as well as the measurement of blood pressure, include assessment of carotid and

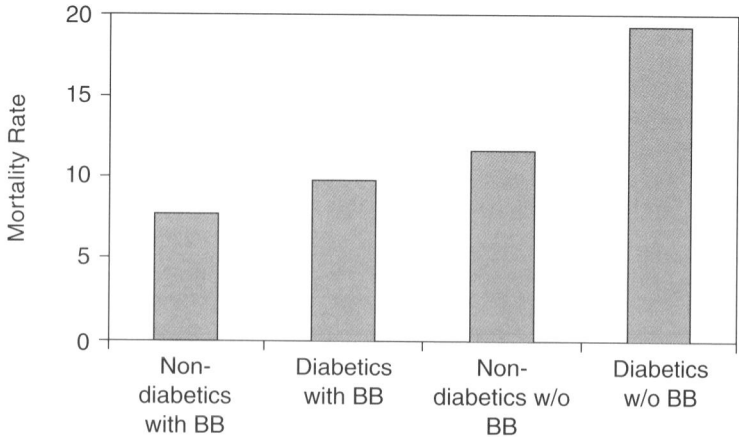

Figure 25.6. The effect of beta-blockers on mortality following a myocardial infarction. Reproduced from Kendall[117].

peripheral arteries for bruits that indicate stenosis of these vessels, a marker for coronary artery disease. An electrocardiogram can help detect the presence of ischemia or infarction in some patients and can also reveal left ventricular hypertrophy, which has been shown to be associated with increased morbidity and mortality in diabetic patients. The presence of micro- or macroalbuminuria should be actively sought as it portends a poor prognosis in diabetic patients with coronary artery disease. A noninvasive test such as a echocardiogram or radionuclide ventriculography may help detect systolic or diastolic left ventricular dysfunction, regional wall motion abnormality indicative of coronary atherosclerosis and, with an echocardiogram, identify left ventricular hypertrophy. Stress testing for myocardial ischemia should be performed in accordance with the American College of Cardiology/ American Heart Association guidelines[108].

MANAGEMENT OF CARDIOVASCULAR DISEASE IN PATIENTS WITH DIABETES

MEDICAL MANAGEMENT

Early and comprehensive medical intervention in patients with existing coronary artery disease has been shown to decrease the incidence of myocardial infarction, increase survival, improve quality of life and decrease the need for invasive therapies such as coronary angioplasty or bypass surgery. The higher mortality and morbidity in diabetic patients mandates an aggressive approach to secondary prevention in those with known coronary artery disease. The general comprehensive guidelines proposed by ACC/AHA for the management of patients with known coronary artery disease for risk reduction should be applied to diabetic patients (Table 25 1)[19,109,110].

ANTIPLATELET AGENTS

The role of aspirin as a secondary prevention therapy following a myocardial infarction (mi) has been well established. In 19791 patients reviewed by the Antiplatelet Therapy Trialists, aspirin begun following myocardial infarction led to a 12% reduction in deaths, a 31% reduction in reinfarction and a 42% reduction in nonfatal stroke, with an overall cardiovascular event risk reduction of 25%[111]. Low to medium doses (75–325 mg/day) appear to be as effective as high doses (1200 mg/day) and have less incidence of gastrointestinal side-effects[111]. Infarction in patients on chronic therapy are more likely to be smaller and non-Q wave[112]. Increased platelet reactivity that not only promotes progression of atherosclerosis and the development of occlusive thrombus at the site of plaque rupture has been demonstrated in diabetic patients[50-52].

Table 25.1. Ways of improving outcome in diabetic patients with known coronary artery disease.

1. Control of hypertension.
2. Stopping smoking.
3. Aspirin 325 mg orally once a day.
4. Clopidogrel 75 mg once a day for aspirin intolerance.
5. Oral anticoagulation for increased risk of embolization from left ventricle or left atrium (those with severe LV dysfunction after MI, persistent atrial fibrillation and/or demonstrated mural or left atrial thrombus). Target INR 2 to 3.
6. Betablockers (preferably beta1-selective agents; avoid beta-blockers with intrinsic sympathomimetic activity).
7. Angiotensin converting enzyme (ACE) inhibitors especially in patients with congestive heart failure and/or left ventricular ejection fraction <35%, but preferably in all patients to prevent and/or slow the progression of nephropathy.
8. Lipid lowering agents in patients with LDL >130 mg %, target LDL <100 mg %.
9. Better glycemic control.
10. Avoidance of calcium channel blockers (CCBs), except in those patients who have preserved left ventricular function and in whom beta-blockers are contraindicated.
11. Diet counseling.
12. Physical activity and weight management.

Thus, even in the absence of targeted randomized trials of aspirin for secondary prevention in diabetics with coronary artery disease, the use of aspirin should be extended to this group of high-risk patients with myocardial infarction. However, the Second International Study of Infarct Survival 2 (ISIS-2) showed no reduction in mortality in diabetic patients with acute myocardial infarction who received 160 mg of aspirin per day[113]. This is probably due to the fact that there is markedly heightened platelet activation, and the dose of aspirin necessary for therapeutic benefit is higher than 160 mg per day. Patients with diabetes and coronary artery disease should thus receive at least 325 mg of aspirin a day. Part of the reluctance to prescribe aspirin may stem from the concern that it may precipitate retinal hemorrhage in diabetics. However, long-term treatment with aspirin (325 mg three times a day) in 267 diabetic patients with early retinopathy resulted in a decrease in the formation of retinal microaneurysm, with not a single case of retinal bleeding[114].

Ticlopidine, an ADP-receptor antagonist, has been shown to be more effective than placebo in reducing vascular death or MI at six months in patients with unstable angina[115]. However, two serious side-effects, reversible neutropenia and thrombotic thrombocytopenic purpura (TTP) have limited the widespread use of this drug for secondary prevention[109].

Clopidogrel, an ADP-receptor antagonist similar to ticlopidine, was tested versus ASA in the CAPRIE (Clopidogrel versus Aspirin in Patients at Risk of Ischemic Events) trial in patients with vascular disease, stroke or MI within the last six months. Patients treated with clopidogrel had a lower risk of ischemic stroke, MI or vascular death compared with those that were treated with ASA[116]. There was no report of TTP in this trial and the incidence of neutropenia was similar for clopidigrel and ASA. Thus, clopidogrel at a dose of 75 mg once a day is recommended for those patients with an allergy or intolerance to aspirin, and for those with recurrent symptoms while on ASA[109,110].

Oral anticoagulants, on the other hand, are indicated for patients at risk of embolization from left ventricular or left atrial clot (those with severe left ventricular dysfunction, persistent atrial fibrillation and/or demonstrated mural or left atrial thrombus). The recommended target international normalized ratio (INR) for such patients is two to three[109].

BETA-BLOCKERS

Beta-blocker therapy has been shown to reduce reinfarction and sudden death in diabetic patients to a greater extent than in nondiabetic patients[117,118]. The pooled data from early treatment of myocardial infarction with beta-blockers indicates a 13% mortality reduction in all patients versus a 37% mortality reduction in diabetic patients[117,119–123]. Long-term studies show mortality reductions of 33% in all patients treated with beta-blockers and 48% in patients with diabetes[122]. Similarly, there was a 21% reduction in the rates of reinfarction in patients without diabetes treated with beta-blockers compared to a 55% reduction in similarly treated diabetic patients[124]. Beta-blockers may theoretically inhibit catecholemine-induced glycogenolysis and glucose metabolization, leading to prolonged hypoglycemia in patients with diabetes. These agents also may attenuate reflex tachycardia and mask warning symptoms due to hypoglcemia, worsen claudications and dyslipidemia, increase fatigue and depression and decrease libido. However, these effects are much less noticeable in patients treated with beta1-selective agents than in those treated with nonselective agents[125,126]. Furthermore, the incidence of hypoglycemia has not been reported to increase among diabetic patients treated with beta-blockers after myocardial infarction[127,128]. While clinicians should be aware of this potential danger, this should not preclude them from using beta-blockers (preferably beta1-selective agents) in these patients[109,110].

ANGIOTENSIN CONVERTING ENZYME INHIBITORS

Angiotensin converting enzyme (ACE) inhibitors (ACEI) have been shown in several randomized clinical trials to be beneficial in secondary prevention after acute myocardial infarction in patients with or without systolic left ventricular dysfunction. They decrease symptoms due to heart failure, reduce

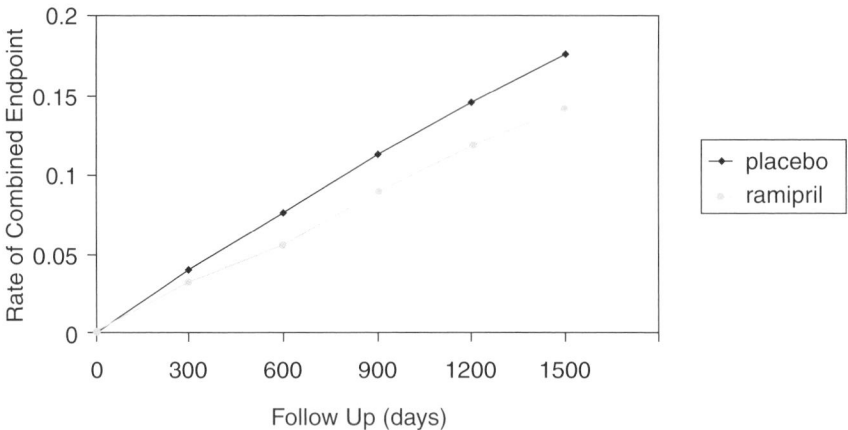

Figure 25.7. The effect of ramipril on outcomes in diabetics with preserved LV function. Reproduced from HOPE Investigators[190].

recurrent ischemia and infarction, prevent hospitalization and improve survival rates[129–132]. Furthermore, by reducing blood pressure, they may reduce the risk of stroke. They have also been shown to prevent the development and delay the progression of diabetic nephropathy[133,134]. Few studies have addressed the role of ACEI in secondary prevention in diabetic patients with coronary artery disease. In a retrospective analysis of diabetic patients with acute myocardial infarction enrolled in the GISSI-3 Study, the use of the ACEI lisinopril was associated with a significant six-week mortality reduction, 27% in type 2 diabetics (OR 0.71, CI 0.54–0.95) and 44% in type 1 diabetics (OR 0.51, CI 0.31–0.81)[135]. Similarly, in a recent large randomized trial in high-risk patients with preserved left ventricular function (80% with coronary artery disease), the use of the ACEI ramipril was associated with a significant reduction in the composite outcome of myocardial infarction, stroke or death in diabetic patients as compared to placebo[136]. Thus, ACEI are currently recommended for all diabetics with hypertension, left ventricular dysfunction or congestive heart failure, and after large anterior wall myocardial infarction[19,109]. In patients who are intolerant or allergic to ACEI, ACE-receptor blockers should be used as alternative agents.

CONTROL OF HIGH BLOOD PRESSURE

As noted above, hypertension worsens the effects of diabetes on cardiovascular morbidity and mortality and increases the risk of diabetic nephropathy. Thus, every effort should be made to decrease high blood pressure in diabetic patients, with a goal of under 135/85 mmHg. While achievement of ideal body weight, exercise and salt restriction should be the first steps toward achieving this goal, it often requires the use of an antihypertensive agent. ACEI should be considered the first agents of choice in diabetics because of their potential beneficial effect on diabetic nephropathy. Other agents such as calcium channel blockers or beta-blockers may also be used, especially if there are other indications for these drugs.

LIPID-LOWERING, CALCIUM CHANNEL BLOCKERS, STOPPING SMOKING, WEIGHT REDUCTION AND PHYSICAL ACTIVITY

These topics are covered in detail elsewhere in this book, and readers are recommended to refer to the appropriate chapters. A few general comments are in order, here, however. Aggressive attempt at lowering LDL cholesterol (when necessary with the use of drugs) to less than 100 should be the primary objective[137]. Statins are the first line of therapy to achieve this goal. If tryglycerides are persistently elevated to above 200 mg/dl, consideration should be given to adding a fibrate to achieve the secondary goal of triglyceride levels of less than 200 mg/dl. Careful monitoring is needed when using a combination of fibrate and statin because of the rare but catastrophic occurrence of life-threatening rhabdomyolysis[138]. Nicotinic acid is effective in normalizing both the lipid and hemostatic derangement associated with dyslipidemia. Thus, it lowers triglycerides, LDL cholesterol, Lp (a) lipoprotein, fibrinogen and plasminogen activator inhibitor-1 1 levels, and increase HDL cholesterol[139,140]. Niacin may exacerbate hyperglcemia in patients with overt type 2 diabetes[141], but this can usually be managed by adjusting the therapy for hyperglycemia. Many studies have supported the beneficial effects of lipid-lowering therapies in improving outcomes in diabetic patients with known coronary artery disease[142–144].

Assessment of calcium channel blockers (CCBs) have yielded mixed results, with no conclusive support for their use[145–148]. Currently, their use is recommended for the control of hypertension or as an anti-ischemic therapy in patients with preserved left ventricular systolic dysfunction in whom beta-blockers are contraindicated. Short-acting dihydropyridines should be avoided in all patients[109]. Similarly, stopping smoking, weight reduction and regular physical exercise all reduce morbidity and mortality in diabetic patients with coronary artery disease and are recommended for all[19].

CONTROL OF HYPERGLYCEMIA

Whether or not tight control of increased blood sugar improves morbidity and mortality related to microvascular complications such as retinopathy and nephropathy, there is a lack of conclusive evidence of its beneficial effects in reducing macrovascular complications, especially cardiovascular events[149,150].

The Diabetes Control and Complications Trial (DCCT) trial showed that major macrovascular events were twice as common in diabetics who received conventional therapy than in those in the intensive-treatment group, although this difference was not statistically significant (p = 0.08)[149]. The United Kingdom Prospective Diabetes Study (UKPDS) in type 2 diabetic patients showed similar improvement on microvascular events, but not in macrovascular complications with intensive-blood sugar control[150]. Data from the Stockholm Diabetes Intervention Study demonstrated that tight control delays the development of ateroclerosis in type 1 diabetic patients[151]. The DIGAMI Study randomized patients with suspected myocardial and hyperglycemia on admission, to receive insulin glucose infusion for 24 hours followed by subcutaneous insulin four times daily for three or more months, or to usual care. Those patients receiving the insulin-glucose infusion without previous insulin treatment showed a significant reduction in one year mortality compared to the usual care group (8.6% versus 18%, p = 0.02)[152].

Metformin has been found to be almost as effective as sulphonylurea in reducing elevated blood sugars. The UKPDS study showed that the metformin-treated group experienced a 36% reduction in all-cause mortality in comparison with the groups receiving sulfonylurea or insulin therapy[150].

Troglitazone, a thiazolidenedione, lowers glucose levels by improving insulin sensitivity in skeletal muscle, liver and adipose tissue, and corrects the fundamental defect of type 2 diabetes mellitus (insulin resistance). It is shown to be as effective as sufonylurea therapy in early studies to lower blood glucose. In addition, it lowers tryglceride levels by approximately 20% and increases HDL by 8%. A few fatal cases of hepatic toxicity were reported in patients who were not monitored[153,154]. Despite its potential hepatotoxicity, troglitazone is currently being widely used to treat hyperglycemia, with careful monitoring for this side-effect[154]. New drugs of the same class, rosiglitazone and pioglitazone, may have less potential hepatotoxicity. Several concerns have been raised about the use of sufonylureas and its cardiovascular effects, namely increased propensity for dysrhythmias, induction of vasoconstriction, increased insulin levels, possible increases in body-weight, decreases in ischemic preconditioning, and worsening of vascular reactivity[155–158]. Despite this, recent trials have failed to demonstrate any increase in cardiac events with these agents[150].

REPERFUSION THERAPY IN PATIENTS WITH ACUTE MYOCARDIAL INFARCTION

Following an acute myocardial infarction, diabetics continues to have mortality rates that are 1.5 to 2 times higher than those for nondiabetics, even in the thrombolytic era[159–162]. However, diabetic patients with acute myocardial infarction treated with thrombolytic therapy have similar reductions in

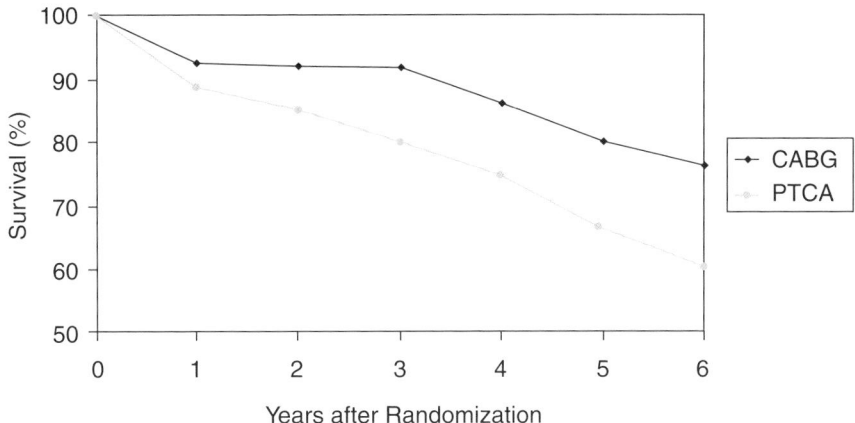

Figure 25.8. Survival in diabetics and modes of revascularization. Reproduced from BARI Investigators[183].

mortality as nondiabetic patients. An overview of thrombolytic trials revealed a slight, but non-significant, 21.7% reduction in 35-day mortality in diabetics as compared to 14.3% in nondiabetics treated with fibronolytic therapy after acute myocardial infarction[113,159,163]. Although there have been case reports of retinal hemorrhage in diabetic patients treated with thrombolytic therapy[164], no significant increase in the risk of retinal or other bleeding or hemorrhagic stroke has been observed with the use of fibrinolytic agents[113,159,163]. Similarly, in a recent report from the GUSTO trial, a combination of aspirin plus thrombolytic therapy was not associated with an increased incidence of retinal hemorrhage[165].

In the Primary Angioplasty in Myocardial Infarction (PAMI) study, in-hospital mortality in diabetics randomized to receive tissue plasminogen activator therapy was 20.8% versus 0% in those randomized to have primary PTCA (percutaneous transluminal coronary angioplasty) (p = 0.01). Similarly, the rate of death or reinfarction was higher in diabetics treated with thrombolytic than with primary angioplasty (25% versus 4%; p = 0.03)[166]. Similarly, the use of primary stenting in diabetic patients with acute myocardial infarction has been shown to improve outcomes[167,168]. All these studies have a small number of patients. Thus, on the basis of the available data, diabetics with acute myocardial infarctions should receive prompt reperfusion therapy.

CORONARY REVASCULARIZATION

Diabetic patients have similar successes with angioplasty as nondiabetics[169]. However, restenosis rates are higher in diabetics (reported as between 47–71%) as compared to nondiabetics (30–45%), thus requiring additional revascularization procedures and increasing late mortality[170–173]. The use of newer devices such as atherectomy, stents or excimer lasers[174–177] has failed to have any major role in decreasing the high restenosis rates reported with balloon angioplasty, although one recent study showed a lower restenosis rate with stents than with balloon angioplasty[178]. The use of platelet glycoprotein IIb/IIIa inhibitor (abciximab) with stenting was recently shown to result in a significant reduction in the six-month rates of death, MI and target vessel revascularization when compared with stent–placebo, or balloon–abximab combinations[179].

Diabetic patients undergoing coronary artery bypass grafting (CABG) have similar relief of symptoms as nondiabetic patients[180–182]. However, long-term survival continues to be poor in diabetics as compared to nondiabetic patients[180–182]. Surgical bypass grafting may often not be feasible in all patients with diabetes, however it is usually effective in achieving more complete revascularization.

Survival has shown to be better in diabetics who have coronary artery disease using CABG than with percutaneous transluminal coronary angio-plasty. In the Bypass Angioplasty Revascularization Investigation (BARI), the five year survival rate among diabetic patients was significantly better after CABG (81%) than after angioplasty (65%, p = 0.003)[183]. The survival advant-age related to CABG was dependent on the use of internal mammary arteries in the diabetic subgroup[183]. While some other studies have confirmed the advantage of CABG over coronary angioplasty in diabetic patients[184–186], other studies have shown similar outcomes[187,188]. Currently, CABG is the preferred strategy for revascularization in patients with multivessel coronary disease, but a subgroup of patients with discrete lesions that can be completely revascu-larized with angioplasty may do equally well with percutaneous interventions.

REFERENCES:

1. Kannel WB, McGee DL (1979) Diabetes and cardiovascular disease: the Framingham Study. *JAMA* **241**: 2035–2038.
2. Wilson PW, D'Agostino RB, Levy D, Belanger AM, Silbershatz H, Kannel WB (1998) Prediction of coronary heart disease using risk factor categories. *Circulation* **97**: 1837–1847.
3. Wilson PW. Diabetes mellitus and coronary heart disease (1998) *Am. J. Kidney Dis.* **32**: S89–S100.
4. Barrett–Connor E, Orchard TJ. Diabetes in America: Diabetes Data Compiled 1984. Bethesda, Md: US Department of Health and Human Services; 1985: XVI1–XVI41. NIH Publication 85–1468.
5. American Diabetes Association (1993) Consensus Statement: Role of cardio-vascular risk factors in prevention and treatment of macrovascular disease in diabetes. *Diabetes Care* **16**: 72–78.

6. Barrett-Connor E, Orchard T (1985) Insulin dependent diabetes mellitus and ischemic heart disease. Diabetic Care **8**: 65–70.
7. Fein FS (1982) Heart disease in diabetes. *Cardiovasc Rev & Rep* **3**: 877–893.
8. Stone PH, Muller JE, Hartwell T, York BJ, Rutherford JD, Parker CB, Turi ZG, Straus HW, Willerson JT, Robertson T (1989) The MILIS Study Group. The effect of diabetes mellitus on prognosis and serial left ventricular function after acute myocardial infarction: contribution of both coronary artery disease and diastolic left ventricular dysfunction to adverse prognosis. *Am. J. Cardiol.* **14**: 49–57.
9. Smith JW, Marcus FI, Serokman R (1984) Prognosis of patients with diabetes mellitus after acute myocardial infarction. *Am. J. Cardiol* **54**: 718–721.
10. Fein F, Scheuer J (1990) Heart disease in diabetes mellitus: theory and practice. In: Rifkin H, Porte D Jr. (eds.) *Diabetes Mellitus: Theory and Practice*. New York: Elsevier, 812–823.
11. Robertson W, Strong J (1968) Atherosclerosis in persons with hypertension and diabetes mellitus. *Lab. Invest.* **18**: 538–551.
12. Hamby R, Sherman L, Mehta J, Aintablian A (1976) Reappraisal of the role of diabetic state in coronary artery disease. Chest **70**: 251–257.
13. Waller B, Palumbo P, Roberts W (1980) Status of coronary arteries at necropsy in diabetes mellitus with onset after age 30 years. *Am. J. Med.* **69**: 498–506.
14. Dortimer AC, Shenoy PN, Shiroff RA, Leaman DM, Babb JD, Liedtke AJ, Zelis R (1978) Diffuse coronary artery disease in diabetics – facts or fiction? *Circulation* **57**: 133–136.
15. Zarich S, Nesto R (1989) Diabetic cardiomyopathy. *Am. Heart J.* 118: 1000–1012.
16. Muller DC, Elahi D, Tobin JD, Andres R (1996) The effect of age on insulin resistence and secretion: a review. Semin Nephrol **16**: 289–298.
17. Cappuccio FP, Cook DG, Atkinson RW, Strazzullo P (1997) Prevalence, detection, and management of cardiovascular risk factors in different ethnic groups in South London. Heart **78**: 555–563.
18. Prevalence of diagnosed diabetes among American Indians/Alaskan Natives in the United States, 1996. MMWR (1998) **47**: 901–904.
19. Grundy SM, Benjamin IJ, Burke GL, Chait A, Eckel RH, Howard BV, Mitch W, Smith SC JR, Sowers JR (1999) Diabetes and cardiovascular disease. A Statement for Health Professionals From American Heart Association. *Circulation* **100**: 1134–1146.
20. Davies MJ, Bland JM, Hangartner JR, Angelini A, Thomas AC (1989) Factors influencing the presence or absence of acute coronary artery thrombi in sudden ischemic death. *Eur. Heart J.* **10**: 203–208.
21. Assmann G, Schulte H (1988) The prospective Munster (PROCAM) study: prevalence of hyperlipidemia in persons with hypertension and/or diabetes mellitus and the relationship to coronary heart disease. *Am. Heart J.* **116**: 1713–1724.
22. Reaven GM, Lithell H, Landsberg L (1996) Hypertension and associated metabolic abnormalities: the role of insulin resistance and the sympatho-adrenal system. *N. Engl. J. Med.* **334**: 374–381.
23. Jensen T, Borch-Johnsen K, Kofoed-Enevoldsen A, Deckert T (1987) Coronary heart disease in young type I diabetic patients with and without diabetic nephropathy: incidence and risk factors. *Diabetologia* **30**: 144–148.
24. Davies M, Thomas A (1985) Plaque fissuring-the cause of acute myocardial infarction, sudden ischemic death and crescendo angina. *Br. Heart J.* **53**: 363–373.
25. Expert Panel on Detection, Evaluation, and Treatment of High Blood Cholesterol in Adults. National Cholesterol Education Program. Second Report of the Expert

Panel on Detection, Evaluation, and Treatment of High Blood Cholesterol (Adult Treatment Panel II). *Circulation* (1994) **89**: 1333–1445.

26. Grundy SM, Wilhelmsen L, Rose G, Campbell RW, Assman G (1990) Coronary heart disease in high-risk populations: lessons from Finland. *Eur. Heart J.* **11**: 462–471.

27. Goldstein JL, Hobbs HH, Brown MS (1985) Familial hypercholesterolemia. In Scriver CR, Beaudet AL, Sly W, Valle D (eds) *The Metabolic and Molecular Basis of Inherited Diseases*. New York: McGraw Hill, 1981–2030.

28. Austin MA, King M-C, Vranizan KM, Krauss RM (1990) Atherogenic lipoprotein phenotype: a proposed genetic marker for coronary heart disease risk. *Circulation* **82**: 495–506.

29. Grundy SM (1997) Small LDL. Atherogenic dyslipidemia, and the metabolic syndrome. *Circulation* **95**: 1–4.

30. Grundy SM (1998) Hypertriglyceridemia, atherogenic dyslipidemia, and the metabolic syndrome. *Am. J. Cardiol* **81**: 18B–25B.

31. Mostaza JM, Vega GL, Snell P, Grundy SM (1998). Abnormal metabolism of free fatty acids in hypertriglyceridemic men: apparent insulin resistance of adipose tissue. *J. Intern. Med.* **243**: 265–274.

32. Austin MA, Breslow JL, Hennekens CH, Buring JE, Willett WC, Krauss RM (1988). Low-density lipoprotein subclass patterns and risk of myocardial infarction. *JAMA* **260**: 1917–1921.

33. Lamarche B, Tchernof A, Moorjani S, Cantin B, Dagenais GR, Lupien PJ, Despres JP (1997). Small dense lipoprotein particles as a predictor of risk of ischemic heart disease in men: prospective results from the Quebec Cardiovascular Study. *Circulation* **95**: 69–75.

34. Kannel W (1985). Lipids, diabetes, and coronary heart disease: insights from the Framingham Study. *Am. Heart J.* **110**: 1100–1107.

35. Brand W, Abbott R, Kannel W (1989). Diabetes, intermittent claudication, and the risk of cardiovascular events *Diabetes* **38**: 504–509.

36. Reaven GM (1996). Insulin resistance and its consequences: non-insulin-dependent diabetes mellitus and coronary heart disease. In: LeRoith D, Taylor SI, Olefsky JM, eds. *Diabetes Mellitus: A Fundamental and Clinical Text*. Philadelphia, PA: Lippinscott-Raven, pp. 509–519.

37. Warram JH, Martin BC, Krowleski AS, Soeldner JS, Kahn CR (1990). Slow glucose removal rate and hyperinsulinemia precede the development of type II diabetes in offspring of diabetic parents. *Ann. Intern. Med.* **113**: 909–915.

38. Perseghin G, Price TB, Petersen KF, Roden M, Cline GW, Gerow K, Rothman DL, Shulman GI (1996). Increased glucose transport-phosphorylation and muscle glycogen synthesis after exercise training in insulin resistant subjects. *N. Engl. J. Med.* **335**: 1357–1362.

39. Rowe JW, Minaker KL, Pallota JA, Flier JS (1995). Characterization of the insulin-resistance of aging. *J. Clin. Invest.* **96**: 88–98.

40. Serrano-Rios M, Perez A, Saban-Ruiz J (1986). Cardiac complications in diabetes. World Book of Diabetes in Practice, Vol. 2. Princeton, NJ: Elsevier, pp. 169–178.

41. Moy CS, LaPorte RE, Dorman JS, Songer TJ, Orchard TJ, Kuller LH, Becker DJ, Drash AL (1990). Insulin-dependent diabetes mellitus mortality: the risk of cigarette smoking. *Circulation* **82**: 37–43.

42. Gall MA, Rossing P, Skott P, Damsbo P, Vaag A, Bech K, Dejgaard A, Lauritzen M, Lauritzen E, Hougaard P (1991). Prevalence of micro- and macroalbominuria, arterial hypertension, retinopathy and large vessel disease in European type 2 (non-insulin-dependent) diabetic patients. *Diabetologia* **34**: 655–661.

43. Mogensen CE (1984). Microalbuminuria predicts clinical protenuria and early mortality in maturity-onset diabetes. *N. Engl. J. Med.* **310**: 356–360.
44. Mattock MB, Morrish NJ, Viberti G, Keen H, Fitzgerald AP, Jackson G (1992). Prospective study of microalbuminuria as a predictor of mortality in NIDDM. *Diabetes* **41**: 736–741.
45. Krolewski AS, Kosinski EJ, Warran JH, Leland OS, Busick EJ, Asmal AC, Rand LI, Christlieb AR, Bradley RF, Kahn CR (1987). Magnitude and determinants of coronary artery disease in juvenile-onset, insulin-dependent diabetes mellitus. *Am. J. Cardiol.* **59**: 750–757.
46. Borch-Johnsen K, Kreiner S (1987). Proteinuria: Value as predictor of cardio-vascular mortality in insulin-dependent diabetes mellitus. *Br. Med. J.* **294**: 1651–1654.
47. Manske CL, Wilson RF, Wang Y, Thomas W (1992). Prevalence of, and risk factors for, angiographically determined coronary artery disease in type I diabetic patients with nephropathy. *Arch. Intern. Med.* **152**: 2450–2455.
48. MacRury S, Lowe G (1990). Blood rheology in diabetes mellitus. *Diabetic Med.* **7**: 285–291.
49. Rosove M, Harrison F, Harwig M (1984). Plasma B-thromboglobulin, platelet factor 4, fibrinopeptide A, and other hemostatic functions during improved short-term glycemic control in diabetes mellitus. *Diabetes Care* **7**: 174–179.
50. Breddin H, Krzywanek H, Althoff P, Schoffling K, Uberla K (1985). PARD: platelet aggregation as a risk factor in diabetes: results of a prospective study. *Horm. Metab. Res.* **15**(suppl.):63–68.
51. Sagel J, Colwell J, Crook L, Laimins M (1975). Increased platelet aggregation in early diabetes mellitus. *Ann. Intern. Med.* **82**: 733–738.
52. Ostermann H, van de Loo J (1986). Factors of the hemostatic system in diabetic patients. *Hemostasis* **16**: 386–416.
53. Ziboh V, Maruta H, Lord J, Cagle WD, Lucky W (1979). Increased biosynthesis of thromboxane A2 by diabetic platelets. *Eur. J. Clin. Invest.* **9**: 223–228.
54. Butkus A, Skrinska A, Schumacher O (1980). Thromboxane production and platelet aggregation in diabetic subjects and clinical complications. *Thromb. Res.* **19**: 211–223.
55. Davi G, Catalano I, Averna M, Notarbartolo A, Strano A, Ciabattoni G, Patrono C (1990). Thromboxane biosynthesis and platelet function in type II diabetes mellitus. *N. Engl. J. Med.* **322**: 1769–1774.
56. Stubbs M, Jimenez A, Yamane M (1990) *et al.* Platelet hyper-reactivity in diabetics: relation to the time of onset of myocardial infarction. *Am. J. Cardiol.* **15**: 119A.
57. Hjalmarson A, Gilpin M, Nicod P, Dittrich H, Henning H, Engler R, Blacky AR, Smith SC Jr, Ricou F, Ross J Jr (1989). Differing circadian patterns of symptom onset in subgroups of patients with acute myocardial infarction. *Circulation* **80**: 267–275.
58. ISIS-2 Collaborative Group (1992). Morning peak in the incidence of myocardial infarction: experience in the ISIS-2 trail. *Eur. Heart J.* **13**: 594–598.
59. Ganda OP, Arkin CF (1992). Hyperfibrinogenemia: An important risk factor for vascular complications in diabetes. *Diabetes Care* **15**: 1245–1250.
60. Stehouwer CDA, Nauta JJP, Zeldenrust GC, Hackeng WH, Donker AJ, den Ottolander GJ (1992). Urinary albumin excretion, cardiovascular disease, and endothelial dysfunction in non-insulin dependent diabetes mellitus. *Lancet* **340**: 319–323.
61. Conlan MG, Folsom AR, Finch A, Davis CE (1993). Association of factor VIII and von Willebrand factor with age, race, sex and risk factors for atherosclerosis:

the Atherosclerosis Risk in Communities (ARIC) Study. *Thromb. Haemost.* **70**: 380–385.

62. Badawi H, El-Sawy M, Mikhail M, Nomeir AM, Tewfik S (1970). Platelets, coagulation and fibrinolysis in diabetic and non-diabetic patients with quiescent coronary heart disease. *Angiology* **21**: 511–519.

63. Wingard DL, Barrett-Connor EL, Sheidt-Nave C, McPhillips JB (1993). Prevalence of cardiovascular and renal complications in older adults with normal or impaired glucose tolerance or NIDDM: a population based study. *Diabetes Care* **16**: 1022–1025.

64. Margolis JR, Kannel W, Feinlieb M, Dawber TR, McNamara PM (1973). Clinical features of unrecognized myocardial infarction – silent and symptomatic. *Am. J. Cardiol* **32**: 1–7.

65. Niakan E, Harati Y, Rolak LA, Comstock JP, Rokey R (1986). Silent myocardial infarction and diabetic cardiovascular autonomic neuropathy. *Arch. Intern. Med.* **146**: 2229–2230.

66. Cabi HS, Roberts WC (1982). Quantitative comparison of extent of coronary narrowing and size of healed myocardial infarct in 33 necropsy patients with clinically recognized and in 28 patients with clinically unrecognized ('silent') previous myocardial infarction. *Am. J. Cardiol* **50**: 677–681.

67. Murray D, O'Brien T, Mulrooney R, O'Sullivan DJ (1990). Autonomic dysfunction and silent myocardial ischemia on exercise testing in diabetes mellitus. *Diabetic Med.* **7**: 580–584.

68. Ambepitya G, Kopelman PG, Ingram B, Swash M. Mills PG, Timmis AD (1990). Exertional myocardial ischemia in diabetes: a quantitative analysis of anginal perceptual threshold and the infuence of autonomic function. *J. Am. Coll. Cardiol.* **15**: 72–77.

69. Faerman I, Faccio E, Milei J, Nunez R, Jadzinsky M, Fox D, Rapaport M (1977). Autonomic neuropathy and painless myocardial infarction in diabetic patients: histolic evidence of their relationship. *Diabetes* **26**: 1147–1158.

70. Lloyd-Mostyn R, Watkins P (1975). Defective innervation of heart in diabetic autonomic neuropathy. *Br. Med. J.* **25**: 15–17.

71. Nesto R, Phillips R (1986). Asymptomatic myocardial ischemia in diabetic patients. *Am. J. Med.* **80**(suppl 4C):40–47.

72. Soler NG, Bennet MA, Pentecost BL, Fitzgerald MG, Malins JM (1975). Myocardial infarction in diabetics. *Q. J. Med.* **173**: 125–132.

73. Stalhandske EJ, Mehta RH, McCargar PA, Eagle KA (1998). Quality of care and outcomes after acute myocardial infarction in elderly diabetic patients: the Michigan Cooperative Cardiovascular Project experience. *Circulation* **98**: I-195.

74. Uretsky BF, Farquhar DS, Berezin AF, Hood WB Jr (1977). Symptomatic myocardial infarction without chest pain: prevalence and clinical course. *Am. J. Cardiol* **40**: 498–503.

75. Fava S, Azzopardi J, Agius-Muscat H (1997). Outcome of unstable angina in patients with diabetes mellitus. *Diabet. Med.* **14**: 209–213.

76. Savage MP, Krolewski AS, Kemien GG, Lebeis MP, Christlieb AR, Lewis SM (1988). Acute myocardial infarction in diabetes mellitus and significance of congestive heart failure as a prognostic factor. *Am. J. Cardiol.* **62**: 665–669.

77. Jaffe AS, Spadaro J, Schectman K, Roberts R, Geltman EM, Sobel BE (1984). Increased congestive heart failure after myocardial infarction of modest extent in patients with diabetes mellitus. *Am. Heart J.* **108**: 1–7.

78. Czyzk A, Krolewski A, Szablowska S, Alot A, Kopezynski J (1980). Clinical course of myocardial infarction among diabetic patients. *Diabetes Care* **4**: 526–529.

79. Rytter L, Troelsen S, Beck-Nielsen H (1985) . Prevalence and mortality of acute myocardial infarction in patients with diabetes. *Diabetes Care* **8**: 230–234.
80. Partamian JO, Bradley RF (1965). Acute myocardial infarction in 258 cases of diabetes: immediate mortality and five year survival. *N. Engl. J. Med.* **273**: 455–461.
81. Hands ME, Rutherford JD, Muller JE, Davies G, Stone PH, Parker C, Braunwald E (1989). The in-hospital development of cardiogenic shock after acute myocardial infarction: incidence, predictors of occurrence, outcome and prognostic factors. *J. Am. Coll. Cardiol.* **14**: 40–46.
82. Fava S, Azzopardi J, Muscat HA, Fenech FF (1993). Factors that influence outcome in diabetic subjects with myocardial infarction. *Diabetes Care* **16**: 1615–1618.
83. Iwasaka T, Takahashi N, Nakamura S, Suigiura T, Tarumi N, Kimura Y, Okubo N, Taniguchi H, Matsui Y, Inada M (1992). Residual left ventricular function after acute myocardial infarction in NIDDM patients. *Diabetes Care* **15**: 1522–1526.
84. Takashi N, Iwasaka T, Sugiura T, Hasegawa T, Tarumi N, Kimura Y, Kurihara S, Onoyama H, Inada M (1989). Left ventricular regional function after acute myocardial infarction in diabetic patients. *Diabetes Care* **12**: 630–632.
85. Ettinger PO, Regan TJ (1989). Cardiac disease in diabetes. *Postgrad. Med.* **85**: 848–855.
86. van Hoeven KH, Factor SM (1990). A comparison of pathological spectrum of hypertensive, diabetic, and hypertensive-diabetic heart disease. *Circulation* **82**: 848–855.
87. Spector KS (1998). Diabetic cardiomyopathy. *Clin. Cardiol.* **21**: 885–887.
88. Kannel WB, Hjortland M, Castelli WP (1974). Role of diabetes in congestive heart failure: The Framingham Study. *Am. J. Cardiol* **34**: 29–34.
89. Coughlin SS, Pearle DL, Baughman KL, Wasserman A. Tefft MC (1994). Diabetes mellitus and risk of idiopathic dilated cardiomyopathy: The Washington *Diabetes Care* Dilated Cardiomyopathy Study. Ann Epidemiol **4**: 67–74.
90. Rubler S, Dlugash J, Yucheoglu YJ, Kumral T, Branwood AW, Grishman A (1972). New type of cardiomyopathy associated with diabetic glomerulosclerosis. *Am. J. Cardiol.* **30**: 595–602.
91. Fischer V, Barner H, Lewis L (1979). Capillary basal laminar thickness in diabetic human myocardium. *Diabetes* **28**: 713–719.
92. Factor S, Okun E, Minase T (1980). Capillary microaneurysms in human diabetic heart. *N. Engl. J. Med.* **302**: 384–388.
93. Regan T, Ettinger P, Kahn MI, Jesrani MU, Oldewutrel HA, Ettinger PO (1974). Altered myocardial function metabolism in chronic diabetes mellitus without ischemia in dogs. *Cir. Res.* **35**: 222–237.
94. Galderisi M, Anderson KM, Wilson PWF, Levy D (1991). Echocardiographic evidence of a distinct diabetic cardiomyopathy: the Framingham Heart Study. *Am. J. Cardiol* **68**: 85–89.
95. Vered Z, Buttler S, Segal P, Liberman D.Yerushalmi Y, Berezin M, Neufeld HN (1984) Exercise-induced left ventricular dysfunction in young men with asymptomatic diabetes mellitus (diabetic cardiomyopathy) *Am. J. Cardiol* **54**: 633–637.
96. Mustonen JN, Uusitupa MIJ, Laakso M, Vanninen E, Lansimies E, Kuikka JT, Pyorala K (1994) Left ventricular systolic function in middle-aged patients with diabetes mellitus. *Am. J. Cardiol* **73**: 1202–1208.
97. Shapiro LM, Leatherdale BA, Mackinnon J, Fletcher RF (1981). Left ventricular function in diabetes mellitus II: Relation between clinical features and left ventricular function. *Br. Heart J.* **45**: 129–132.

98. Pfeiffer MA, Weinberg CR, Cook DL, Reenan A, Halter JB, Ensinck JW, Porte D Jr (1984). Autonomic neural dysfunction in recently diagnosed diabetic patients. *Diabetic Care* **7**: 447–453.

99. Ziegler D, Dennehl K, Volksw D, Muhlen H. Spuler M, Gries FA (1992). Prevalence of cardiovascular autonomic dysfunction assessed by spectral analysis and standing tests of heart rate variability in newly diagnosed IDDM patients. *Diabetes Care* **15**: 908–911.

100. Kahn J, Zola B, Juni JE, Vinik AI (1986). Decreased exercise heart rate and blood pressure response in diabetic subjects with cardiac autonomic neuropathy. *Diabetes Care* **9**: 389–394.

101. Hilsted J, Galbo H, Christensen N (1979). Impaired cardiovascular responses to graded exercise in diabetic autonomic neuropathy. *Diabetes Care* **28**: 313–319.

102. Almog C, Pik A (1978). Acute myocardial infarction as a complication of diabetes mellitus. *JAMA* **239**: 2782–2784.

103. Ewing D, Campbell I, Clarke B (1976). Mortality in diabetic autonomic neuropathy. *Lancet* **1**: 601–603.

104. Ewing D, Boland O, Neilson JM, Cho CG, Clarke BF (1991). Autonomic neuropathy, QT interval lengthening, and unexpected deaths in male diabetic patients. *Diabetologia* **34**: 182–185.

105. Bellavere F, Ferri M, Guarini L, Bax G, Piccoli A, Cardone C, Fedele D (1988). Prolonged QT period in diabetic autonomic neuropathy: a possible role in sudden cardiac death? *Br. Heart J.* **59**: 379–383.

106. Jermendy G, Toth L, Voros P, Koltai MZ, Pogatsa G (1991). Cardiac autonomic neuropathy and QT interval length. A follow-up study in diabetic patients. *Acta Cardiologica* **46**: 189–200.

107. Ewing D, Campbell I, Clarke B (1980). Assessment of cardiovascular effects in diabetic autonomic neuropathy and prognostic implications. *Ann. Intern. Med.* **92**: 308–311.

108. Gibbons RJ, Balady GJ, Beasly JW, Bricker JT, Duvernoy WF, Froelicher VF, Mark DB, Marwick TH, McCallister DB, Thompson PD, Winters WL Jr, Yanowitz FG, Ritchie JL, Cheitlin MD, Eagle KA, Gardner TJ, Garson A Jr. Lewis RP, O'Rourke RA, Ryan TJ (1997). ACC/AHA Guidelines for Exercise Testing: Executive Summary. A report of the American College of Cardiology/American Heart Association Task Force on Practice Guidelines (Committee on Exercise Testing). *Circulation* **96**: 345–354.

109. Ryan TJ, Antman EM, Brooks NH, Califf RM, Hillis LD, Hiratzka LF, Rapaport E, Riegel B, Russell RO, Smith SC Jr (1999). 1999 Update: ACC/AHA Guidelines for the management of patients with acute myocardial infarction: A report of the ACC/AHA Task Force on Practice Guidelines (Committee on Management of Acute Myocardial Infarction). *Circulation* **100**: 1016–1030.

110. Mehta RH, Eagle KA (1998). Secondary prevention in acute myocardial infarction. *Br. Med. J.* **316**: 838–842.

111. Antiplatelet Trialist Collaboration: Collaborative overview of randomized trial of antiplatelet therapy. I. Prevention of death, myocardial infarction, and stroke by prolonged antiplatelet therapy in various categories of patients. *BMJ* (1994) **308**: 81.

112. Col NF, Yarzebski J, Gore JM, Alpert JS, Goldberg RJ (1995). Does aspirin consumption affect the presentation or severity of acute myocardial infarction? *Arch. Intern. Med.* **155**: 1386.

113. ISIS-2 (Second International Study of Infarct Survival) Collaborative Group. Randomized trial of intravenous streptokinase, oral aspirin, both, or neither

among 17,187 cases of suspected acute myocardial infarction: ISIS–2. *Lancet* (1988) **2**: 349–360.
114. DAMAD Study Group (1989). Effect of aspirin alone and aspirin plus dipyridamole in early diabetic retinopathy. *Diabetes* **38**: 491–498.
115. Balsano F, Rizzon P, Violi F, Scrutinio D, Cimminiello, C, Aguglia F, Pasotti C, Rudelli G (1990). Antiplatelet treatment with ticlopidine in unstable angina: a controlled multicenter trial: the Studio Della Ticlopidina nell'Angina Instabile Group. *Circulation* **82**: 17–22.
116. A randomized, blinded, trial of clopidogrel versus aspirin in patients at risk of ischemic events (CAPRIE). CAPRIE Steering Committee. *Lancet* (1996) **93**: 683–688.
117. Kendall MJ, Lynch KP, Hjalmarson A, Kjekshus J (1995). Beta-blockers and sudden cardiac death. *Ann. Intern. Med.* 358–367.
118. Tse WY, Kendall M (1994). Is there a role for beta-blockers in hypertensive diabetic patients? *Diabetic Med.* **11**: 137–144.
119. The First International Study of Infarct Survival (ISIS-1) Study Group (1986). Randomized trial of intravenous atenolol among 16,027 cases of suspected acute myocardial infarction: ISIS-1. *Lancet* **2**: 57–66.
120. The Trial Research Group (1985). Metoprolol in acute myocardial infarction (MIAMI) A randomized placebo-controlled international trial. *Eur. Heart J.* **6**: 199–226.
121. Herlitz J, Elmfeldt D, Holmberg S, Malek I, Nyberg G. Pennert K, Ryden L, Swedberg K, Vedin A, Waagstein F (1984). Goteborg Metoprolol Trial: mortality and causes of death. *Am. J. Cardiol* **53**: 9D–14D.
122. Gullestad L, Kjekshus J (1992). Myocardial disease in diabetes mellitus. *Tidsskr Nor Laegeforen* **112**: 1016–1019.
123. Kjekshus J, Gilpin E, Cali G, Blackey AR, Henning H, Ross J Jr (1990). Diabetic patients and beta-blockers after acute myocardial infarction. *Eur. Heart J.* **11**: 43–50.
124. Gundersen T, Kjershus J (1983). Timolol after myocardial infarction in diabetic patients. *Diabetes Care* **6**: 285–290.
125. Lager I, Blohme G, Smith U (1979). Effect of cardio-selective and non-selective beta-blockade on the hypoglycemic response in insulin-dependent diabetics. *Lancet* **1**: 458–462.
126. Rosenson RS (1993). The truth about beta-blocker adverse effects-depression, claudication and lipids. *J. Ambul. Monitoring* **6**: 163–171.
127. The Norwegian Multicenter Study Group (1981). Timolol induced reduction in mortality and reinfarction in patients surviving acute myocardial infarction. *N. Engl. J. Med.* **304**: 801–807.
128. The BHAT Study Group (1982). A randomized trial of propranolol in patients with acute myocardial infarction. Mortality results. *JAMA* **247**: 1707–14.
129. Pfeffer MA, Braunwald E, Moye LA, Basta L, Brown EJ Jr, Cuddy TE, Davis BR, Geltman EM, Goldman S, Flaker GC (1992). Effect of captopril on mortality and morbidity in aptients with left ventricular dysfunction after myocardial infarction: results of the Survival and Ventricular enlargement Trial. *N. Engl. J. Med.* **327**: 669–677.
130. Yusuf S, Pepine CJ, Garces C, Pouleur H, Salem D, Kostis J. Benedict C, Rousseau M, Bourassa M, Pitt B (1992). Effect of enalapril on myocardial infarction and unstable angina in patients with low ejection fractions. *Lancet* **340**: 1173–1178.

131. The Acute Infarction Ramipril Efficacy (AIRE) Study Investigators (1993). Effect of ramipril on mortality and morbidity of survivors of acute myocardial infarction with clinical evidence of heart failure. *Lancet* **342**: 821–828.

132. Garg R, Yusuf Y (1995). Overview of randomized trials of angiotensin-converting enzyme inhibitors on mortality and morbidity in patients with heart failure. *JAMA* **273**: 1450–1456.

133. Lewis EJ, Hunsicker LG, Bain RP, Rohde RD (1993). Effect of angiotensin-converting enzyme inhibition on diabetic nephropathy. *N. Engl. J. Med.* **329**: 1456–1462.

134. Ravid M, Savin H, Jutrin I, Bental T, Katz B, Lishner M (1993). Long-term stabilizing effect of angiotensin-converting enzyme inhibition on plasma creatinine and on proteinuria in normotensive type II diabetic patients. *Ann. Intern. Med.* **118**: 577–81.

135. Zuanetti G, Latini R, Maggioni AP, et al. (1996) on behalf of GISSI-3 Investigators. Prognosis of diabetic patients after myocardial infarction: Effect of early treatment with ACE-inhibitors, *J. Am. Coll. Card.* **27**: 319A.

136. The Heart Outcomes Prevention Evaluation Study Investigators (2000). Effects of an angiotensin-converting-enzyme inhibitor, ramipril, on cardiovascular events in high-risk patients. *N. Engl. J. Med.* **342**: 145–153.

137. Expert Panel on Detection Evaluation and Treatment of High Blood Cholesterol in Adults: Summary of the second report of the National Cholesterol Education Program Expert Panel on Detection, Evaluation and Treatment of High Blood Cholesterol in Adults (Adult Treatment Panel II). *JAMA* (1993) **269**: 3015–3023.

138. Pierce LR, Wysowski DK, Gross TP (1990). Myopathy and rhabdomyolysis associated with lovastatin-gemfibrozil combination therapy. *JAMA* **264**: 71–75.

139. O'Keefe JH, Harris WS (1997). Nicotinic acid – the underused ally in the fight against coronary disease. *J. Cardiovasc. Risk* **4**: 161–163.

140. Johansson JO, Egberg N, Asplund-Carlson A (1997). Nicotinic acid treatment shifts the fibrinolytic balance favorably and decreases plasma fibrinogen in hypertriglyceridemic men. *J. Cardiovasc. Risk* **4**: 165–171.

141. Garg A, Grundy SM (1990). Nicotinic acid as therapy for dyslipidemia in non-insulin-dependent diabetes mellitus. *JAMA* **264**: 723–726.

142. Pyorala K, Pedersen TR, Kjekshus J, Faergeman O, Olsson AG, Thorgeirsson G (1997). Cholesterol lowering with simvastatin improves prognosis of diabetic patients with coronary heart disease. A subgroup analysis of the Scandinavian Simvastatin Survival Study. *Diabetes Care* **20**: 614–620.

143. Sacks FM, Pfeffer MA, Moye LA, Rouleau JL, Rutherford JD, Cole TG, Brown L, Warnica JW, Arnold JM, Wun CC, David BR, Braunwald E (1996). The effect of pravastatin on coronary events after myocardial infarction in patients with average cholesterol levels. *N. Engl. J. Med.* **335**: 1001–1009.

144. Tonkin A, Aylward P, Colquhoun D, et al. (1998) Prevention of cardiovascular events and death with pravastatin in patients with coronary artery disease and a broad range of initial cholesterol levels. *N. Engl. J. Med.* **339**: 1349–1357.

145. Furberg CD, Psaty BM, Meyer JV (1995). Nifedipine: dose-related increase in mortality in patients with coronary heart disease. *Circulation* **92**: 1326–1331.

146. Estacio RO, Schrier RW (1998). Antihypertensive therapy in type II diabetes: implications of appropriate blood-pressure control in diabetes (ABCD) trial. *Am. J. Cardiol* **82**: 9R–14R.

147. Tuomilehto J, Rastenyte D, Birkenhager WH, Thijs L, Antikainen R, Bulpitt CJ, Fletcher AE, Forette F, Goldhaber A, Palatini P, Sarti C, Fagard R (1999).

Effects of calcium channel blockade in older patients with diabetes and systolic hypertension. *N. Engl. J. Med.* **340**: 677–684.

148. Sowers JR (1998). Comordity of hypertension and diabetes: the Fosinopril versus Amlodipine Cardiovascular Events Trial (FACET). *Am. J. Cardiol* **82**: 15R–19R.

149. The Diabetes Control and Complication Trial Research Group (1993). The effect of intensive treatment of diabetes on the development and progression of long-term complications in insulin-dependent diabetes mellitus. *N. Engl. J. Med.* **329**: 977–986.

150. United Kingdom Prospective Diabetes Study (UKPDS) Group (1998). Intensive blood-glucose control with sulphonylureas or insulin compared with conventional treatment and risk of complications in patients with type II diabetes (UKPDS 33). *Lancet* **352**: 837–853.

151. Jensen-Urstad KJ, Reichard PG, Rosfors JS, Lindblad LE, Jensen-Urstad MT (1996). Early atherosclerosis is retarded by improved long-term blood glucose control in patients with IDDM. *Diabetes* **45**: 1253–1258.

152. Malmberg K, Ryden L, Efendic S, Herlitz J, Nicol P, Waldenstrom A, Wedel H, Welin L (1995). On behalf of the DIGAMI Study Group. Randomized trial of insulin-glucose infusion followed by subcutaneous insulin treatment in diabetic patients with acute myocardial infarction (DIGAMI Study): effects on mortality at one year. *J. Am. Coll.Cardiol.* **26**: 57–65.

153. Schwartz S, Raskin P, Fonseca V, Graveline JF (1998). (Troglitazone and Exogenous Insulin Study Group). Effect of trpglitazone in insulin-treated patients with type II diabetes mellitus. *N. Engl. J. Med.* **338**: 861–866.

154. Watkins PB, Whitcomb RW (1998). Hepatic dysfunction associated with troglitazone [letter]. *N. Engl. J. Med.* **338**: 916–917.

155. Leibowitz G, Cerasi E (1996). Sulphonylurea treatment on NIDDM patients with cardiovascular disease: a mixed blessing? Diabetologia **39**: 503–514.

156. Baker JE, Curry BD, Olinger GN, Gross GJ (1997). Increased tolerance of the chronically hypoxic immature heart to ischemia: contribution of the KATP channel. *Circulation* **95**: 1278–1285.

157. Smits P, Thien T (1995). Cardiovascular effects of sulphonylurea derivatives: implications for the treatment of NIDDM? *Diabetologia* **38**: 116–121.

158. O'Keefe JH, Blackstone EH, Sergeant P, McCallister BD (1998). The optimal mode of coronary revascularization for diabetics: a risk-adjusted long-term study comparing coronary angioplasty and coronary bypass surgery. *Eur. Heart. J.* **19**: 1696–1703.

159. Granger CB, Califf RM, Young S, Candela R, Samaha J, Worley S, Kereiakes DJ, Topol EJ (1993). Outcomes of patients with diabetes mellitus and acute myocardial infarction treated with thrombolytic agents: the Thrombolysis and Acute Myocardial Infarction (TAMI) Study Group. *J. Am. Coll. Cardiol.* **21**: 920–925.

160. Barbash GI, White HD, Modan M, Van de Werf F (1993). Investigators of the International Tissue Plasminogen Activator/Streptokinase Mortality Trial. Significance of diabetes mellitus in patients with acute myocardial infarction receiving thrombolytic therapy. *J. Am. Coll. Cardiol.* **22**: 707–713.

161. Zuanetti G, Latini R, Maggioni AP, Santoto L, Franzosi MG (1993). Infuence of diabetes on mortality in acute myocardial infarction: data from GISSI 2 study. *J. Am. Coll. Cardiol.* **22**: 1788–1794.

162. Lee KL, Wood LH, Topol EJ, Weaver WD, Betriu A, Col J, Simoons M, Aylward P, Van de Werf F, Califf RM (1995) for the GUSTO-I Investigators.

Predictors of 30-day mortality in the era of reperfusion for acute myocardial infarction. *Circulation* **91**: 1659–1668.

163. Fibrinolytic Therapy Trialist (FTT) Collaborative Group (1994). Indications for fibrinolytic therapy in suspected acute myocardial infarction: Collaborative overview of early mortality and major morbidity results from all randomized trials of more than 1000 patients. *Lancet* **343**: 311–322.

164. Carmelli B, Transcesci B, Jr. Gebara OC, de Sa LC, Pileggi FJ (1991). Retinal hemorrhage after thrombolytic therapy. *Lancet* **337**: 1356–1357.

165. Mahaffey KW, Granger CB, Toth CA, White HD, Stebbins AL, Barbash GI, Vahanian A, Topol EJ, Califf RM (1997). Diabetic retinopathy should not be a contraindication to thrombolytic therapy for acute myocardial infarction: review of ocular hemorrhage incidence and location in the GUSTO-I trial. *J Am Coll Cardiol* **30**: 1606–1610.

166. Stone GW, Grines CL, Browne KF, et al. (1995) Does primary angioplasty improve the prognosis of patients with diabetes and acute myocardial infarction? *J. Am. Coll. Cardiol.* **25**: 401A.

167. Wilson SH, Velianou JL, Caplice NM, et al. (1999) Coronary stent placement is associated with improved outcomes in diabetics with acute myocardial infarction treated with primary percutaneous coronary intervention. *Circulation* **100**: I-365.

168. McGarvey JFX, Johnson JD, Souther J, et al. (1999) Coronary stenting reduces mortality in diabetics with acute myocardial infarction:six-month follow-up in the 500 patient propective PAMI-no SOS Registry. *Circulation* I-139.

169. Stein B, Weintraub WS, Gebhart SP, Cohen Bernstein CL. Grosswald R, Liberman HA. Douglas Js Jr. Morris DC. King SB 3rd (1995). Influence of diabetes mellitus on early and late outcome after percutaneous transluminal coronary angioplasty. *Circulation* **91**: 979–989.

170. Holmes DR, Viestra RE, Smith HC, Vetrovec GW, Kent KM, Cowley MJ, Faxon DP, Gruentzig AR, Kelsey SF, Detre KM (1984). Restenosis after percutaneous transluminal coronary angioplasty (PTCA): a report from PTCA Registry of National Heart, Lung, and Blood Institute. *Am. J. Cardiol* **53**: 77C–81C.

171. Weintraub WS, Kosinki AS, Brown CL 3rd, King SB 3rd (1993). Can restenosis after coronary angioplasty be predicted from clinical variables? *J. Am. Coll. Cardiol.* **21**: 6–14.

172. Vandormael MG, Deligonul U, Kern MJ, Harper M, Presant S, Gibson P, Galan K, Chaitman BR (1987). Multilesion coronary angioplasty: Clinical and angiographic outcome. *J. Am. Coll. Cardiol.* **10**: 246–252.

173. Lambert M, Bonan R, Cote G, Crepeau, J, de Guise P, Lesperance J, David PR, Waters DD (1988). Multiple coronary angioplasty: A model to discriminate systemic and procedural factors related to restenosis. *J. Am. Coll. Cardiol.* **12**: 310–314.

174. Warth DC, Leon MB, O'Neil W, Zacca N, Polissar NL, Buchbinder M (1994). Rotational atherectomy multicenter registry: Acute results, complications and six-month angiographic follow-up in 709 patients. *J. Am. Coll. Cardiol.* **24**: 641–648.

175. Carozza JP, Kuntz RE, Fishman RF, Baim DS (1993). Restenosis after arterial injury caused by coronary stenting in patients with diabetes mellitus. *Ann. Intern. Med.* **118**: 344–349.

176. Wong SC, Baim DS, Schatz RA, Teirstein PS, King SB 3rd, Curry RC Jr, Heuser RR, Ellis SG, Cleman MW, Overlie P (1995). Immediate results and late

outcome after stent implantation in saphenous vein graft lesions: the multicenter US Palmaz–Shatz experience. *J. Am. Coll. Cardiol.* **26**: 704–712.

177. Rabbani LE, Edelman ER, Ganz P, Selwyn AP, Loscalzo J, Bittl JA (1994). Relation of restenosis after excimer laser angioplasty to fasting insulin levels. *Am. J. Cardiol* **73**: 323–327.

178. Van Belle E, Bauters C, Hubert E, Bodart JC, Abolmaali K, Meurice T, McFadden EP, Lablanche JM, Bertrand ME (1997). Restenosis rates in diabetic patients: a comparison of coronary stenting and balloon angioplasty in native coronary vessels. *Circulation* **96**: 1454–1460.

179. Marso SP, Lincoff AM, Ellis SG, Bhatt DL, Tanguay JF, Kleiman NS, Hammond T, Booth JE, Sapp SK, Topol EJ (1999). Optimizing the percutaneous interventional outcomes for patients with diabetes mellitus: results of the EPISTENT (Evaluation of Platelet IIb/IIIa Inhibitor for Stenting trial) diabetic Substudy. *Circulation* **100**: 2477–2484.

180. Barzilay JJ, Kronmal RA, Bittner V, Eaker E, Evans C, Foster ED (1994). Coronary artery disease and coronary artery bypass grafting in diabetic patients aged >65 years (Report from Coronary Artery Surgery Study Registry). *Am. J. Cardiol.* **74**: 334–339.

181. Morris JJ, Smith LR, Jones RH, Glower DD, Morris PB, Muhlbaier LH, Reves JG, Rankin JS (1991). Influence of diabetes and mammary artery artery grafting on survival after corornary bypass. *Circulation* **84**: III-275–III-284.

182. Lawrie G, Morris G, Glaeser D (1986). Influence of diabetes mellitus on the results of coronary artery bypass surgery. *JAMA* **256**: 2967–2971.

183. The Bypass Angioplasty Revascularization Investigation (BARI) Investigators (1996). Comparison of bypass surgery with angioplasty in aptients with multivessel disease. *N. Engl. J. Med.* **335**: 217–225.

184. CABRI Trial Participants (1995). First year of results of CABRI (Coronary Angioplasty versus Bypass Revascularization Investigation). *Lancet* **346**: 1179–1184.

185. Gum PA, O'Keefe JH, Borkon AM, Spertus JA, Bateman TM, McGraw JP, Sherwani K, Vacek J, McCallister BD (1997). Bypass surgery versus coronary angioplasty for revascularization of treated diabetic patients. *Circulation* **96**: II7–II10.

186. O'Keefe JH, Blackstone EH, Sergeant P, McCallister BD (1998). The optimal mode of coronary revascularization for diabetics; a risk-adjusted long-term study comparing coronary angioplasty and coronary bypass surgery. *Eur. Heart J.* **33**: 119–124.

187. Barsness GW, Peterson ED, Ohman EM, Nelson CL, Delong ER, Reves JG, Smith PK, Anderson RD, Jones RH, Mark DB, Califf RM (1997). Relationship between diabetes mellitus and long-term survival after coronary bypass and angioplasty. *Circulation* **96**: 2551–2556.

188. King SB, Lembo NJ, Weintraub WS, Kosinski AS, Barnhart HX, Kutner MH, Alazraki NP, Guyton RA, Zhao XQ (1994). (Emory Angioplasty versus Surgery Trial [EAST]). A randomized trial comparing coronary angioplasty with coronary bypass surgery. *N. Engl. J. Med.* **331**: 1044–1050

189. Duell PB (1999). Diabetes Mellitus. In: Betteridge DJ, ed. Lipoproteins in Health and Disease. Neew York, NY: Oxford University Press; 897–929.

190. Heart Outcomes Prevention Evaluation (HOPE) Study Investigators (2000). Effects of ramipril on cardiovascular and microvascular outcomes in people with diabetes mellitus: results of the HOPE study and MICRO-HOPE substudy. *Lancet* 355: 253–259.

26

Treatment of Cerebrovascular Disease

SUSAN L. HICKENBOTTOM

University of Michigan Health System, Ann Arbor, Michigan, USA

Stroke is an international problem that creates tremendous personal and economic burdens. Approximately 4.6 million deaths from stroke occur each year, making stroke the second most common cause of death worldwide[1]. Population-based studies in Europe, the USA, Australia and Asia have estimated overall stroke incidence rates to range from 200/100 000 to 500/100 000[2-4]. Caring for stroke is an expensive undertaking. Stroke accounts for almost 5% of all health service costs in the UK[5]. In 1997, the estimated direct cost for acute care of stroke was found to be £1.1–1.6 million/100 000 population per year[6]. In the USA, the total cost for stroke has been estimated at US$41 billion per year, which includes both direct costs for hospitalization and indirect costs such as lost productivity at work[7].

Cerebrovascular disease has been recognized as a complication of diabetes mellitus but, until recently, surprisingly little information regarding the specific epidemiology and pathophysiology of diabetes and stroke has been available. Over the past several years, new information about the nature of stroke in diabetes and potential treatment strategies has become available. Better understanding of the epidemiology, pathophysiology and clinical features of cerebrovascular disease in the diabetic patient can assist physicians in the appropriate management of this condition.

The Evidence Base for Diabetes Care. Edited by R. Williams, W. Herman, A.-L. Kinmonth and N. J. Wareham.

EPIDEMIOLOGY

ISCHEMIC STROKE

Multiple epidemiological studies have demonstrated that diabetes is an independent risk factor for ischemic stroke, with the vast majority focusing on type 2 diabetes. Table 26.1 outlines prospective studies that have shown an increased relative risk for stroke in diabetic populations. The Framingham study initially revealed that the incidence of ischemic stroke was 2.5–3.5 times higher in diabetic patients[8]. Later adjustments for the influence of cofactors such as age, systolic blood pressure, antihypertensive therapy, cigarette smoking, ischemic cardiovascular disease and atrial fibrillation still found diabetes to be an independent risk factor for stroke[9]. The Honolulu Heart Program demonstrated that diabetic men were almost 2.5 times as likely to suffer a stroke than men without diabetes[10]. More recent large-scale prospective studies from the UK and USA have also demonstrated diabetes to be an independent risk factor for stroke with similar relative risks as the older studies[11,12]. Differences in relative risks between the studies can be explained by differences in definition of diabetes used, type of stroke examined and specific population differences, such as geographic location, race/ethnic mix, age and sex. In retrospective case-control studies, diabetes has also been found to be an independent risk factor for stroke. One study of 1444 ischemic stroke patients found the odds ratio for stroke in the setting of diabetes to be 1.7 (95% confidence interval (CI), 1.2–2.4)[13]. Similar risks for transient ischemic attack (TIA) were also identified[14]. Using these data, the investigators estimated the population-attributable risk (PAR) of stroke from diabetes to be 5% (95% CI, 2–9)[15]. In this model, diabetes appeared to be a less potent risk factor for ischemic stroke than cigarette smoking, ischemic heart disease or hypertension, for which PARs ranged from 12–26%. These findings have mirrored results from prospective studies, which have also found diabetes to be a less marked risk factor than those outlined above[16].

A relatively new development in this arena is the investigation of the relationship between hyperglycemia, glucose intolerance, hyperinsulinemia and the incidence of ischemic stroke in nondiabetic patients. Data regarding these possible risk factors for stroke are conflicting. Some studies demonstrate a positive association, though not always statistically significant, between ischemic stroke and: (1) hyperglycemia[17,18]; (2) glucose intolerance[19–21]; and (3) hyperinsulinemia[12,22]. Other studies have shown no independent association between these factors and stroke: (1) hyperglycemia[11]; (2) glucose intolerance[23]; and (3) hyperinsulinemia[11,17,24.] Criticisms of the studies that showed a positive association between these factors and stroke have included small numbers of subjects evaluated, the inclusion of subjects with subclinical diabetes, and demonstration of increased risk only at the extreme end of the

Table 26.1. Relative risk of stroke in diabetic persons according to prospective studies (Modified from Lukovits *et al.* 1999, with permission)

Location	Author	N	% diabetic	Sex	Stroke type	Relative risk
Framingham, MA	D'Augustino et al. 1994	2372 3362	10.6 7.9	men women	all (and TIA)	1.41 (0.97–2.04) 1.75 (1.25–2.45)
Rochester, MN	Davis et al. 1987	686 938	13.8 combined	men women	ischemic	2.6 (CI not reported) n.s.
MRFIT sites	Stamler et al. 1993	347978	1.5	men	fatal	2.8 (2.0–3.7)
Finland	Tuomilehto et al. 1996	8077 8572	4.6 18.8	men women	fatal	3.35 (1.96–5.43) 4.89 (2.83–8.45)
Honolulu, HI	Abbott et al. 1987	7598	9.1	men	ischemic	2.45 (1.73–3.47)
Rancho Bernardo, California	Barrett-Connor et al. 1988	1729 2049	11.2 6.1	men women	all	1.7 (1.0–2.9) 1.3 (0.7–2.5)
Finland	Kuuisisto et al. 1994	470 828	15.7 18.8	men women	all	1.36 (0.44–4.18) 2.25 (1.65–3.06)
United Kingdom	Wannamethee et al. 1999	7735	5.4	men	all	2.27 (1.23–4.20)
ARIC sites	Folsom et al. 1999	15792	10	both	ischemic	3.70 (2.7–5.1)

Figures in parentheses indicate 95% confidence intervals. n.s = not statistically significant; MRFIT = Multicenter Risk Factor Intervention Trial, ARIC = Atherosclerosis Risk in Communities; TIA = transient ischemic attack.

distribution of the population. Further large-scale studies will need to be done to establish the actual relationship between glucose intolerance/hyperinsulinemia and the risk of ischemic stroke.

Few studies have specifically addressed the relationship between type 1 diabetes and stroke. A prospective study of patients who had type 1 diabetes for more than 40 years reported a 10% incidence of stroke and 7% mortality from stroke[25]. Review of death certificates in the UK found similar rates of death attributable to type 1 diabetes[26].

HEMORRHAGIC STROKE

While there is strong evidence that diabetes is an independent risk factor for ischemic stroke, the few epidemiologic studies examining its relationship with hemorrhagic stroke have demonstrated a negative association. In the general population, stroke results from ischemic infarction approximately 80% of the time and from cerebral hemorrhage approximately 20% of the time. However, in the Rochester Epidemiolgic Project, ischemic stroke accounted for just over 88% of all strokes among diabetics[27]. Primary intracerebral hemorrhage (ICH) occurred six times less frequently in the Copenhagen Stroke Project[28]. The risk of ICH was not significantly increased in the Honolulu Heart Program[29]. In the only study to examine the association between diabetes and subarachnoid hemorrhage, (the University of Iowa–Cooperative Aneurysm Study), a negative correlation was demonstrated[29].

PATHOPHYSIOLOGY

PATHOLOGICAL CHANGES

Autopsy studies have demonstrated a greater frequency of cerebral infarction in diabetic individuals[30–33]. These studies found a much higher frequency of small vessel ischemic disease of the penetrating arteries supplying the basal ganglia, thalamus, pons and cerebellum, resulting in 'lacunar' infarction. Smaller autopsy series have not reported an association between diabetes alone and lacunar infarction, but do note the association between diabetes, hypertension and lacunar disease[34]. Other studies have also noted the potentially synergistic effect of hypertension and diabetes on the cerebral vasculature[35–37]. Histopathologic changes seen in cerebral small vessels in diabetics include endothelial proliferation and 'hyaline arteriosclerosis', or 'lipohyalinosis'[130,38]. This condition affects the small penetrating arteries in the brain, in which medial smooth muscle first hypertrophies and is then replaced by extracellular and plasma proteins, eventually leading to vessel occlusion and the production of small, deep lacunar infarcts. There is much less information available on large vessel atherosclerotic disease in the diabetic population. Certainly, systemic atherosclerotic disease occurs earlier and more commonly in diabetics and advances more rapidly, but there has been little pathological documentation of such changes in the cerebral circulation. Some autopsy studies have found large vessel cerebral occlusive disease to be more frequent in diabetics, while others have not[30,37]. With regard to hemorrhagic stroke, autopsy studies found it to be uncommon in diabetics, mirroring the results of epidemiologic studies[30,31,33,39].

PHYSIOLOGICAL CHANGES

Numerous investigators have also speculated that other pathogenic factors may be at play in cerebral ischemia in the diabetic patient. Hyperglycemia itself is a major determinant of diabetic complications, as has been discussed earlier in this text. In the setting of acute ischemic stroke, hyperglycemia may arise as the result of underlying diabetes, or serum glucose may increase from physiologic stress, or both. However, many authors argue that hyperglycemia arises independently of the stress response and thus may be seen to a greater degree in diabetics[40–42].

Animal models of focal ischemia indicate that hyperglycemia increases the extent of ischemic brain damage in some settings[43–46]. There are several possible explanations for worsening of ischemic damage in the presence of hyperglycemia. Under hypoxic conditions, elevated serum glucose levels result in increased anaerobic metabolism, lactic acid production and cellular acidosis, which causes damage to neurons, glial cells and vascular tissue[47–50]. Moreover, hyperglycemia increases the risk for cerebral edema formation[51]. The extracellular concentrations of the excitatory neurotransmitters, glutamate and aspartate, are elevated in the presence of hyperglycemia and hypoxia[52]. These neurotransmitters initiate an extensive cascade of neurotoxic biochemical steps, including increased intracellular calcium levels and free radical production[53]. Finally, animal models have demonstrated that hyperglycemia promotes the development of hemorrhagic transformation of ischemic infarcts[54]. Retrospective case-control and case series of human subjects have also reported an association between elevated blood glucose and/or history of diabetes and hemorrhagic transformation of ischemic infarcts[55,56].

Pathogenic factors other than hyperglycemia may also contribute to cerebrovascular disease in the diabetic patient, and are outlined in Table 26.2. These mechanisms are not mutually exclusive and many may play a role in worsening ischemic damage from stroke in the diabetic patient.

OUTCOME OF STROKE IN DIABETES

Diabetic patients have worse outcome from stroke when it occurs, perhaps because of the pathophysiological derangements described above. Mortality is

Table 26.2. Factors that may promote ischemic cerebrovascular disease in the diabetic patient

Endothelial dysfunction	Cohen 1993
	Dandona *et al.*1978
	Johnstone *et al.*1993
Platelet dysfunction	Colwell *et al.*1983
	Davi *et al.*1990
Hyperviscosity/hypercoaguability	Barnes *et al.*1977
	Biller and Love 1993
Decreased fibrinolytic activity	McGill *et al.*1994
Excessive production of advanced glycation end-products (AGEs)	Lyons 1993
	Wolffenbuttel and van Haeften 1995
Upregulation of immediate-early genes	Koistinaho *et al.*1999

increased both in patients with previously diagnosed diabetes[28,57,58]. and in those with acute hyperglycemia[11,42]. Recovery is also poorer and proceeds more slowly in those with diabetes or hyperglycemia[48,59,60]. A recent meta-analysis of 20 studies concluded that hyperglycemia is associated with increased 30-day mortality and with worse functional outcome one year following stroke[61].

TREATMENT

PRIMARY STROKE PREVENTION

Clearly, the best way to decrease the burden created by stroke is to prevent it from occurring in the first place. Primary stroke prevention in diabetic patients is achieved through risk factor modification, which has been addressed in previous chapters. It is important to emphasize here, though, that well-established modifiable risk factors for stroke should be sought in the diabetic patient and treated according to established guidelines. These risk factors include hypertension, ischemic cardiac disease, atrial fibrillation (AF), hyperlipidemia and cigarette smoking[62]. An excellent review of guidelines for the prevention of first stroke has been published by the National Stroke Association[63]. Patients should also be questioned for a history of focal neurologic symptoms suggestive of TIA or stroke, which would then place them in the category of secondary prevention.

Unlike the other risk factors listed above, nonvalvular AF has not traditionally been associated with diabetes. Nevertheless, the United Kingdom Prospective Diabetes Study identified AF as the risk factor most strongly identified with stroke in patients newly diagnosed with diabetes; diabetics with AF were eight times more likely to suffer a stroke than those in sinus rhythm[64]. If AF is detected, patients at high risk for thromboembolism should be started on long-term anticoagulation with warfarin with goal International Normalized Ratio (INR) of 2.0–3.0, presuming they have no obvious contraindications to anticoagulation. The Stroke Prevention in Atrial Fibrillation III trial classified patients at high risk if they had congestive heart failure or left ventricular fraction shortening of less than 25%, had previous evidence of thromboembolism, had systolic blood pressure greater than 160 mmHg or were over 75 years of age[65]. The trial was terminated early after patients receiving adjusted-dose warfarin demonstrated a significantly lower annual rate of ischemic stroke and systemic embolism than those treated with aspirin and low, fixed-dose warfarin (1.9% versus 7.9%, respectively) with no difference in the rate of major bleeding events. For patients with none of these risk factors, the risk for stroke from AF is relatively low and these patients can be managed with aspirin alone[66].

Finally, it should be noted that although aspirin has conclusively been found to be beneficial in the primary prevention of ischemic heart disease, it has never been demonstrated to be effective in the primary prevention of ischemic stroke[67,68]. Some studies raised the concern for increased rates of intracranial hemorrhage in patients receiving aspirin[68,69]. However, studies of antiplatelet agent use in diabetics suggest no increased risk for cerebrovascular hemorrhage[70,71]. As such, the American Diabetes Association recommends the use of low-dose enteric coated aspirin (81–325 mg) as safe and effective therapy for patients over the age of 30 with diabetes who also have other risk factors for vascular disease, including family history of coronary heart disease, hypertension, cigarette smoking, obesity and dyslipidemia[72].

SECONDARY STROKE PREVENTION

Once stroke or TIA has occurred, emphasis shifts to preventing recurrent stroke. Diabetic patients appear to be at higher risk of stroke recurrence. Short-term (30-day) stroke recurrence has been found to be more frequent in diabetics than non-diabetics (4.88% versus 2.65%, respectively)[73]. Other studies have documented increased long-term recurrence rates in diabetics, with relative risk ratios approximately 1.7 when compared to non-diabetics[74–76]. Hyperglycemia at the time of hospitalization for acute ischemic stroke has also been found to lead to increased risk for stroke recurrence[77]. One relatively large population-based study did not demonstrate an increased risk of stroke recurrence in diabetics, but subjects in this study maintained good glycemic control following the initial event[78].

Certainly, risk factor modification as recommended for the primary prevention of stroke should also be pursued in secondary stroke prevention. Detailed descriptions of interventions for glycemic control, hypertension, hyperlipidemia, tobacco use and physical inactivity and adiposity are left to other chapters. In addition to risk factor modification, specific pharmacologic and/or surgical interventions can be implemented to prevent stroke recurrence.

PHARMACOLOGIC INTERVENTION

Antiplatelet agents

Until recently, aspirin was the only antiplatelet agent available for secondary stroke prevention. Now, several others – ticlopidine, clopidogrel and dipyridamole – have also been found to be effective in preventing stroke and other vascular events in patients with cerebrovascular disease. Few of the antiplatelet trials have analyzed specific benefits for diabetic patients, but data regarding diabetics will be discussed below, where it is available. Otherwise, results from secondary prevention trials in the general stroke population will have to be applied to the management of the diabetic patient.

Aspirin: In the Antiplatelet Trialists' (APT) metanalysis of 145 randomized trials of antiplatelet therapy in non-diabetic and diabetic patients who had already had a major vascular event, the odds reduction for stroke or vascular death attributable to aspirin therapy alone was 25%[79]. This study also analyzed differences in response to antiplatelet agents by age, sex and various risk factors. No difference in response was detected in diabetics as compared to non-diabetics. In a smaller metanalysis of 10 APT trials which evaluated the benefit of aspirin alone in patients with prior stroke or TIA as entry criteria, aspirin reduced the odds for stroke, MI or vascular death by only 16%[80]. Nonetheless, aspirin currently remains the standard initial medical treatment for the secondary prevention of stroke, given its low rate of side-effects and low cost[62]. Further trials may help to delineate specific high-risk stroke populations who might benefit more from the selection of alternate antiplatelet agents as an initial step in secondary stroke prevention.

The optimal dose of aspirin for the stroke prevention remains somewhat controversial, with doses in randomized clinical trials ranging from 30–1300 mg daily. Only two trials performed head-to-head comparison of different aspirin doses, and neither demonstrated any difference in efficacy based on aspirin dose[81,82]. Furthermore, meta-analysis across all trials of aspirin for secondary stroke prevention has not demonstrated differences in efficacy between high-dose (900–1500 mg/day), medium-dose (300 mg/day) and low-dose (50–75 mg/day) regimens[83]. More favorable side-effect profiles have been seen with low to medium doses, with fewer bleeding events and far fewer gastrointestinal events[83]. Thus, current guidelines for the use of aspirin in secondary stroke prevention recommend doses of between 50–325 mg daily[84].

Ticlopidine: Ticlopidine is a thienopyridine that inhibits platelet aggregation induced by adenosine phosphate. Two randomized trials have evaluated ticlopidine for secondary stroke prevention. In the Ticlopidine Aspirin Stroke Study (TASS), patients with TIA or minor stroke received ticlopidine, 250 mg twice daily, or aspirin, 650 mg twice daily.(Hass *et al.* 1989) The risk for non-fatal stroke or death was 17% in the ticlopidine arm and 19% in the aspirin arm; a small but significant reduction. *Post hoc* analysis of the TASS data examined patient baseline characteristics to determine if treatment effect differed in various subgroups[85]. This analysis indicated diabetics requiring medical treatment had fewer strokes when treated with ticlopidine (9.4% as compared to 17.2% with aspirin). However, caution must be used when applying these results clinically, since the analysis was not preplanned and included only a small number of patients.

The Canadian American Ticlopidine Study (CATS) compared ticlopidine, 250 mg twice daily, with placebo in patients with major stroke, and demonstrated an absolute risk reduction of 4% for stroke, MI and vascular death in patients treated with ticlopidine (10.8% versus 15.3% with placebo)[86]. Taken together, these trials show that ticlopidine significantly reduced the risk for stroke and other vascular outcomes in patients with cerebrovascular disease, and TASS demonstrated superiority over aspirin, perhaps with additional benefits seen in diabetic patients treated with ticlopidine.

In both trials, however, side-effects of diarrhea and rash were more common in the ticlopidine-treated group and about 4% were unable to tolerate the drug. Severe neutropenia occurred in about 1% of patients receiving ticlopidine, which resulted in recommendations for frequent blood-count monitoring during the first three months of therapy. More recently, 60 cases of thrombotic thrombocytopenic purpura associated with ticlopidine use have been reported[87]. Ticlopidine's poor side-effect profile and the introduction of newer antiplatelet agents with similar efficacy but minimal adverse effects have led to a substantial reduction in its use for secondary stroke prevention.

Clopidogrel: Clopidogrel is a new thienopyridine with a similar mechanism of action as ticlopidine. The Clopidogrel versus Aspirin in Patients at Risk of Ischemic Events (CAPRIE) trial found that the annual combined risk for MI, ischemic stroke or vascular death was 5.32% in clopidogrel-treated patients (75 mg/day) and 5.83% in patients receiving 325 mg of aspirin daily[88]. The absolute risk reduction of 0.5% for combined vascular end-points was small but statistically significant. However, for the over 6400 patients entered into CAPRIE with a stroke as the qualifying event, no statistically significant difference was seen between the treatment groups in the rates of combined end-point (MI, stroke or vascular death). Safety and side-effect profiles were similar for aspirin and clopidogrel. *Post hoc* analysis of the CAPRIE data has been performed to look for additional benefit over aspirin in high-risk patients, but no such analysis specifically examining diabetic patients has been done to date.

Dipyridamole: Dipyridamole is a platelet adhesion inhibitor that is postulated to work through interaction with adenosine uptake and inhibition of thromboxane A_2. Until recently, no trials had shown benefit for dipyridamole use in secondary stroke prevention. The Antiplatelet Trialists' meta-analysis found no significant difference in stroke prevention between treatment with dipyridamole and treatment with aspirin, in either diabetic or non-diabetic patients, although both agents were superior to placebo[79]. In the European Stroke Prevention Study (ESPS), 216 diabetic patients were treated with dipyridamole and aspirin had a statistically insignificant reduction in the risk of stroke, all cerebrovascular events and death when compared to placebo[89]. In the VA Cooperative Study, 231 diabetic patients with recent gangrene and amputation were treated with dipyridamole and aspirin and had a lower incidence of stroke and TIA than the placebo group, but no reduction in primary vascular end-points, and a higher mortality rate[90]. More recently, the second European Stroke Prevention Study (ESPS 2) randomized patients with TIA or stroke to one of four treatment arms: placebo, aspirin alone (25 mg twice daily), dipyridamole alone (modified-release formula, 200 mg twice daily) or a combination of aspirin and modified-release dipyridamole[91]. Risk of stroke or death was reduced by 13% with aspirin alone, by 16% with dipyridamole alone, and by 24% with the combination therapy, all of which were statistically significant results. No specific subgroup analysis of diabetics has been performed on the ESPS 2 data.

ORAL ANTICOAGULANT AGENTS

As with many of the antiplatelet agents, little is known about the specific role of warfarin in secondary stroke prevention in the diabetic patient. Thus, results from studies of general stroke populations will have to be applied to those with diabetes. The most extensive studies of warfarin for stroke prevention have been done in patients with non-valvular AF, and the recommendations for the use of warfarin for primary stroke prevention in the setting of AF, outlined above, should be applied to secondary prevention as well. Other indications for warfarin in stroke prevention have been less well studied, such as following MI[92], with intracranial atherosclerotic disease[93] or with hypercoaguable states[94]. Prospective data are needed before firm treatment recommendations can be made in these clinical settings.

The use of warfarin as compared to aspirin in the general stroke population has been evaluated in a double-blind controlled trial that randomized patients to either low-dose aspirin (30 mg/day) or relatively high-dose warfarin (INR 3.0–4.5)[95]. This trial was terminated prematurely because of significant excess in major bleeding complications in the warfarin-treated group. The results of this trial clearly indicate that warfarin therapy with an INR between 3.0–4.5 is unsafe for secondary prevention in the general stroke population, and should not be used in diabetic patients. A large multicenter randomized trial is underway to investigate the safety and efficacy of moderate dose warfarin (INR 1.4–2.8) as compared to 325 mg of aspirin daily in secondary prevention in the general stroke population (the Warfarin–Aspirin Recurrent Stroke Study). A prospective multicenter, randomized trial of warfarin compared to aspirin in patients with symptomatic intracranial cerebrovascular disease has also begun, and may be of particular importance in diabetic patients, who may be at higher risk of intracranial atherosclerosis.

SURGICAL INTERVENTION

In addition to risk factor modification and pharmacologic therapy, carotid endarterectomy (CEA) may also play a role in secondary stroke prevention in selected patients. Two large randomized clinical trials, the North American

Symptomatic Carotid Endarterectomy Trial (NASCET) and the European Carotid Surgery Trial (ECST) have demonstrated marked benefits of CEA in preventing recurrent ipsilateral stroke in symptomatic patients with moderate to severe carotid stenosis[96-98]. The NASCET enrolled patients with 30–99% symptomatic carotid stenosis. In patients with severe (70–90%) stenosis, a dramatic reduction was found in the rate of ipsilateral stroke for patients undergoing CEA and medical treatment as compared to those receiving medical therapy alone (9% versus 26% at two years, respectively). The ECST found similar results, although the degree of stenosis for which benefit was documented was somewhat higher (80%). Differences in the outcomes of the two trials are partly explained by the different methods used to calculate degree of stenosis. More recently, the NASCET has also demonstrated a less robust, but statistically significant, benefit for CEA in patients with moderate (50–69%) carotid stenosis: a 15.7% rate of ipsilateral stroke over five years among patients treated surgically versus 22.2% in medically managed patients. Patients with less than 50% stenosis did not benefit from CEA.

While lacunar infarction is thought to be most common in diabetic patients, extracranial carotid disease may also contribute to cerebrovascular disease among diabetics. A prospective study of diabetic patients, revealed that greater than 50% stenosis was detected in 8.2% of diabetic patients, compared to 0.7% of matched controls[99]. Other studies have also documented the association between diabetes and angiographically documented extracranial carotid artery occlusion[100,101]. However, care should be taken in pursuing CEA in some diabetic patients. *Post hoc* subgroup analysis performed on NASCET patients with moderate (50–69%) stenosis revealed that those with diabetes were less likely to benefit from CEA than those without diabetes. Moreover, studies of patients undergoing endarterectomy have shown that diabetics may have increased postoperative mortality, mainly due to higher rates of MI[102].

A possible alternative to CEA is carotid angioplasty and stenting (CAS). To date, only anecdotal experience with this technique has been reported, but a randomized trial comparing CEA and CAS, the Carotid Revascularization Endarterectomy versus Stent Trial (CREST), is now underway.

ACUTE STROKE TREATMENT

Fundamentals of management

In general, the work-up and treatment of acute stroke in the diabetic patient do not differ greatly from that in the non-diabetic patient. Basic management of the patient with acute stroke begins in the emergency department. The patient should have a rapid evaluation to ensure adequate airway, breathing and circulatory status. Vital signs, including temperature, pulse, blood pressure and oxygen saturation should be monitored frequently. Endotracheal intubation and mechanical ventilation should be instituted in those patients unable to protect the airway or in those with poor ventilatory drive. Patients with stable respiratory function may receive supplemental oxygen to maintain adequate tissue saturation, since hypoxia may further worsen ischemia[103]. Rapid determination of blood glucose level should be made in all acute stroke patients to rule out hypo- or hyperglycemia as a cause of neurologic deficit. This is especially important in diabetic patients who are more predisposed to develop these metabolic abnormalities. Other laboratory work-ups include a complete blood count, chemistry profiles and coagulation studies. A toxicology profile may be ordered in young patients and any others suspected of illicit drug use. An electrocardiogram should be obtained to assess for evidence of arrhythmia or cardiac ischemia; if clinically indicated, a serum cardiac ischemia profile may be ordered. A sample emergency department protocol for the initial management of acute ischemic stroke is provided in Table 26.3.

Treatment of hypertension in acute stroke remains controversial. Mild to moderate elevation of blood pressure is common in the first hours after acute stroke and gradually resolves without intervention[104,105]. Normal cerebral autoregulation is disrupted in acute ischemia with cerebral perfusion in the ischemic areas dependent on systemic arterial pressure[106]. Overly aggressive blood pressure reduction to normotensive levels may worsen the ischemic insult; as such, recent evidence-based guidelines recommend minimal or no initial treatment of mild to moderate hypertension in the setting of acute ischemic stroke[107]. Antihypertensive therapy may be considered, however, in

Table 26.3. Emergency department protocol for the initial management of presumed acute ischemic stroke.

1. Obtain vital signs including temperature, pulse, blood pressure and oxygen saturation; continue to monitor every 15 minutes.
2. Begin continuous cardiac and oxygen saturation monitoring.
3. Ensure adequate airway/respiratory status:
    a. Intubate and initiate mechanical ventilation if necessary.
    b. Otherwise, begin oxygen at 2 liters per minute via nasal cannula.
4. IV access: 0.9 normal saline at 50 cc/hr; saline lock in opposite arm.
5. STAT laboratory studies:
    a. Serum glucose (may be done at bedside).
    b. Complete blood count with platelet count.
    c. Chemistry profile.
    d. Coagulation studies (prothrombin time, activated partial thromboplastin time).
    e. Urine pregnancy test for females of childbearing age.
    f. Urine toxicology screen.
6. Establish patient's weight (measure or estimate).
7. Obtain IV pump for possible infusion.
8. Order STAT head CT without contrast.
9. No aspirin or other antiplatelet agents, heparins or warfarin to be given to potential thrombolytictherapy patients.

specific clinical settings: prior to and following thrombolytic therapy, in the presence of myocardial ischemia or aortic dissection, or in the setting of hypertensive encephalopathy.

As these general steps are undertaken, specific evaluation for stroke can also begin. History should be obtained to establish time of stroke onset and to elucidate any factors that would preclude treatment with thrombolytics or other agents. Medical history and physical examination, including a careful cardiovascular exam, may suggest stroke etiology. Finally, emergent neuro-imaging with computed tomography (CT) should be performed to evaluate for the presence of intracerebral hemorrhage (ICH) and for signs of early cerebral edema.

Acute Treatment of Hyperglycemia

Between 25–50% of acute stroke patients present with hyperglycemia[40,108], and many investigators have questioned whether treatment of hyperglycemia in this setting might improve outcome. Studies of insulin treatment in animal models of focal ischemia demonstrate its mitigating effects on infarct volume and neuronal cell loss, both with administration before and after induction of ischemia[109]. In several models of focal ischemia, concomitant administration of glucose negated most of the neuroprotective effect of insulin, arguing that almost all the benefit gained from insulin results from reduction of peripheral glucose rather than a primary neuroprotective effect[110]. Moreover, it was shown in a cat model of focal ischemia that infarct size decreases when normoglycemia is attained, but increases with hypoglycemic blood glucose levels[45]. Thus, results from animal stroke models indicate that if insulin is to be used to treat hyperglycemia in acute stroke, normoglycemia is the optimal goal.

Hyperglycemia has also been found to be a marker for mortality in diabetics with acute myocardial infarction, and a randomized trial in diabetics with myocardial infarction demonstrated that insulin-glucose treatment was safe to use in hyperglycemic patients and also decreased relative mortality rates by 29% (18.6% in the treated group versus 26% in the placebo group)[111,112]. Until recently, no similar intervention with insulin-glucose therapy for hyper-glycemia in the setting of acute ischemic stroke had been attempted. In 1999, the results of the Glucose Insulin in Stroke Trial (GIST) were published[113]. This controlled pilot safety trial randomized 53 acute ischemic stroke patients who presented within 24 hours of symptom onset and had mild to moderate hyperglycemia (plasma glucose 7.0–17.0 mmol/L) to receive either a glucose potassium insulin (GKI) infusion or placebo infusion of 0.9% normal saline over 24 hours. Patients were excluded if they had cardiac failure, renal failure, severe anemia, radiographic evidence of pneumonia, coma, previous disabling stroke, hemorrhagic stroke or previously diagnosed insulin-treated diabetes mellitus (type 1 or 2). Treatment consisted of a combined infusion of 500 mL 10% dextrose with 16 units of human insulin and 20 mmol potassium chloride, with administration according to a specific protocol based on serum glucose values. Plasma glucose samples were obtained every eight hours and standard bedside glucose strip testing every two hours, unless serum glucose levels fell below 4 mmol/L, in which case monitoring was performed more frequently. Clinical outcomes were assessed using two stroke outcome scales; assessments were not performed in blinded fashion. Fifty patients were included in the final analysis after three were excluded for protocol enrollment violations; 25 patients were in the treatment group and 25 in the placebo group. No significant differences existed between the two groups at baseline.

The main objective of the trial was to assess the feasibility and safety of using a GKI infusion in this acute stroke population. The GKI protocol was not followed accurately in the first two GKI treated patients, but all subsequent patients were treated accurately. The concentration of insulin in the GKI had to be changed at least once in 23 of the 25 GKI patients, with a mean number of changes at 2.5 times (range 1–6). Four of the GKI group required a single dose of 10 mL 50% glucose for persistent, asymptomatic low test-strip glucose values, and only one additional patient required similar intervention for symptomatic hypoglycemia, which resolved promptly with treatment. Plasma glucose levels were non-significantly lowered in the GKI group throughout the infusion period. Four-week mortality in the GKI group was seven (28%), as compared to eight (32%) in the placebo group. There was no statistical difference between the groups in outcome at any time period, although the study was not powered to detect such differences. This study demonstrated that administering a 24-hour infusion of GKI was feasible and safe in patients with mild to moderate hyperglycemia in the setting of acute ischemic stroke. Larger randomized trials will need to be undertaken to determine the effectiveness of such therapy in improving outcome from stroke.

Thrombolytic Therapy

Thrombolytic therapy can reestablish cerebral perfusion via recanalization of acutely occluded arteries and may be delivered either intravenously or intra-arterially. To date, only one thrombolytic agent has been approved for use in acute ischemic stroke. In 1996, the US Food and Drug Administration (FDA) approved recombinant tissue plasminogen activator (rt-PA) for use in specific acute ischemic stroke patients. The approval was based largely on the results of the National Institute of Neurological Disorders and Stroke (NINDS) rt-PA Stroke Study[114]. Briefly, this was a multicenter randomized double-blind, placebo-controlled trial of 624 patients who presented within three hours of symptom onset. Patients were randomized to receive either IV rt-PA (0.9 mg/kg, maximum dose 90 mg) or placebo. Primary end-points included 'favorable' outcome (minimal or no disability) as measured on four different outcome scales three months after stroke. Significantly improved outcome on all four scales was documented for the rt-PA treated group, with an 11–13% absolute and 30–50% relative increase in favorable outcome and an odds ratio of 1.7 (95% confidence interval, 1.2–2.8, p = 0.008) Treatment with rt-PA was of benefit in all stroke subtypes, including lacunar infarct. While there was a statistically significant increase in the rate of symptomatic ICH in the first 36 in the rt-PA group (6.4% versus 0.6% for the placebo group, p <0.001), there was no difference in mortality between the two groups at three months. Following approval of rt-PA in the USA, both the Stroke Council of the American Heart Association and the American Academy of Neurology have issued practice guidelines for the use of rt-PA in acute ischemic stroke, and these documents outline in detail the inclusion/exclusion criteria for treatment, protocols for delivering the drug and for monitoring and treating hypertension in the setting of thrombolytic therapy[115,116]. In 1997, the NINDS t-PA Stroke Study Group published subgroup analysis from the initial study[60]. Multivariate analysis revealed that diabetes was independently associated with a worse three-month outcome, but that diabetics treated with rt-PA did better than those in the placebo group. This argues that all eligible acute stroke patients in the USA, including diabetics, should receive IV rt-PA for acute ischemic stroke. The risk for treatment-associated ICH may be higher in diabetics and those patients who present with hyperglycemia. A recent retrospective study of 138 patients who had received rt-PA for acute ischemic stroke indicated that elevated baseline serum glucose was an independent predictor of symptomatic ICH, as was a history of diabetes[117]. However, the authors acknowledge that further study of this phenomenon must be made before changes in the recommendations for rt-PA use will be made.

The results of European trials of rt-PA for acute ischemic stroke are conflicting. The initial European Cooperative Acute Stroke Study (ECASS) used a higher dose of rt-PA and a longer six-hour time window for administration; this trial revealed significantly increased ICH rates and no benefit to rt-PA therapy, but results were compromised by a large percentage of protocol violations[118]. Retrospective analysis of the ECASS intention-to-treat population using the dichotomized NINDS endpoints did reveal statistically significant improvement in the rt-PA treated group three months after stroke[119], as did *post hoc* analysis of the ECASS cohort treated within three hours of symptom onset[120]. The ECASS II study was subsequently undertaken using the lower dose of rt-PA used in the NINDS trial but maintaining the six-hour time window[121]. Like ECASS I, this trial did not demonstrate improved outcome in the rt-PA treated group at three months, although only 158 of the 800 patients were enrolled within three hours of symptom onset. Symptomatic ICH rates were similar to those seen in the NINDS trial. No subgroup analysis of diabetic patients was performed for either ECASS trial. As a result of the conflicting results of these trials, no specific recommendations can be made regarding the use of rt-PA in acute stroke patients, or in diabetic stroke patients specifically, outside the USA.

Several new therapies remain under investigation both in the USA and internationally. Two have completed phase III trials with promising results: intra-arterial pro-urokinase[122] and an IV defibrinogenating agent, ancrod[123]. However, both trails await further scrutiny prior to approval for use in acute ischemic stroke. Neither trial included pre-planned analysis of diabetic sub-populations.

Other acute stroke therapies

A detailed description of other reperfusion, antithrombotic and anticoagulant therapies available for the treatment of acute ischemic stroke is beyond the scope of this chapter. No subgroup analysis of diabetic patients has been performed in these various trials, and further discussion would provide no specific additional information about the acute management of stroke in the diabetic patient. Readers interested in other management therapies available to the general stroke patient are referred to a recent review article on the subject[124].

REFERENCES

1. Hankey GJ (1999) Stroke: how large a public health problem, and how can the neurologist help? *Arch. Neurol.* **56**: 748–754.
2. Broderick J, Brott T, Kothari R, Miller R, Khoury J, Pancioli A, Gebel J, Mills D, Minneci L, Shulka R (1998) The Greater Cincinnati/Northern Kentucky Stroke Study. Preliminary first-ever and total incidence rates of stroke among blacks. *Stroke* **29**: 415–421.
3. Brown RD, Whisnant JP, Sicks JD, O'Fallon WM, Wiebers DO (1996) Stroke incidence, prevalence and survival: secular trends in Rochester, Minnesota, through 1989. *Stroke* **27**: 373–380.
4. Sudlow CLM and Warlow CP, for the International Stroke Incidence Collaboration (1997) Comparable studies of the incidence of stroke and its pathological types. Results from an international collaboration. *Stroke* **28**: 491–499.
5. Isard PA and Forbes JF (1992) The cost of stroke to the National Health Service in Scotland. *Cerebrovasc. Dis.* **2**: 47–50.
6. Currie CJ, Morgan CL, Gill L, Stott NCH, Peters JR (1997) Epidemiology and costs of acute hospital care for cerebrovascular disease in diabetic and nondiabetic populations. *Stroke* **28**: 1142–1146.
7. American Heart Association (AHA) (1997) *Heart and Stroke Statistical Update.* AHA, Dallas, TX.
8. Kannel WB and McGee DL (1979) Diabetes and cardiovascular disease: The Framingham Study. *JAMA* **241**: 2035–2038.

9. Dandona P, James IM, Newburg PA, Wollard ML, Beckett AG (1978) Cerebral blood flow in diabetes mellitus: evidence of abnormal cerebrovascular reactivity. *Br. Med. J.* **2**: 325–326.

9. D'Augustino RB, Wolf PA, Belanger AJ, Kannel WB (1994) Stroke risk profile: adjustment for antihypertensive medication. *Stroke* **25**: 40–43.

10. Abbott RD, Dunanue RP, MacMahon SW, Reed DM, Yano K (1987) Diabetes and the risk of stroke: The Honolulu Heart Program. *JAMA* **257**: 949–952.

11. Wannamethee SG, Perry IJ, Shaper AG (1999) Nonfasting serum glucose and insulin concentrations and the risk of stroke. *Stroke* **30**: 1780–1786.

12. Folsom AR, Rasmussen ML, Chambless LE, Howard G, Cooper LS, Schmidt MI, Heiss G (1999) Prospective associations of fasting insulin, body fat distribution, and diabetes with risk of ischemic stroke. *Diabetes Care* **22**: 1077–1083.

13. Whisnant JP, Wiebers DO, O'Fallon DM, Sicks JD, Frye RL (1996) A population-based model of risk factors for ischemic stroke: Rochester, Minnesota. *Neurology* **47**: 1420–1428.

14. Whisnant JP, Brown RD, Petty GW, O'Fallon WM, Sicks JD, Wiebers DO (1999) Comparison of population-based models of risk factors for TIA and ischemic stroke. *Neurology* **53**: 532–536.

15. Whisnant JP (1997) Modeling of risk factors for ischemic stroke: The Willis Lecture. *Stroke* **28**: 1839–1844.

16. Davis PH, Dambrosia JM, Schoenberg DG, Pritchard BS, Lillienfeld AM, Whisnant JP (1987) Risk factors for ischemic stroke: a prospective study in Rochester, Minnesota. *Ann. Neurol.* **22**: 40–43.

17. Burchfiel CM, Curb JD, Rodriguez BL, Abbott RD, Chiu D, Yano K (1994) Glucose and 22-year stroke incidence: The Honolulu Heart Program. *Stroke* **25**: 951–957.

18. Haheim LL, Holme I, Hjermann I, Lenen P (1995) Non-fasting glucose and the risk of fatal stroke in diabetic and non-diabetic subjects: 18-year follow-up of the Oslo study. *Stroke* **26**: 774–777.

20. Fuller JH, Shipley MJ, Rose G, Jarrett RJ, Keen H (1983) Mortality from coronary heart disease and stroke in relation to degree of glycaemia: The Whitehall Study. *BMJ* **287**: 861–867.

21. Sandercock PAG, Warlow CP, Jones LN, Starkey IR (1989) Predisposing factors for cerebral infarction: the Oxfordshire Community Stroke Project. *BMJ* **298**: 75–80.

22. Kuusisto J, Mykkanen L, Pyorala K, Laakso M (1994) Non-insulin dependent diabetes and its metabolic control are important predictors of stroke in elderly subjects. *Stroke* **25**: 1157–1164.

23. Qureshi AI, Giles WH, Croft JB (1998) Impaired glucose tolerance and the likelihood of nonfatal stroke and myocardial infarction. The third National Health and Nutrition Examination Survey. *Stroke* **29**: 1329–1332.

24. Pyorala M, Miiettinen H, Laakso M, Pyorala K (1998) Hyperinsulinemia and the risk of stroke in healthy middle-aged men: the 22-year follow-up results of the Helsinki Policemen Study. *Stroke* **29**: 1860–1866.

25. Deckert T, Poulsen JE, Larsen M (1978) Prognosis of diabetics with diabetes onset before the age of thirty–one. I. Survival, causes of death, and complications. *Diabetologia* **14**: 363–370.

26. Tunbridge WMG (1981) Factors contributing to deaths of diabetics under 50 years of age. *Lancet* **2(8246)**: 569–572.

27. Roehmholdt ME, Palumbo PJ Whisnant JP, Elveback LR (1983) Transient ischemic attack and stoke in a community-based diabetic cohort. *Mayo Clin. Proc.* **58**: 56–58.

28. Jorgensen HS, Nakayama H, Ranschou HO, Olsen TS (1994) Stroke in patients with diabetes: The Copenhagen Stroke Study. *Stroke* **25**: 1977–1984.
29. Adams HP, Patman SF, Kassell NF, Torner JC (1984) Prevalence of diabetes mellitus among patients with subarachnoid hemorrhage. *Arch. Neurol.* **41**: 1033–1035.
30. Alex M, Baron EK, Goldenberg S, Blumenthal HT (1962) An autopsy study of cerebrovascular accident in diabetes mellitus. *Circulation* **25**: 663–673.
31. Aronson SM (1973) Intracranial vascular lesions in patients with diabetes mellitus. *J. Neuropathol. Exp. Neurol.* **32**: 183–196.
32. Bell ET (1952) A postmortem study of vascular disease in diabetics. *Arch. Pathol.* **53**: 444–455.
33. Peress NS, Kane WC, Aronson SM (1973) Central nervous system findings in a tenth decade autopsy population. *Prog. Brain. Res.* **40**: 473–483.
34. Lodder J and Boiten J (1993) Incidence, natural history, and risk factors in lacunar infarction. In *Advances in Neurology, Volume 62: Cerebral Small Artery Disease* (eds Pullicino P, Caplan LR and Hommel M), Raven Press: New York, pp. 218–219.
35. Arboix A, Marti-Vilalta JL, Garcia JH (1990) Clinical study of 227 patients with lacunar infarcts. *Stroke* **21**: 842–847.
36. Lammie GA, Brannan F, Slattery J, Warlow C (1997) Nonhypertensive cerebral small vessel disease. An autopsy study. *Stroke* **28**: 2222–2229.
37. Lukovits TG, Mazzone T, Gorelick PB (1999) Diabetes mellitus and cerebrovascular disease. *Neuroepidemiol.* **18**: 1–14.
38. Garcia and Anderson (1991)
39. Kane WC and Aronson SM (1970) Cerebrovascular disease in an autopsy population. 3. Diminished frequency of cerebral hemorrhage in diabetics. *Trans. Amer. Neur. Assoc.* **95**: 266–268.
40. Scott JF, Robinson GM, French JM, O'Connell JE, Alberti KGMM, Gray CS (1999) Prevalence of admission hyperglycemia across clinical subtypes of acute stroke. *Lancet* **353**: 376–377.
41. van Kooten F, Hoogerbrugge N, Naarding P, Koudstaal PJ (1993) Hyperglycemia in the acute phase of stroke is not caused by stress. *Stroke* **24**: 1129–1132.
42. Weir CJ, Murray GD, Dyker AG, Lees KR (1997) Is hyperglycemia an independent predictor of poor outcome after acute stroke? Results of a long-term follow-up study. *BMJ* **314**: 1303–1306.
43. Venables G, Miller SA, Gibson G, Hardy J, Strong A (1985) The effects of hyperglycaemia on changes during reperfusion following focal cerebral ischaemia in cats. *J. Neurol. Neurosurg. Psychiatry* **48**: 663–669.
44. Voll C and Auer R (1988) The effect of postischemic glucose levels on ischemic brain damage in the rat. *Ann. Neurol.* **24**: 638–644.
45. deCourten-Myers GM, Kleinholz M, Wagner KR, Myers RE (1994) Normoglycemia (not hypoglycemia) optimizes outcome from middle cerebral artery occlusion. *J. Cereb. Blood Flow Metab.* **14**: 227–236.
46. Kawai N, Keep RF, Betz Al (1997) Hyperglycemia and the vascular effects of cerebral ischemia. *Stroke* **28**: 149–154.
47. Collins RC, Dobkin BH, Choi DW (1989) Selective vulnerability of the brain: new insights into the pathophysiology of stroke. *Ann. Intern. Med.* **110**: 992–100.
48. Pulsinelli W, Levy DE, Sigsbee B, Scherer P, Plum F (1983) Increased damage after ischemic stroke in patients with hyperglycemia with or without established diabetes mellitus. *Am. J. Med.* **74**: 540–543.
49. Rehcrona S, Rosen I, Siesjo BK (1981) Brain lactic acidosis and ischemic cell damage: biochemistry and neurophysiology. *J. Cereb. Blood Flow Metab.* **1**: 297–311.

50. Smith ML, Von Hanwehr R, Siesjo BK (1986) Changes in extra and intracellular pH in the brain during and following ischemia in hyperglycemic and in moderately hypoglycemic rats. *J. Cereb. Blood Flow Metab.* **6**: 574–583.
51. Berger L and Hakim AM (1986) The association of hyperglycemia with cerebral edema in stroke. *Stroke* **17**: 865–871.
53. Hickenbottom SL and Grotta JC (1998) Neuroprotective therapy. *Semin. Neurol.* **18**: 485–492.
53. Rothman SM and Olaney JW (1986) Glutamate and the pathophysiology of hypoxic-ischemic brain damage. *Ann. Neurol.* **19**: 105–111.
54. deCourten-Myers GM, Kleinholz M, Holm P, Schmitt G, Wagner KR, Myers RE (1992) Hemorrhagic infarct conversion in experimental stroke. *Ann. Emerg. Med.* **21**: 120–125.
55. Beghi E, Boglium G, Cavaletti G, Sanguineti I, Tagliabue M, Agostoni F, Macchi I (1989) Hemorrhagic infarction: risk factors, clinical and tomographic features, and outcome: a case-control study. *Acta. Neurol. Scand.* **80**: 226–231.
56. Broderick JP, Hagen T, Brott T, Tomsick T (1995) Hyperglycemia and hemorrhagic transformation of cerebral infarcts. *Stroke* **26**: 484–487.
57. Tumilehto J, Rastenyte D, Jousilihti P, Sarti C, Vartiainen E (1996) Diabetes mellitus as a risk factor for death from stroke: prospective study of the middle-aged Finnish population. *Stroke* **27**: 210–215.
58. Webster P (1980) The natural history of stroke in diabetic patients. *Acta Med Scand*, **207**, 417–424.
59. Bruno A, Biller J, Adams HP, Clarke WWR, Woolson RF, Williams LS, Mansen MD, for the Trial of ORG 10172 in Acute Stroke Treatment (TOAST) Investigators (1999) Acute blood glucose level and outcome from ischemic stroke. *Neurology*, **52**: 280–284.
60. The NINDS t-PA Stroke Study Group (1997) Generalized efficacy of t-PA for acute stroke: subgroup analysis of the NINDS t-PA Stroke Trial. *Stroke* **28**: 2119–2125.
61. Capes SE (1999) How critical is blood glucose to the outcome of stroke? *Neurol. Rev.* **7**: 26–30.
62. Chaturvedi S, Hickenbottom S, Levine S (1999) Ischemic stroke prevention. *Curr. Treatment Options Neurol.* **1**: 113–125.
63. Gorelick PB, Sacco RL, Smith DB, Alberts M, Mustone-Alexander L, Rader D, Ross JL, Raps E, Ozer MN, Brass LM, Malone ME, Goldberg S, Booss J, Hanley DF, Toole JF, Greengold NL, Rhew DC (1999) Prevention of a first stroke: a review of guidelines and a multidisciplinary consensus statement from the National Stroke Association. *JAMA* **281**: 1112–1120.
64. Davis TME, Millns H, Stratton IM, Holman RR, Turner RC (1999) Risk factors for stroke in type 2 diabetes mellitus: United Kingdom Prospective Diabetes Study (UKPDS) 29. *Arch. Int. Med.* **159**: 1097–1103.
65. Stroke Prevention in Atrial Fibrillation Investigators (1996) Adjusted-dose warfarin versus low-intensity, fixed-dose warfarin plus aspirin for high-risk patients with non-valvular atrial fibrillation: Stroke Prevention in Atrial Fibrillation III randomised clinical trial. *Lancet* **348**: 633–638.
66. The SPAF III Writing Committee for the Stroke Prevention in Atrial Fibrillation Investigators (1998) Patients with nonvalvular atrial fibrillation at low risk of stroke during treatment with aspirin: Stroke Prevention in Atrial Fibrillation Study. *JAMA* **279**: 1273–12777.
67. Peto R, Gray R, Collins R, Wheatley K, Hennekens C, Jamrozik K, Warlow C, Hafner B, Thompson E, Norton S (1988) Randomised trial of prophylactic daily aspirin in British male doctors. *BMJ* **296**: 313–316.

68. Steering Committee of the Physicians' Health Study Research Group (1989) Final report on the aspirin component of the ongoing Physicians' Health Study. *N. Engl. J. Med.* **321**: 129–135.

69. He J, Whelton PK, Vu B, Klag MJ (1998) Aspirin and risk for hemorrhagic stroke: a meta-analysis of randomized controlled trials. *JAMA* **280**: 1930–1935.

70. Colwell JA (1997) Aspirin therapy in diabetes. *Diabetes Care* **20**: 1767–1771.

71. Colwell JA (1999) Aspirin and the risk of hemorrhagic stroke. *JAMA* **282**: 731–733.

72. American Diabetes Association (1997) Aspirin therapy in diabetes. *Diabetes Care* **20**: 1772–1773.

73. Sacco RL, Foulkes MA, Mohr JP, Worf PA, Hier DB, Price TR (1989) Determinants of early recurrence of cerebral infarction: the Stroke Data Bank. *Stroke* **20**: 983–989.

74. Burn J, Dennis M, Bamford J, Sandercock P, Wade D, Warlow C (1994) Long-term risk of recurrent stroke after a first-ever stroke: the Oxfordshire Community Stroke Project. *Stroke* **25**: 333–337.

75. Hier DB, Foulkes MA, Swiontoniowski M, Sacco RL, Goerlick PB, Mohr JP, Price TR, Wolf PA (1991) Stroke recurrence within two years after ischemic infarction. *Stroke* **22**: 155–161.

75. Petty GW, Brown RD, Whisnant JP, Sicks JD, O'Fallon WM, Wiebers DO (1998) Survival and recurrence after first cerebral infarction: a population-based study in Rochester, Minnesota, 1975–1989. *Neurology* **50**: 208–216.

77. Sacco RL, Shi T, Zamanillo MC, Kargman DE (1994) Predictors of mortality and recurrence after hospitalized cerebral infarction in an urban community: the Northern Manhattan Stroke Study. *Neurology* **44**: 626–634.

78. Lai SM, Alter M, Firday G, Sobel E (1994) A multifactorial analysis of risk factor for recurrence of ischemic stroke. *Stroke* **25**: 958–962.

79. Antiplatelet Trialists' Collaboration (1994) Collaborative overview of randomised trials of antiplatelet therapy. I. Prevention of death, myocardial infarction, and stroke by prolonged antiplatelet therapy in various categories of patients. *BMJ* **308**: 81–106.

80. Algre A and van Gijn J (1996) Aspirin at any dose above 30 mg offers only modest protection after cerebral ischaemia. *J. Neurol. Neurosurg. Psychiatry* **56**: 17–25.

81. The Dutch TIA Trial Study Group (1991) A comparison of two doses of aspirin (30 mg vs. 283 mg a day) in patients after a transient ischemic attack or minor ischemic stroke. *N. Engl. J. Med.* **325**: 1261–1266.

82. UK-TIA Study Group (1991) United Kingdom Transient Ischemic Attack (UK-TIA) aspirin trial: final results. *J. Neurol. Neurosurg. Psychiatry* **54**: 1044–1054.

83. Albers GW and Tijssen JGP (1999) Antiplatelet therapy: new foundations for optimal treatment decisions. *Neurology,* **53(Supp. 4)**, S25–S31.

84. FDA monograph (1998) Internal analgesic, antipyretic, and antirheumatic drug products for over-the-counter human use; final rule for professional labeling of aspirin, buffered aspirin, and aspirin in combination with antacid drug products. *Federal Registrar* **63(205)**: 56802–56819.

85. Gent M, Blakely JA, Easton JD, Ellis DJ, Hachinski VC, Harbison JW, Panak E, Roberts RS, Sicurella J, Turpie AGG and the CATS Group (1989) The Canadian American Ticlopidine Study (CATS) in thromboembolic stroke. *Lancet* **1**: 1215–1220.

85. Grotta JC, Norris JW, Kamm M and the TASS Baseline and Angiographic Data Subgroup (1992) Prevention of stroke with ticlopidine: who benefits most? *Neurology* **42**: 111–115.

87. Bennett CL, Weinberg PD, Rozenberg-Ben-Dror K, Yarnold PR, Kwaan HC, Green D (1998) Thrombotic thrombocytopenic purpura associated with ticlopidine. A review of 60 cases. *Ann. Intern. Med.* **128**: 541–544.

88. CAPRIE Steering Committee (1996) A randomized, blinded, trial of clopidogrel versus aspirin in patients at risk of ischaemic events (CAPRIE). *Lancet* **348**: 1329–1339.

89. Sivenius J, Laakso M, Riekkinen P, Smets P, Lowenthal A (1992) European Stroke Prevention Study: effectiveness of antiplatelet therapy in diabetic patients in secondary prevention of stroke. *Stroke* **23**, 851–854.

90. Colwell JA, Bingham SF, Abraira C, Anderson JW, Comstock JP, Kwaan HC and the Cooperative Study Group (1986) Veterans Administration Cooperative Study on antiplatelet agents in diabetic patients after amputation for gangrene. II. Effects of aspirin and dipyridamole on atherosclerotic vascular disease rates. *Diabetes Care* **9**: 140–148.

91. Diener HC, Chnha L, Forbes J, Sivenius P, Smets P, Lowenthal A (1996) European Stroke Prevention Study 2. Dipyridamole and acetylsalicylic acid in the secondary prevention of stroke. *J. Neurol. Sci.* **143**: 1–13.

92. Azar AJ, Koudstaal PJ, Wintzen AR, van Bergen PF, Jonker JJ, Deckers JW (1996) Risk of stroke during long-term anticoagulant therapy in patients after myocardial infarction. *Ann. Neurol.* **39**: 301–307.

93. Chimowitz MI, Kokkinos J, Strong J, Brown MB, Levine SR, Silliman S, Pessin MS, Weichel E, Sila CA, Furlan AJ, Kargman DE, Sacco Rl, Wityk RJ, Ford G, Fayad PB for the Warfarin-Aspirin Symptomatic Intracranial Disease Study Group (1995) The Warfarin-Aspirin Symptomatic Intracranial Disease Study. *Neurology* **45**: 1488–1493.

94. Khamashta MA, Cuadrado MJ, Mujic F, Taub NA, Hunt BJ, Hughes GRV (1994) The management of thrombosis in the antiphospholipid antibody syndrome. *N. Engl. J. Med.* **332**: 993–997.

95. The Stroke Prevention in Reversible Ischemia Trials (SPIRIT) Study Group (1997) A randomized trial of anticoagulants versus aspirin after cerebral ischemia of presumed arterial origin. *Ann. Neurol.* **42**: 857–865.

96. Barnett HJM, Taylor DW, Eliasziw M, Fox AJ, Ferguson GG, Haynes RB, Rankin RN, Clagett GP, Hachinski VC, Sackett DL, Thorpe KE, Meldrum HE for the North American Symptomatic Carotid Endarterectomy Trial Collaborators (1998) Benefit of carotid endarterectomy in patients with symptomatic moderate or severe stenosis. *N. Engl. J. Med.* **339**: 1415–1425.

97. European Carotid Surgery Trialists' Collaborative Group (1998) Randomised trial of endarterectomy for recently symptomatic carotid stenosis: final results of the MRC European Carotid Surgery Trial (ECST). *Lancet* **351**: 1379–1387.

98. North American Symptomatic Carotid Endarterectomy Trial Collaborators (1991) Beneficial effect of carotid endarterectomy in symptomatic patients with high-grade carotid stenosis. *N. Engl. J. Med.* **325**: 445–453.

99. Kuebler TW, Bendick PJ, Fineberg SE, Markand ON, Norton JA, Vinicor FN, Clark CM (1983) Diabetes mellitus and cerebrovascular disease: prevalence and associated risk factors in 482 adult diabetic patients. *Diabetes Care* **6**: 274–278.

100. Bogousslavsky J, Regli F, Van Melle G (1985) Risk factors and concomitants of internal carotid artery occlusion or stenosis. *Arch. Neurol.* **42**: 864–867.

101. Yasaka M, Yamaguchi T, Shibiri M (1993) Distribution of atherosclerosis and risk factors in atherothrombotic occlusion. *Stroke* **24**: 206–211.

102. Campbell DR, Hoar CS, Wheelock FC (1984) Carotid artery surgery in diabetic patients. *Arch. Surg.* **119**: 1405–1407.

103. Kwiatkowsi TG and Libman RB (1997) Emergency strategies. In *Primer on Cerebrovascular Diseases* (eds Welch KMA, Caplan LR, Ries DJ, Siesjo BK, Weir B), Academic Press: San Diego, p. 672.

104. Broderick J, Brott T, Barsan W, Haley ED, Levy D, Marler J, Sheppard G, Blum C (1993) Blood pressure during the first minutes of focal cerebral ischemia. *Ann. Emerg. Med.* **22**: 1438–1444.

105. Harper G, Castleden CM, Potter JF (1994) Factors affecting changes in blood pressure after acute stroke. *Stroke* **25**: 1726–1729.

106. Powers W (1993) Acute hypertension after stroke: the scientific basis for treatment decisions. *Neurology* **43**: 461–467.

107. Adams HP, Brott T, Crowell R, Furaln AJ, Gomez CR, Grotta J, Helgason CM, Marler JR, Woolson RF, Zivin JA, Feinberg W, Mayberg M (1994) AHA Medical/Scientific Statement – Guidelines of management of patients with acute ischemic stroke: a statement for healthcare professionals from a special writing committee of the Stroke Council, American Heart Association. *Stroke* **25**, 1901–1914.

108. Scott J, O'Connell J, Gray C (1997) Hyperglycaemia after acute stroke: participants required for trial of treatment with glucose and insulin. *BMJ* **315**: 811(letter).

109. Auer RN (1999) Insulin, blood glucose levels, and ischemic brain damage. *Neurology* **51(Suppl. 3)**: S39–S43.

110. Hamilton MG, Tranner BI, Auer RN (1995) Insulin reduction of cerebral infarction due to transient focal ischaemia. *J Neuro Surg* **82**: 262–268.

111. Malmberg K, Ryden L, Efendic S, Herlitz J, Nicol P, Waldenstrom A, Wedel H, Welin L (1995) Randomized trial of insulin-glucose infusion followed by subcutaneous insulin treatment in diabetic patients with acute myocardial infarction (DIGAMI study). Effects on mortality at one year. *J. Am. Coll. Cardiol.* **26**: 57–65.

112. Malmberg K, Norhammar A, Wedel H, Ryden L (1999) Glycometabolic state at admission: important risk marker of mortality in conventionally treated patients with diabetes mellitus and acute myocardial infarctions. Long-term results from the Diabetes and Insulin-Glucose Infusion in Acute Myocardial Infarction (DIGAMI) study. *Circulation* **99**: 2626–2632.

113. Scott JF, Robinson GM, French JM, O'Connell JE, Alberti KGMM, Gray CS (1999) Glucose potassium insulin infusions in the treatment of acute stroke patients with mild to moderate hyperglycemia. The Glucose Insulin in Stroke Trial (GIST). *Stroke* **39**: 793–799.

114. The National Institute of Neurologic Disorders and Stroke (NINDS) rt-PA Stroke Study Group (1995) Tissue plasminogen activator for acute ischemic stroke. *N Engl J Med*, **333**, 1581–1587.

115. Adams HP, Brott T, Furlan AJ, Gomez CR, Grotta J, Helgason CM, Kwiatkowski T, Lyden PD, Marler JR, Torner J, Feinberg W, Mayberg M, Thies W (1996) Guidelines for thrombolytic therapy for acute stroke: a supplement for the guidelines for the management of patients with acute ischemic stroke. A statement for healthcare professionals from a special writing group of the Stroke Council of the American Heart Association. *Stroke*, **27**, 1711–1718.

116. Report of the Quality Standards Subcommittee of the American Academy of Neurology (1996) Practice advisory: thrombolytic therapy for acute ischemic stroke – summary statement. *Neurology* **47**: 834–839.

117. Demchuk AM, Morgenstern LB, Krieger DW, Chi TL, Hu W, Wein TH, Hardy RJ, Grotta JC, Buchan AM (1999) Serum glucose level and diabetes predict tissue

plasminogen activator-related intracerebral hemorrhage in acute ischemic stroke. *Stroke* **30**: 34–39.

118. The European Cooperative Acute Stroke Study (ECASS) (1995) Intravenous thrombolysis with recombinant tissue plasminogen activator for acute hemispheric stroke. *JAMA* **274**: 1017–1025.

119. Hacke W, Bluhmki E, Steiner T, Tatlisumark T, Mahagne MH, Sacchetti ML, Meier D (1998) Dichotomized efficacy end points and global end-point analysis applied to the ECASS intention-to-treat data set: post hoc analysis of ECASS I. *Stroke* **29**: 2073–2075.

120. Steiner T, Bluhmki E, Kaste M, Toni D, Trouillas P, von Kummer R, Hacke W (1998) The ECASS 3-hour cohort. Secondary analysis of ECASS data by time stratification. ECASS Study Group. European Cooperative Acute Stroke Study. *Cerebrovasc Dis.* **8**: 198–203.

121. Hacke W, Kaste M, Fieschi C, von Kummer R, Davalos A, Meier D, Larrue V, Bluhmki E, Davis S, Donnan G, Schneider D, Diez-Tejedor E, Trouillas P (1998) Randomised, double-blind, placebo-controlled trial of thrombolytic therapy with intravenous alteplase in acute ischemic stroke. (ECASS II). Second European-Australian Acute Stroke Study Investigators. *Lancet* **352**: 1245–1251.

122. Furlan AJ, Higashida R, Wechsler L, Gent M, Rowley H, Kase C, Pessin M, Ahuja A, Cahallan F, Clark WM, Silver F, Rivera F, for the PROACT Investigators (1999) Intra-arterial prourokinase for acute ischemic stroke. The PROACT II study: a randomized controlled trial. *JAMA* **282**: 1999.

123. Sherman DG, for the STAT Writers Group (1999) Defibrinogenation with Viprinex™ (ancrod) for the treatment of acute ischemic stroke. *Stroke* **30**: 234 (abstract).

124. Hickenbottom SL and Barsan WG (2000) Acute stroke therapy. *Neurol. Clincs North Amer.* in press.

27

Treatment of Peripheral Vascular Disease

ALLEN D. HAMDAN and FRANK B. POMPOSELLI JR.

Harvard Medical School,Boston, USA

INTRODUCTION

More than half of all lower limb amputations in the USA are performed on persons with diabetes even though the diabetic population accounts for less than 5% of the total population[1]. In addition, more than 50% of diabetic amputees require subsequent amputation of the contralateral limb within four years of the original operation[2]. The treatment of diabetics with complications of peripheral vascular disease is a major health care problem.

PATHOGENESIS

MACROCIRCULATION

The pattern of atherosclerotic occlusion commonly found with diabetes involves the tibial and peroneal arteries, but spares both the superficial femoral artery as well as the arteries of the foot, especially the dorsalis pedis artery[3]. In general, patients without diabetes tend to have more proximal disease affecting the distal aorta, iliac and femoral arteries. The propensity toward tibial/peroneal involvement (crural disease) in diabetes mellitus was noted in prospective studies of amputation specimens[4]. and more recently by arteriography[5]. One of the early impediments to attempts at extreme distal reconstruction in diabetes probably resulted from the initial suggestions that there was an occlusive lesion in the microcirculation (so-called small vessel disease) that would prevent tissue perfusion[6]. Subsequent prospective studies have

The Evidence Base for Diabetes Care. Edited by R. Williams, W. Herman, A.-L. Kinmonth and N. J. Wareham.
© 2002 John Wiley & Sons, Ltd

failed to confirm the existence of such a lesion. Noninvasive vascular evaluation of diabetic and nondiabetic patients presenting with foot ulceration confirmed that there was no evidence of higher vascular resistance[7].

Although stenosis or occlusion of large vessels in diabetics may occur in different locations than in nondiabetics, the gross histology of the plaque is the same. However, the function of the endothelial cell may be altered, accounting for the possible acceleration of vascular disease in diabetics. One of the earliest findings in the progression to atherosclerosis is endothelial dysfunction. This can be seen even before plaques develop. Known diabetics have impaired vasdodilatory capabilities of their macrocirculation. Even patients with occult diabetes have impaired vascular reactivity which normalizes on treatment with an oral hypoglycemic agent. Further evidence for dysfunction of the vessel wall in diabetics is that even in healthy subjects, simple ingestion of a glucose load impairs endothelial-dependent vasodilatation in the brachial artery[8]. Thus, diabetics may have endothelial cell dysfunction superimposed upon developing or pre-existing atherosclerosis due to long-term hyperglycemia.

MICROCIRCULATION

Although there is not a prerequisite occlusion of the microcirculation in diabetic feet, there clearly are changes that alter the pathobiology of the diabetic foot. These changes occur with or without ischemia, although they can become more pronounced with progression of ischemia. There is evidence for thickening of capillary basement membrane[9]. The capillary basement membrane is key in the exchange of nutrients and metabolic products between the capillary lumen and the interstitium. The chemical structure of the membrane is altered by glycosylation, causing cross-linking of proteins and a decrease in the number of highly charged sulfur groups[10]. This may explain why molecules such as albumin leak through the capillary membrane in diabetics. There is no impairment in oxygen diffusion and in fact diabetics with foot ulceration have higher levels of transcutaneous PO_2 than nondiabetics[11]. Further evaluation of the microanatomy reveals more tortuous capillaries in diabetics, appearing as tufts instead of the typical simple hairpin loops. In addition, with ischemia, there is less recruitment of new capillaries into the circulation[12].

POLYNEUROPATHY

Polyneuropathy has a major effect on the complications seen in patients with diabetes. Neuropathy afflicts at least 50% of patients, with an increase to 80% in those with foot lesions. Its course is progressive without spontaneous remissions. The cause is not completely known but is likely due to metabolic defects secondary to hypoglycemia and nerve hypoxia. It has been shown that there is reduced endoneurial blood flow and increased vascular resistance. Further evaluation of diabetic neuropathy has implicated the role of endo- thelial cell dysfunction. Diabetics with neuropathy have a reduction in endothelial-dependent vasodilatation at the foot level. This occurs with or without concomitant macrovascular disease. The inability to maximally vaso- dilate in these patients correlates with reduced expression of endothelial nitric oxide synthetase. A very interesting finding was that patients with diabetes and no neuropathy had preservation of endothelial-dependent vasodilatation, emphasizing the important role of neuropathy in the pathogenesis of vascular disease[13].

The other ways that neuropathy affects the diabetic foot are dependent on the nerve type involved. Intrinsic muscle atrophy from motor neuropathy leads to characteristic foot deformities (claw) creating pressure points under the metatarsal heads, tips of the toes, etc. Sensory neuropathy diminishes awareness of pressure-related trauma or other injuries to the skin, establishing a portal for entry for bacteria. Autonomic neuropathy leads to loss of sweat and oil gland production, resulting in skin that dries and fissures. In addition, the alterations in autonomic function can impair distal perfusion by arteriovenous shunting of blood around the capillary bed, leading to an increase in non- nutritive blood flow. Finally, the neurogenic inflammatory response mediated by fine sensory C-fibers and neurokinins is blunted. Thus, the usual signs and symptoms of early infection are absent. Under these circumstances, profound deep tissue infections can occur before a diagnosis is made.

To assess the role of ischemia in the maintenance or progression of diabetic neuropathy we looked at the effects of revascularization on the diabetic extremity. Reversal of hypoxia via peripheral bypass halted the progression of diabetic neuropathy but did not reverse the process. Control limbs (no operation) showed a decrease in nerve conduction velocity of 2 m/s per year while those after revascularization showed no deterioration[14]. This provides evidence that local tissue hypoxia is involved in the progression of neuropathy.

Thus pathogenic changes in the macro- and microcirculation as well as the development of polyneuropathy account for the complex pathobiology and clinical presentation of the diabetic foot. Successful management of the ischemia, and limb salvage, requires a clinical care plan that addresses all aspects of the underlying pathology.

PRINCIPLES OF THERAPY

As described above, the pathobiology of the diabetic foot can be complex. However, following some basic principles in caring for these patients can lead to successful results.

1. Prompt and thorough drainage of infection and debridement of obviously necrotic tissue. This is the first order of business in the management of any diabetic foot problem, even in the face of ischemia. Aggressive evaluation for 'pockets' of infection in the foot is key since, as noted above, all the standard signs of infection seen in nondiabetics may be blunted. One sign, however, that is often present is either an increase in glucose levels or in the insulin requirements on an acute basis. Several debridements may be necessary, over the course of a few days, before the sepsis is controlled. Due to the neuropathy, some or all of the debridements may be performed without need for local anesthesia.

2. Always evaluate for ischemia even when infection and neuropathy are present. Often, because an ulcer is located in a typical location, beneath the metatarsal head, it is referred to as 'neuropathic'. Under these circumstances, the single most important observation is the presence or absence of a clearly palpable dorsalis pedis or posterior tibial artery pulse at the ankle. If these pulses are not palpable, a bedside Doppler exam allows for further evaluation and sometimes location of the vessel. If there is no pulse in the foot then in most instances arteriography will be needed. Noninvasive tests may be of additional help, especially for baseline information. However, the presence or absence of a clearly palpable pulse is a highly effective guide. It is important to remember that ankle-brachial indices can be inaccurate in diabetics because of the false elevation due to noncompressible calcified vessels. Pulse volume recording as a noninvasive test is much more accurate in this patient population.

3. The arteriogram must be conducted so the status of the foot arteries is determined even if the tibial and peroneal arteries are occluded. A common mistake is to terminate the arteriogram once the occluded tibial vessels are encountered, on the presumption that all distal vessels are occluded. The use of intra-arterial digital subtraction arteriography has greatly simplified the imaging of the distal ankle and foot vessels in these patients[15]. Adequate hydration prior to the arteriogram will help diminish contrast-induced renal failure, particularly in patients with diabetes who have pre-existing renal insufficiency.

4. Arterial reconstruction should then be performed to restore maximum perfusion to the foot. The decision on the most suitable distal vessel is determined by the arteriogram as well as the available conduit.

5. Secondary revisions or closure of the open foot lesion after revascularization can usually be carried out as a separate procedure. This might involve further debridement, toe amputations, occasional transmetatarsal amputation, local flaps and, rarely, free flaps. With the fully vascularized foot, even in the presence of diabetes, all of the options become available.

Only within the broader context of understanding can distal bypass be used effectively. The clinician dealing with these patients must understand that the operation is only part of the overall surgical care necessary to obtain limb salvage. If the operation is approached as a technical exercise without proper attention to the role of infection and neuropathy, the results will be compromised.

PATIENT SELECTION

Once a patient has been evaluated through the aforementioned protocol and a patent dorsalis pedis artery or tibial vessel is identified, consideration may be given to a bypass. It is, of course, important that the site of the anastomosis be free of necrosis or active infection. Other than that, patients with necrosis of the forefoot or plantar aspect of the foot or heel are all suitable for reconstruction. The details of the arteriogram are important. Calcifications may be seen on the plain films of the leg including the dorsalis pedis artery in the foot. This observation, however, should not be regarded as a contraindication to an attempt at arterial reconstruction, as the calcification does not imply an occlusive lesion. Distal lower extremity arteriography has been greatly enhanced by the widespread use of digital subtraction technology. This makes it possible for the angiographer to observe distal vessels over an extended time course following contrast injection and capture the best images for hard copy. Both anteroposterior and lateral foot views must be included with the infrageniculate portion of the arteriogram in order to obtain as complete a picture as possible of the location of all stenoses and occlusions. The foot views should be obtained without excessive plantar flexion, as this can stop flow in the dorsalis pedis, and it may not be visualized. The pattern of occlusive disease on a given arteriogram may present several options for arterial reconstruction. Our goal is to restore palpable foot pulses whenever possible. When bypasses into the tibial or popliteal arteries will not achieve this goal, we preferentially extend bypass to the foot, usually to the dorsalis pedis artery. Although this is our preferred approach, we will alter the plan based on individual factors, such as conduit availability and extent of infection.

TECHNICAL CONSIDERATIONS

At this time, autogenous vein is the only appropriate conduit for bypass to the dorsalis pedis or tibial arteries. Beyond this, however, there is room for a great deal of flexibility on the part of the surgeon. Our experience has indicated that the outcome of bypass is not influenced by the use of *in situ*[16], reversed, translocated[17] or nonreversed vein grafts. Each of these techniques has specific advantages that apply to different technical situations.

As noted earlier, in patients with diabetes, the superficial femoral artery is often spared and the occlusion is confined to the tibial and peroneal vessel segments. Under these circumstances the superficial femoral or popliteal artery can be used for inflow source. This would be uncommon in a patient without diabetes. This results in a shorter vein graft and avoids the need for groin incisions, which can be a source of major morbidity, especially in obese patients. Several studies have reported excellent long-term patency with lower-extremity vein grafts originating from the popliteal artery, showing that concerns about progression of atherosclerotic disease in the superficial femoral artery as a cause of graft failure are unjustified[18,19]. An easily palpable popliteal pulse on physical examination, coupled with an angiogram, is a perfectly adequate assessment. Since the vein graft is going to a small artery with a relatively limited outflow bed, the increased flow demand on the popliteal artery is limited.

With a complete angiogram of the lower extremity circulation, it is often possible to choose an outflow artery that will restore a palpable foot pulse. As a consequence of compromised biology in the diabetic foot, as a general rule, it is desirable to restore maximum perfusion to the foot. This can usually be accomplished by a bypass to the anterior or posterior tibial artery that is continuous with the foot, or with a bypass directly to a foot artery, most often the dorsalis pedis. Bypass grafts to an isolated popliteal segment or to the peroneal artery will improve circulation to the foot but will not restore maximum perfusion. In particular, some debate has centered on the choice between the peroneal artery or dorsalis pedis for a vein graft when both are patent[20]. Our preference is for the dorsalis pedis, since it is easily accessible, provides maximum perfusion to the foot, and provides equivalent if not better patency[21]. However, bypass to the dorsalis pedis is unnecessary when a more proximal bypass will restore foot pulses, and it should not be done when there is inadequate high-quality autogenous vein conduit to reach the foot.

SPECIAL SITUATIONS

It is very common for diabetics to present with foot ischemia in the context of an acute infection. We evaluated the complexity and high cost of treating those patients in which pedal bypass was carried out in the face of serious infections. Fifty-six patients were examined. Control of sepsis required pre-operative debridement or open amputation in 25 cases and delayed bypass about 11 days. After bypass, 12.5% developed serious infections, one of which resulted in death. Postbypass foot procedures were needed in 36 cases, and total stay was about 30 days. In addition, 20 patients required 35 readmissions for related foot problems that delayed ultimate healing an average of 5.5 months. In spite of these problems, graft patency and limb salvage were

91.8% and 97.8% at three years[22]. This emphasizes the amount of time and patience that is required to salvage functional limbs in some of these patients. A successful bypass is only a small part of the total treatment.

RESULTS OF REVASCULARIZATION

From 1985 to 1992 we performed 384 consecutive bypass grafts to the dorsalis pedis artery in 367 patients, accounting for about 25% of our infrainguinal bypasses in diabetics. In 275 cases the dorsalis pedis artery was the only available outflow target and in 109 others pedal bypasses were done in preference to an isolated popliteal segment or a distal peroneal artery. Twenty-nine bypasses failed within 30 days for a 30-day graft failure of 7.5%, but the majority were successfully revised. However, in those who failed early and were not amenable to revision, the amputation rate was 80%. The perioperative mortality was 1.8% with a 5.4% rate of myocardial infarction (MI). In follow-up ranging from one to 83 months (mean 20 months) primary and secondary patency at five years were 68% and 82%[23]. Limb salvage at five years was 87%. Similarly, grafts with inflow arising from the common femoral, and more distally, demonstrated no difference. All patients had bypass delayed until active spreading infection was controlled, which averaged about five days. No patient lost a potentially salvageable limb during this time delay. Bypass to the dorsalis pedis artery can be performed with a high rate of success and low mortality, certainly equivalent to that achieved with other lower extremity grafts.

SUMMARY

Improvements in angiography and in the results of distal reconstruction have established extreme distal autogenous vein reconstruction to the foot vessels as a safe and effective treatment for limb-threatening ischemia. This has proven especially important for patients with diabetes mellitus who are most likely to require these procedures due to the predilection of atherosclerotic lesions to involve the crural vessels with relative sparing of the foot vessels, especially the dorsalis pedis artery. Bypass grafts to the dorsalis pedis artery currently constitute approximately 25% of all lower extremity arterial reconstruction in our patients with diabetes. Our increased use of this procedure has correlated almost precisely with a decline in the incidence of all levels of amputations in our practice[24]. Success with this operation requires a familiarity with all techniques for autogenous vein reconstruction. Because nearly all the patients undergoing dorsalis pedis bypass have diabetes, a thorough understanding of the pathobiology of diabetic foot problems is also essential for success. A carefully planned approach including prompt control of infection, complete arteriography and arterial reconstruction to maximize foot perfusion affords a likelihood of successful limb salvage in diabetics, that should equal or exceed that in nondiabetics.

REFERENCES

1. Reiber GE (1994) Who is at risk of limb loss and what to do about it? *J. Rehabil. Res. Dev.* **31**: 357–62)
2. Ebskov B, Josephsen P (1980) Incidence of reamputation and death after gangrene of the lower extremity. *Prosthet. Orthotics Int.* **4**: 77–80.
3. Conrad MC (1967) Large and small artery occlusion in diabetics and nondiabetics with severe vascular disease. *Circulation* **36**: 83–91.
4. Strandness DE Jr., Priest RE, Gibbons GE (1964) Combined clinical pathological study of diabetic and nondiabetic peripheral arterial disease. *Diabetes* **13**: 366–72.
5. Menzoian JO, Lamorte WW, Paniszyn CC, McBride KJ, Sidawy AN, LoGerfo FW, Connors ME, Doyle JE Symptomatology and anatomic patterns of peripheral vascular disease: Differing impact of smoking and diabetes. *Ann. Vasc. Surg.* **3**: 224–228.
6. Goldenberg SG, Alex M, Joshi RA, Blumenthal HT (1959) Nonatheromatous peripheral vascular disease of the lower extremity in diabetes mellitus. *Diabetes* **8**: 261–73.
7. Irwin ST, Gilmore J, McGrann S, Hood J, Allen JA (1988) Blood flow in diabetics with foot lesions due to small vessel disease. *Br. J. Surg.* **75**: 1201–06.
8. Akbari CM, Saouaf R, Barnhill DF, Newmman, PA, Lo Gerfo FW, Veves A (1998) Endothelium-dependent vasodilatation is impaired in both microcirculation and macrocirculation during acute hyperglycemia. *J. Vasc. Sur.* **28**: 687–94)
9. Siperstein MD, Unger RH, Madison LL (1968) Studies of muscle capillary basement membranes in normal subjects, diabetic and prediabetic patients. *J. Clin. Invest.* **47**: 1973–1999.
10. Brownlee M, Cerami IA, Vlassara H (1988) Advanced glycosylation end products in tissue and the biochemical basis of diabetic complications. *N. Engl. J. Med.* **318**: 1315–21.
11. Wyss CR, Matsen FA, Simmons CW, Burgess EM (1964) Transcutaneous oxygen tension measurements on limb of diabetic and nondiabetic vascular disease. *Diabetes* **13**: 366–372.
12. Katz MA, McNeill G (1987) Defective vasodilation response to exercise in cutaneous precapillary vessels in diabetic humans. *Diabetes* **36**: 1386–96.
13. Veves A, Akbari CM, Primavera J,Donaghue VM, Zacharoulis D, Chrzan JS, DeGirolami U, Lo Gerfo FW, Freeman R (1998). Endothelial dysfunction and the expression of endothelial nitric oxide synthetase in diabetic neuropathy, vascular disease and foot ulceration. *Diabetes* **47**: 457–63.
14. Akbari CM, Gibbons GW, Habershaw GM, Lo Gerfo, FW, Venes A (1997). The effect of arterial reconstruction on the natural history of diabetic neuropathy. *Arch. Surg.* **132**: 148–152.
15. Blakeman BM, Littooy FM, Baker WH (1986) Intra-arterial digital subtraction angiography as a method to study peripheral vascular diseases. *J. Vasc. Surg.* **4**: 168–73.

16. Leather RP, Powers SR, Karmody AM. (1979) A reappraisal of the in situ saphenous vein arterial bypass: its use in limb salvage. *Surgery* **86**: 453–61.
17. Thompson RW. Mannick JA, Whittemore AD (1987) Arterial reconstruction at divers sites using nonreversed autogenous vein. *Ann. Surg.* **205**: 747–51.
18. Veith FJ, Gupta SK, Samson RH, Flores SW, Janko G, Scher LA (1981) Superficial femoral and popliteal arteries as inflow site for distal bypasses. *Surgery* **90**: 980–90.
19. Sidawy AN, Menzoian JO, Cantelmo NL, LoGerfo FW (1986). Effect of inflow and outflow sites on the results of tibioperoneal vein grafts. *Am. J. Surg.* **152**: 211–24.
20. Plecha EJ, Seabrook GR, Bandyk DF, Towne JB (1993) Determinants of successful peroneal artery bypass. *J. Vasc. Surg.* **17**: 97–106.
21. Schneider JR, Walsh DB, McDaniel MD, Zwolek RM, Besso SR, Cronenwett JL. (1993) Pedal bypass versus tibial bypass with autogenous vein: a comparison of outcome and hemodynamic results. *J. Vasc. Surg.* **17**: 1029–40.
22. Tannebaum GA, Pomposelli FB Jr., Marcaccio EJ, Gibbons GW, Campbell DR, Freeman DV, Miller A, Lo Gerfo FW (1992) Safety of vein bypass grafting to the dorsalis pedis artery in diabetic patients with foot infections. *J. Vasc. Surg.* **15**: 982–88.
23. Pomposelli FB Jr., Marcaccio EJ, Gibbons GW, Campbell DR, Freeman DV, Burgess AM, Miller A, Lo Gerfo FW (1995) Dorsalis pedis arterial bypass: durable limb salvage for foot ischemia in patients with diabetes mellitus. *J. Vasc. Surg.* **21**: 35–45.
24. LoGerfo FW, Gibbons GW, Pomposelli FB Jr., Campbell DR, Miller A, Freeman DV, Qvist WC (1992) Trends in the care of the diabetic foot: expanded role of arterial reconstruction. *Arch. Surg.* **127**: 617–21.

28

Epidemiology of Diabetic Foot Ulcers and Amputations: Evidence for Prevention

GAYLE E. REIBER and WILLIAM R. LEDOUX

VA Puget Sound, Seattle, WA, USA

INTRODUCTION

Diabetes mellitus affects millions of people around the world with devastating complications. In the USA, 6% of the population (17 million people) have diagnosed or undiagnosed diabetes[1]. The 1996 global estimate of 135 million people with diabetes is projected to increase to 300 million by the year 2025[2]. Many people with diabetes develop complications including cardiovascular disease, renal failure and lower-limb complications, including foot ulcers and amputations.

Foot ulcers are lesions that include loss of the epithelium and may extend into the dermis and deeper layers, sometimes involving bone and muscle.

Amputation is the removal of a terminal, nonviable portion of a limb.

The annual incidence of foot ulcers ranges from 1.0–4.1% while the cumulative lifetime incidence is approximately 15%[3–8]. Foot ulcers may become complicated by infection or gangrene, and ultimately result in amputation.

Studies report foot ulcers preceded 71–84% of nontraumatic amputations in persons with diabetes[9–10]. In 1997, 68% of US amputations were performed in persons with diabetes. Only 47% of people with diabetes had high-level (transtibial or transfemoral) amputations compared to 70% in people without diabetes (Table 28.1)[11,12]. Incidence of lower extremity amputation among people with diabetes ranges from 2.1–13.7 per 1000[13–20].

The purpose of this chapter is to review the analytic or experimental studies, concerning risk factors and causal pathways for ulcers and amputations in

The Evidence Base for Diabetes Care. Edited by R. Williams, W. Herman, A.-L. Kinmonth and N. J. Wareham.
© 2002 John Wiley & Sons, Ltd

Table 28.1. Number and percentage of US amputation discharges by diabetes status and amputation level (1997).

	Nationwide inpatient survey	Veterans Health Administration	Total	Percent
Diabetes				
Minor amputations[1]	46 680	1987	48 667	53
Major amputations[2]	41 661	1678	43 339	47
Sub total	88 341	3665	92 006	68
No Diabetes				
Minor amputations[1]	12 128	574	12 702	30
Major amputations[2]	28 574	1405	29 979	70
Sub total	40 702	1997	42 681	32
Total	129 043	5644	134 687	100

[1]Toe, ray, metatarsal or Syme amputation
[2]Transtibial or transfemoral amputation

Sources: US Nationwide Inpatient Sample[11], Veterans Health Administration Patient Treatment File[12].
Adapted from Reiber[21]. Reproduced with permission of JRRD, Department of Veterans Affairs.

people with diabetes and to present evidence-based interventions on their prevention. The evidence reviewed for this chapter includes patient education, foot-related self-management, foot examinations, therapeutic footwear and system changes to foot health care delivery. We performed keyword searches on 'patient education', 'self management education', 'foot examinations', 'therapeutic footwear' and 'systems of care changes'. The results from this literature search were restricted to articles that used human subjects and were published in the English language between 1986 and 2001. Only articles describing an intervention to address the outcome ulcer or amputation were selected.

RISK FACTORS FOR ULCERS AND AMPUTATIONS

ULCERS

Each year, foot ulcers develop in about 1.0–4.1% of adults with diabetes[3–8]. While comprehensive surveillance of all outpatient foot ulcers is limited to managed care systems with sophisticated data management systems, surveillance of US hospital discharges for foot ulcers is available from the National Hospital Discharge Survey (NHDS) and Nationwide Inpatient Sample (NIS). Demographic characteristics were collected from 1983 to 1990 from the NHDS to identify foot ulcer discharges[22]. The data indicate that the highest percentage of discharges for foot ulcers was in patients aged 45–64, while patients under age 45 had the lowest percentage of discharges. When age was standardized, males had a higher discharge rate than females for all years. Considerable variation occurred among white and nonwhite persons, although rates were not uniformly higher in either group.

Multivariate analyses were employed in several analytic studies to identify independent risk factors for diabetic foot ulcers. Table 28.2 shows the most commonly reported factors include long duration of diabetes, neuropathy and peripheral vascular disease. Several studies also reported a significantly elevated ulcer risk associated with poor glycemic control, foot deformity, increased plantar pressure, low HDL, prior foot ulcer and prior amputation.

Long duration of diabetes was a common, although not uniform, risk factor for foot ulcers[6,7,23–28]. The development of peripheral neuropathy, which has been associated with hyperglycemia, was reduced by 69% in the Diabetes Control and Complications Trial (DCCT)[29]. This trial also demonstrated that intensive treatment of hyperglycemia over an average of six years reduced the risk of developing retinopathy by 76% and microalbuminuria by 34% in patients without vascular pathology at baseline.

Several of the measures used to quantify peripheral neuropathy were found to independently predict foot ulcers. Two studies found a positive relationship between insensitivity to the Semmes–Weinstein 5.07 mm (10 g) monofilament and ulcers[24,28]. However, the study by Abbott[23] reported no relationship between the monofilament test and foot ulcers, but found that both vibration perception threshold and reflex/muscle strength score were significantly related to ulcer development. Other neuropathy risk factors significantly associated with foot ulcers included the neuropathy disability score[7], absent light touch sensation[6] and impaired pain perception[6].

High plantar pressure has also been linked to ulcer development. In a prospective study of people with diabetes attending a diabetes foot clinic, Veves *et al.*[30] used a modified neuropathic deficit score (NDS) to define neuropathy (reduced or absent reflexes and reduced or absent sensation to pain, touch and vibration) in a study of 58 neuropathic and 28 non-neuropathic subjects. Plantar pressure was measured at baseline and again after an average of 35 months. Incidence of neuropathic ulcers was noted. At baseline, 53% of neuropathic and 43% of non-neuropathic patients exhibited high plantar pressure. After follow-up 34% of neuropathic and 4% of non-neuropathic patients with high pressures developed foot ulcers. However, 55% of diabetic neuropathic patients with high foot pressures did not develop neuropathic ulcers, suggesting that high plantar pressure and insensitivity alone are not sufficient to predict ulcer development.

In a prospective study investigating the relationship between plantar pressure and ulcer development, 248 patients from three large diabetic foot centers were evaluated for peripheral neuropathy, joint mobility, peak plantar pressure and vascular status (Pham H *et al.* 2000). Multivariate analyses were conducted to identify ulcer risk factors. After an average of 30 months follow-up, ulcers

Table 28.2. Selected analytical studies of risk factors for diabetic foot ulcers.

Reference, analysis	Study design, diabetes type	Long DM duration	Neuropathy (monofilament, reflex, vibration, or neurologic summary score)	Low AAI, TcPO$_2$ or absent pulses	High HbA$_{1c}$	Deformity	Smoking	Ulcer	Amputation
								History	
Abbott et al. (1998)[23] Cox regression	RCT Patients with VPT ≥ 25; type 1 = 255 type 2 = 780	0	0 Monofilament + VPT + Reflex	Exclusion criteria			Exclusion criteria	Exclusion criteria	Exclusion criteria
Boyko et al. (1999)[24] Cox regression	Cohort Veterans type 1 = 48 type 2 = 701	0	+ Monofilament	+ AAI + TcPO$_2$	0	+ Charcot	0	+	+
Kumar et al. (1994)[7] Logistic regression	Cross-sectional 811 type 2 from UK general practices	+	+ NDS	+					
Litzelman et al. (1997)[25] Generalized estimation equations	RCT 352 type 2	0	+	0	0		0	+	+

Table 28.2. contd.

Reference, analysis	Study design, diabetes type	Long DM duration	Neuropathy (monofilament, reflex, vibration, reflex or neurologic summary score)	Low AAI, TcPO$_2$ or absent pulses	High HbA$_{1c}$	Deformity	Smoking	History Ulcer	History Amputation
Moss *et al.* (1999)[26] Logistic regression	Cohort 2990 patients with early and late-onset diabetes	Borderline older			+		Borderline young		
Pham *et al.* (2000)[27] Logistic regression	Cohort type 1 = 49 type 2 = 199	Control variable	+NDS +VPT 0 Monofilament	Control variable				0	
Rith-Najarian *et al.* (1992)[28] Chi square	Cohort 358 type 2 Chippewa Indians	+	+ Monofilament			0			
Walters *et al.* (1992)[6] Logististic regression	Cohort 10 UK general practices, 1077 type 1 = 212, type 2 = 865	+	+ Absent light touch + Impaired pain perception 0 VPT	+ Absent pulses			0		

AAI = ankle-arm index; DM = diabetes mellitus; HbA$_{1c}$ = hemoglobin A$_{1c}$; NDS = neuropathy disability score; RCT = randomized control trial; TcPO$_2$ = transcutaneous oxygen tension; VPT = vibration perception threshold. Blank cell = not studied; + = statistically significant finding; 0 = no statistically significant finding.

Reproduced with permission from *The Diabetic Foot*, eds J. H. Bowker and M. A. Pfeifer, pp. 13–32. 2001. Copyright © 2001 Mosby.

had developed in 29% of patients. Persons who ulcerated had significantly more neuropathy and significantly higher foot pressures.

The association between peripheral vascular disease and foot ulcer was ascertained using several measures: (1) the ankle-arm index (AAI) (suggesting impaired large vessel perfusion), (2) low transcutaneous oxygen tension (TcPO$_2$) (indicating diminished skin oxygenation) and (3) absent peripheral pulses. In a cohort study, both AAI and TcPO$_2$ were significant ulcer predictors[24]. Absent pulses[6,7] and a history of revascularization (angioplasty or bypass surgery)[7] have also been identified as independent risk factors associated with foot ulcers.

Smoking was not found to be a statistically significant risk factor for foot ulcers in most studies[6,7]. However, Moss[5] reported a borderline significant finding in persons diagnosed with early onset diabetes. Smoking is one of the major alterable risk factors implicated in atherosclerosis development in nondiabetic patients, along with lipoprotein abnormalities and high blood pressure. These three risk factors are assumed to be similarly atherogenic in persons with diabetes[31-33]. Despite the fact that smoking has not been conclusively linked to ulcer development in persons with diabetes, it is a significant risk factor for many other adverse health outcomes[5].

High levels of glycosylated hemoglobin (HbA$_{1c}$) were reported as an ulcer risk factor in only one of three studies addressing this parameter[24-26]. A history of ulcers and a history of amputation were commonly associated with risk for ulcer[5,24,25,27].

The risk of foot ulcer was shown to be proportional to the number of risk factors in a case-control study of Pima Indians[34]. Persons with diabetes who had any risk factor (peripheral neuropathy, peripheral vascular disease, bony deformities and a history of foot ulcers) were 2.1 (95% CI, 1.4–3.3) times more likely to develop an ulcer than the control subjects, persons with two risk factors were 4.5 (95% CI, 2.9–6.9) times more likely, and persons with three or four risk factors were 9.7 (95% CI, 6.3–14.8) times more likely to develop a foot ulcer.

AMPUTATIONS

Nontraumatic lower limb amputation hospital discharge rates obtained from the US NHDS from 1983 to 1996 demonstrate the effect of age, gender and race[35]. The highest amputation discharge rates were in patients 75 years of age or older. After controlling for age, males had an increased hospital discharge amputation rate across all years. Similarly, age-standardized comparisons of African-Americans and whites showed higher amputation discharge rates in African-Americans in each year studied.

As with ulcers, several studies employed multivariate analyses to explore the risk factors associated with amputation (Table 28.3). Eight rigorous analytic studies were selected for inclusion in this chapter to identify the amputation risk factors.

Long-term duration of diabetes was found to be statistically significantly related to amputation in five of the eight studies[13,17,34,36,37]; two others found no relationship[27,38], and the last study included duration as a control variable[40].

Peripheral neuropathy, diagnosed using the methods described above, was a significant independent risk factor in all of the studies measuring this variable[13,17,34,36–39]. Lack of protective sensation results in diminished patient awareness of painful and potentially harmful stimuli.

Peripheral vascular disease, also diagnosed with methods described previously, was found to be an independent risk factor in all of the studies making direct lower limb assessments[17,34,38,39]. Circulatory problems may also contribute to faulty wound healing[40].

Findings implicating high blood pressure as a risk factor for lower limb amputation were inconsistent. Three studies reported systolic, diastolic or elevations of both systolic and diastolic blood pressure as independent risk factors for amputation[27,36,37]. However, none of these studies also used a direct measure of peripheral vascular disease. Aspirin use was identified as a significant protective factor decreasing amputation risk[26].

High fasting plasma glucose or glycosylated hemoglobin was a statistically significant risk factor for amputation in most studies[13,17,27,34,36,37,39]. Poor glycemic control has been shown to increase the risk of neuropathy.

A history of retinopathy was found to be a risk factor for amputation in most studies[13,17,27,34,36,37,39]. Retinopathy is thought to reflect the extent of microvascular disease, and may be a proxy measure for diabetes severity[36].

A history of ulcers was found to increase the risk of amputation in three of the four studies that examined this parameter[27,34,38]. Other significant risk factors for amputation included use of insulin[36,38], elevated cholesterol[17,36], the presence of urinary proteins[17] and a prior history of amputation[38]. In two studies assessing the case-control impact of prior patient education on amputation risk, findings were mixed. There was a significant protective effect in one study[39] and no significant finding in another[36].

CAUSAL PATHWAYS TO ULCERS AND AMPUTATIONS

Consideration of the causes of ulcers and amputations is important in determining prevention strategies for persons with diabetes. Elucidating causal pathways is a way to link responsible events and contributing pathophysiological factors to foot ulcers and amputation. The causal pathway, adapted from Rothman and Pecoraro *et al.*, as shown in Figure 28.1, is a set of minimal conditions and events accumulating over time that inevitably pro-

Table 28.3. Selected analytical studies of risk factors for diabetic foot amputation.

Reference, analysis	Study design, diabetes type	Long DM duration	Neuropathy (monofilament, reflex, vibration)	PVD, AAI, TcPO$_2$ or pulses	HBP	High HbA$_{1c}$	History			
							Smoking	Ulcer	Retinopathy	Pt Ed
Alder et al. (1999)[38] Survival analysis	Cohort 776 veterans type 1 = 51 type 2 = 725	0	+	+		0	0	+		
Lee et al. (1993)[36] Survival analysis	Cohort 875 type 2 Oklahoma Indians	+			+SBP Male +DBP Female	+ Male	0	0	+	
Lehto et al. (1996)[17] Univariate and multivariate regression	Cohort 1044 type 2, Finland	+	+	+	0	+	0		+	
Mayfield et al. (1996)[34] Logistic regression	Retrospective case-control 244 type 2 Pima Indians	+	+	+	0	+	0	+	+	
Moss et al. (1999)[27] Logistic regression	Cohort 2990 early and late onset, WI, US	0			+DBP	+	+ Younger	+	+	

Table 28.3. contd.

Reference, analysis	Study design, diabetes type	Long DM duration	Neuropathy (monofilament, reflex, vibration)	PVD, AAI, TcPO$_2$ or pulses	HBP	High HbA$_{1c}$	Smoking	History Ulcer	Retinopathy	Pt Ed
Nelson et al. (1988)[13] Stratified	Cohort 4399 Pima Indians, Arizona, US type 2	+	+	+[1]	0	+	0		+	+
Reiber et al. (1992)[39] Logistic regression	Prospective case-control and 316 type 1 and 2 veterans	Control variable	+	+	0	+	0		+	+
Selby and Zhang (1995)[37] Logistic regression	Nested retrospective case-control type 1 = 9, type 2 = 390, 29 undetermined HMO	+	+		+SBP	+	0		+	

[1] Medial arterial calcification

AAI = ankle-arm index; DBP = diastolic blood pressure; DM = diabetes mellitus; HbA$_{1c}$ = hemoglobin A$_{1c}$; HBP = high blood pressure; Pt Ed = patient outpatient education; PVD = peripheral vascular disease; SBP = systolic blood pressure; TcPO$_2$ = transcutaneous oxygen tension.
Blank cell = not studied; + = statistically significant finding; 0 = no statistically significant finding.
Reproduced with permission from *The Diabetic Foot*, eds J. H. Bowker and M. A. Pfeifer, pp. 13–32, 2001. Copyright © 2001 Mosby.

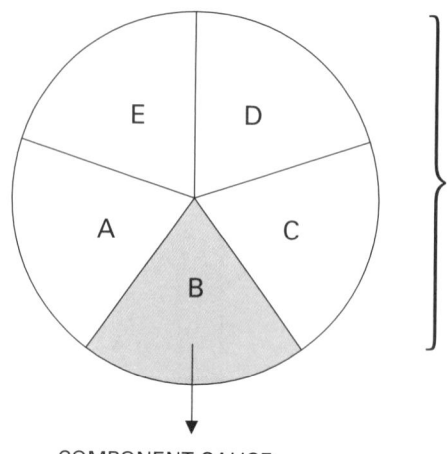

SUFFICIENT CAUSE:

– Inevitably produces the effect

– Restricted to the minimal number of component causes required for causation

COMPONENT CAUSE:

– Not sufficient in itself

– Removal or blocking renders action of other components insufficient

Figure 28.1. The sufficient and component causes of diabetic foot ulcers. A to E represent component causes that are not sufficient in and of themselves but, together, they inevitably produce the effect. Adapted from Rothman[41] and Pecoraro *et al.*[9] Reprinted with permission from Diabetes Care Vol. 22, 1999; 157–162. Copyright © 1999 American Diabetes Association.

duce a disease, with none of the conditions or events being superfluous[41]. A component cause is not sufficient to cause the outcome by itself, but is required to complete the causal chain in one or more distinct pathways. By removing just one of the components from a causal pathway, the effect of the disease can be delayed or prevented[41]. The ulcer or amputation outcome results from an accumulation of component causes or through one sufficient cause[9,42].

ULCERS

Reiber *et al.* conducted a study of the causal pathways leading to foot ulcer[42]. Data on important anatomic (structural foot deformity, including hammer toes, claw toes, hallux valgus or prominent metatarsal heads), pathophysiological (peripheral neuropathy, peripheral ischemia, infection, edema and callus formation) and environmental (minor foot trauma) variables were collected on 92 patients with incident ulcers from Manchester, England and 56 patients from Seattle, Washington State, USA with ages ranging from 30 to 85 years.

Five investigators independently reviewed each subject's data and determined the component causes that were present. Results were tabulated and consensus was achieved by all investigators using a modified Delphi process[43]. There were 32 unique component cause pathways, but only two causes were sufficient in and of themselves; trauma alone gave rise to ulcers in nine patients (6%) and edema was a sufficient cause in one (<1%). When the frequency of component causes was tabulated, the triad of the most prevalent causes leading to ulcer was neuropathy (78%), minor trauma (77%) and foot deformity (63%) (Table 28.4 and Figure 28.2).

AMPUTATIONS

Pecoraro *et al.*[9] investigated the causal pathways to diabetic amputation in 80 consecutive veterans aged 30 to 85 years who required a lower extremity amputation for reasons other than trauma. Again using Rothman's model of causation, component causes suggested by previous literature on diabetes and amputations were used, namely: neuropathy, ischemia, infection, wound healing failure, cutaneous ulcer, gangrene and minor trauma[42]. Specific pathways were identified using prospectively collected objective and subjective data. Objective measures in agreement with clinical observations were used to assign neuropathy and ischemia. The presence of ulcers, and gangrene, was determined by physical examination. Major infection was determined by physical examination, microbiological cultures and/or pathology and radiology reports indicative of osteomyelitis. Wound healing failure was indicated if there was no healing after six weeks and this was judged significant by the investigator. Minor trauma was assigned as a cause based on the patient interview and if the investigator judged it to have led to subsequent pathological events. Using a modified Delphi process, unanimous consensus was achieved by the investigators in assigning component or sufficient causes.

Table 28.4. The frequency of component causes present in studies of foot ulcers and amputations.

Component causes	Ulcers (%)[42]	Amputations (%)[9]
Peripheral neuropathy	78	61
Callus	30	
Deformity	63	
Peripheral ischemia	35	46
Infection	1.0	59
Edema	37	
Minor trauma	77	81
Ulceration		84
Faulty wound healing		81
Gangrene		55

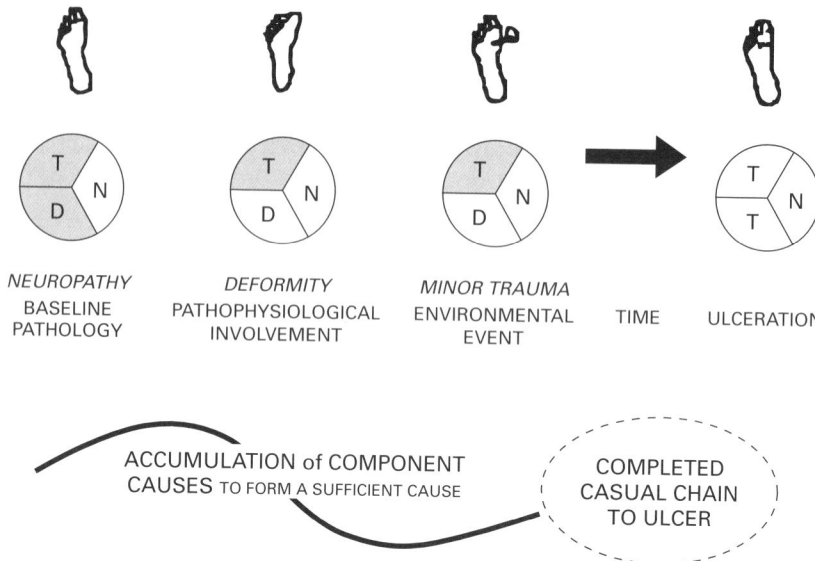

Figure 28.2. The most common causal pathway (neuropathy, deformity and minor trauma) to diabetic foot ulceration. Adapted from Reiber *et al.*[42] Reprinted with permission from *Diabetes Care*, Vol. 22, 1999; 157–162. Copyright © 1999 American Diabetes Association.

There were 23 unique causal pathways. The percentage of each component involved in amputations ranged from 46% with ischemia to 84% with ulcers (Table 28.4). A triad of component causes (minor trauma, cutaneous ulcer and subsequent failure to heal) was present in 72% of all amputations.

EVIDENCE-BASED RESEARCH: FINDINGS FOR INTERVENTIONS THAT PREVENTED ULCERS AND AMPUTATIONS

FOOT-RELATED SELF-MANAGEMENT EDUCATION

Malone *et al.* demonstrated that a simple education program can be used to lower the incidence of lower extremity ulcers and amputations in patients with diabetes (Table 28.5)[44]. Veterans with uninfected foot ulcers were prospectively randomized into two groups: group 1, education (103 patients, 203 limbs) and group 2, no education (100 patients, 193 limbs). Patients from both groups received the same clinical care, except for a one-hour education class, which consisted of slides depicting infected and amputated limbs and a set of patient care instructions. Following the class, no other education was provided. Follow-up averaged 13.2 months for the education group and 9.2 months for the control group. There was a significant reduction in both ulcers and amputations in comparing the group receiving education compared to the control group.

In an Australian population, Barth and colleagues[45] provided 14 hours of education over three days to all patients with diabetes. The intervention group in this study (n = 32) received an additional nine hours of content on foot care in four sessions held over one month. Differences in foot care problems including foot ulcers were significantly lower in the intervention group at one month, but not at three or six months.

Bloomgarden and colleagues[46] randomized 749 patients requiring insulin treatment to either a special diabetes education group or to a control group. While the primary study aim was a reduction in HbA_{1c}, a secondary aim was reduction of foot lesions. Among the 266 participants who completed the study (average 1.5-year follow-up), there were no significant differences in the frequency of foot lesions between the intervention and control groups.

FOOT EXAMINATIONS

The effectiveness of foot examinations in reducing the risk of diabetic amputation was studied by Mayfield *et al.*[49] in a case-control study of 61 patients who developed ulcers and 183 controls who did not (Table 28.6)[43]. Patients' preventive foot examinations over a three year period were classified into three-groups: (1) A visual scan to check for breaks in the skin; (2) A comprehensive exam which included a visual exam plus an evaluation for bony deformity, neurological status and vascular status; and (3) A therapeutic exam, conducted when a preventive procedure such as callus removal was performed. Persons requiring the fourth type of foot exam, a treatment examination for foot ulcers and lesions, were excluded from this analysis. The odds ratio 0.55 (95% CI, 0.2–1.7, p = 0.31) suggested a protective effect from preventive foot exams, yet the confidence interval included 1.

In a randomized clinical trial in Finland, groups were randomized to podiatric foot care, counseling and primary prevention or regular care and written foot care instruction. After a seven-year follow-up interval there were no statistically significant reductions in ulcers or amputations[48].

THERAPEUTIC FOOTWEAR

Litzelman analyzed the population in her randomized controlled trial (RCT) using generalized estimation equation techniques. Only the prescription of specialized shoes was significantly associated in the model with foot ulcer development[49].

Uccioli *et al.* explored the efficacy of therapeutic shoes in preventing reulceration in people with diabetes (Table 28.7)[50]. Patients (n = 69) with

Table 28.5. Effectiveness of foot-related patient self-management education and foot examinations in reducing foot ulcers and amputations.

Reference, analysis	Study design, diabetes type	Intervention (Groups/Arms/ Comparisons)	Prevent Ulcer	Prevent LEA
Patient foot self-management education				
Barth et al. (1991)[42] Multiple linear regression	Prospective intervention Volunteers with type 2 diabetes	Intervention group = 32 (normal plus intensive education); normal education (14 hours over3 days) plus 4 specialfoot care sessions over4 weeks (additional 9 hours); provided in groups of 8–10 persons. Control group = 38 (normal education)	Reduction in foot problems at 1 month, $p < 0.006$, but no reduction at 6 months. Foot problems included foot ulcer	
Bloomgarden et al. (1987)[43] Analysis of variance	RCT. 266 type 1 patients	Intervention group received 9 education sessions and control groups received usual care	Nonsignificant differences in foot lesions including ulcers	
Malone et al. (1989)[41] Chi-square corrected for continuity	RCT. 203 veterans, randomized into two groups. Diabetes type not stated	Group 1: education (n = 90, with 177 limbs) and group 2: no education (n = 92, with 177 limbs)	Invention group had 8/177 ulcers; control group had 26/177 ulcers, $p \leq 0.005$	Intervention group had 7/177 amputations; Control group had 21/177 amputations, $p \leq 0.025$

Table 28.6. Effectiveness of foot-related patient self-management education and foot examinations in reducing foot ulcers and amputations.

Reference, analysis	Study design, diabetes type	Intervention (Groups/Arms/ Comparisons)	Prevent Ulcer	Prevent LEA
Foot examinations				
Hamalainen *et al.* (1998)[48]	RCT. Type 1 and type 2 diabetes	Intervention group (n = 267): podiatric care with counseling and primary prevention. Control group (n = 263): written instructions. 1166 preventive foot exams over 3 years (foot scans, comprehensive examinations and therapeutic examination)	Nonsignificant difference	Nonsignificant difference
Mayfield *et al.* (2000b)[47] Logistic regression	Case-control Pima Indians 61 cases, 183 controls type 2			Benefit of one or more foot exams on amputation risk OR = 0.55 (CI 0.2–1.7). Foot exams may or may not decrease LEA in Pima Indians

previous ulcers or those at risk for developing ulcers were randomized into two groups: group 1 (n = 36) wore ordinary, nontherapeutic shoes while group 2 (n = 33) wore therapeutic shoes with custom-molded insoles. Ulcer relapses occurred in 58.3% of the group with their own shoes, but only occurred with 27.7% of the patients with therapeutic shoes. The odds ratio was 0.26 (95% CI 0.2–1.54, p = 0.009) and suggesting a protective association between the use of therapeutic shoes and ulcer development, despite the wide confidence interval which included 1.

Reiber *et al.* conducted a randomized clinical trial of 400 men and women from two Western Washington health care organizations[51]. Participants were randomized into one of three study groups. Group 1 (n = 121) wore study shoes and customized, medium-density cork inserts with a closed cell neoprene cover. Group 2 (n = 119) wore study shoes and noncustomized medium-density polyurethane inserts with a nylon cover, and the controls in group 3 (n = 160) wore their own footwear. Two-year cumulative reulceration incidence across groups 1, 2 and 3 was low: 15%, 14% and 17% respectively. Patients in study shoes did not have a significantly lower risk of reulceration compared to controls: group 1, Risk Ratio (RR) 0.88, (CI 0.51–1.52); group 2, RR 0.85 (CI 0.48–1.48). All ulcer episodes in study shoes and 88% in nonstudy shoes occurred in patients with insensate feet. The authors concluded that the study shoes and custom cork or polyurethane inserts conferred no significant ulcer reduction benefit compared to control patients' footwear. This study suggests that careful attention to foot care by providers may be more important than therapeutic footware. The study did not negate the possibility that special footwear is beneficial in patients with diabetes who do not receive such close attention to foot care by their providers.

Edmonds *et al.*[52] studied 239 ulcer patients with either ischemic (n = 91) or neuropathic (n = 148) ulcers. Subjects were either given therapeutic and custom shoes or wore their own footwear. Among the neuropathic group, 121 subjects reulcerated after an average follow-up time of 26 months. The reulceration rates were 26% among the therapeutic footwear group and 83% among those who wore their own footwear. However, these findings may have been influenced by the inclusion of subjects with severe foot deformities.

SYSTEMS OF CARE CHANGES

Systems approaches have been used to improve health care outcomes in a variety of health care settings (Table 28.8)[53,54]. Components for an optimal system for chronic illness care have been identified as (1) coordinated community resources and politics; (2) health care system organization; (3) patient self-management support; (4) provider decision support; (5) health system delivery design; and (6) clinical information systems. Within an

Table 28.7. The effectiveness of therapeutic footwear in reducing foot ulcers and amputations.

Author, analysis	Study design, diabetes type	Intervention (Groups/Arms/ Comparisons)	Prevent Ulcer	Prevent LEA
Edmonds *et al.* (1986)[52] Descriptive analysis	Descriptive 148 patients with foot ulcers and sensory loss. type 1 = 86 type 2 = 62	Footwear (n = 86), no footwear (n = 35) follow-up averaged 26 months	26% reduction in footwear group, 83% reulceration in own footwear group	Pre-post amputation reduction noted of 50%
Litzelman *et al.* (1997)[49] Generalized estimation equations	RCT. 352 type 2 patients	Physician education and reminders, patient education, system interventions	Special shoes OR = 2.19 (CI 1.07–4.49)	
Reiber et al.[51] Chi-square, Fisher's exact test	RCT. 400 men and women with type 1 and 2 diabetes and a history of foot ulcers from Western Washington health care organizations. type 1 = 20 type 2 = 380	Group 1 = 3 pair study shoes and custom inserts Group 2: 3 pair study shoes and polyurethane inserts Group 3 (controls): own footwear All participants received slippers Two-year follow-up	Ulcer rates comparing study shoes and cork inserts to controls RR = 0.88 (CI 0.51–1.52) Ulcer rate comparing study shoes and polyurethane inserts to controls RR = 0.85 (CI 0.48–1.48) There was no significant reduction in ulcers	
Uccioli *et al.* (1995)[50] Chi-square	RCT. 69 diabetic patients (type 1 = 17, type 2 = 52) with previous ulcers or high risk of developing ulcers.randomized from two Italian teaching hospitals	Group 1 (n = 36): own, non-therapeutic shoes Group 2 (n = 33): therapeutic shoes with custom-molded insoles. One-year follow-up	Reulceration with intervention shoes = 27.7% versus 58.3% in own footwear. OR = 0.26 (CI 0.2 – 1.54), p = 0.009	

Table 28.8. The impact of changes in foot care in health care systems on ulcers and amputations in people with diabetes.

Author, analysis	Study design, diabetes type	Intervention (Groups/Arms/Comparisons)	Prevent Ulcer	Prevent LEA
Carrington et al. (2001)[60]	Retrospective. 143 unilateral amputees Diabetes type not stated	Intervention group: foot care program based on critical pathway plus lower limb assessment, podiatric care and education. Control group: lower limb assessment		15.4% amputations in intervention group, 14% in matched controls. No significant difference
Dargis et al. (1999)[56] Analysis of variance	Nonrandomized two-year prospective study of patients with diabetes and prior ulcer. Intervention = 56 patients. Control = 89 patients from other geographic areas type 1 = 31, type 2 = 114	Intervention group received multidisciplinary team foot care; control group received regular care	Significant reduction in reulceration between groups (30.4% versus 58.4%); $p < 0.001$	
Edmonds et al. (1986)[52] Descriptive analysis	Descriptive. 148 patients with neuropathic foot ulcers	Average 26 months follow-up; comprehensive team foot care (inpatient and outpatient); footwear	Reulceration in 26% patients in special shoes and 83% in own shoes	Pre-post amputation reduction noted of 50%
Larsson et al. (1995)[10] Mann–Whitney, Chi-square	Retrospective. 224 126 residents of Lund or Orup Districts, Sweden, with an estimated 2.4% diabetic subjects	Multidisciplinary team to diagnose/prevent/ treat diabetic foot ulcers	Not assessed	Decrease in amputations from 7.9/1000 in 1982 to 4.1/1000 in 1993

Table 28.8. contd.

Litzelman et al. (1993)[25] Chi-square	Randomized clinical trial. 396 type 2 patients in intercity clinic	*Patient interventions*: foot care education group with education, behavioral contracting, phone and postcard prompts *Physician interventions*: practice guidelines, information on amputation risk factors, foot care practice and prompts.	Patients increased self-foot care behaviors. Prevented minor lesions. Better ulcer detection and documentation in intervention group	Intervention = 0.5%. Control = 2.0%. p = 0.20
McCabe et al. (1998)[57] Chi-square	Prospective. 2001 patients Diabetes type not stated	Intervention group (n = 1000): for foot screening, exam, 128 high-risk patients in foot protection program, control group (n = 1000): routine care, two-year follow-up	Nonsignificant difference	Nonsignificant difference for minor amputation. Significant reduction in major amputation
Patout et al. (2000)[58]	Pre-post intervention historic controls. 197 patients with type 1 or 2 diabetes	Foot outcomes one-year pre- and post-LEAP program. Program provided components including risk-stratified, case-managed education, foot care, footwear	Decreased foot ulcer days, hospitalizations, emergency room visits and antibiotics for foot ulcers	Decreased lower limb amputations
Rith-Najarian et al. (1998)[59]	Cohort. 639 American Indians, Minnesota, 98% type 1	Staged diabetes management		Amputation reduction from 29/1000 to 21/1000 to 15/1000 (~50%)

organization, the ideal foot care system would provide cost-effective care to maintain patient function and quality of life and prevent or delay the development of ulcers and amputation. Foot care systems often include multidisciplinary health professionals working as a team headed by a 'champion'.

The influence of systems of care has been addressed in several historic and analytic studies published since the mid-1980s. Edmonds and colleagues designed and implemented a specialized foot clinic to manage patients with diabetes from a large referral area in South London. Over a three-year period this multidisciplinary group demonstrated a high frequency of ulcer healing and a reduction in major amputations[52].

A population-based Swedish retrospective study addressed the impact of a multidisciplinary program for foot care persons with diabetes[10]. Larsson and colleagues noted the total incidence of amputation in persons with diabetes decreased from 7.9 to 4.1/1000 over an 11-year interval. This success was attributed to the combination of increased availability of preventive foot care and footwear, a prompt and coordinated evaluation and follow-up of foot problems, increased use of noninvasive vascular testing, greater use of peripheral vascular procedures and strict criteria for amputation level. Falkenberg describes similar successes by a multidisciplinary team, also in Sweden[57].

In Lithuania, Dargis and colleagues[56] allocated 56 patients residing in one city to multidisciplinary foot care team follow-up, while 89 patients living in 13 other geographic areas received standard care. The foot care intervention included multidisciplinary foot care, footwear, foot care education and re-education on foot problems every three months. After two years follow-up, there were significantly fewer recurrent ulcers in the intervention group than the standard treatment group (30% versus 58%).

McCabe and colleagues[57] selected 2001 people with diabetes and allocated them into two groups. The 1000 people targeted for intervention received foot screening which yielded 128 high-risk patients who were then enrolled in a foot protection program. Clinical and administrative data for the control group was used for comparison. After a two-year follow-up, no significant differences were reported in minor amputation, but a significant reduction was reported in major amputations.

Litzelman and colleagues[25] targeted an intercity population of 395 patients with type 2 diabetes with a multifaceted intervention. Participants received education prior to initiating a behavioral contract for self-foot care. Study staff provided support and reminders. Providers received practice guidelines, foot care flowsheets and prompts to stimulate routine foot examination and education. After a one-year intervention, there was a statistically significant decrease in serious foot lesions between the intervention and control groups. The providers were significantly more likely to examine feet, document foot findings and refer patients for podiatric services.

Patout and colleagues[58] instituted a foot care program and followed 197 patients with diabetes for one year. A decrease in foot ulcer days, hospitalizations and emergency room visits was observed over the year they were in the lower extremity amputation prevention program, compared to their experience in the year prior to the program.

Beginning in 1985, Rith-Najarian and colleagues in Minnesota, USA followed a cohort of 639 American Indians with diabetes[59]. After instituting a staged diabetes management program that included foot evaluations and foot care, a 50% reduction in amputations was documented (29/1000 to 15/1000).

Carrington and colleagues[60] targeted patients with a prior unilateral amputation. A special foot care program was provided to 143 people based on critical pathways which included physical assessment, podiatric care and education. There were 148 matched controls who did not receive this special program. After a two-year follow-up, there were no significant differences in reamputation frequency between the intervention group and their matched controls.

SUMMARY AND CONCLUSIONS

In summary, prospective research on foot ulcers and amputations in persons with diabetes has identified risk factors common to both conditions: longer diabetes duration, impaired glycemic control, peripheral neuropathy and peripheral vascular disease. Preventive intervention strategies have been explored and the most promising include patient self-management, education and alterations in systems of care. These strategies have statistically significantly reduced both ulcers and amputations. The effect of two additional preventative strategies, namely foot examinations and therapeutic footwear, is less conclusive, but still may be beneficial in some populations.

ACKNOWLEDGMENTS

This research was supported by the Department of Veterans Affairs, Veterans Health Administration and Health Services Research and Development (project number RCS98-353) and Rehabilitation Research and Development Service (project number A0806C).

REFERENCES

1. http://www.Diabetes.org (2002).
2. King H, Aubert RE and Herman WH (1998) Global burden of diabetes, 1995–2025: prevalence, numerical estimates, and projections. *Diabetes Care* **21**, 1414–1431.
3. Palumbo PJ and Melton LJ (1985) Peripheral vascular disease and diabetes. In *Diabetes in America* (ed. MI Harris), NIDDR: pp. 401–408.
4. Borssen B, Bergenheim T and Lithner F (1990) The epidemiology of foot lesions in diabetic patients aged 15–50 years. *Diabetic Medicine* **7**, 438–444.

5. Moss SE, Klein R and Klein BEK (1992) The prevalence and incidence of lower-extremity amputation in a diabetic population. *Archives of Internal Medicine* **152**, 610–616.
6. Walters DP, Gatling W, Mullee MA and Hill RD (1992) The distribution and severity of diabetic foot disease: A community study with comparison to a non-diabetic group. *Diabetic Medicine* **9**, 354–358.
7. Kumar S, Ashe HA, Parnell LN, Fernando DJ, Tsigos C, Young RJ, Ward JD and Boulton AJ (1994) The prevalence of foot ulceration and its correlates in type 2 diabetic patients: A population-based study. *Diabetic Medicine* **11**, 480–484.
8. Ramsey SD, Newton K, Blough D, McCulloch DK, Sandhu N, Reiber GE and Wagner EH (1999) Incidence, outcomes, and cost of foot ulcers in patients with diabetes. *Diabetes Care* **22**, 382–387.
9. Pecoraro RE, Reiber GE and Burgess EM (1990) Pathways to diabetic limb amputation. Basis for prevention. *Diabetes Care* **13**, 513–521.
10. Larsson J, Apelqvist J, Agardh CD and Stenstrom A (1995) Decreasing incidence of major amputation in diabetic patients: A consequence of a multidisciplinary foot care team approach? *Diabetic Medicine* **12**, 770–776.
11. AHRQ (2000) Nationwide Inpatient Sample.
12. Mayfield JA, Reiber GE, Maynard C, Czerniecki JM, Caps MT and Sangeorzan BJ (2000) Trends in lower limb amputation in the Veterans Health Administration, 1989–1998. *Journal of Rehabilitation Research & Development* **37**, 23–30.
13. Nelson RG, Gohdes DM, Everhart JE, Hartner JA, Zwemer FL, Pettitt DJ and Knowler WC (1988) Lower-extremity amputations in NIDDM. 12-year follow-up study in Pima Indians. *Diabetes Care* **11**, 8–16.
14. Siitonen OI, Niskanen LK, Laakso M, Siitonen JT and Pyorala K (1993) Lower-extremity amputations in diabetic and nondiabetic patients. A population-based study in eastern Finland. *Diabetes Care* **16**, 16–20.
15. Humphrey LL, Palumbo PJ, Butters MA, Hallett JW Jr., Chu CP, O'Fallon WM and Ballard DJ (1994) The contribution of non-insulin-dependent diabetes to lower-extremity amputation in the community. *Archives of Internal Medicine* **154**, 885–892.
16. Humphrey AR, Dowse GK, Thoma K and Zimmet PZ (1996) Diabetes and nontraumatic lower extremity amputations. Incidence, risk factors, and prevention – a 12-year follow-up study in Nauru. *Diabetes Care* **19**, 710–714.
17. Lehto S, Ronnemaa T, Pyorala K and Laakso M (1996) Risk factors predicting lower extremity amputations in patients with NIDDM. *Diabetes Care* **19**, 607–612.
18. Trautner C, Haastert B, Giani G and Berger M (1996) Incidence of lower limb amputations and diabetes. *Diabetes Care* **19**, 1006–1009.
19. Van Houtum WH and Lavery LA (1996) Outcomes associated with diabetes-related amputations in the Netherlands and in the state of California, USA. *Journal of Internal Medicine* **240**, 227–231.
20. Morris AD, McAlpine R, Steinke D, Boyle DI, Ebrahim AR, Vasudev N, Stewart CP, Jung RT, Leese GP, MacDonald TM and Newton RW (1998) Diabetes and lower-limb amputations in the community. A retrospective cohort study. DARTS/ MEMO Collaboration. Diabetes Audit and Research in Tayside Scotland/ Medicines Monitoring Unit. *Diabetes Care* **21**, 738–743.
21. Reiber GE (2002) Epidemiology and health care costs of diabetic foot problems. In *The Diabetic Foot: Medical and Surgical Management* (eds A. Veves, JM Giurini and FW LoGerfo), Humana Press, Totowa, NJ, pp. 35–58.
22. Reiber GE, Boyko EJ and Smith DG (1995) Lower extremity foot ulcers and

amputations in diabetes. In *Diabetes in America* (ed. MI Harris, NIDDK-Washington, D.C. Pub No. 95–1468, pp. 409–428.

23. Abbott CA, Vileikyte L, Williamson S, Carrington AL and Boulton AJ (1998) Multicenter study of the incidence of and predictive risk factors for diabetic neuropathic foot ulceration. *Diabetes Care*, **21**, 1071–1075.

24. Boyko EJ, Ahroni JH, Stensel V, Forsberg RC, Davignon DR and Smith DG (1999) A prospective study of risk factors for diabetic foot ulcer. The Seattle Diabetic Foot Study. *Diabetes Care* **22**, 1036–1042.

25. Litzelman DK, Slemenda CW, Langefeld CD, Hays LM, Welch MA, Bild DE, Ford ES and Vinicor F (1993) Reduction of lower extremity clinical abnormalities in patients with non-insulin-dependent diabetes mellitus. A randomized, controlled trial. *Annals of Internal Medicine* **119**, 36–41.

26. Moss SE, Klein R and Klein BEK (1999) The 14-year incidence of lower-extremity amputations in a diabetic population–The Wisconsin Epidemiologic Study of Diabetic Retinopathy. *Diabetes Care* **22**, 951–959.

27. Pham H, Armstrong DG, Harvey C, Harkless LB, Giurini JM and Veves A (2000) Screening techniques to identify people at high risk for diabetic foot ulceration: A prospective multicenter trial. *Diabetes Care* **23**, 606–611.

28. Rith-Najarian SJ, Stolusky T and Gohdes DM (1992) Identifying diabetic patients at high risk for lower-extremity amputation in a primary health care setting. A prospective evaluation of simple screening criteria. *Diabetes Care* **15**, 1386–1389.

29. Diabetes Control and Complications Trial Study Group (1993) The effect of intensive treatment of diabetes on the development and progression of long term complications in insulin dependent diabetes mellitus. *New England Journal of Medicine* **329**, 997–968.

30. Veves A, Murray HJ, Young MJ and Boulton AJ (1992) The risk of foot ulceration in diabetic patients with high foot pressure: A prospective study. *Diabetologia* **35**, 660–663.

31. Gordon T and Kannel WB (1972) The Framingham Study: Predisposion to atherosclerosis in the head, heart and legs. *Journal of the American Medical Association* **221**, 661–666.

32. Jarrett RJ and Deen H (1975) Diabetes and atherosclerosis. In *Complications of Diabetes*. (eds H Keen and RJ Jarrett) London: Edward Arnold, pp. 179–204.

33. Kannel WB and McGee DL (1979) Diabetes and cardiovascular disease: The Framingham study. *Journal of the American Medical Association* **241**, 2035–2038.

34. Mayfield JA, Reiber GE, Nelson RG and Greene T (1996) A foot risk classification system to predict diabetic amputation in Pima Indians. *Diabetes Care* **19**, 704–709.

35. Reiber GE (2001) Epidemiology of foot ulcers and amputations in the diabetic foot. In *The Diabetic Foot* (eds JH Bowker and MA Pfeifer, Mosby, St. Louis, pp. 13–32.

36. Lee JS, Lu M, Lee VS, Russell D, Bahr C and Lee ET (1993) Lower-extremity amputation. Incidence, risk factors, and mortality in the Oklahoma Indian Diabetes Study. *Diabetes* **42**, 876–882.

37. Selby JV and Zhang D (1995) Risk factors for lower extremity amputation in persons with diabetes. *Diabetes Care* **18**, 509–516.

38. Adler AI, Boyko EJ, Ahroni JH and Smith DG (1999) Lower-extremity amputation in diabetes. The independent effects of peripheral vascular disease, sensory neuropathy, and foot ulcers. *Diabetes Care*, **22**, 1029–1035.

39. Reiber GE, Pecoraro RE and Koepsell TD (1992) Risk factors for amputation in patients with diabetes mellitus. A case-control study. *Annals of Internal Medicine* **117**, 97–105.

40. IWGDF (1999) International consensus on the diabetic foot, International Working Group on the Diabetic Foot, 1–96.
41. Rothman KJ (1976) Reviews and commentary: Causes. *American Journal of Epidemiology*, **104**, 587–592.
42. Reiber GE, Vileikyte L, Boyko EJ, del Aguila M, Smith DG, Lavery LA and Boulton AJ (1999) Causal pathways for incident lower-extremity ulcers in patients with diabetes from two settings. *Diabetes Care* **22**, 157–162.
43. Linstone HA and Turoff M (1975) In *The Delphi Method: Techniques and Applications*. Reading, MA: Addison-Welsey.
44. Malone JM, Snyder M, Anderson G, Bernhard VM, Holloway GA Jr. and Bunt TJ (1989) Prevention of amputation by diabetic education. *American Journal of Surgery* **158**, 520–523; discussion 523–524.
45. Barth R, Campbell LV, Allen S, Jupp JJ and Chisholm DJ (1991) Intensive education improves knowledge, compliance and foot problems in type 2 diabetics. *Diabetic Medicine* **8**, 111–117.
46. Bloomgarden ZT, Karmally W, Metzger JM, Brothers M, Nechemias C, Bookman J, Faierman D, Fellner FG, Rayfield E and Brown V (1987) Randomized, controlled trial of diabetic patient education: improved knowledge without improved metabolic status. *Diabetes Care*, **10**, 263–272.
47. Mayfield JA, Reiber GE, Nelson RG and Greene T (2000) Do foot examinations reduce the risk of diabetic amputation? *Journal of Family Practice* **49**, 499–504.
48. Hamalainen H, Ronnemaa T, Toikka T and Liukkonen I (1998) Long-term effects of one year of intensified pediatric activities on foot-care knowledge and self-care habits in patients with diabetes. *Diabetes Educator* **24**, 734–740.
49. Litzelman DK, Marriott DJ and Vinicor F (1997) The role of footwear in the prevention of foot lesions in patients with NIDDM. Conventional wisdom or evidence-based practice? *Diabetes Care* **20**, 156–162.
50. Uccioli L, Faglia E, Monticone G, Favales F, Durola L, Aldeghi A, Quarantiello A, Calia P and Menzinger G (1995) Manufactured shoes in the prevention of diabetic foot ulcers. *Diabetes Care* **18**, 1376–1378.
51. Reiber GE, Smith DG, Wallace C, Sullivan K, Hayes S, Vath C, Maciejewski M, Yu O and Heagerty PJ, LeMaster J (2002) Effect of therapeutic footwear on foot reulceration in patients with diabetes. A randomized controlled trial. *JAMA* **287**, 2552–2558.
52. Edmonds M, Blundell M and Morris M (1986) Improved survival of the diabetic foot. *Quarterly Journal of Medicine* **60**, 763–771.
53. Wagner EH, Austin WM and Von Korff M (1996) Organizing care for patients with chronic diseases. *Milbank Quarterly* **74**, 511–544.
54. Berwick DM (1998) Developing and testing changes in delivery of care. *Annals of Internal Medicine* **128**, 651–656.
55. Falkenberg M (1990) Metabolic control and amputations among diabetics in primary health care – a population-based intensified programme governed by patient education. *Scandinavian Journal of Primary Health Care* **8**, 25–29.
56. Dargis V, Pantelejeva O, Johushaite A, Vileikyte L and Boulton AJM (1999) Benefits of a multidisciplinary approach in the management of recurrent diabetic foot ulceration in Lithuania. *Diabetes Care* **22**, 1428–1431.
57. McCabe CJ, Stevenson RC and Dolan AM (1998) Evaluation of a diabetic foot screening and protection programme. *Diabetic Medicine* **15**, 80–84.
58. Patout CA Jr., Birke JA, Horswell R, Williams D and Ceriise FP (2000) Effectiveness of a comprehensive diabetes lower-extremity amputation prevention program in a predominantly low-income African-American population. *Diabetes Care* **23**, 1339–1342.

59. Rith-Najarian S, Branchaud C, Beaulieu O, Gohdes D, Simonson G and Mazze R (1998) Reducing lower-extremity amputations due to diabetes. Application of the staged diabetes management approach in a primary care setting. *Journal of Family Practice* **47**, 127–132.
60. Carrington AL, Abbott CA, Griffiths J, Jackson N, Johnson SR, Kulkarni J, Van Ross ER and Boulton AJ (2001) A foot care program for diabetic unilateral lower-limb amputees. *Diabetes Care* **24**, 216–221.

29

Can Established Diabetic Complications be Reversed? The Evidence for Secondary Prevention

KEN SHAW

Academic Department of Diabetes and Endocrinology, Portsmouth NHS Hospitals Trust, Portsmouth, UK

Prevention of long-term complications is a major consideration in the management of diabetes, striving towards a quality of life and life expectancy comparable to that of the general population. For many people with diabetes, development of complications is not inevitable and great strides have been made in the primary prevention of such, particularly within the spectrum of microvascular disorders. Yet, for various reasons, many people still develop distressing consequences of diabetes which significantly contribute to premature morbidity and mortality and which, once established, often progress inexorably. Can this progression be contained or, indeed, can such complications be reversed (secondary prevention)?

The July 2000 issue of the popular journal *Scientific American* included an article[1]. on the topic of 'AGE Breakers' ('Rupturing the body's sugar-protein bonds might turn back the clock'). Specific reference was made to the premature acceleration of the aging process in diabetes, through deposition of advanced glycation end products (AGEs) leading to tissue damage including thickening of arteries and stiffening of myocardium. The prospect that drugs could be developed with the potential of 'breaking this molecular glue' offers encouragement for the future. The AGE-receptor is relatively ubiquitous, promising potential future modification by pharmacological inhibition of advanced glycation. Already agents such as aminoguandine and pyridoxamine

The Evidence Base for Diabetes Care. Edited by R. Williams, W. Herman, A.-L. Kinmonth and N. J. Wareham.
© 2002 John Wiley & Sons, Ltd

are being investigated but unfortunately such therapy is still on the distant horizon and other therapeutic strategies still need to be addressed.

Such treatments do depend on the particular complication concerned and the causative factors that are thought to contribute to their development. Therapeutic options for the secondary prevention of complications in diabetes involve multifactorial considerations. Genetic factors are in part likely to determine susceptibility of individuals to complications. These cannot presently be modified, although the expression of such may be attenuated by adjustment of lifestyle e.g. by weight reduction, healthy eating, physical exercise, not smoking etc. Various risk factors make their own individual contributions to the causation of complications, and the outcome of treatment interventions will depend on which risk factor is targeted. Often the result is an interrelated complexity of several simultaneous risk factors, making it difficult to determine the precise consequences of treatment intervention.

In as much as hyperglycaemia has been identified as an independent risk factor in its own right, the restoration of sustained normoglycaemia from pancreatic transplantation should indicate to what extent drug treatment of hyperglycaemia might be expected to diminish or delay progression of established complications. The evidence base is still uncertain. Again it would seem as though complications in early stages may be modified, but more advanced tissue damage is less reversible. Pancreas transplantation and consequent normoglycaemia may neither reverse nor prevent progression of advanced diabetic retinopathy[2]. and indeed accelerated progression of retinopathy can be an observed phenomenon with intensified metabolic control. Similar results have been reported in respect of diabetic nephropathy with failure of pancreas transplantation to reverse established lesions within five years of normoglycaemia. However longer-term normoglycaemia over 10 years following pancreas transplantation has been linked with improvements in advanced structural changes within the diabetic kidney[13], with observed lessening of glomerular and tubular basement membrane thickening and mesangial expansion. This late improvement may reflect the slow dynamics of the glycosylation process and show that normalising glycosylated matrix may require many years to take effect.

Currently, the evidence that normoglycaemia (as achieved by pancreas transplantation) can reverse established complications is uncertain. By extrapolation, it may therefore be unreasonable and unduly optimistic to expect prescribed hypoglycaemic therapy alone, with its inevitable imperfect suboptimal control, either with tablets or with insulin, to have a significant impact on the complications of diabetes once tissue damage has reached a point of advanced structural change. The state of pancreatic islet cell transplantation is promising[14]. but there are as yet no adequate long-term observations in respect of reducing the progression, let alone reversal, of established complications.

So is there evidence that earlier intervention has a better prospect of lessening complications? Prior to DCCT (Diabetes Control and Complications Trial), the evidence that early complications in type 1 diabetes could be ameliorated by intensive treatment was hotly debated[15]. Neither multiple insulin injection therapy nor continuous insulin-pump treated patients had been associated with convincing improvements in microvascular dysfunction, and furthermore in respect of retinopathy a worsening of condition may be observed during the first two years following more intensified intervention.

It was on the basis of these unanswered questions concerning prevention of complications (both primary and secondary) that DCCT proceeded. Thus this major study[16]. of type 1 diabetic patients treated over a mean of 6.5 years has become the primary reference source for the evidence that intensive treatment of diabetes can beneficially influence the progression of long-term complications. A secondary-intervention cohort was recruited from patients with one to 15 years of type 1 diabetes, with established early complications described as 'very mild to moderate' non-proliferative retinopathy and incipient nephropathy with urinary albumin excretion >40 mg but mg/24 hours to <300 mg. In this group, intensified therapy was associated with reduced progression of retinopathy by 54% and more severe retinopathy was reduced by 47%. A similar outcome was observed for microalbuminuria. DCCT showed that the progression of established complications could be reduced by intensive treatment, but the reduction was less than that achieved with the primary prevention cohort. The earlier commencement of treatment, the better the prospect of preventing progression.

It is interesting to observe that these benefits have been sustained for at least four years after completion ('close-out') of the main study, despite approximation of glycaemic control between the two groups (conventional and intensive), again indicating that intervention during the early stages of developing complications may be particularly important in securing good long-term outcomes[7].

The question as to whether intensive glycaemic control reduces microvascular complications in patients with type 2 diabetes has been extensively debated; but current consensus does provide reasonable support that good glycaemic control is beneficial in respect of the three main microangiopathies[18]. The landmark UKPDS study specifically addressed the relationship of blood glucose control and the future occurrence of long-term complications[9]. The positive results reported are now well known and widely quoted as the evidence-based reference source for aggressive glycaemic intervention in the treatment of type 2 diabetes. The results appear good in the context of trial outcome measures, but two comments need to be made. First, the UKPDS data has been presented in terms of relative risk reduction which looks impressive, but it is still disappointing to note that disease progression in the majority of the intensively treated group still continued with the passage of time. In support of the overall positive conclusions, UKPDS patients were recruited at a relatively early stage in their diabetes (fasting blood glucose >6 mmols/l) and the mean haemoglobin A_{1C} levels, even in the conventionally treated groups, were much less than commonly observed in an everyday diabetes clinic, which might have lessened greater potential differences between the two compared groups. The second consideration is to note that most of the evidence from UKPDS associating hyperglycaemia and microvascular complications in type 2 diabetes relates to primary rather than secondary prevention. The initial development of microangiopathies may well be significantly reduced by good early glycaemic control. The evidence that the progression of more established complications may be ameliorated is much less certain, an observation that most would find consistent with clinical experience.

Thus limited observations from pancreas transplantation and data from the two landmark studies of DCCT for type 1 diabetes and UKPDS for type 2 diabetes offer indications and some encouragement that tight glycaemic control may benefit microvascular complications, but probably with most benefit during early stages and least benefit once complications are fully established.

INDIVIDUAL COMPLICATIONS

Diabetic foot disease can account for serious and tragic consequences, including loss of limb. Treatment involves multifaceted therapies, but results are still inconclusive. The effectiveness of intervention in the management of diabetic foot ulceration has been reviewed[10] with good evidence that the amputation rates of high-risk cases can be reduced by a foot protection programme, including identification of those at high risk, followed by referral to specialist foot care clinics providing education, podiatry and individualised footwear. The evidence base for specific local treatments for diabetic foot ulcers, however, is still lacking, particularly regarding the multiple antibiotic regimens that are often employed. Growth factors, G-CSF, other topical agents and hyperbaric oxygen still require further research. A further critical appraisal of the evidence for effective treatment of diabetic foot ulceration[11] has again highlighted the relative paucity of sound objective outcome data, commenting that randomised control trials with cost–benefit analysis are urgently needed. Much still needs to be done in terms of specific therapies, but it is good to note that improved pathways of care with multidisciplinary involvement are proving effective and offering real opportunities to lessen the potentially tragic consequences of diabetic foot disease.

The natural history of *diabetic nephropathy* appears to have changed, at least in the Western world[12]. Substantial reductions in the incidence of end-stage renal failure have been reported in Scandinavia and in the UK, although the burden continues with the increasing prevalence of diabetes, particularly type 2. This reduction is likely to reflect improved management and treatment regimens. DCCT[6] has shown reduced progression of microalbuminuria in early nephropathy (type 1) by intensified insulin treatment, but glycaemic control is less effective in more advanced renal failure, when other interventions become more important. A number of meta-analyses of the beneficial effects of antihypertensive drug treatments on renal function have been reviewed[13], and have concluded that ACE-inhibitors offer particular benefits for people with diabetic renal disease or microalbuminuria, even when normotensive. Of other potential interventions some evidence has been found that dietary protein restriction may slow progression to renal failure in type 1 diabetics but not in type 2, whilst no conclusive evidence has been found in respect of lipid reduction. Tight blood pressure control is the most beneficial treatment for all stages of nephropathy, and is cost-effective.

The risk of developing *retinopathy* directly correlates with the degree of hyperglycaemia and duration of disease. Visually threatening proliferative retinopathy remains a high risk for type 1 diabetes with long-standing poor control. DCCT showed that this could be reduced, but as retinopathy becomes established, tight glycaemic control becomes less effective and may well aggravate progression for some time. The possibility that ACE-inhibitors might limit progression of retinopathy in patients with type 1 diabetes has been suggested from the EUCLID study[14] but the study group commented that further control trials are needed before changes in clinical practice are advocated. The results of smoking cessation and treatment of systolic hypertension are less certain.

The evidence base for retinal screening is established[15] offering a potential substantial impact in the prevention of new blindness[16] through the confirmed and highly successful application of laser photocoagulation therapy developing visually threatening retinopathy is detected[17]. Several methods of screening (direct ophthalmoscopy by clinician or optometrist; retinal photography) are available, but the evidence is currently insufficient to make recommendations as to which is best[15]. This depends on local circumstances.

If the evidence for secondary prevention of established diabetic microvascular complications would seem lacking, that for *macrovascular disease* is even more equivocal. The combination of research evidence and clinical observation has enabled promotion and implementation of better treatment strategies to improve diabetes control for type 1 and type 2 patients, with a consequent reduction in primary development of long-term microvascular disorders. This significant epidemiological change has exposed a different pattern of diabetic complications, with macrovascular disease becoming the more prevalent clinical problem and greater therapeutic challenge. Hyperglycaemia contributes as an independent risk factor to development of large vessel disease but so far there is very limited evidence that intensive glycaemic control reduces adverse cardiovascular outcome[18].

This is particularly so for type 1 diabetes. As with microvascular disease, the main reference source remains the DCCT[6] where no detectable treatment-related differences in rates of macrovascular events were observed in the study groups either with intensive or conventional treatment. Intensive insulin therapy was associated with a relative risk reduction of 41% for all major cardiovascular events, but this was not statistically significant, again illustrating the limitations of interpreting data in relative terms. The relative youth of patients in the trial (mean age 27 years) for both primary and secondary prevention cohorts militated against a likely impact, particularly in respect of coronary disease within the 6.5-year time period. Surrogate markers of potential coronary heart disease were studied in the trial with no evidence of change in blood pressure but with some improvement in total cholesterol and LDL cholesterol concentrations. Unfortunately data in respect of macrovascular progression in the four-year post-DCCT study[7] were not given. There is no clear-cut evidence that established coronary heart disease in type 1 diabetes can be significantly ameliorated by aggressive glycaemic intervention.

The observations arising from Diabetes Mellitus Insulin-Glucose Infusion in Acute Myocardial Infarction Study Group(DIGAMI)[18] of benefits following acute myocardial infarction await further validation. Immediate and continued insulin usage appeared to offer the prospect of more prolonged survival at three years, but the two groups (insulin versus non-insulin) were not sufficiently distinct in characteristics and other possible contributory factors could not be excluded. DIGAMI-2 is currently in progress and may answer some of the outstanding questions.

The evidence base for cardiovascular prevention in type 2 diabetes is not that much better. UKPDS just failed to demonstrate a significant influence of glycaemic control on coronary outcome (16% relative risk reduction of myocardial infarction). Overall a reduction of haemoglobin A_{1c} from 9% to 8% appeared to reduce the risk of myocardial infarction by 18%. On a numbers needed to treat (NNT) basis, 37 patients would need treatment over 10 years to prevent one myocardial infarction, and 167 patients need to be treated in order to prevent one stroke. The prospect of improving coronary risk by tight glycaemic control appears tantalisingly close, but in reality it is still to be established. When considering a cardiovascular 30% risk reduction over 10 years, other interventions to prevent a vascular event may be superior when assessed on a NNT basis, e.g. aspirin 15.2; stopping smoking 17.4; blood pressure control NNT 15.9, compared to glycaemic control 20.8[19]. Having said that, risk may be multiplicative: from UKPDS a haemoglobin A_{1c} >8% plus systolic blood pressure >150 mmHg increases mortality risk 11-fold. Hence, total rather than individual risk factor intervention needs to be considered.

Thus it can be understood that vascular disease in diabetes arises from a complexity of multifactorial predisposing factors including genetic susceptibility, metabolic dysfunction and lifestyle issues. This risk is particularly associated with the concept of insulin resistance, which is well recognised in type 2 diabetes, but probably a common occurrence in type 1 diabetes as well[20], and suspected clinically in the presence of concomitant hypertension, hyperlipidaemia, obesity and high insulin dosage. Although weight reduction in obese patients and increased physical exercise should lessen coronary risk as well as improving insulin sensitivity the evidence of benefit for diabetes has not been established. This contrasts with the considerable evidence emerging that other risk factor intervention can have substantial beneficial effects in those at risk.

What of specific risk factor interventions? *Dyslipidaemia,* disturbance of lipid and lipoprotein metabolism, commonly occurs in diabetes and almost certainly contributes to the pathogenesis of vascular complications. Such abnormalities show considerable variation, often in parallel with varying levels of glycaemic control. No consistent abnormality is observed with regard to total cholesterol for either type 1 or type 2 diabetes, but with type 2 diabetes in particular, low HDL lipoprotein-cholesterol is frequently detected, and hypertriglyceridaemia is characteristic, often preceding diagnosis and providing a predictive indication of diabetes to come.

The benefits of therapeutic lipid intervention in the prevention of coronary heart disease in the population as a whole is now well established. It could be anticipated that such benefit would also be expected in the diabetes subpopulation; possibly to a greater extent. In a secondary prevention trial, the sub-group analysis of the Scandinavian Simvastatin Survival Study[21] concluded that cholesterol lowering with simvastatin improved the prognosis of diabetic patients with coronary heart disease. Benefit was expressed in terms of improved relative risk over a 5.4 year median follow-up, observing a 57% reduction in total mortality and a 45% reduction in major coronary heart disease events. In view of the high risk of coronary heart disease in diabetes, the authors suggested that the absolute clinical benefit achieved by cholesterol lowering may be greater in diabetic than in non-diabetic patients with coronary heart disease.

Confirmation of these findings was also provided by the Cholesterol and Recurrent Events (CARE) Trial[22] in which diabetic patients with prior myocardial infarction and treated with pravastatin over five years experienced a 25% relative risk reduction in all CHD event end-points. A more detailed review of various intervention trials (statin and fibrates) has been provided by Watts[23]. Substantial evidence exists that cholesterol reduction significantly reduces the risk of coronary disease and related events, and this evidence would support the conclusion that high-risk groups such as type 2 diabetics will gain most from treatment intervention. The interesting concept is that all type

2 diabetics should be managed as secondary prevention irrespective of preceding coronary history, following the observation that the predicted mortality risk of a person with type 2 diabetes without a prior coronary event is comparable to that of a non-diabetic person who has sustained a myocardial infarction[24]. If patients with type 2 diabetes are to be considered in the context of secondary prevention, irrespective of previous coronary history, then targeting a similar total cholesterol of <5 mmol/l as for non-diabetics with previous history of a coronary event would mean that almost 75% of type 2 patients with diabetes would be candidates for statin therapy.

For *hypertension* in diabetes, the clear benefits of antihypertensive treatment in respect of micro/macroproteinuria and nephropathy in type 1 diabetes contrasts with the benefits of blood pressure (BP) control of large vessel disease, where the situation is less clear. Much data concerning blood pressure management in type 2 diabetes exists, but there has never been a primary prospective randomised placebo control trial of the treatment of hypertension among type 2 diabetes patients[25]. However, current consensus from sub-group analyses of large blood pressure intervention trials interprets the evidence as being overwhelmingly supportive of good blood pressure control being beneficial in respect of major cardiobascular system outcomes. UKPDS[9] demonstrated that lowering an elevated blood pressure had a major impact on the subsequent development of myocardial infarction, congestive cardiac failure and stroke, much more defined than the outcome data from glycaemic control. In UKPDS, beta-blockers were seemingly as effective as ACE-inhibitors, suggesting that it was the lowering of the blood pressure itself, rather than the means of doing so, that was the beneficial factor. Many intervention trials have been published with particular implications for the treatment of type 2 diabetes. These various studies all indicate benefit in terms of cardiovascular outcomes, but from differing perspectives[26]. The Hypertension Optimal Treatment (HOT) Study[27] observed that aggressive blood pressure lowering with a calcium channel blocker (CCB) (felodipine) was associated with decreased CVS events (particularly stroke), but could not exclude influence from other combined therapeutic agents. The Appropriate BP control in Diabetes Trial (ABCD)[28] favoured ACE-inhibitor therapy (enalapril) and raised the possibility that a dihydropyridine CCB (nisoldipine) might actually aggravate adverse CVS outcome. All of the four main classes of antihypertensive drugs – thiazide diuretics, CCBs, ACE-inhibitors and beta-blockers – have supporting evidence of efficacy[29] but, as Padfield has argued[25], a number of questions remain. The desirable blood pressure target end-point has yet to be determined; what drug combinations are most effective? (UKPDS showed that multiple therapies were often required). Is it simply blood pressure reduction that is effective, or are there differences in outcome between the different classes of hypotensive agents and indeed within each class of drugs as well? Are there benefits from lowering a normal blood pressure?

The Heart Outcomes Prevention Evaluation (HOPE) Study[30] is a good example of how additional questions can be raised even with the most encouraging of observed outcome results. The main HOPE Study recruited patients with existing evidence of coronary heart disease but excluded those with heart failure or significant left ventricular dysfunction. The multicentre randomised double-blind study of the ACE-inhibitor ramipril at a dose of up to 10 mgs/day for an average of 4.5 years included a diabetic sub-group. Reported separately as the Micro HOPE Study[31], type 2 diabetic patients with presumed high likelihood of silent coronary heart disease were recruited on the basis of diabetes plus one or more cardiovascular risk factor such as hyperlipidaemia, hypertension, cigarette smoking or microalbuminuria. Evaluation included not only future cardiovascular events but also the risk of progression from microalbuminuria to overt nephropathy.

An independent data safety and monitoring panel recommended the conclusion of the trial after 4.5 years, when significant outcome differences were observed between ramipril- and placebo-treated groups for primary (myocardial infarction, stroke, CVS death) and secondary (total mortality, overt nephropathy, heart failure and unstable angina) end-points. Clinical outcomes included relative risk reduction by 25% for combined primary end-points; by 22% for myocardial infarction; by 33% for stroke and by 37% for CVS deaths, all of statistical significance. The implications of these results have been reviewed[32] including comment that application of the HOPE Study inclusion criteria in clinical practice would result in virtually all diabetic subjects over the age of 55 meriting the addition of an agent such as ramipril to their existing therapy.

Interpretation of the study poses some difficulties. How was the benefit achieved? There was no change in glycosylated haemoglobin A_{1C} levels and, hence, improved glycaemic control was an unlikely factor. The mean difference in blood pressure (10/5 mm Hg) was relatively small, which suggests that other factors could be exerting the apparent beneficial effect. These have yet to be determined, but could include direct vascular and endothelial protective effects, improvements in myocardial perfusion, and other possibilities. Unfortunately interpretation of results is further confounded by a relatively high drop-out rate (circa one in three) for both ramipril-treated and placebo-treated patients. Furthermore, despite the high CVS risk of recruited patients, other therapies potentially influencing outcome e.g. concomitant beta-blockers, lipid-lowering drugs, aspirin etc. were very variable and, in general, underprescribed.

Trials such as Micro HOPE provide a considerable thought-provoking exercise. Striking outcome results still need careful consideration and reflection before they are implemented in clinical practice. Conservative Clinicians often require more convincing, particularly when mechanisms of effect are uncertain or other confounding variables may be operative. This was a high-risk population. Can the conclusions be extrapolated to type 2 diabetic patients without other risk factors coming into play? Are the results a class drug effect and if so can they reasonably be expected with other ACE-inhibitors? What about angiotensin receptor antagonists? On an evidence-based principle, these questions remain to be answered.

This chapter has shown that complications of diabetes, once established are not easily reversed. Ideally, understanding the causes of complications will lead to effective therapies in the primary prevention of all unwanted long-term consequences of diabetes. Much has been achieved, particularly in reducing the risk of microvascular dysfunction, and there is real optimism for the future. Secondary prevention is much more difficult, and depends on how far tissue damage has progressed. It may be unrealistic to expect advanced structural change to regress, and the progress that has been made is disappointing. To some extent, the relatively limited benefit of intensified glycaemic control in respect of secondary prevention is thwarted by the current imperfect means of enabling normalisation of blood glucose levels. We still await the time when more physiological control can be achieved.

Complications are associated with several other considerations, and attention to these individual risk factors can make a significant difference. An individual analysis of how much can be achieved from each specific intervention can be discouraging, but taking a global perspective can be much more optimistic. Perhaps the greatest benefits are already being achieved by improvements in delivery and pathways of care, where the management of the patient involves not only treatment interventions but also a wider range of educational initiatives and psychosocial understanding.

REFERENCES

1. Melton I (2000) Age breakers. *Scientific American* **283**: 12.
2. Ramsey RC, Goetz FRC Switzerland DER, Maver SM, Robinson LL, Cantrill HL, Knobloch WH, Najaran JS (1988) Progression of diabetic retinopathy after pancreas transplantation for insulin – dependent diabetes mellitus. N. Eng. J. Med. **318**: 208–214.
3. Floretto P, Steffes MW, Sutherland DER, Goetz FC, Maver M (1998) Reversal of lesions of diabetic nephropathy after pancreas transplantation. *N. Eng. J. Med.* **339**: 69–75.
4. Shariro AMJ, Lakey JRT, Ryan EA, Korbutt GS, Toth E, Warnock GL (2000) Islet cell transplantation in seven patients with type 1 diabetes mellitus using a glucocorticoid free immunsuppressing regimen. *N. Eng. J. Med.* **343**: 230–237.
5. The DCCT Research Group (1988) Are continuing studies of metabolic control and microvascular complications in Insulin-dependent diabetic mellitus justified? *N. Eng. J. Med.* **318**: 246–249.
6. Diabetes Control and Complications Trial Research Group (1993) The effects of intensive treatment of diabetes and the development and progression of long-term complications in insulin-dependent diabetes mellitus. *N. Eng. J. Med.* **329**: 977–986.

7. The Diabetes Control and Complications Trial/Epidemiology of Diabetic Treatments and Complications Research Group (2000) Retinopathy and nephopathy in patients with type 1 diabetes four years after a trial of intensive therapy. *N. Eng. J. Med.* **342**: 381–389.

8. Herman WH (1999) Glycaemic control in diabetes: clinical evidence. *BMJ* **319**: 104–106.

9. UKPDS Group (1998) Intensive blood glucose control with sulphonylureas or insulin compared with conventional treatment and risk of complication in patients with type 2 diabetes (UKPDS 33) *Lancet* **352**: 837–853.

10. The University of York NHS Centre for Reviews and Dissemation (1999) Complication of diabetes: management of foot ulcers. *Effective Healthcare* **5**: 6–11.

11. De P, Scharpello JHB (1999) What is the evidence for effective treatment of diabetic foot ulceration? *Pract. Diab. Int.* **16**: 179–184.

12. Bojestig M, Arnquist HJ, Hermansson E, Karlberg BE, Ludvigsson J (1994) Declining incidence of nephopathy in insulin-dependent diabetes mellitus. *N. Eng. J. Med.* **300**: 15–18.

13. The University of York NHS Centre for Reviews and Dissemination (2000) Complication of diabetes: renal disease and promotion of self-management. *Effective Health Care* **6**: 1–11.

14. Chaturvedi N, Sjolie A, Stephenson JM and the EULID Study Group (1998) Effect of lisinopril on progression of retinopathy in normotensive people with type 1 diabetes. *Lancet* **351**: 28–31.

15. The University of York NHS Centre for Reviews and Dissemination (1999) Complications of diabetes: screening for retinopathy. *Effective Health Care* **5**: 1–6.

16. Rohan TE, Frost CD, Walt NJ (1989) Prevention of blindness by screening for diabetic retinopathy: a quantitative assessment. *BMJ* **299**: 1198–1201.

17. Diabetic Retinopathy Study Research Group (1998) Photocoagulation treatment of diabetic retinopathy: clinical application of DRS findings. *Opthalmology* **116**: 297–303.

18. Malmberg K and DIGAMI (Diabetes mellitus insulin glucose infusion in acute myocardial infarction) study group (1997) Prospective randomised study of intensive insulin treatment on long-term survival after acute myocardial infarction in patients with diabetes mellitus. *BMJ* **314**: 1512–1515.

19. Yudkin J (1999) Proceedings of Annual Professional Conference, British Diabetic Association, Glasgow.

20. Williams KV, Erby JR, Becker D, Arslanian S, Orchard TJ (2000) Can clinical factors estimate insulin resistance in type 1 diabetes? *Diabetes* **49**: 626–632.

21. The Scandinavian Simvastatin Survival Study (45) Group (1997) Cholesterol lowering with simvastatin improves progress of diabetic patients with coronary heart disease. *Diabetes Care* **20**: 614–620.

22. Goldberg RB, Mellies MJ, Sacks FM, Moye LA, Howard BV, Howard WJ, Davis BR, Cole TG, Pfeiffer MA, Braunwald E (For the CARE Investigation) (1998) Cardiovascular events and the reduction with pravastatin in diabetic and glucose-intolerant myocardial infarction survivors with average cholesterol levels. *CIRCULATION* **98**: 2513–2519.

23. Watts GF (2000) Coronary disease, dyslipidaemia and Clinical Trials in type 2 diabetes. *Pract. Diab. Int.* **17**: 54–59.

24. Haffner SM, Lehto S, Ronnemaa T, Pyoralda K, Laakso M (1998) Mortality from coronary disease in subjects with type 2 diabetes and in non-diabetic subjects. *N. Eng. J. Med.* **339**: 229–234.

25. Padfield PL (2000) Managing blood pressure in type 2 diabetes mellitus (Leader). *Practical Diabetes International* **17**–35.

26. Jermus G, Chattington P (1999) Management of hypertension in patients with diabetes. In *Diabetes and Cardiovascular Complications* (ed. PG McNally) Science Press, pp. 59–71.

27. Hanson L, Zanchetti A, Carruthers SG (1998) Effects of intensive blood pressure lowering and low-dose aspirin in patients with hypertension: the hypertension optimal treatment (HOT) randomised trial. *Lancet* **351**: 1755–1762.

28. Estacio RO, Jeffers BW, Hiatt WR, Biggerstaff SL, Gifford N, and Schrier, R (1998) The effects of nisoldipine as compared with enalapril on cardiovascular outcomes in patients with non-insulin-dependent diabetes hypertension. *N. Eng. J. Med.* **338**: 645–652.

29. McKnight JA (2000) Managing blood pressure in type 2 diabetes mellitus. *Practical Diabetes International* **17**: 49–53.

30. The Heart Outcomes Prevention Evaluation (HOPE) Study Investigation (2000) Effects of the angiotensin-converting enzyme inhibitor ramipril on cardiovascular events in high-risk patients. *N. Eng. J. Med.* **342**: 145–153.

31. Heart Outcomes Prevention Evaluation (HOPE) Study Investigation (2000) Effects of ramipril on cardiovascular and microvascular outcome in people with diabetes mellitus: results of the HOPE study and micro-HOPE study. *Lancet* **355**: 253–259.

32. Fisher M, Kennon B (2000) The HOPE study: practical implications for people with diabetes. *Practical Diabetes International* **17**: 191–194.

Part VIII

DELIVERY OF CARE

30

What is the Evidence that Increasing Participation of Individuals in Self-management Improves the Processes and Outcomes of Care?

DEBRA ROTER and ANN-LOUISE KINMONTH

Johns Hopkins School of Public Health, Baltimore, MD 21205, USA

Dept. of Public Health and Primary Care, University Forvie Site,
Cambridge CB2 2SR, UK

Assessing the needs of patients with a chronic disorder such as diabetes, and choice of treatment options, has traditionally relied on the judgement of physicians. A cultural shift is currently occurring in medical care in parallel with that in society in general. This questions whether the physician's judgement alone is either a sufficient or an adequate basis for deciding between treatment options[1]. One argument put forward is that physician-centred decision making is associated with poor compliance among patients with diabetes. In contrast, increasing patient participation in self-care and medical consultation is argued to lead to better adherence to agreed treatment decisions, and better clinical outcomes[2,3].

Effective management of diabetes is complex; it demands not only changes in behaviours in the medical sphere through, for example, regular glucose testing and taking of medications, but also the adoption of healthy lifestyle behaviours, including diet, exercise, safety precautions and other preventive self-care actions[3]. These behaviours appear relatively independent; effective self-management in one area is not necessarily predictive of effective performance in others[2-4]. Indeed, patients appear to engage in a process of decision-making that often involves trading off behaviour in one sphere against others.

The Evidence Base for Diabetes Care. Edited by R. Williams, W. Herman, A.-L. Kinmonth and N. J. Wareham.
© 2002 John Wiley & Sons, Ltd

Insight into the nature of patient decision-making regarding the management of diabetes has been hampered by a traditionally narrow approach to assessment of patient compliance. Many authors acknowledge that the term compliance, which has been used historically to characterize the extent to which a patient is willing to follow a detailed set of procedures or medical guidelines, including medication prescriptions, connotes patient passivity[5-7]. Patient compliance is consistent with a biomedical paradigm that devalues independent patient judgement and sees failures to comply as the result of patient incompetence, deviance or irresponsibility. In reaction to the authoritarian and directive tone of 'compliance', some investigators have suggested 'adherence' as a less imposing alternative semantic, carrying a suggestion of active cooperation[6,7].

The difference in terms, however, is subtle and the change has not been widely adopted by researchers in the field[5-7]. A more substantive departure from the directive terminology of compliance or adherence, which is more in keeping with an emphasis on patient autonomy in treatment decision-making, is evident in increasing reference to patient self-care or self-management activities[2,3]. Self-management approaches reflect involvement of patient judgements and values within the context of daily living to inform how a comprehensive treatment plan can be best agreed and implemented. This approach has been pioneered in the diabetes literature, where a consideration of the broader life context within which treatment decisions must be carried out is especially relevant[2,3]. Consistent with this self-management perspective, the American and British Diabetes Associations (Diabetes UK) now refer to diabetes education as diabetes self-management education, and the American Academy of Diabetes Educators refers to diabetes education as 'an interactive, collaborative, ongoing process'[8]. Since semantics can have so powerful a role in shaping and focusing debate and in providing a guide to how social reality is interpreted, understood and acted upon, self-management will be used in the remainder of this chapter to reflect active patient engagement in making decisions about the management plan, and carrying out the planned treatment behaviours and activities.

Several meta-analytic reviews of diabetes-related intervention studies (or a diabetes subset of chronic disease studies) have been conducted over the past 10 years[9-11]. There is considerable agreement that educational programmes confer benefits on patients across a range of outcomes. Effect sizes were often largest for self-reported measures, including knowledge, diet and exercise change, and smaller for more objectively measured outcomes such as increasing skills, weight change and control of blood glucose. The Brown meta-analysis[9] estimated a small effect size (as measured by a Cohen's d) for educational interventions, of 0.41 for HbA_{1c} and somewhat smaller effects for other measures (Cohen's d = 0 .35 for blood glucose concentrations and 0.27 for psychological outcomes). An exception to this pattern of results was a large knowledge effect (Cohen's d = 1.0) produced by the interventions. In the meta-analysis by Roter *et al.* of compliance-specific interventions[10], the effect size for the subset of diabetes studies for effects on HbA_{1C} and blood glucose was moderate in magnitude (Cohen's d = 0.56). A notably stronger effect was evident for compliance indicators measured through pill count and pharmacy record review (Cohen's d = 1.0) and, as in the Brown study, for knowledge (Cohen's d = 0.8).

The effects evident in the reviews, however, may not be long-lasting. In addition to finding similar short-term estimates as those reported by Brown[9] and Roter[10], Padgett[11] calculated effect sizes over time. She found that an effect size of 0.36 for HbA_{1C} at six months following interventions fell to virtually zero (0.03) by 12 months; effects on blood glucose concentration measures were reduced also falling from 0.58 at six months to 0.20 at 12 months. Only psychological and knowledge effect sizes were maintained at moderate levels over time.

Interpretation of these findings is problematic, however, because of wide-spread methodological weaknesses in individual studies. Evidence from randomized controlled trials is limited. Sampling and recruitment strategies were rarely reported, studies were often small and of short duration (the majority being less than 15 weeks long), few studies referred to a theoretical or conceptual framework for the intervention or provided a sufficiently detailed description of the intervention to make replication possible, and measures of intervention effect were poorly described, developed, or validated[12, 13].

The focus of reported diabetes interventions appears primarily cognitive (instruction alone or in combination with behavioural training in diet, exercise and/or self-monitoring techniques) or behavioural (characterized by behaviour modification or social learning strategies). A few studies address techniques such as relaxation and biofeedback therapies or psychodynamic counselling; even fewer address patient empowerment and activation strategies (see below). Importantly, interventions based on ideas of informed choice and acquiring skills of self-management including group work, the addition of audiovisual aids, and behavioural and social learning approaches, were more effective than narrowly didactic approaches[9–12].

Other factors that contribute to self-management of diabetes are beliefs and personal models of the disease, motivation, and social and environmental factors that include support resources as well as barriers.[14] Sociodemographic characteristics are poor predictors of which patients will follow management recommendations and which will not. There is no consistent relationship between gender, education, income, intelligence, general knowledge about health and illness and personality type and adherence to medical regimes[3,7,12,14].

Conscious decisions to forgo self-management activities are much more complex and less responsive to traditional interventions than inadvertent errors[2–7]. As noted earlier, patients often only selectively, partially or erratically engage in medical and lifestyle activities recommended by their physician. It is the domain of patient decision-making which ignores, delays, minimizes or curtails responses to medication and lifestyle recommendations that poses the greatest challenges to successful self-management of diabetes.

There are two promising sources of evidence, however, to guide practice in supporting improved self-management among people with diabetes. The first, already referred to, is the application of understandings from psychology to inform patient education strategies. These span both the cognitive field, using techniques to test and strengthen motivations to act, and the behavioural field, to support the implementation of chosen activities and build them into habits.[14,15,16,17,18] The second lies in the growing recognition of the importance of the nature of the patient–practitioner relationship within which the educational strategy is applied. Increasing patient engagement in the communication process may be an important vehicle through which treatment decisions are made, and subsequently applied. Much of the supportive evidence for this contention was synthesized in Stewart's review of analytic and randomized controlled trials of physician–patient communication, in which a health-related outcome was reported[19]. The nature and process of communication in the consultation was found to influence patient outcomes, particularly emotional distress, but also symptom resolution, functional status and physiology including blood pressure and blood glucose. Characteristics of the consultation linked to positive health and treatment outcomes included patients asking questions, agreeing about the nature of the problem and the need for follow-up, and perceiving that a full discussion of the problem had taken place; practitioners answering patients' questions with clear information, asking questions about the patients' ideas, concerns and expectations, and showing empathy.

This chapter reviews the evidence linking levels of patient engagement in medical visit communication and self-management to diabetes-related outcomes. It defines the principles emerging from this evidence, to inform better clinical practice.

THE PATIENT PARTICIPATION CONTINUUM IN COMMUNICATION

A common point of departure for studies linking patient and physician communication to clinical outcomes is some measure of patient engagement in the dialogue of the visit. A critical reading of this literature can distinguish three levels of patient engagement: patient participation, patient activation, and patient empowerment.

Patient participation: The first level of engagement is simple participation in the medical dialogue. This can be defined as any patient or physician strategy that facilitates the inclusion of the patient's perspective or the patient's preferences into the medical plan, primarily through facilitated disclosure of the patient's illness narrative[2]. The primary vehicle for enhanced patient participation is the use of patient-centred interviewing skills[20,21]. Patients may participate in the dialogue by simply telling their story. At its most basic level, feeling listened to and heard is a fundamental function of the therapeutic relationship. As expressed by George Engel in recognizing the patient's power in telling his story ' ... interpersonal engagement required in the clinical realm rests on complementary and basic human needs, especially the need to know and understand and the need to feel known and understood'[22].

The power of disclosing relevant life experiences, perspectives and preferences is not only in being validated and feeling known, but also in the power of one's narrative to act as a vehicle of self-reflection. Within this context, the patient is transformed from a reporter of symptoms to a 'co-investigator' of his health problems[23]. The critical communication skills that facilitate active patient participation in the medical visit include those originally derived from the psychotherapy literature and applied to interviewing skills: data gathering, relationship building and partnering skills[24]. At its most elementary level, patient participation in the medical visit can be seen as reactive; physicians enquire and patients respond. Data-gathering skills reflect a variety of questioning behaviours that are varied in both form and content. Restricted opportunities for patient participation in the visit are provided through closed-ended questions, to which the patient provides direct answers. The transformation from restricted to full participation is contingent on broadening the parameters of elicitation so that patients can fully and most meaningfully tell their story. Open questions, by their very nature, allow more room for patient discretion in response than closed-ended questions. Questions about things patients know and care about and that are relevant to daily experience and context potentially enhance the relevance and the meaning of disclosure.

Relationship-building skills, including emotional support, empathy, reassurance and personal regard create an atmosphere that facilitates open and sensitive disclosure by optimizing rapport and trust.

Partnership skills also make it easier for a patient to tell his story by actively facilitating patient input through prompts and signals of interest, interpretations, paraphrases, requests for opinions and probes for understanding. In addition, patients may be encouraged to more actively participate in the visit by having the physician assume a less dominating relationship stance. This includes lowered verbal dominance, for example, by listening more and talking less, using head nods and eye contact and forward body lean to signal interest.

Attempting to understand the use and consequence of patient-centred skills for patient activation, Street undertook a descriptive study of natural communication patterns in which patient participation in the medical dialogue could be linked to metabolic control[25]. For this study, following an initial educational programme, audiotape recordings were made of consultations between newly diagnosed diabetic patients and nurses during a session to review strategies for managing diabetes and progress and problems related to metabolic control. Patients of nurses with a participatory style, facilitating patient input into medical dialogue and limiting the use of controlling communication, experienced better metabolic control than patients of 'take charge' nurses (that is, those who issued directives, recommendations and orders, interrupted the patient, disagreed with the patient, or changed a patient-initiated topic).

It was suggested that a controlling communication style may inhibit patients' ability to convey the full spectrum of their concerns and communicate their illness narrative; that is, to tell the story of their illness and engage in the process of reflection and understanding. This includes raising concerns of a psychosocial and emotional nature and becoming actively involved in problem-solving for disease management. A controlling style may act to depersonalize both the visit and the therapeutic regimen. A somewhat similar conclusion was drawn by a group of Finnish researchers who found, in a cross-sectional study, that patient reports of a positive doctor–patient relationship (for example, taking notice of the patient as an individual) correlated with tighter metabolic control[26].

Patient activation: At a second level, patient activation heightens patient engagement from disclosure to a process of exploration and enquiry into the conditions and circumstances that may contribute to the medical problem or may be useful in treatment and management[21]. The medical dialogue provides the vehicle of patient activation in agenda setting, question asking and joint problem-solving.

Active involvement in the dialogue transforms the patient role from reactive to proactive, with patients taking the initiative in assuring that their agenda is presented and their needs met. Activation interventions have generally included guides or algorithms given directly to patients by a researcher, or via trained practitioners. They aim to help patients identify, phrase and rehearse questions, concerns and issues to be included in the agenda of the visit[27]. Physicians can be taught to assist patients by providing full and relevant information and counselling, by the use of partnership-building skills, including the solicitation of patient questions, expectations, preferences and probing the patient's explanatory framework, or by engaging in a process of negotiation and problem-solving related to treatment and lifestyle regimens, which values individual context as well as population-based evidence. A particularly important partnership-building behaviour is simply not to interrupt. In observational studies physicians frequently interrupt patients, on average after less than 25 seconds after beginning the statement of their primary problem. The interruption moves to follow up the first, but not necessarily most important, stated concern[28,29].

The first of the studies to link glycosylated haemoglobin, as a measure of diabetic control to active patient engagement in medical visit communication was the seminal work of Greenfield and colleagues[30]. This and subsequent trials are summarized in Table 30.1 and described below. These researchers conducted an experimental intervention which was designed to improve information-seeking skills so that patients could interact more effectively and in a more participatory manner with their physician. Patients who attended two university hospital outpatient clinics were enrolled in the study and randomly assigned to intervention or comparison groups. The first of these clinics was exclusively devoted to diabetes treatment, and administered by the Endocrinology Division in the Department of Medicine, while the second was a general medical clinic.

During the 20 minutes immediately preceding the medical visit on two consecutive visits, experimental group patients were approached by a clinic assistant who did the following things to develop patient activation:

1. Reviewed the patient's medical record with the patient.

2. Acquainted the patient with how his or her disease was treated at that clinic.

3. Helped patients identify relevant medical decisions likely to arise during the upcoming visit, with special emphasis on treatment issues that could be affected by their lifestyle and preferences.

4. Taught the patient several skills designed to increase involvement in the doctor–patient interaction. These skills were not elaborate. Patients were encouraged to ask questions, recognize relevant medical decisions, and negotiate these decisions, with physicians. Assistants also coached patients in the use of simple techniques for overcoming common barriers to discussing issues with physicians including embarrassment, fear of appearing foolish, forgetting to bring up an issue, and intimidation by the physician.

The control group of patients received an 'attention control' intervention comprising 20 minutes of standardized educational materials on diabetes. The investigators then tape-recorded visits by both experimental and control patients, and gathered post-visit questionnaires from patients and doctors, including a mailed questionnaire 12 weeks later. The audiotapes showed that the 'activated' patients were 30% more active in the conversation with the doctor than attention-controls.

Not only did patients in the intervention group talk more with their providers, they were more assertive, controlling the consultation more than the comparison group, and eliciting twice the number of factual statements from their providers, so that the talk was more explicitly related to the

Table 30.1. Randomized control trials of patient activation/empowerment (in chronological order).

Study, Author (ref), year, country, setting, diabetes type	Randomized participants N. age, gender, baseline HbA$_{1c}$	Intervention (I) and Control (C) • no. evaluated (N), • delivery • duration • type	Process Measures and direction of effect*	Outcome Measures and direction (effect size)	Design issues: Length of follow-up from baseline, % attrition > <30% Notes
Greenfield[30], 1988 USA OPD Mixed type 1, type 2 Established diabetes	N = 73 Mean age 50 years (±14) F: 50% HbA$_{1c}$ (NR 4.0–6.8%) 10.5±2.0%	I: N = (33) • to patients • 2 × 20 min • patient activation pre-consultation C: N = (26) • attention control – standardized education	Audiotape of consultation: • conversational acts (+) • question asking (0) • controlling acts (+) • information eliciting (+) Questionnaire: • patient satisfaction (0) • knowledge (0)	HbA$_1$ (+) (0.72) Functional status (+) Health-related quality of life (+)	12 weeks <30% *Small study with short follow-up*
Rost[31], 1991 USA Hospital Mixed type 1, type 2 Established diabetes	N = 61 Mean age 40 years (±15) F: 60% HbA$_{1c}$ (NR 4.4–6.3%) 13.2 ± 3.5%	I: N = (23) • to patients • 3 day evaluation + educational programme; 45 min patient activation, 1 hour self-administered booster, post-discharge (adapted from Greenfield) C: N = (29) • to patients • 3 day evaluation + educational programme only.	Audiotape of question asking at discharge (+) Questionnaires: • patient involvement (0) • patient satisfaction (0) • patient knowledge (0) • practitioner satisfaction at discharge (0)	HbA$_{1c}$ (0) Functional status: physical (+) psychological (0)	16 weeks <30% *Block randomization by week of admission, with allocation concealment Small study with short follow-up*

Table 30.1. contd.

Study	Participants	Intervention	Measures	Results	Notes
Anderson[39], 1995 USA Diabetes education centre volunteers Mixed type 1, type 2 Established diabetes	N = 46 Mean age 50 years F: 70% HbA$_{1c}$ (NR 4–8%) 11.3 ± 3%	I: N = (23) • to patients • 6 × 2 hr • empowerment programme over 6 weeks C: N = (22) • waiting list controls	Questionnaires: • self-efficacy scales (+) • diabetes attitudes scales (+)	HbA$_{1c}$ (+) (0.27)	12 weeks <30% *Small study among motivated volunteers Randomization by patient*
Pill[40], 1998 UK General practice Type 2 Established diabetes	N = 190 Mean age 58 years (±9.4) F: 50% HbA$_{1c}$ (NR 5.7–8%) 11.6 ± 11.2%	I: N = (77) • to practitioners • 3 + hours • patient activation skills and materials C: N = (88) usual practice	Audiotapes of practitioners' competence (+) Questionnaires: • application of intervention by practitioners: 19% at two years	HbA$_{1c}$ (0) (−0.17) BP (0) BMI (0) Functional status (0)	18 months <30% *Randomization by practice* (I: N = 15, C: N = 14)
Kinmonth[41], 1998 UK General practice Type 2 Newly diagnosed diabetes	N = 360 Mean age 57 years (30–71 y) F: 41% HbA$_{1c}$ NR 4.7–6.8% (at outcome) 7.1, range 4.2–14.0%	I: N = (142) • to practitioners • 1.5 days • patient activation skills and materials, Diabetic Association guidelines and materials C: N = (108) • Diabetic Association guidelines + materials only	Questionnaires: • patient ratings of communication (+) • satisfaction with treatment (+) • wellbeing (+) • knowledge of selfcare B (−) • lifestyle change (0)	HbA$_{1c}$ (0) (0.05) BP (0) BMI (−) Triglyceride (−) Functional Status (0)	12 months >30% *Randomization by practice* (I: N = 21, C: N = 20)

+ = significant difference in favour of intervention, $p<0.05$ 0 = no significant difference.   − = significant difference in favour of control.

patient's agenda for improving health. However, this process did not lead to any differences between groups in satisfaction, or knowledge of diabetes.

Activated patients were found to have lower HbAl levels at follow-up than the comparison group, allowing for baseline. They also reported significantly fewer physical limitations in the weeks that followed the visit, including fewer days off work and less limitation on their ability to perform other important social roles.

In an exploration of the relationships between patient behaviour during the visit and HbAl, significant correlations were found between the number of conversational acts (Pearsons $r = -0.29$, p<0.001), number of controlling acts ($r = -0.38$, p<0.001), effective information elicitation ($r = -0.51$, p<0.01) and subsequent HbAl. In a regression analysis of predictors of functional limitation at follow-up, four variables explained 66% of the variance: the intervention, functional limitation at baseline, HbAl at follow-up and number of diabetic complications. This strongly suggests that the intervention had an effect not mediated through blood glucose or disease severity alone. The authors propose that an increased sense of control gained from the intervention may alter the way individuals perceive their health status and their physical limitations[30].

In a replication of this study, conducted in a hospital setting, Rost and colleagues[31] attempted to further specify the intervention's effective element by distinguishing participation in decision-making from increased information seeking. They also explored the pathways by which the intervention might influence metabolic control and functional status. The investigators replicated the links between patient activation in information seeking and improved physical functioning at four months, using a validated measure[32]. They demonstrated no significant impact of the intervention on glycosylated haemoglobin (baseline levels of 13% (±3.5) I and 13.5% (±3.6) C falling at four months in both groups to 11.8% (±3.0) and 12.4% (±3.3) respectively). Among the 37 patients with audiotapes available, those in the experimental group asked significantly more questions at discharge than did those in the control group (7.8 I versus 3.1 C, F = 18.41, P <0.001, in an analysis of covarience controlling for number of questions asked at the admission interview). Moreover, in a subsequent exploratory analysis the perception of patients that they were successful in question asking predicted improved glycosylated haemoglobin at four months (p = 0.05).

There was greater support for the link between question asking and subsequent metabolic control than for involvement in decision making. However, patient decision making was somewhat idiosyncratically defined as the frequency of patient requests, disagreements and interruptions rather than factors relating to, for example, choice of personally important goals and individual steps to their achievement. Pathways to improved outcomes were explored but remained unclear; there was no evidence that the functional status improvements associated with the intervention were mediated by increases in patient recall or understanding of information, satisfaction with care or the satisfaction of the treating physicians.

Patient empowerment: The final step, empowerment, implies the ability to take thoughtful action on one's own behalf[33]. While physicians have long recognized the importance of patients taking responsibility for behaviours affecting health, there has been relatively little attention paid to the extent to which they themselves facilitate this process. A contribution in this regard has been made by the Medical Outcomes Study (MOS)[34]. This prospective cohort study surveyed over 7000 patients after visits with 300 physicians to determine the extent to which the patients reported having been offered choice, control and responsibility over treatment decisions. Physician practice and patient experience in terms of shared decision-making were found to vary widely. Most notably, physicians with primary care or interviewing skills training were reported to be more facilitative of active patient engagement in the decision-making process than were other physicians. While the MOS study did not identify particular facilitative skills for participatory decision-making, other observational studies have found that physicians trained in interviewing skills differed from other physicians in key ways: trained physicians were more likely to engage in discussion of psychosocial issues, be emotionally support-ive, ask questions in an open manner, ask for patient opinion, be skilled in interpersonal communication, be psychologically-minded and be less verbally dominant.[35,36,37]

In using these communication skills for empowerment, the physician's communication role is to provide an atmosphere in which confidence and competence is built, emotional support given, and in which support for choice, control and responsibility for health behaviour is recognized and reinforced[21].

Taking an empowerment approach, Langewitz and associates[38] in Switzerland, and Anderson and colleagues in the USA[39] designed programmes to build patients' competence and confidence to effectively self-manage their diabetes. While not directly equivalent to one another in content, the programmes do have a common theme of promoting patient competence for decision making and treatment self-management. The Langewitz programme provided patients with more sophisticated knowledge regarding insulin requirements in relation to different glucose challenges. This went beyond conventional approaches to insulin therapy and enabled individuals to take informed control of their insulin regimen. An important element of the training programme was its focus on the importance of patient autonomy in self-management of insulin therapy. The Anderson programme also emphas-ized diabetes management, but included biomedical as well as psychological and social coping.

The Langewitz study investigated 43 patients with long-standing type 1 diabetes (mean age 33 ± 10 y, mean duration of diabetes 15 ± 10 y) to see whether an empowering approach to insulin self management improved the doctor–patient relationship, quality of life or metabolic control[38]. A 'before and after' design was used with follow-up at one year. Patients volunteered for the study, and were younger, and with more frequent severe hypoglycaemia than the clinic population as a whole. Indeed, baseline HbA_{1c} was 6.61 ($\pm$1.46)% leaving little room for improvement, which was however significant four months after treatment (6.29 $\pm$ 1.01%, p <0.05) but not at one year. Improvements were found at one year in the doctor–patient relationship, patient satisfaction, reductions in depression and anxiety in general and particularly a reduction in worry about diabetes, in association with a reduction in frequency of severe hypoglycaemic attacks. Patients reported increasing closeness to their doctors and loss of hierarchical distance. The main advantage they reported of training in insulin management was a greater freedom to choose the time to eat. The authors point out that metabolic control did not deteriorate in this group, despite patients' greater autonomy in self-care, and called for randomized trials of the 'empowerment' approach to self-care.

Anderson and colleagues provided a randomized evaluation of their empowerment programme, with a focus on self-efficacy and its component skills[39]. These included the ability to identify areas of satisfaction and dissatisfaction related to living with diabetes, to identify and achieve personal goals, to use problem-solving to eliminate barriers to these goals, to cope with the emotional aspects of living with diabetes, to manage stress, to attain appropriate social support, to strengthen motivation to act, and to make cost–benefit decisions about planned behaviours. These skills draw strongly on the social cognitive literature[15,16]. Forty-six volunteers, mainly overweight, well educated women, who already felt comfortable living with diabetes, were randomized to immediate programme attendance, or waiting list control, after a full induction into the study design and intervention approach. Participants were asked to complete experiential worksheets, attend six sessions and participate in group discussions. At 12 weeks from baseline, the intervention group demonstrated a significantly greater improvement in glycosylated haemoglobin than the control group (intervention 11.75 $\pm$ 3.01% to 11.02 $\pm$ 2.89%; control 10.82 $\pm$ 2.94% to 10.87 $\pm$ 2.59%, p = 0.05). Self-efficacy was significantly increased among the intervention group in terms of setting goals, managing stress, obtaining social support and making self-care treatment decisions. There was also a significant reduction in the perceived impact of diabetes and negative attitudes towards diabetes among the intervention group.

Two subsequent trials in the UK, among individuals with type 2 diabetes, have built on the earlier trials reported from the USA, using larger study populations, and longer follow-up periods[40,41].

Pill et al.[40] devised an intervention for general practitioners and nurses, drawing on elements of patient participation, activation and empowerment facilitation. Simple visual aids were designed to assist clinicians in encouraging active patient participation. The core message was that individual patients should be encouraged to air personal concerns about their condition, to choose particular areas of lifestyle and self-management they felt most relevant for discussion, test out their readiness to change behaviour and, if appropriate, set personal goals. The intervention was provided by a multidisciplinary team at practice visits of an hour each, continuing until practitioners felt competent to deliver the programme in consultations. Halfway through the study 71% of practitioners reported using the materials frequently. However, at two years, less than 20% reported using the intervention systematically with patients. Lack of application may explain the lack of effect on glycosylated haemoglobin, measures of health status, wellbeing, satisfaction with treatment and attitudes to diabetes.

The study group was not dissimilar from those in the USA trials in terms of relatively poor diabetic control, and the study had greater power to detect differences. Problems with assay changes during the study may have compromised the measures of metabolic control, but the main difference between this and the more successful USA trials could be the attempt to deliver the programme through education of practitioners and routine practice rather than through expert coaching of patients themselves.

A similar approach was taken in the study by Kinmonth and colleagues[41], but this time among patients with newly diagnosed type 2 diabetes. Nurses and GPs were trained in groups. In the first half-day they were given evidence for a patient-centred approach and taught how to offer to patients a booklet 'Diabetes in Your Hands' to encourage patients to ask questions and prepare their agenda before consultations, and an insert of possible concerns for people with diabetes, including diabetic complications. Nurses then attended a full day of skills training, learning to elicit and listen well to the patient agenda, negotiate behaviour change, and use a framework for supporting individual choice and change, using the stages of change model[42], with a focus on identifying individual costs and benefits of choices before providing tailored lifestyle advice[43]. Patients attending trained, compared with untrained, practitioners, reported (at the end of their first year with diabetes) better communications with their doctors (OR 2.8; 95% CI 1.8–4.3), greater treatment satisfaction (OR 1.6; 1.1–2.5) and wellbeing (difference in means (d) 2.8; 0.4–5.2). There were no differences between groups in self-reported diet or exercise. However, knowledge scores of critical/self-care issues were lower in the intervention group (d = -2.74; -0.23 to –5.25) and their body mass index was significantly higher (d = 2.0; 0.3–3.8) as were triglyceride concentrations (d = 0.4 mmol/l; 0.07–0.73 mmol/l. HbA_{1c} levels were not significantly improved in the intervention group, achieved control being good in both groups.

As in the study by Pill *.et al.*, nurses became less keen on the approach over time, and were frustrated by time constraints[44]. Patients diagnosed later in the study were less likely to recognize the materials than those diagnosed earlier.

The less impressive effect sizes in this study compared with those in the USA may again relate to the indirect delivery of the intervention to patients via training of their practitioners. Practitioners appeared to find it easier to learn data gathering, relationship and partnering skills, rather than to integrate these with patient education and counselling, negotiation and joint problem solving[43].

EFFECTIVE COMMUNICATION PATHWAYS

The communication studies described were built upon a foundation of patient–physician collaboration and partnership. However the causal pathways linking these approaches to the improvements in process and outcomes demonstrated remain unclear. A direct pathway explaining these results might propose that information leads to more informed, appropriate and efficacious action; a better educated patient will have the capacity to comply more fully with medical recommendations. Alternatively, one might speculate that the interventions leading to better perceived communication with practitioners and less hierarchical relationships might increase patient satisfaction and lead to higher levels of commitment to the doctor–patient relationship, and subsequently to the therapeutic plan.

The very complexity of the interventions evaluated and the limits of the measures employed constrain conclusions. However, neither the Greenfield *et al.*[30] nor Rost *et al.*[31] studies found that activated patients scored any higher in recall or understanding of diabetes-related information, and in the Kinmonth[41] study knowledge of self-care was greatest among patients consulting practitioners without additional training in patient-centred care. Nor did patients in the intervention groups of Greenfield and Rost report greater satisfaction than those in the comparison groups, despite better metabolic control or functional status. Some other mechanism must have been at work in these studies.

Patient activation may have acted as a vehicle for increased self-efficacy and 'internality training'. Enhanced internal locus of control provides a plausible mechanism by which improved metabolic control and functional status are achieved; internality may result directly in health benefits by inspiring greater patient initiative in responsible health behaviors (appointment keeping and conscientious adherence to regimes) but also indirectly as an effective coping mechanism for the anxiety and uncertainty associated with illness. Simply feeling that one's health is not beyond one's control may, in and of itself, reduce stress and improve metabolic processes and functional status. Neither of these explanations are necessarily linked to patient satisfaction or improved understanding of the underlying mechanisms and rationale of the therapy[21].

The Greenfield[30] and Anderson[39] studies paid particular attention to the management of negative emotions about either diabetes itself, or about consultations about diabetes and its care, such as fear, anxiety and embarrassment. Both demonstrated improvements in metabolic control. In the Anderson study an emphasis on psychosocial coping was associated with increased self-efficacy in stress management and obtaining social support, plausibly mediating the improvements in attitude to diabetes, reduction in impact of the disease on life, and positive metabolic outcomes.

The balance of evidence from the studies reviewed suggests that when the physician is patient-centred (and non-controlling), when patients are verbally active overall, especially in information-seeking, and when the patient is empowered to make treatment decisions, self-reported health and functional status and metabolic control are improved. The dissonant findings in the Kinmonth study[41] deserve some comment in this regard. Despite the intervention proving successful in improving patients' views of communication with their practitioners, with patients reporting greater satisfaction with treatment and wellbeing at one year compared with controls, their disease status was worse, with significantly greater weight gain and higher triglycerides, while their HbA_{1c} was not significantly improved. The more successful interventions appeared to pay greater attention to patient education and counselling about the disease than was achieved in the Kinmonth study, drawing attention to the importance of practitioners not losing the focus on disease management while attempting to achieve the benefits of more patient-centred consulting.

There are also noteworthy differences between the activation interventions of Greenfield and Rost and the empowerment interventions of Anderson and Langewitz. Activation focuses on encouraging patients to work through their physicians in eliciting information and establishing a partnership, while the empowerment programmes directly provide patients with the capacity to act independently of the physician if need be. While both approaches may act to enhance internality (and achieve the benefits described earlier), activation may put strains on the patient–physician relationship by linking the patient's success at partnering to the physician's receptivity. Empowerment, however, may act to 'level the playing field' to some extent by providing patients with skills in self-management, thus diminishing the usual layman–professional gap. This may, in fact, act to optimize patient–physician relations by equipping the patient with the 'wherewithall' to assume a collaborative relationship.

Despite the small number of trials in this area, and their methodological limitations, sufficient evidence is available to justify the planning of further evaluations of very clearly defined interventions, perhaps integrating the well operationalized interventions from the patient–practitioner literature with the more strongly theorized models of behavioural choice and change from psychology. The gap between the apparent efficacy of interventions aimed directly at patients to activate or empower and of those applied through practitioner training programmes, with their worryingly weak application over time, is a particular challenge.

TRANSLATING RESEARCH RESULTS TO CLINICAL PRACTICE

The foundation of patient-centred skills are those core communication elements which allow the physician to partner, inform, activate and support their patients[20]. In operational terms, this means the application of several critical principles of good communication[45].

The first of these is to hear the patient's perspective. Too often, treatment discussions begin (and end) in focusing on identifying the 'right' drug or therapy. A more fruitful search, however, might be for a better understanding of the patient. Patients often have very specific ideas regarding the cause of their medical problems and what might help. By probing the patient's perspective and determining what the patient knows, believes and expects in terms of treatment, the physician or nurse can gain insight into anxieties and motivation, and possibly any idiosyncratic or contradictory explanatory framework held by the patient.

Key questions that are useful for eliciting the patient's perspective include: 'What do you think caused it?', 'What do you think will help?', 'What do you want me to do?'

A second principle is to provide information that is useful and relevant. A singularly consistent finding in studies of providers and patients conducted over the past 25 years has been that patients want as much information as possible from their provider. Unfortunately, the provision of information unrelated to the patients' position has not been shown to be very effective in improving processes or outcomes of care. The patient is often considered devoid of knowledge and experience, an empty vessel into which directives, advice and rules for living are poured. The alternative is to start where the patient is by asking, 'What do you already know about your diabetes?'

Even well-informed patients are surprised by informational gaps they discover when attempting to articulate what they know and understand about their condition and its treatment. This process allows for a tailored approach to patient education in which new information is presented in such a way that misinformation may be corrected, informational gaps filled, and an assessment of the patient's fund of knowledge made more accurate.

Before a provider can assume that a patient has integrated new information in a way that has meaning for a daily routine, specific checks for accuracy must be made. The most straightforward of these is to directly ask the patient to repeat back the information given. This again provides the opportunity to correct misinformation and misinterpretations and reinforce an accurate report.

A third principle is the need to negotiate a plan and anticipate problems. In most instances, a range of treatment goals and options are reasonable. Often, however, decisions are made unilaterally by the provider when patient input could be elicited and accommodated. To the extent to which patients' preferences and concerns can be accommodated (these may include physical, social, emotional and financial considerations) and regimens tailored, the data suggest that the likelihood of success is increased. Of course, not all aspects of the treatment regimen are open to negotiation, and these must be clear. However, a surprisingly high level of control over the regimen may be afforded the patient without compromising good medicine, as demonstrated by Rost *et al.*[31] Examples of negotiation include: 'I need to know if you can live with what we discussed.' 'Do you think you will have any trouble with anything we talked about – anything at all?', 'What do you think would work for you? Any ideas? What else could we try?'

A fourth principle is the need to offer ongoing monitoring of compliance and compliance difficulties; problems should be expected even in patients with well established regimens. It is critical to monitor compliance at every visit, but in ways that allow a patient to admit to non-compliance without feeling a failure. Framing compliance monitoring questions in a way that allows for an acceptable negative answer, for instance, 'Most people have some trouble; what kinds of problems have you been having?' has been a successful strategy in facilitating open and honest patient disclosure of compliance problems.

This leads to the next principle: finding problems and renegotiating solutions. Once compliance difficulties are established, the problems need to be specified and addressed. Misunderstandings and misinformation can be corrected with the use of simple direct language and written aids. Unanticipated side-effects, cost, forgetting and simple demotivation may be dealt with through problem-solving. For instance, the following may be helpful: 'What is it about the diet that is most troublesome?', 'What do you think would work?', 'What one thing are you willing to try?'

Finally, the last communication principle is to provide emotional support to the patient. Although patients certainly want as much information as possible from their doctors and nurses, the evidence suggests that information is not all that patients need for effective participation in self-care. Physicians are not simply expert consultants, although they are that; the physician or nurse is also someone to whom people go when they are particularly vulnerable. It is important that they are able to respond to patients' emotions and provide support, reassurance, partnership and respect to assure commitment to the therapeutic relationship as well as motivation for compliance with therapeutic regimen[45].

Words that may be helpful in this context include: 'This must be hitting you pretty hard', 'Anyone would feel overwhelmed by it all at first', 'I'm here to help you through; we'll work it out together', 'I'm sure we'll be able to get this under control'.

While medicine has always sought to serve patients' needs, it has relied upon physicians to define those needs. The broadening definition of quality in medical care of the past decade, which includes providers' interpersonal skills, calls for systematic efforts to incorporate the patient's perspective into medical care at all levels. Exactly how to achieve this, and which of the many facets of patient-centred care can be cost-effectively operationalized in modern medical practice, and by what kinds of practitioner, remain questions for research.

REFERENCES

Portions of this article were presented at the 5th International Symposium on Type 2 Diabetes, Copenhagen, December 7-8, 1998.

1. Maloney T, Paul B (1993) Rebuilding public trust and confidence, (eds) Gerteis M, Edman-Levitan S, Daley J, Delbanco T). *Through the Patient's Eyes: Understanding and promoting Patient-centered Care*. San Francisco, CA: Jossey-Bass.
2. Golin CE, DiMatteo MR, Gelberg L (1996) The role of patient participation in the doctor visit: Implications for adherence to diabetes care. *Diabetes Care* **19**: 1153-1164.
3. Glasgow RE (1991) Compliance to diabetes regimens: Conceptualization, complexity and determinants. In *Patient Compliance in Medical Practice and Clinical Trials* (eds Cramer JA, Spiker B), New York: Raven Press.
4. Rogers PG, Bullman WR (1995) Prescription medicine compliance: A review of the baseline of knowledge. A report of the National Council on Patient Information and Education. *J. Pharmacoepidemiology* **2**: 3-36.
5. Cramer JA (1992) Overview of methods to measure and enhance patient compliance. In *Patient Compliance in Medical Practice and Clinical Trials* (eds Cramer JA and Spilker B), ibid, pp. 3–11.
6. Probstfield JL (1992) Clinical trial prerandomization compliance (Adherence) Screen. In *Patient Compliance in Medical Practice and Clinical Trials* (eds Cramer JA and Spilker B), ibid, pp. 323–333.
7. DiMatteo, MR, DiNicola, DD (1982) *Achieving Patient Compliance*. New York: Pergamon Press.
8. American Association of Diabetes Educators (2000) The 1999 scope of practice for diabetes educators and the standards of practice for diabetes educators. *Diabetes Educator* **26**(1): 25–31.
9. Brown SA (1990) Studies of educational interventions and outcomes in diabetic adults: A meta-analysis revisited. *Patient Educ. Couns.* **16**: 189–215.
10. Roter, DL, Hall, JA, Merisca, R, Ruehle, B, Cretin D, Svarstad, B. (1998) Effectiveness of interventions to improve patient compliance: A meta-analysis. *Medical Care* **36**: 1138–1161.
11. Padgett D, Mumford E, Hynes M, Carter R (1988) Meta-analysis of the effects of educational and psychosocial interventions on management of diabetes mellitus. *J. Clin. Epidemiol.* **41**: 1007.

12. Griffin S, Kinmonth A-L, Skinner C, Kelly J (1998) Educational and psychosocial interventions for adults with diabetes. British Diabetic Association Report, British Diabetic Association, London

13. Fain JA, Nettles A, Funnell MM, Prochownik DC (1999) Diabetes patient education research: An integrative literature review. *Diabetes Educator* **25**(6): 7–15.

14. Glasgow RE, Fisher EB, Anderson BJ, LaGreca A, Marrero D et al. (1999) Behavioral science in diabetes. *Diabetes Care* **22**: 832–843.

15. Bandura A (1997) *Self-Efficacy: The Exercise of Control*. New York: Freeman.

16. Sutton S (1998) Predicting and explaining intentions and behaviour: how well are we doing? *J. Appl. Soc. Psychol.* **28**: 1317–38

17. Gollwitzer PM, Brandstatter V (1997) Implementation intentions and effective goal pursuit. *J. Personality and Social Psychology* **73**: 186–199.

18. Pearce S, Wardle J (1989) *The Practice of Behavioural Medicine*. The British Psychological Society, Oxford Science Publications.

19. Stewart MA (1996) Effective physician–patient communication and health outcomes: A review. *Canadian Med. Assoc. J.* **152**: 1423–1433.

20. Roter DL (2000) The enduring and evolving nature of the patient-physician relationship. *Patient Educ. Couns.* **39**: 5–15.

21. Roter DL (2000) The medical visit context of treatment decision-making and the therapeutic relationship. *Health Exp*.**3**: 17–25.

22. Engel GL (1988) How much longer must medicine's science be bound by a seventeenth-century world view? In White, K (ed.) *The Task of Medicine: Dialogue at Wickenburg*. Menlo Park, CA: The Henry J. Kaiser Family Foundation.

23. Wallerstein N, Bernstein E (1988) Empowerment education: Freire's ideas adapted to health education. *Health Education Quarterly* **15**: 379–394.

24. Lazare A, Putnam SM, Lipkin, M (1995) Three functions of the medical interview. In *The Medical Interview: Clinical Care, Education, and Research* (eds Lipkin M, Putnam S, Lazare A), New York: Springer-Verlag, pp. 3–19.

25. Street RL Jr, Piziak VK, Carpenter WS et al. (1993) Provider-patient communication and metabolic control. *Diabetes Care* **16**: 714–721.

26. Viinamaki H, Niskanen L, Korhonen T et al. (1993) The patient–doctor relationship and metabolic control in patients with type 1 (insulin-dependent) diabetes mellitus. *Intl. J. Psychia. in Med.* **23**: 265–274.

27. Roter, DL (1977) Patient participation in the patient–provider interaction: the effects of patient question-asking on the quality of interaction, satisfaction and compliance. *Health Educ. Mono.* **50**: 281–315.

28. Beckman HB, Frankel, RM, Darnley J (1984) The effect of physician behavior on the collection of data. *Ann. Int. Med.* **101**: 692–6.

29. Marvel MK, Epstein RM, Flowers K, Beckman HB (1999) Soliciting the patient's agenda: Have we improved? *JAMA* **281**: 283–7.

30. Greenfield S, Kaplan SH, Ware JE (1988) Expanding patient involvement in care – effects on blood sugar control and quality of life in diabetes. *J. Gen. Intern. Med.* **3**: 448–457.

31. Rost KM, Flavin KS, Cole K et al. (1991) Change in metabolic control and functional status after hospitalization: impact of patient activation intervention in diabetic patients. *Diabetes Care* **14**: 881–889.

32. Jette AM, Davies AR, Cleary PD, Calkins DR, Rubenstein LV, Fink A, Kosecoff J, Young RT, Brook RH, Delbanco TL (1986) The functional status questionnaire: reliability and validity when used in primary care. *J. Gen. Intern. Med.* **1**: 143–9

33. Freire P (1983) *Education for Critical Consciousness*. New York: Continuum Press.

34. Kaplan SH, Greenfield S, Gandek B, Rogers W, Ware JE (1996) Characteristics of physicians with participatory decision-making styles. *Ann. Int. Med.* **124**: 497–504.
35. Roter DL, Hall JA, Kern DE, Barker LR, Cole KA, Roca RP (1995) Improving physicians' interviewing skills and reducing patients' emotional distress: a randomized clinical trial. *Arch. Int. Med.* **155**: 1877–1884.
36. Levinson W, Roter D (1993) The effects of two continuing medical education programs on communication skills of practicing primary care physicians. *J. Gen. Int. Med.* **8**: 318–324.
37. Roter DL, Cole KA, Kern DE, Barker LR, Grayson M (1990) An evaluation of residency training in interviewing skills and the psychosocial domain of medical practice. *J. Gen. Int. Med.* **5**: 347–454
38. Langewitz W, Wossmer B, Iseli J et al. (1997) Psychological and metabolic improvement after an outpatient teaching program for functional intensified insulin therapy (FIT) *Diabetes Res. and Clin. Pract.* **37**: 157–164.
39. Anderson RM, Funnell MM, Butler PM et al. (1995) Patient empowerment: results of a randomized controlled trial. *Diabetes Care* **18**: 943–9.
40. Pill R, Stott NCH, Rollnick SR, Rees M (1998) A randomised controlled trial of an intervention designed to improve the care given in general practice to type II diabetic patients: patient outcomes and professional ability to change behaviour. *Fam. Pract.* **15**: 229–235
41. Kinmonth AL, Woodcock A, Griffin S, Spiegal N, Campbell MJ (1998) Randomised controlled trial of patient-centred care of diabetes in general practice: impact on current wellbeing and future disease risk. *Brit. Med. J.* **317**: 1202–8.
42. Prochasca JO, DiClemente CCD (1984) *The trans theoretical approach: crossing traditional boundaries of therapy.* Homewood, IL: Dow Jones Irwin.
43. Kinmonth A-L, Spiegal N, Woodcock AJ (1996) Developing a training programme in patient-centred consulting for evaluation in a randomised controlled trial: Diabetes Care from Diagnosis in British Primary Care. *Patient Educ. Couns.* **29**: 75–86.
44. Woodcock AJ, Kinmonth A-L, Campbell MJ, Griffin SJ, Spiegal NM (1999) Diabetes care from diagnosis: effects of training in patient centred care on beliefs, attitudes and behaviour of primary care professionals. *Patient Educ. Couns.* **37**: 65–79.
45. Roter, DL, Hall, JA (1992) *Doctors Talking to Patients/Patients Talking to Doctors: Improving Communication in Medical Visits.* Westport, CT: Auburn House.

31

Promoting Self-management in Primary Care Settings: Limitations and Opportunities: A Commentary

MICHAEL G. GOLDSTEIN

Bayer Institute for Health Care Communication, West Haven, Connecticut, USA

In Chapter 30, Drs Roter and Kinmonth review research evidence that links efforts to promote patient self-management with the outcomes of diabetes care. As they note, research in this area is exceedingly difficult to evaluate. Studies vary widely across several domains, including the definition and conceptualization of self-management; the populations of patients and providers studied; the type of study (e.g. observational, intervention trial with a pre-post design; randomized controlled trial (RCT)); the level at which the patient self-management intervention was delivered (e.g. patients, clinicians); and the type of outcomes studied (e.g. processes of care, glucose control, quality of life, functional status).

Although Roter and Kinmonth's review confirms a strong positive relationship between patient activation and empowerment and diabetes outcomes, almost all of this evidence is based on observational studies. Only five RCTs were identified by the authors; three testing interventions that were directed at patients[1-3], and two that tested educational interventions for clinicians to help them to implement patient activation or empowerment interventions with their patients[4,5]. Although the three RCTs that targeted patients produced positive outcomes, the two that tested interventions aimed at clinicians produced rather disappointing results. As Roter and Kinmonth imply in the concluding section of their chapter, there is a considerable gap between what we know about how to activate and empower patients to enhance diabetes care and

The Evidence Base for Diabetes Care. Edited by R. Williams, W. Herman, A.-L. Kinmonth and N. J. Wareham.
© 2002 John Wiley & Sons, Ltd

what we know about how to translate, apply and disseminate these research findings within real-world practice settings. Until this gap is filled, research evidence from the provider–patient communication literature, cited by Roter and Kinmonth and elsewhere[6-10], and emerging evidence from efforts to improve the processes and outcomes of chronic disease care[11-15] can inform efforts to disseminate patient activation and empowerment interventions. To promote the translation of research results into clinical practice, Roter and Kinmonth offer several critical principles for effective clinician–patient communication. These principles, which are based on their review of the literature and patient-centered models of care[16], are listed in Table 31.1. In the following pages, I will briefly review additional evidence that might inform and guide translation efforts. I will conclude by offering additional recommendations for implementing interventions to promote self-management in health care settings.

As noted by Roter and Kinmonth, three RCTs that tested the efficacy of self-management interventions produced positive outcomes[1-3]. Roter and Kinmonth suggest that these patient activation and empowerment interventions improved outcomes by increasing patient self-efficacy and 'internality'. Internality is defined by the authors as an internal locus of control that results in health benefits 'by inspiring greater patient initiative in responsible health behaviors' and 'by helping patients to cope with the anxiety and uncertainty associated with illness' (Chapter 30). Indeed, increases in self-efficacy were linked to empowerment and improved outcomes in one of the RCTs[3]. Clement, in a previous review of diabetes self-management education, concluded that diabetes self-management education is effective only when behavior change strategies are extensively used[17]. Clement also concluded that self-management education is *most* effective when coupled with expert adjustment of medication and reinforcement of learned behaviors by the health care provider[17]. Moreover, a large body of behavioral science research in diabetes, reviewed recently by Glasgow and colleagues[11], has demonstrated a strong relationship between patient participation in diabetes self-management and several psychological constructs including self-efficacy, empowerment, behavioral intentions and problem-solving or coping skills. Elements that address these constructs will likely enhance the effectiveness of diabetes self-management interventions.

Table 31.1. Principles of good communication (from Chapter 30).

- Hear the patients perspective.
- Provide information that is useful and relevant.
- Negotiate a plan and anticipate problems.
- Offer ongoing monitoring of compliance and compliance difficulties.
- Find problems and renegotiate solutions.
- Provide emotional support.

Three other promising approaches to promoting changes in health behavior have recently been applied to diabetes self-management: self-determination theory[18], the transtheoretical model of change[19] and motivational interviewing[20,21]. Self-determination theory is a theory of human motivation that is built around the distinction between motivations that are autonomous versus controlled[22]. A prospective study by Williams and colleagues[22] confirmed positive relationships between patients' perceptions of autonomy support (a concept similar to empowerment), patients' motivation to self-regulate glucose level, perceived competence (a concept similar to self-efficacy) and improvements in HbA_{1c} values. Williams has operationally defined autonomy support as actively engaging the patient, understanding her perspective and feelings, providing relevant information and advice, and offering treatment options[22]. Williams also specifies that autonomy-supportive providers offer advice and treatment options 'without pressure or demand' in a noncontolling nonauthoritarian way[22].

The transtheoretical model of change[19] is based on empirical evidence that individuals progress through a series of stages when making lifestyle changes: precontemplation (unaware of a problem or no plan to change in the foreseeable future); contemplation (ambivalent about changing with no commitment to change); preparation (intends to take action within the next month and has made some changes in the past year); action (has made commitment to change and is actively attempting to make behavior change); and maintenance (has successfully made change but still needs to monitor behavior to prevent slips and relapse). Although originally applied to specific problematic health behaviors such as tobacco use, alcohol abuse and sedentary behavior, the transtheoretical model has also been applied to more complex clusters of health behaviors such as dietary behavior and diabetes self-management[23-25]. Individuals at different stages of change utilize different behavioral and experiential change strategies and appear to respond best to interventions that are linked to these strategies[23,26,27]. The transtheoretical model has become increasingly popular in health promotion, although there is limited evidence for the differential effectiveness of interventions that are matched versus mismatched to the patient's stage of change[28]. Meanwhile, strategies for counseling patients with diabetes in the precontemplation and contemplation stages might appropriately include providing personalized information and feedback about the impact of diabetes on specific symptoms that are already of concern to the patient; helping the patient to assess how he feels about himself as a person with diabetes; and offering to help with problems that are barriers to change[29]. Action-oriented counseling strategies might include assisting patients to develop and implement a plan, teaching skills, providing direct services (e.g. medication, dietary counseling, an exercise prescription), and referring them for further education, screening or treatment. By recognizing that many patients are in the early stages of change and not ready to take action, clinicians may revise their expectations and goals and redefine success as moving patients along the continuum of stages of change, rather than as reaching desirable final outcomes, such as a HbA_{1c} below 7%[29]. This orientation may help providers to reduce their own frustration about facilitating patient behavior change and thus address an important barrier to delivering self-management interventions. Despite the limited evidence, the transtheoretical model and, more specifically, tailoring of counseling to the patient's readiness for change, has been integrated into several widely disseminated health behavior counseling strategies, such as the 5As approach to health behavior counseling, adopted by the United States Public Health Service's Treating Tobacco Use and Dependence Guideline[30].

Motivational interviewing[20,21] is an approach to patient counseling that is compatible with self-determination theory[22] and closely aligned with patient-centered approaches[16,31,32] and the transtheoretical model[33]. Rollnick and Miller have defined motivational interviewing as 'as a directive, client-centered counseling style for eliciting behavior change by helping clients to explore and resolve ambivalence'[34]. Motivational interviewing was developed primarily for treatment of problematic alcohol use and substance abuse disorders, and most of the evidence for its effectiveness is based on trials in patients with these disorders[35]. However, it is now increasingly being applied to other behaviors, including diabetes self-management[35,36]. Miller and Rollnick[20] describe five general principles which underlie this approach: (1) Express empathy; (2) Develop discrepancy; (3) Avoid argumentation; (4) Roll with resistance; and (5) Support self-efficacy. *Empathic warmth* is perhaps the most important element of motivational interviewing[35]. This style involves the use of open-ended questions, reflective listening, legitimization of patients' feelings and validating the patients' freedom to change or not change without judging. Ambivalence is acknowledged as a normal part of the change process[20]. *Developing discrepancy* is accomplished by raising patients' awareness of the consequences of their present behavior and highlighting the discrepancy between their present behavior and their own important personal goals. Wherever possible, patients are encouraged to identify their own reasons for change. The clinician should *avoid argumentation*, since arguments are counterproductive and often lead to defensiveness and increased resistance. *Rolling with resistance* involves backing off when the patient expresses resistance, by acknowledging that change is difficult while also inviting the patient to consider new information or perspectives without imposing the clinician's ideas. The clinician *supports self-efficacy* by helping the patient to build on past successes and by offering a range of alternative approaches and choices for taking the next step.

Brief versions of motivational interviewing have been developed for use by clinicians in primary care and other health care settings[21,37,38]. These versions emphasize strategies to build rapport (i.e. reflective listening and empathy) and assessment of patients' stage of change and two specific dimensions of motivation: (1) *conviction or importance* regarding the need for change; and (2) *confidence or self-efficacy* about taking action. Assessment is followed by tailoring of counseling to address patients' levels of conviction and confidence. For patients with low conviction, counseling strategies include providing information and feedback (with patients' permission), exploration of ambivalence, and providing a menu of options for treatment of follow-up. Patients not ready for change are encouraged to continue to think about the possibilities for change and are offered help when they are ready to take action. For patients with low confidence, strategies include: reviewing past experience, especially successes; teaching problem-solving and coping skills; and encouraging small steps that are likely to lead to initial success. (See Table 31.2 for a summary of these strategies). Note that these strategies encompass many of the principles of good communication recommended by Roter and Kinmonth, and that they are also consistent with findings from research on self-management education, patient-centered care, self-determination theory, the transtheoretical model, and motivational interviewing.

As previously noted, the two RCTs reviewed by Roter and Kinmonth that tested self-management interventions aimed at clinicians produced rather disappointing results[4,5]. Both of these studies evaluated the effects of educational programs for clinicians that were based on a patient-centered model of care[16]. Both trials also trained intervention clinicians to utilize a counseling strategy based at least in part on the transtheoretical model[19] and the study conducted by Pill and colleagues also included training in brief motivational interviewing techniques[21,39]. The negative outcomes of these two trials is

Table 31.2. Principles of patient-centered counseling.

Assess (before telling)
- Strive to understand the patient's perspective (experience, feelings, ideas, function, expectations).
- Assess readiness, conviction and confidence

Build rapport
- Reflective listening.
- Express empathy.
- Provide support.

Tailor counseling: match to readiness, conviction and confidence
For low conviction:
- Provide information and feedback (with permission).
- Explore ambivalence.
- Provide a menu of options, and support choice and autonomy.
For low confidence:
- Review successful past experience.
- Teach problem-solving and coping skills.
- Encourage small steps.

particularly disappointing in light of evidence of the effectiveness of primary care clinician-delivered patient-centered counseling approaches that have emerged from research conducted outside diabetes care. Ockene and colleagues have demonstrated the effectiveness of clinician-delivered patient-centered counseling in promoting smoking cessation[40], reducing problematic alcohol consumption[41] and reducing dietary fat consumption and promoting weight loss[42]. Our own research has demonstrated that a patient-centered approach to delivering physical activity counseling is associated with short-term, but not long-term, changes in motivational readiness to engage in regular physical activity[43]. These investigators have also demonstrated that clinicians who received training in patient-centered counseling increased their knowledge, skill and confidence in providing patient-centered counseling to their patients[32,44-46]. However, the actual delivery of patient-centered counseling to patients during these trials was dependent on the use of system-based interventions to prompt clinicians in the intervention conditions to counsel patients and provide associated print materials[47-49].

How might one understand the negative findings of the two diabetes care RCTs in light of several positive trials of patient-centered counseling interventions in other areas? As Roter and Kinmonth have noted, both diabetes care trials reported that clinicians in the intervention groups varied considerably in their implementation of the intervention protocols, especially over the course of the intervention period[4,5,50,51]. For example, after two years of the three-year intervention period, only 19% of the clinicians in the intervention arm of the Pill and colleagues study continued to systematically apply the method[4]. Based on observations and interviews with participating nurses assigned to the intervention condition, Pill and colleagues conclude that a substantial subgroup of the nurses had trouble applying the patient-centered approach and 'letting go' when patients' diabetic control was poor[50]. Kinmonth and colleagues reach a similar conclusion, though they also cite perceived time constraints among the intervention clinicians as another important mediator of the lack of an effect of the intervention[5,51].

Although the conclusions reached by the investigators to explain the lack of intervention effect on patient outcomes are plausible, another important reason is the relative paucity of system-based interventions that were included as elements of the interventions. As noted above, education/training programs to promote behavioral counseling are most effective when they are combined with system-based strategies that assess patient needs, prompt the clinician to intervene, provide guidelines for the clinician and resources for the patient, and provide reinforcement to the clinician through feedback or reimbursement[42,48,49]. These findings are consistent with what we have learned, more generally, about how to change and maintain clinicians' practice behaviors[12,52-54].

Perhaps the most important advance in recent years in our understanding of the forces that influence the delivery of care is the emergence of a model and set of principles for effective chronic illness care[12,13,15,55,56]. A key characteristic of an effective chronic disease program is one which does not rely on individual clinicians or educators to remember to deliver a service or implement correctly, but creates an environment that supports and reinforces self-management and collaborative care[12].

In 1999, the National Institute of Diabetes and Digestive and Kidney Diseases (NIDDK) convened a conference on Behavioral Research and Diabetes. The planning committee for this conference created four work groups to review the status of current research in specific areas and make recommendations for future research. The work group that focused on health care delivery identified several key characteristics of effective diabetes management programs[12]. These characteristics are reproduced in Table 31.3. In addition to highlighting the importance of incorporating the patient as an active participant in patient-centered collaborative goal-setting and self-management, characteristics of an effective disease management program include the use of information systems to identify and track patients, reminder systems to prompt clinicians and patients, team development to coordinate care and share responsibility, and system redesign to plan office visits, implement follow-up procedures and proactively reach out to patients[12]. Most of these characteristics were derived from the Chronic Illness Care Model developed by Edward Wagner and staff at the Improving Chronic Illness Care initiative based at the MacColl Institute for Healthcare Innovation in Seattle, Washington, USA[13,15,56].

If one contrasts the key elements of an effective diabetes management program (listed above and in Table 31.3) with the elements of the intervention that were tested in the two primary care-based self-management RCTs, one can identify several potential barriers that may have limited the achievement of positive outcomes (e.g. absence of information systems to remind clinicians to deliver counseling and track patient participation in treatment, limited team coordination). On a positive note, the explication of the Chronic Illness Care Model provides an opportunity to identify innovative ways to integrate self-management interventions, including clinician-delivered patient-centered

Table 31.3. Key characteristics of effective diabetes management programs.*

- Use a population-based system approach.
- Involve proactive contacts, surveillance and reminders.
- Incorporate the patient as an active participant and use patient-centered collaborative goal-setting.
- Implement consistent follow-up procedures.
- Assign responsibilities to nonphysician team members, such as nurse care managers.
- Plan office visits and focus on outcome and outcome-related processes.
- Use clinical information systems, such as diabetes registries and electronic medical records, to improve quality of care.

Reprinted from Glasgow et al., "Report of the Health Care Delivery Work Group: Behavioral Research Related to the Establishment of a Chronic Disease Model for Diabetes Care", Diabetes Care 24:124-130, 2001.

counseling approaches, into health care settings. As suggested by the NIDDK Health Care Delivery Work Group, future studies might include evaluations of self-management interventions that take advantage of technological advances in information systems and provide both patients and clinicians with information gleaned from automated patient assessments performed outside the office setting[12]. This is just one example of an attempt to close the gap between what we know about self-management and individual behavior change and what we know about how to translate, apply and disseminate these research findings within real-world practice settings. The reader is referred to the report of the Work Group for several other recommendations to guide future research efforts toward identifying effective strategies for integrating diabetes self-management strategies into health care settings[12], and to Chapter 32 in this volume for further evidence on delivery of care within practice settings.

REFERENCES

1. Greenfield S et al. (1988) Patients' participation in medical care: effects on blood sugar control and quality of life in diabetes. *J. Gen. Intern. Med.* **3**(5): 448-57.
2. Rost KM et al. (1991) Change in metabolic control and functional status after hospitalization. Impact of patient activation intervention in diabetic patients. *Diabetes Care* **14**(10): 881–9.
3. Anderson R et al. (1995) Patient empowerment: Results of a randomized controlled trial. *Diabetes Care* **18**(7): 943–949.
4. Pill R et al. (1998) A randomized controlled trial of an intervention designed to improve the care given in general practice to type II diabetic patients: patient outcomes and professional ability to change behaviour. *Fam. Pract.* **15**(3): 229–35.
5. Kinmonth AL et al. (1998) Randomised controlled trial of patient-centred care of diabetes in general practice: impact on current wellbeing and future disease risk. The *Diabetes Care* From Diagnosis Research Team. *BMJ* **317**(7167): 1202–8.
6. Stewart MA (1995) Effective physician-patient communication and health outcomes: a review [see comments]. *CMAJ* **152**(9): 1423–33.
7. Anderson L (1990) Health-care communication and selected psychosocial correlates of adherence in diabetes management. *Diabetes Care*, **13**(Suppl. 2): 66–76.
8. Hall JA, Roter DL, and Katz NR (1988) Meta-analysis of correlates of provider behavior in medical encounters. *Med. Care.* **26**(7): 657–75.
9. Roter D.L. and J.A. Hall (1994) Strategies for enhancing patient adherence to medical recommendations. *JAMA* **271**(1): 80.
10. Roter D, and Hall J (1992) *Doctors Talking with Patients/Patients Talking with Doctors: Improving Communication in Medical Visits.* Westport, CT: Auburn House.
11. Glasgow RE et al. (1999) Behavioral science in diabetes. Contributions and opportunities. *Diabetes Care* **22**(5): 832–43.
12. Glasgow RE et al. (2001) Report of the health care delivery work group: behavioral research related to the establishment of a chronic disease model for diabetes care. *Diabetes Care* **24**(1): 124–30.
13. Wagner EH et al. (2001) Quality improvement in chronic illness care: a collaborative approach. *Jt. Comm. J. Qual. Improv.* **27**(2): 63–80.

14. Wagner EH, Austin BT and Von Korff M (1996) Improving outcomes in chronic illness. *Manag. Care Q*. **4**(2): 12–25.
15. Von Korff M, et al. (1997) Collaborative management of chronic illness. *Ann. Intern. Med*. **127**(12): 1097–102.
16. Stewart M et al. (1995) *Patient-Centered Medicine: Transforming the Clinical Method*. Thousand Oaks, CA: Sage.
17. Clement S (1995) Diabetes self-management education. *Diabetes Care* **18**(8): 1204–14.
18. Deci EL and Ryan RM (1985) *Intrinsic Motivation and Self-Determination in Human Behavior*. New York: Plenum.
19. Prochaska JO and DiClemente CC (1986) Towards a comprehensive model of change. In T*reating Addictive Disorders: Processes of Change* (eds W.R. Miller and N. Heather). New York: Plenum Press.
20. Miller WR and Rollnick S (1991) *Motivational Interviewing: Preparing People to Change Addictive Behavior*. New York: Guilford.
21. Rollnick S, Heather N and Bell A (1992) Negotiating behaviour change in medical settings: The development of brief motivational interviewing. *J. Mental Health* **1**: 25–37.
22. Williams GC, Freedman ZR and Deci EL (1998) Supporting autonomy to motivate patients with diabetes for glucose control. *Diabetes Care* **21**(10): 1644–51.
23. Prochaska JO et al. (1994) Stages of change and decisional balance for 12 problem behaviors. *Health Psychol*. **13**(1): 39–46.
24. Ruggiero L et al. (1997) Diabetes self-management. Self-reported recommendations and patterns in a large population. *Diabetes Care* **20**(4): 568–76.
25. Trigwell P, Grant PJ and House A (1997) Motivation and glycemic control in diabetes mellitus. *J. Psychosom. Res*. **43**(3): 307–15.
26. Prochaska JO, DiClemente CC and Norcross JC (1992) In search of how people change. Applications to addictive behaviors. *Am. Psychol*. **47**(9): 1102–14.
27. Prochaska JO et al. (2001) Evaluating a population-based recruitment approach and a stage-based expert system intervention for smoking cessation. *Addict. Behav*. **26**(4): 583–602.
28. Sutton S (2000) A Clinical review of the transtheoretical model applied to smoking cessation. In: *Understanding and Changing Health Behaviour; from Health Beliefs to Self-Regulation* (eds P. Norman, C. Abrahan and M. Conner) Reading: Harwood Academic Press.
29. Prochaska JO and Goldstein MG (1991) Process of smoking cessation. Implications for clinicians. Clin. Chest. Med. **12**(4): 727–35.
30. Fiore M et al. (2000) Treating Tobacco Use and Dependence, Clinical Practice Guideline US Department of Health and Human Services, Public Health Service: Rockville, MD.
31. Rogers C (1959) A theory of therapy, personality, and interpersonal relationships as developed in the client-centered framework. In *Psychology, The Study of a Science: Formulations of the Person and the Social Context*, (ed. E. Koch). New York: McGraw-Hill, pp. 184–256.
32. Ockene JK et al. (1988) A residents' training program for the development of smoking intervention skills. *Arch. Intern. Med*. **148**(5): 1039–45.
33. Prochaska JO and DiClemente CC (1983) Stages and processes of self-change of smoking: toward an integrative model of change. *J. Consult. Clin. Psychol*. **51**(3): 390–5.
34. Rollnick S and Miller WR (1995) What is motivational interviewing? *Behav. Cognitive Psychotherapy* **23**: 325–334.

35. Miller WR (2000) Rediscovering fire: small interventions, large effects. *Psychol. Addict. Behav.* **14**(1): 6–18.
36. Smith DE et al. (1997) Motivational interviewing to improve adherence to a behavioral weight-control program for older obese women with NIDDM: A pilot study. *Diabetes Care* **20**: 54–54.
37. Rollnick S, Mason P and Butler C (1999) *Health Behavior Change: A Guide for Practitioners* Edinburgh: Churchill Livingstone.
38. Keller V and White M (1997) Choices and changes: A new model for influencing patient health behavior. *JCOM* **4**(6): 33–36.
39. Stott NC et al. (1995) Innovation in clinical method: diabetes care and negotiating skills. *Fam. Pract.* **12**(4): 413–8.
40. Ockene JK et al. (1991) Increasing the efficacy of physician-delivered smoking interventions: a randomized clinical trial. *J. Gen. Intern. Med.* **6**(1): 1–8.
41. Ockene JK et al. (1999) Brief physician- and nurse practitioner-delivered counseling for high-risk drinkers: does it work? *Arch. Intern. Med.* **159**(18): 2198–2205.
42. Ockene I et al. (1999) Effect of physician-delivered nutrition counseling training and an office-support program on saturated fat intake, weight, and serum lipid measurements in a hyperlipidemic population. *Arch. Intern. Med.* **159**: 725–731.
43. Goldstein M. et al. (1999) Physician-based physical activity counseling for middle-aged and older adults: A randomized trial. *Ann. Behav. Med.* **21**(1): 40–47.
44. Ockene JK et al. (1995) Physician training for patient-centered nutrition counseling in a lipid intervention trial. *Prev. Med.* **24**(6): 563–70.
45. Ockene JK et al. (1997) Provider training for patient-centered alcohol counseling in a primary care setting. *Arch. Intern. Med.* **157**(20): 2334–41.
46. Pinto BM et al. (1998) Acceptability and feasibility of physician-based activity counseling: The PAL project. *Am. J. Prev. Med.* **15**(2): 95–102.
47. Ockene I et al. (1996) Effect of training and a structured office practice on physician-delivered nutrition counseling: The Worcester Area trial for counseling in hyperlipidemia (WATCH). *Am. J. Prev. Med.* **12**: 252–258.
48. Ockene J et al. (1997) Synthesis of lessons learned from cardiopulmonary preventive interventions in healthcare practice settings. *Ann. Epidemiol.* **S7**: S32–S45.
49. Ockene JK and Zapka J (1997) Changing provider behaviour: provider education and training. *Tot. Control* **6**(Suppl. 1): S63–7.
50. Pill R. et al. (1999) Can nurses learn to let go? issues arising from an intervention designed to improve patients' involvement in their own care. *J. Adv. Nurs.* **29**(6): 1492–9.
51. Woodcock AJ et al. (1999) Diabetes care from diagnosis: Effects of training in patient-centred care on beliefs, attitudes and behavior of primary care professionals. *Patient Educ. Couns.* **37**: 65–79.
52. Davis DA et al. (1995) Changing physician performance. A systematic review of the effect of continuing medical education strategies. *JAMA* **274**(9): 700–5.
53. Greco P (1993) Changing physicians' practices. *NEJM* **329**: 1271–1274.
54. Kottke T, Brooks S and Hagen P (1999) Counseling: Implementing our knowledge in a hurried and complex world. *Am. J. Prev. Med.* **17**(4): 295–298.
55. Glasgow R et al. (2000) A social-ecologic approach to assessing support for disease self-management: The chronic illness resources survey. *J. Behav. Med.*
56. Wagner E, Austin B and von Korf M (1996) Organizing care for patients with chronic illness. *Milbank Quarterly* **74**(4): 511–544.

32

Delivering Care to the Population

SIMON GRIFFIN AND RHYS WILLIAMS

University of Cambridge, Institute of Pbulic Health, Cambridge CB2 2SR, UK
Nuffield Institute of Health, Leeds LS2 9PL, UK

This chapter draws upon the analysis contained in three previously published reviews together with observations and recommendations from more recent articles on delivering diabetes care to populations. The three reviews deal with interventions to improve the management of diabetes in primary care, out-patient and community settings[1], a meta-analysis of randomised control trials of general practice diabetes care[2] and a review of shared (hospital and primary care) largely focused on the UK[3]. From these a synthesis is provided of existing knowledge on the most effective means of delivering diabetes care to populations, and recommendations are made for future studies in this area. These reviews deal almost exclusively with studies from developed countries simply because these countries, at the moment, provide almost all the available analytical studies of the delivery of diabetes care to the population. More recently, the needs of chronically ill people on a global scale are being addressed[4] and it has been pointed out that, for non-communicable diseases in general, including diabetes[5], 'many health care providers are ill-equipped to manage [them] effectively, and many governments cannot cope with the escalating disease burden and costs'.

PRIMARY CARE – STRENGTHS AND WEAKNESSES

The ideal primary care service offers 'first contact, continuous, comprehensive and co-ordinated care to individuals and populations [ideally] undifferentiated by gender, disease, organ system or social status'[6]. Primary care is widely

The Evidence Base for Diabetes Care. Edited by R. Williams, W. Herman, A.-L. Kinmonth and N. J. Wareham.

perceived to be the rational core of an efficient, equitable and effective health service in both developed and developing nations[7].

Many features of primary care are particularly suited to meet the clinical needs of people with diabetes[3]. For example, in systems such as that in the UK and many Western European nations, primary care provides open access, free at the point of delivery and a generalist approach well suited to initial diagnosis over a whole range of conditions. It also has, at its heart, a preventive approach with, in the best organised practices, registers of people with long-term conditions so that periodic recall and review may be organised on a population basis. In the ideal situation, primary care is local and convenient, provides 24 hour cover and takes a holistic approach, with the primary care team aware of and sensitive to family circumstances and effects.

This encouraging picture is balanced, however, by certain obstacles to the delivery of effective primary care[3]. These include the need for the care team to be alert to non-specific presentations which may be missed in a complex clinical situation. These complex care needs may be best provided by the specialist team in a hospital setting with extensive diagnostic and therapeutic back-up. Also, many of the advantages listed in the previous paragraph rely on *well organised* primary care. Without appropriate infrastructure and organisation, patients needs may remain unidentified and the individuals may be lost to surveillance. When more specialised skills are needed for such surveillance, these may be lacking or may have deteriorated with infrequent use. (Examples within the field of diabetes care are fundoscopy skills and the knowledge and confidence to make changes in treatment, such as the initiation of insulin therapy.) Lack of sufficient time to devote to individual patients and to continuing education for primary care professionals can lead to less effective care and professional discontent.

One of the most important functions of general practitioners is as co-ordinators of continuous and comprehensive care. In this role they are well suited to offer, or to ensure referral to, a structured programme of clinical surveillance based on registers, recall and regular review, and to call on the wide range of specialist agencies available in the community or hospital sectors to support the diabetes patient in self-care.

A number of characteristics of the nature and current epidemiology of diabetes and the evolution of health care systems have contributed to a recent increase in the involvement of primary care. Among these is the recognition that effective clinical surveillance leading to near normal control of blood glucose and blood pressure are associated with better outcomes and that continuing patient education, self-care and family support are likely to enhance such control. Diabetes epidemiology is changing such that incidence rates and prevalence are rising, especially in children and some minority groups. These changes, coupled with severe pressures on resources, are leading to overcrowded hospital clinics, some of which are, in any case, difficult for patients to access. These difficulties in access will be particularly severe in scattered rural communities, in countries without affordable transport systems and for people who are economically disadvantaged or disabled in some way.

Patient preferences also have an influence, with some, though by no means all, favouring the convenience and familiarity of their local primary care setting as opposed to the less comforting atmosphere of the hospital. In addition to this, depending on the means by which health care is funded in different countries, patients may be unable to afford hospital treatment even if they can physically access it. For a variety of reasons, many of them also economic, policy makers have lately favoured a devolution of care away from secondary to primary care with chronic disease management schemes and financial incentives to widen the role of primary care teams in this area of practice.

Recognition of the widening role of the general practitioner in diabetes care has occurred in parallel with the developing role of the practice nurse and community diabetes specialist nurse, podiatrist and dietician. Where these specialist skills are available in the community they can be brought together into a community-based team joined, in some instances, by hospital-based physicians, clinical biochemists and other specialists on an 'outreach' basis. The current concept of the 'extended diabetes team' embraces professionals based in either primary care, secondary care or both.

THE NATURE OF CURRENTLY AVAILABLE EVIDENCE

Randomised trials of health care delivery are uncommon, largely because the interventions being evaluated are usually complex. In his systematic review, published in 1998[2], Griffin set out to identify and evaluate all published randomised trials of hospital versus general practice care for people with diabetes, to compare the effectiveness of general practice and hospital care through the use of meta-analysis of the identified trials and to explore variations in the findings of the individual trials. He identified only a few trials which met the inclusion criteria.

Details of the search strategies used can be found in the original publication[2]. In brief, the medical subject heading 'diabetes' was combined with a number of others (e.g. 'family practitioner', 'family medicine', 'primary care' etc.) to identify all relevant studies in all languages. A wide range of databases was used (Embase, CRIB, Dissertation Abstracts, the UK National Research Register, Medline, Cinahl, Psychlit and Healthstar). These automated searches were combined with manual searches for further trial references. Studies were included in which people with diabetes (type 1 or type 2) were randomly allocated to hospital or general practice or 'shared care' for routine review and surveillance for complications, regardless of the quality of allocation concealment or choice of outcome measures.

The combined searches identified over 1200 studies but only six (Table 32.1) met the inclusion criteria. These were based in the UK (four trials) or Australia. All six trials employed satisfactory randomisation of individual subjects, however they were of short duration, only one lasting more than two years[8]. One of these trials was published almost 20 years ago. The most recent of them was published in 1994.

On aggregate, 1058 people seen in hospital diabetes clinics were eligible and agreeable to randomisation to continuing hospital outpatient review or follow-up in the community, either by their family doctor alone or as part of a shared care scheme. The organisation of care for the hospital outpatient group was not clearly defined, although the descriptions appear to be broadly similar. All the general practitioners were provided with educational sessions or protocols before the trials. However, the support for care in general practice changed over time.

The two studies published in the 1980s evaluated basic general practice care[8,9]. Two of the more recent studies included computer prompting systems[10,11]. The publication by Hoskins *et al.*[12] compared both basic and prompted general practice care with hospital care and was, therefore, included as two separate studies.

The outcome measures used included process measures (primary care follow-up appointments and reviews, hospital consultations and admissions); morbidity measures (symptoms, weight, blood pressure, blood glucose, HbA_1 etc.), patient satisfaction and diabetes knowledge, and mortality (in all studies except those of Hoskins[12]. The latter study alone included measures of cost.

There was heterogeneity between these trials. In the shared care schemes featuring more intensive support by means of computerised prompting systems[10–12] there was no difference in mortality between those patients randomised to hospital and those randomised to hospital follow-up. Those randomised to primary care tended to have lower values of HbA_1 (a weighted difference in means of -0.28%, 95% confidence interval -0.59 to 0.03). Losses to follow-up were significantly less in the case of prompted general practitioner care (odds ratio 0.37, 95% confidence interval 0.22–0.61). Patients randomised to primary care with less well developed support tended to have worse outcomes that those allocated to hospital follow up in the same study (Figures 32.1 and 32.2).

Thus, these results supported the provision of 'regular prompted recall and review of selected people with diabetes by willing general practitioners'[2]. These were a small number of trials, however, carried out in only two developed countries with comparatively similar systems of health care delivery.

Since the publication of that review, another randomised controlled trial, based in Denmark, has been published[13]. In this study, 311 general practitioners, in 474 general practices, took part in a six-year study which included regular patient follow-up and individual goal-setting supported by the prompt-

Table 32.1. Characteristics of trials of general practice versus hospital care for diabetes (cited in Griffin[2]). Reproduced with permission.

Name Year Reported	Setting	F/up (yrs)	Method of random allocation	Exclusion criteria	N	Type of diabetes	Mean duration of diabetes	Mean age (yrs)	Intervention	Main outcome measures
Porter 1982[9]	Fife, Scotland	2	Opaque sealed envelopes. independently prepared using random number tables	Insulin treatment	197	Type 2 diabetes from hospital clinic	Not stated	Not stated	Routine GP care • diabetes team meetings • record card • recall system for those GPs without one	Symptoms, limb function, fundi, weight, blood pressure, blood glucose, urinalysis, costs, mortality
Hayes and Harris 1984[8]	Cardiff, Wales	5	Independently prepared (MRC*) sealed envelopes	Diabetic complications Serious medical problems	200	Type 2 diabetes from hospital clinic	Not stated	GP** 59.7 H*** 58.4	Routine GP care	Follow-up: reviews and blood tests, HbA1, hospital admissions, mortality
Hurwitz 1993[10]	London, England	2	Random number tables	Diabetic complications Serious medical problems Immobile >80 years Women of childbearing age	181	Type 2 diabetes from hospital clinic	7 years	GP 62.0 H 63.1	Prompted GP care • GP education sessions • structured review form • fundoscopy by optometrists • central computerised recall • patient and GP prompts	Follow up: reviews and blood tests, weight, blood pressure, HbA1, consultation rates, hospital admission, satisfaction, mortality
Hoskins 1993[12]	Sydney, Australia	1	A number (1 to 3) was drawn from a bag by an independent person	Diabetic complications Serious medical problems	134	Type 1 and type 2 diabetes newly referred to hospital clinic	3 years	GP 54 H 52	Prompted GP care • individual management protocols sent to patient and GP • central liaison nurse prompting patient and GP	Follow up: reviews and blood tests, weight, blood pressure, HbA1, costs

Table 32.1. contd.

Hoskins 1993[12]	Sydney, Australia	1	A number (1 to 3) was drawn from a bag by an independent person	Diabetic complications Serious medical problems	137	Type 1 and type 2 diabetes newly referred to hospital clinic	3 years GP 54 H 52	Routine GP care	Follow up: reviews and blood tests, weight, blood pressure, HbA₁, costs
DICE 1994[11]	Grampian, Scotland	2	Opaque sealed envelopes, independently prepared using random number tables	<18 years Planning pregnancy Serious medical problems	274	Type 1 and type 2 diabetes	9 years GP 58.1 H 59.6	Prompted GP care • hospital annual review • guideline and structured review form • central computerised recall • patient and GP prompts	Follow up: reviews and blood tests, blood pressure, body mass index, creatinine, HbA₁, costs, knowledge, psychological tests, mortality

*MRC = Medical Research Council: **GP = patients randomised to general practice care: ***H = patients randomised to hospital care.3

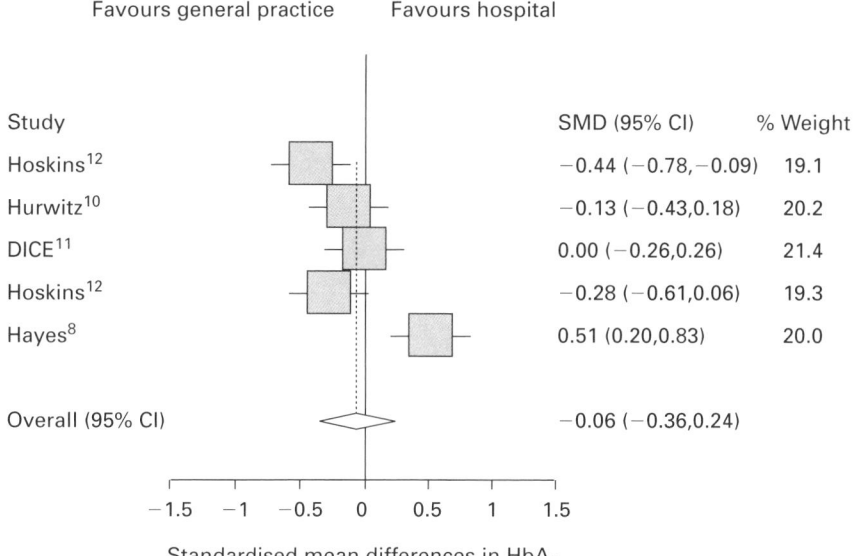

Figure 32.1. Standardised mean differences in HbA_1 (%)[2]. Reproduced with permission.

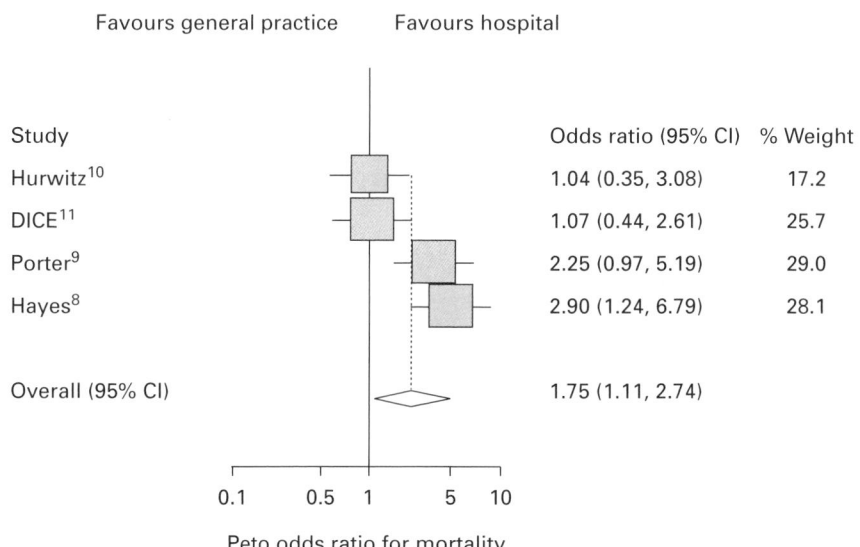

Figure 32.2. Peto odds ratios for mortality in GP and hospital care[2]. Reproduced with permission.

ing of doctors, clinical guidelines, feedback and continuing medical education. The results included significantly lower (at the p <0.001 level) median plasma glucose levels in the intervention group than in the comparison group (7.9 versus 8.7 mmol/l), lower median glycated haemoglobin levels (8.5% versus 9.0%) and lower median systolic blood pressures (145 versus 150 mmHg). The doctors in the intervention group 'arranged more follow-up consultations, referred fewer patients to [hospital] diabetes clinics, and set more optimistic goals'[13].

The trial, though well conducted and exceeding the follow up period of all of the six trials analysed by Griffin[2], 1998, does not allow a judgement to be made as to whether the interventions studied could be introduced throughout primary care in Denmark. The patients selected for the study were a representative sample of patients with diabetes attending these practices, but the practices were not representative of those in Denmark[14]. To what extent these encouraging outcomes can be achieved by less well motivated practices, particularly when such practices are faced with the combination of a rising prevalence of diabetes and limited resources, is not known.

The review by Renders *et al.*,[15] was been conducted within the Effective Practice and Organisation of Care (EPOC) review group of the Cochrane Collaboration[1]. The EPOC search strategy was combined with free-text words and key words regarding 'diabetes' and 'primary care' or 'community care' or 'outpatient care'. The databases searched were Medline (1966 to 2000), Embase (1980 to 2000), Cinahl (1982 to 2000), the EPOC trials register (1999) and the Cochrane Clinical Trials' Register (1999).

The details of the study selection methods are included in the original review[1,15]. In summary, they were studies aimed at evaluating the effectiveness of interventions *directed at health care professionals* who care for patients with type 1 or type 2 diabetes in primary care, outpatient or community settings and which fulfilled certain EPOC quality criteria[1,15]. In order to be included, the studies must have used a 'reliable, objective, predetermined measure of the process of health care or patient outcomes'[15].

The review included 48 publications describing 41 studies. Of these, 27 were randomised controlled trials[10,12,16–40,54], 12 were 'before and after' studes[34,41–51] and two were interrupted time series[52,53]

All of the studies included were regarded as having methodological limitations. Only six of the RCTs were regarded as having adequate methods for the concealment of allocation[10,18,20,35,37,39]. Contamination of the comparison groups was likely in the 15 studies[10,12,16,18,19,26,28–30,32,35,37,41,51,54] in which patients or health care professionals were randomized within a clinic or practice. In a further two studies it was likely that the comparison group also received the intervention (in that, for one of these, both intervention and control clinics were staffed by the same personnel[43] and in the other, a cross-over design was used[23]. Other methodological limitations were observed, such as lack of comparability of intervention and comparison groups, inadequate 'blinding' in the assessment of outcomes, less than satisfactory follow-up of patient outcomes, failure to provide 'intention to treat analysis' or the lack of *a priori* statistical power calculations.

From the detailed results of this review, a number of important conclusions were drawn. First, although complex professional interventions often improved the process of care, the effects on health-related outcomes was unclear, as these were rarely assessed. Significant improvement in patient outcome was reported in only one study[24]. Second (and echoing the earlier results of the Griffin review[2]), process improvements were also observed in studies of organisational interventions which included structured and regular review. A small beneficial effect in glycaemic control was observed in studies in which a nurse[43] or pharmacist[32] assumed part of the physician's role. Third, in studies which combined professional and organisational interventions, features which were associated with improvements in process measures were computer-assisted recall and reminder systems, in combinations with professional interventions[10,48]. The involvement of nurses and the inclusion of patient education were associated with positive effects on patient outcomes[29,37,46,48]. Overall, despite the methodological flaws and inconsistencies which this review described, it seems clear that combinations of professional interventions, organisational interventions, nurse involvement and the incorporation of patient education often *does* make a positive difference in the process of care, and *can* make a positive difference in the outcome of care. The review also makes the point that diabetes care is a good model for the care of many chronic diseases.

Epping-Jordan *et al.*, have drawn attention to the observation[55] that chronic conditions contribute around two-thirds of the global burden of disease worldwide. Much of this burden will fall on the individuals and families who can least afford to bear the direct health care costs and resulting losses of income and on low-income countries who also suffer substantial burdens from communicable disease, and the long-term health effects of physical injuries (for example, those sustained in traffic accidents and resulting from wars and humanitarian disasters). If diabetes care is to be a model for the effective delivery of care to populations then the knowledge base for practice and policy needs to be widened to include countries and health systems that are not represented in the studies and reviews detailed above. Some of these conclusions may be applicable to other countries, many will not be.

REFERENCES

1. Renders CM, Valk GD, Griffin SJ, Wagner EH, van Eijk JTM, Assundelft WJJ (2001) Interventions to improve the management of diabetes mellitus in primary care, outpatient and community settings: a systematic review. *Cochrane Database Syst. Rev.* **1**: CD001481.
2. Griffin S (1998) Diabetes care in general practice: meta-analysis of randomized control trials. *BMJ* **317**: 390–5.
3. Griffin SJ, Kinmonth AL (1997) The management of diabetes by general practitioners and shared care. In Pickup J, Williams G (eds) *Textbook of Diabetes* Vol. 2, 2nd edn. Blackwell Science: Oxford, pp. 80.1–80.2.
4. Wagner EH (2001) Meeting the needs of chronically ill people. *BMJ* **323**: 945–6.
5. Epping-Jordan J, Bengoa R, Kawar R, Sabate E. The challenge of chronic conditions: WHO responds *BMJ* **323**: 947–8.
6. Starfield B, Fox R (1994) Primary care tomorrow. *Lancet* **344**: 1129–33.
7. World Health Organization (1978) Regional Office for Europe. Alma Ata Declaration. WHO Copenhagen.
8. Hayes TM, Harries J (1984) Randomised controlled trial of routine hospital clinic care versus routine general practice care for type II diabetes. *BMJ* **289**: 728–30.
9. Porter AMD (1982) Organisation of diabetic care. *BMJ* **285**: 1121–4.
10. Hurwitz B, Goodman C, Yudkin J (1993) Prompting the clinical care of non-insulin dependent (type II) diabetic patients in an inner city area: one model of community care. *BMJ* **306**: 5624–30.
11. Diabetes Integrated Care Evaluation (DICE) Team (1994) Integrated care for diabetes: Clinical, psychosocial, and economic evaluation. *BMJ* **308**: 1208–12.
12. Hoskins PL, Fowler PM, Constantino M, Forest J, Yue DK, Turtle JR (1993) Sharing the care of diabetic patients between hospital and general practitioners: does it work? *Diab. Med.* **10**: 81–6.
13. Olivarius NdeF, Beck-Nielsen H, Andreasen AH, Horder M, Pedersen PA (2001) Randomised controlled trial of structured personal care of type 2 diabetes mellitus. *BMJ* **323**: 970–5.
14. Griffin SJ (2001) The management of diabetes. *BMJ* **323**: 946–7.
15. Renders CM, Valk GD, Griffin SJ, Wagner EH, van Eijk JTM, Assendelft WJJ (2001) Intervention to improve the management of diabetes in primary care, outpatient, and community settings. *Diab. Care* **24**: 1821–33.
16. Stein GH (1974) The use of a nurse practitioner in the management of patients with diabetes mellitus. *Med. Care* **12**: 885–90.
17. Palmer RH, Louis TA, Hsu LN, Peterson HF, Rothrock JK, Strain R et al. (1985) A randomised controlled trial of quality assurance in sixteen ambulatory care practices. *Med. Care* **23**: 751–70.
18. Smith DM, Norton JA, Weinberger M, McDonald CJ, Katz BP (1986) Increasing prescribed office visits. A controlled trial in patients with diabetes mellitus. *Med. Care* **24**: 189–99.
19. Vinicor F, Cohen SJ, Mazzuca SA, Moorman N, Wheeler M, Keubler T et al. (1987) DIABEDS: a randomized trial of the effects of physician and/or patient education on diabetes patient outcomes. *J. Chronic Dis.* **40**: 345–56.
20. Mazzuca SA, Vinicor F, Einterz RM, Tierney WM, Norton JA, Kalasinski LA (1990) Effects of the clinical environment on physicians' response to postgraduate medical education. *Am. Educ. Res. J.* **27**: 473–88.
21. Rutten G, van Eijk J, de Nobel E, Beek M, van der Velden J (1990) Feasibility and effects of a diabetes type II protocol with blood glucose self-monitoring in general practice. *Fam. Pract.* **7**: 273–8.

22. Carlson A, Rosenqvist U (1991) Diabetes care organization, process, and patient outcomes: effects of a diabetes control program. *Diabetes Educ.* **17**: 42–8.
23. Shultz EK, Bauman A, Hayward M, Holzman R (1992) Improved care of patients with diabetes through telecommunications. *Ann. NY Acad. Sci.* **670**: 141–5.
24. Litzelman DK, Slemenda CW, Langfield CD, Hayes LM, Welch MA, Bilf DE et al (1993) Reduction of lower extremity clinical abnormalities in patients with non-insulin-dependent diabetes mellitus. A randomized, controlled trial. *Ann. Intern. Med.* **119**: 36–41.
25. Lobach DF, Hammond WE (1994) Development and evaluation of a Computer-Assisted Management Protocol (CAMP): Improved compliance with care guidelines for diabetes mellitus. *Proc. Annu. Symp.on Comput. Appl. Med. Care*, 787–91.
26. Mazze RS, Etzwiler DD, Strock E, Peterson K, McClave CR 2nd, Meszaros JF et al. Staged diabetes management. Toward an integrated model of diabetes care. *Diab. Care* **17(Suppl. 1)**: 56–66.
27. Naji S, Cameron I, Russell I, Harvey R, Leng M, McLeod K et al. (1994) Integrated care for diabetes: clinical, psychosocial, and economic evaluation. *BMJ* **308**: 1208–12.
28. Marrero DG, Vandagriff JL, Kronz K, Fineberg NS, Golden MP, Gray D et al. (1995) Using telecommunication technology to manage children with diabetes: the Computer-Linked Outpatient Clinic (CLOC) Study. *Diabetes Educ.* **21**: 313–9.
29. Weinberger M, Kirkman MS, Samsa GP, Shortliffe EA, Landsman PB, Cowper PA et al. (1995) A nurse-coordinated intervention for primary care patients with non-insulin-dependent diabetes mellitus: impact on glycemic control and health-related quality of life. *J. Gen. Intern. Med.* **10**: 59–66.
30. Nilasena DS, Lincoln MJ (1995) A computer-generated reminder system improves physician compliance with diabetes preventive care guidelines. *Proc. Annu. Symp. Comput. Appl. Med. Care*, 640–5.
31. Feder G, Griffiths C, Highton C, Eldridge S, Spence M, Southgate L (1995) Do clinical guidelines introduced with practice-based education improve care of asthmatic and diabetic patients? A randomized controlled trial in general practices in east London. *BMJ* **311**: 1473–8.
32. Jaber LA, Halapy H, Fernet M, Tummalapalli S, Diwakaran H (1996) Evaluation of a pharmaceutical care model on diabetes management. *Ann. Pharmacother.* **30**: 238–43.
33. Ward A, Kamien M, Mansfield F, Fatovich B (1996) Education feedback in the management of type 2 diabetes in general practice. *Educ. Gen. Pract.* **7**: 142–50.
34. de Sonnaville JJ, Bourma M, Colly LP, Devillé W, Wijkel D, Heine RJ (1997) Sustained good glycaemic control in NIDDM patients by implementation of structured care in general practice: 2-year follow-up study. *Diabetologia* **40**: 1334–40.
35. Kinmonth A, Woodcock A, Griffin S, Spiegal N, Campbell MJ (1998) Randomized controlled trial of patient-centred care of diabetes in general practice: impact on current well-being and future disease risk. The Diabetes Care From Diagnosis Research Team. *BMJ* **317**: 1202–8.
36. Pill R, Stott NC, Rollnick SR, Rees M (1998) A randomized controlled trial of an intervention designed to improve the care given in general practice to type II diabetic patients: patient outcomes and professional ability to change behaviour. *Fam. Pract.* **15**: 229–35.
37. Aubert RE, Herman WH, Waters J, Moore W, Suton D, Peterson BL et la. (1998) Nurse case management to improve glycaemic control in diabetic patients in a health maintenance organization. *Ann. Intern. Med.* **129**: 605–12.

38. Halbert RJ, Leung KM, Nichol JM, Legorreta AP (1999) Effect of multiple patient reminders in improving diabetic retinopathy screening: A randomized trial. *Diab. Care* **22**: 752–5.
39. Sadur CN, Moline N, Costa M, Michalik D, Mendlowitz D, Roller S et al. (1999) Diabetes management in a health maintenance organization. Efficacy of care management using cluster visits. *Diab. Care* **22**: 2011–7.
40. Tai SS, Nazareth I, Donegan C, Haines A (1999) Evaluation of general practice computer templates. Lessons from a pilot randomised controlled trial. *Method. Inf. Med.* **38**: 177–81.
41. Boucher BJ, Claff HR, Edmonson M, Evans S, Harris BT, Hull SA et al. (1987) A pilot diabetic support service based on family practice attenders: Comparison with diabetic clinics in East London. *Diab. Med.* **4**: 480–4.
42. Deeb LC, Pettijohn FP, Shirah JK, Freeman G (1998) Interventions among primary-care practitioners to improve care for preventable complications of diabetes. *Diab. Care* **11**: 275–80.
43. Day JL, Metacalfe J, Johnson P (1992) Benefits provided by an integrated education and clinical diabetes centre: a follow-up study. *Diab. Med.* **9**: 855–9.
44. Hartman P, Bott U, Grusser M, Kronsbein P, Jorgens (1995) Effects of peer-review groups on physicians' practice. *Eur. J. Gen. Pract.* **1**: 107–12.
45. Pieber TR, Holler A, Sibenhofer, Brunner GA, Semlitsch B, Schattenberg S et al. (1995) Evaluation of a structured teaching and treatment programme for type 2 diabetes in general practice in a rural area of Austria. *Diab. Med.* **12**: 349–54.
46. O'Connor PJ, Rush WA, Peterson J, Morben P, Cherney L, Keogh C, Lasch S, (1996) Continuous quality improvement can improve glycemic control for HMO patients with diabetes. *Arch. Fam. Med.* **5**: 502–6.
47. Legorreta AP, Peters AL, Ossorio RC, Lopez RJ, Jatulis D, Davidson MB (1996) Effect of a comprehensive nurse-managed diabetes program: an HMO prospective study. *Am. J. Man. Care.* **2**: 1024–30.
48. Peters AL, Davidson MB (1998) Application of a diabetes managed care program. The feasibility of using nurses and a computer system to provide effective care. *Diab. Care* **21**: 1037–43.
49. Taplin S, Galvin MS, Payne T, Coole D, Wagner E (1998) Putting population-based care into practice: real option or rhetoric? *J. Am. Board. Fam. Pract.* **11**: 116–26.
50. Benjamin EM, Schneider MS, Hinchey KT (1999) Implementing practice guidelines for diabetes care using problem-based learning. A prospective controlled trial using firm systems. *Diab. Care* **22**: 1672–8.
51. Branger PJ, van't Hooft A, van der Wouden JC, Moorman PW, van Bemmel JH (1999) Shared care for diabetes: supporting communication between primary and secondary care. *Int. J. Med. Inf.* **53**: 133–42.
52. Sullivan FM, Menzies A (1991) The costs and benefits of introducing a nurse-run diabetic review service into general practice. *Pract. Diab.* **8**: 47–50.
53. Rith-Najarian S, Branchaud C, Beaulieu O, Gohdes D, Simonson G, Mazze R (1998) Reducing lower-extremity amputations due to diabetes. Application of the staged diabetes management approach in a primary care setting. *J. Fam. Pract.* **47**: 127–32.
54. Hawkins DW, Fielder FP, Douglas HL, Eschbach RC (1979) Evaluation of a clinical pharmacist in caring for hypertensive and diabetic patients. *Am. J. Hosp. Pharm.* **36**: 1321–5.
55. Murray CJL, Lopez AD (1996) The global burden of disease. Boston: Harvard School of Public Health.

33

Delivering Care to the Population: A Commentary

URBAN ROSENQVIST

Department of Public Health, Uppsala, Sweden

This commentary chapter clearly demonstrates how difficult it is to translate research into practice. Today, we know that normalized glucose concentration, blood pressure and lipids, as well as regular eye examination and good footwear, all function to significantly lower the risk for late diabetes complication. Yet, how do we make this happen in the real world? After many trials, we concluded that the system of care delivery must be viewed from an entirely new perspective[1].

Patients with diabetes determine their long-term outcome through their daily activities, including controlling their glucose levels, wearing the right shoes, having regular eye examinations and having blood pressure measured daily. If self-care were fully successful, the current burden on the health care system should ease. Patients also have a strong desire to function as active partners whose ideas about their health are taken seriously[2]. So, in my mind the new approach would recognize the central role of the patient and find ways to help the patient carry out her self-managed care.

This new approach would certainly call for more efficient and comprehensive patient education[3]. Home blood glucose measurement would be an excellent teaching aid, and one that can help individuals understand how food and exercise can affect their their diabetes control. A close analysis of the patient's learning process has shown that, in order for learning to take place, staff must help patients to reflect on their situation, and spend less time giving advice[4]. Learning could also be facilitated in group settings where patients can learn from others with similar experiences[5]. It has also been shown that organizations outside the regular health service, and care (e.g. pharmacies) can provide a viable platform for patient learning. Research indicates that patients appreciate such a service, and would recommend it to peers[6].

The Evidence Base for Diabetes Care. Edited by R. Williams, W. Herman, A.-L. Kinmonth and N. J. Wareham.
© 2002 John Wiley & Sons, Ltd

Other branches of the health care service might have to be redesigned in order to fully realize their potential. For instance, eye complications are often not noted by patients themselves, suggesting that a secure follow-up system is needed. It must function over a long period of time and resist fluctuations in funding or organizational support, as well as provide a high-quality service. This might call for a centralized, specialized system to ensure that eye examinations are systematically arranged[7].

How to provide good shoes for patients with impaired sensory functioning of the foot is a demanding challenge. First, patients should be aware of their sensory loss, and second, they must have some guidelines to help them find proper shoes. Unfortunately, the shoes' appeal does not always correspond to how well they fit. Perhaps shop owners could be recruited into a campaign to promote good shoes, where they can prompt elderly customers if they find that they have a sensory dysfunction of the foot. Such a testing procedure could become a routine feature of the salesperson's job.

Nowadays, many patients with diabetes can read and use the Internet to obtain information and support. These patients have often managed their life in critical situations and can fall back on years of experience. Because of their diabetes, some patients tend to hold an overly pessimistic view of life and are not aware of what they could do or what they should ask for from others. Still, their input is of vital importance for the outcome of care and the reduction of costs. The patient also holds the full continuity of care, and the patient is the only person who can mend the defects of care that occur regularly, even in the best systems. Therefore, the accumulated knowledge and unique skills of the patient should be focused on for the health services of the future. This way patients will be able to select those services they need, make comparisons between various services (i.e. function as an informed consumer) and put pressure on these services to adapt them to the patient's individual needs. In the end, this should also benefit those persons who are weaker or less empowered, who could take advantage of other resources, which were previously spent on persons who could perform their self-care more skilfully.

REFERENCES

1. Rosenqvist, U (1995) Diabetes service management training and the need for a patient perspective: a 10-year evolution of training strategies and goals. *Patient Educ. Couns.* **26**(1–3): 209–13.
2. Thorne SE and Paterson BL (2001) Health care professional support for self-care management in chronic illness: insights from diabetes research. *Patient Educ. Couns.* **42**(1): 81–90.
3. Rosenqvist U, Theman J and Assal J-P (1994) The patient's task: new development in diabetes education. TDTL, Diabetes Education Study Group of the European Association for the Study of Diabetes. Geneva: EASD.

4. Saleh Stattin N (2001) Immigrant patients with diabetes: How they understand and learn to manage and live with their diabetes. Thesis, Department of Public Health and Caring Sciences, Uppsala University, Sweden.
5. Sarkadi A and Rosenqvist U (2001) Field test of a group education program for type 2 diabetes: Measures and predictors of success on individual and group levels. *Patient Educ. Couns.* **44**(2): 129–39.
6. Sarkadi A and Rosenqvist U (1999) Study circles at the pharmacy – a new model for diabetes education? *Patient Educ. Couns.* **37**(1): 89–96.
7. Bäcklund LB, Algvere PV and Rosenqvist U (1997) New blindness in diabetes reduced by more than one-third in Stockholm County. *Diabet. Med.* **14**(9): 732–40.

Part IX

CONTINUING EDUCATION

34

Keeping Up To Date Through Lifelong Learning

DAVID PENCHEON and JOHN WRIGHT

Institute of Public Health, Cambridge CB2 2SR, UK

Bradford Hospitals NHS Trust, Bradford BD9 6RT, UK

'The person who qualifies today and stops learning
tomorrow is uneducated the day after'

Anon

'Experience is the process of becoming increasingly
confident with doing things wrong'

Attributed to Michael O'Donnell

INTRODUCTION

Medical knowledge is expanding at an exponential rate and new methods are
needed to stay afloat in this new and stormy sea. The days of omniscient
doctors leaving medical school with their 'bible' to see them through their
professional careers are long gone (if they ever existed). As well as facing
rapidly changing treatments and practice, our minds are not designed, as
CD-ROMs are, to store huge databases of 'answers'. We are human and we
forget. This can have its advantages (grievances, out-of-date medical practice)
but for most health professionals this outcome is not helpful. In order to
address it, the first step we must take is to recognise it and admit it. Like the
recovering alcoholic in admitting a problem, we need to be proud of standing
up and saying 'I don't know'. The alternative – to pretend, to cover up, to bluff
– is no longer an acceptable option.

As well as encouraging health professionals to recognise learning needs and
deal with them, we must also ensure that the environments in which they work

The Evidence Base for Diabetes Care. Edited by R. Williams, W. Herman, A.-L. Kinmonth and N. J. Wareham.
© 2002 John Wiley & Sons, Ltd

are supportive and conducive to learning. This is not just the responsibility of the doctor or nurse. We must move away from an atmosphere of name, shame and blame to one of shared responsibility for the professional, the patient and the organisation.

The professional: Just by reading this sentence we know you are the wrong reader. It is likely that this book will preach to the converted rather than deal with getting concepts and information to those professionals that most need it. Like most continuing professional and medical education, there is a strong element of self-selection. Just as continuing professional education works if you do not want it, and if you do want it you don't need it[1], it is likely that the books we read reflect our own particular interests rather than our educational needs. This becomes almost an inverse need law with professional development – we learn more and more about less and less.

This chapter outlines the three general steps we can take to meet these educational needs:

1. Recognising educational needs. Effective learning will occur when the subject is important and the learning combines reflection with actual experience.

2. Doing something about identified needs. The idea of 'just in time' information conveys the right approach to learning in today's busy health service environments. Rather than be guided by what happens to be on the front page of our favoured professional journal that week, we need to be able to turn everyday problems into clear questions and then to have quick access to reliable information to answer them.

    Information technology (IT) holds great potential for realising this possibility. Many hospitals and general practices already have access to medical and health databases on the wards and in the consultation rooms, via intranet, Internet or CD-ROM. Ensuring access to up-to-date knowledge wherever decisions about patient care are being made (in outpatient departments, on the ward) can be, and should be, an achievable goal over the next 10 years.

3. Having the skills to assess the evidence. We need to know how to read papers, assess their validity and decide what they mean for the patients we see. Hierarchies of evidence provide a welcome move away from the GOBSAT evidence (good old boys sitting around a table) or the 'someone once told me' level of evidence. Published evidence can relate to diagnosis and prognosis for people with diabetes, as can papers that evaluate the clinical and cost-effectiveness of existing treatments and interventions or new interventions (health technology assessments).

At the same time, there is a tension between qualitative and quantitative research. Randomised controlled trials can provide the best, objective evidence of treatments in diabetes. However, care needs to be taken not to focus only on methods which may include only a narrow patient group, and which tend to be dominated by pharmaceutical interventions. Other research methods, such as qualitative research and observational studies, can provide a valuable balance between the internal validity of evidence from a trial and its external validity to everyday clinical practice[2]. It is important to ensure that similar standards of critical appraisal are still applied[3].

This critical eye is not confined to external information. It should also encourage greater reflection and evaluation of our own clinical practice.

The patient: One of the benefits of evidence-based practice is that it is explicit about the basis of clinical decision-making. This allows clinical practice to be more transparent and enables patients to be more involved in the decision-making. For many patients there is no desire to enquire further than, 'what do you think, doctor?' However, we live in an increasingly consumer-focused society and more and more patients want to know more about the health care they receive.

Guidelines provide a clear description of nationally or locally recommended practice, and there is no reason why guidelines cannot be used as the basis of discussion between health professional and patient. Some guidelines are now disseminated into a form that is much more meaningful to patients[4].

Access to good-quality information is important. Many health professionals will already have experienced the competition from Internet sources – patients attending clinic with advice downloaded from the World Wide Web. The development of 'approved' information sources, such as the National Centre for Information Quality and the National Electronic Library for Health (NeLH) in the UK, will contribute greatly to ensuring the accuracy and relevance of health information. Independent evaluation of the quality of information on the Internet, using kite-marks or hallmarks to distinguish valid information from fiction may also be of value[5].

The organisation: The section in this chapter on audit, governance and collaborative learning highlights the importance of the health care organisation, department or team in providing evidence-based health care. The key responsibility of the health care organisation is to provide the environment for lifelong learning and evidence-based practice.

Lifelong learning and quality improvement are not discrete activities to be undertaken in the privacy of your own home. They must be intrinsic to the complete quality improvement process in the workplace. Clinical audit, risk management, research and development, clinical guidelines, evidence-based practice and, patient involvement are all often disparate activities that need to be pulled together for the same common purpose: improving patient care.

We should consider how we can strengthen multidisciplinary working to achieve this, not because this is politically correct, but because this is how we work in reality – as part of a team. Shared goals around patient needs can help break down traditional barriers[6].

As part of a group of health professionals working together we also need to influence our organisation and its use of resources rather than retreat into splendid isolation. This should be about ensuring adequate time to reflect on our practice and agree ways to improve it. It should be about training and ensuring that staff have the opportunity to develop the necessary skills to keep up to date (whether learning how to search the Cochrane Library or how to prescribe a new drug). It should be about meeting future information technology needs. It should also be about non-clinical decision making (management and policy decisions for example) and ensuring that they are preceded by the questions: 'What is the question?' and 'What is the evidence?' just as clinical decisions should be.

WHY IS THERE A SPECIAL NEED TO KEEP UP TO DATE?

Maintaining health and delivering health care effectively depends on a huge body of knowledge that changes daily. We learn of better ways to diagnose and treat. We also learn that traditional methods are less effective than we thought. This body of knowledge increases exponentially with many millions of biomedical papers published each year in many thousands of journals. There is good evidence that professionals are generally not good at keeping up to date; not only do we recommend treatments up to 10 years after they have been shown to be useless, but we fail to recommend treatment up to 10 years after it has been proven beneficial[7]. Professionals, patients and the public need to be continually aware of the rapid change in the knowledge and values that underpin health and health care decision making. Only then will we be better partners in both delivering and receiving the most effective and appropriate care.

This acceleration of knowledge has two important consequences. First, the knowledge that is necessary to practice competently is changing so rapidly that simply staying up-to-date with information just in case one needs it is almost impossible. A hundred years ago, it might have been possible for doctors to learn at medical school most of the knowledge that was known. This would usually have served them and their patients well for the rest of their careers. Second, the needs, demands and expectations of the world around us are also changing rapidly. Professionals are, quite rightly, no longer immune from the critical attitudes and consumerist behaviour of those they purport to serve. Patients and their families have always been best placed to know how a chronic disease such as diabetes affects them *personally*; what is new is the amount of *generalisable* knowledge about diabetes that patients are usefully learning and interpreting.

WHAT IS LIFELONG LEARNING?

How do we develop a process for keeping up to date when the knowledge base is changing and increasing more rapidly every day? Staying aware of the best evidence and best practice is not just a frustrating challenge in the short term; there may be legal consequences for those who are not willing or able to stay abreast.

Traditional continuing medical education (CME) (as defined by attending conferences, accruing CME points etc.) is associated with neither a significant change in behaviour nor an improvement in patient outcomes[8-10]. Changing practice is essentially about changing behaviour. Behaviour is determined more by beliefs than by the internal incorporation of knowledge; a more effective and sustainable approach to keeping up to date must, therefore, address people's beliefs as well as their knowledge[11]. Acknowledging the importance of beliefs and developing a genuine willingness to address them are perhaps the most important steps in keeping up to date. The essential ingredients for lifelong learning are awareness, opportunity and motivation. However, professionals do not always work in an environment in which admitting uncertainty or challenging orthodoxy is either feasible or rewarded.

Continuing medical education is therefore not about exhorting professionals to attend conferences. It is concerned with creating a learning culture in people, in teams, and in organisations. Creating this culture and combining it with simple systems of prompts, rewards and deterrents in clinical practice may do far more to improve patient care than expensive and inefficient hours in darkened lecture theatres[12]. Taking control of your individual learning needs and meeting them systematically and effectively, both in terms of technical skills and knowledge, and in terms of generic skills such as management, personal and team skills, differentiates CME from the broader term of continuing professional development (CPD).

WHY IS LIFELONG LEARNING IMPORTANT?

The rate of increase of medical knowledge means that the only sustainable coping strategy is to supplement our knowledge (i.e. content) with the actual skills (i.e. process) of lifelong learning (i.e. learning how to learn throughout our lives). So much knowledge is being generated (and is *theoretically* available) that we stand no chance of proactively keeping up to date with all that we might need to know, no matter how specialised we are[13].

One sustainable method of using the most up to date knowledge is to find it when it is needed, rather than learning it in case it is needed one day. The former policy needs very good decision support using information technology and good databases (as well as the skills of phrasing questions and searching). The latter system is no longer tenable due to the amount of information currently available and the speed at which it becomes out of date or less generalisable. A 'just in time' approach to finding knowledge needs to supplement our 'just in case' approach.

After learning the basic knowledge and technical skills (e.g. regarding diabetes care), we need to supplement them with:

- the skills of being reflective;
- identifying what needs to be clarified;
- turning problems into questions that are answerable from reliable evidence;
- finding and appraising such evidence;
- implementing what needs to be developed and changed, on the basis of what we find.

Many professionals are already explicitly incorporating evidence into their clinical practice. The rest of us call this approach 'evidence-based practice' as discussed in Chapter 1. Figure 34.1 shows how the world of learning has changed for professionals[14]:

Paradigms in Learning
OLD

- knowing what you *should* know
- much learning "complete" at the end of formal training
- uncertainty discouraged and ignorance avoided
- learning by humiliation; name shame and blame
- sole methods: apprenticeship, learning from accepted wisdom
- finite amount of knowledge to be absorbed
- intuition very powerful
- dominated by knowledge from experience
- fact and *content* based learning
- professionals on top

NEW

- knowing what you *don't* know, (not feeling bad about it) and knowing *how* to find out (or help others to...)
- learning from cradle to grave (life-long learner)
- legitimising uncertainty, learning by questioning
- able to question received wisdom
- turning problems into questions, and to find, appraise, store, and act on experience and evidence to solve them
- complementing experience with knowledge from research
- problem and *process* based learning
- professionals on tap

Figure 34.1. How the world of learning has changed for professionals[14].

WHY IS BEING A LIFELONG LEARNER AND DEVELOPING EVIDENCE-BASED PRACTICE CHALLENGING?

There are at least four important problems with our personal knowledge base and related professional attitudes and behaviour.

- Much of what we think is correct may not be.
- We may be unaware of better practice.
- We may feel defensive about our own uncertainty and threatened by the knowledge of others (researchers, professional bodies, colleagues or patients).
- We may have very little training in generating questions, searching for evidence, critical appraisal and changing our practice (and that of our colleagues).

To be a lifelong learner, we need to appreciate these problems, learn to live with our own uncertainties without being paralysed by them, and to develop ways of dealing with them constructively, both as individuals and as teams.

The first step involves being able to reflect on one's personal knowledge and practice. No two professionals have exactly the same approach to managing diabetes, for example. This is only important when people become fixed and unjustifiably confident about their beliefs and practice[9]. Natural variation in knowledge, belief and clinical practice is only a problem when we are not prepared to learn from it (e.g. by observing and analysing the differences systematically, and carefully measuring processes and outcomes). Figure 34.2 shows the classic progress over time of competence and insight. Having insight

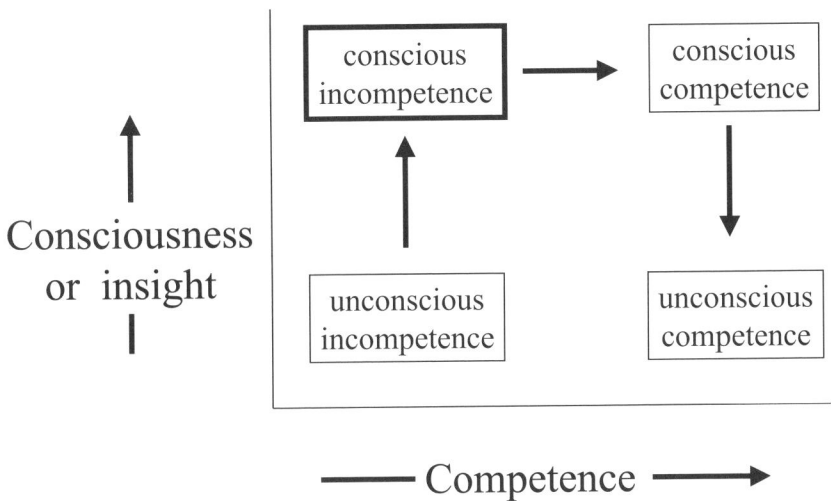

Figure 34.2. Competence/consciousness.

into one's uncertainty is the essential first step to identifying (and hence meeting) important learning needs.

Lifelong learning is an attitude before it is a skill. There is little point in trying to develop the skills if the fundamental attitude is not in place.

After coping with these shifts in attitudes, the next task is to be able turn everyday problems in the home, surgery, clinic or laboratory into questions that are phrased in such a way that they suggest the search strategy of any evidence that might address the issue. Details of these techniques can be found in an increasing number of texts[16-18].

AUDIT, GOVERNANCE AND PROFESSIONAL RESPONSIBILITY TO KEEP UP TO DATE

Clearly everyone has a responsibility and an interest in keeping up to date. In the world of diabetes care and prevention, there are three groups of people for whom this is particularly important. The methods, reasons and consequences of staying abreast of knowledge may differ for these three groups, especially through the newer opportunities of electronic communications[19]:

- people whose prime responsibility is professional provision of care;
- people who spend most of their time conducting research into diabetes;
- people (and their families and carers) who live with diabetes.

Establishing criteria and meeting standards in these criteria have been the classic ways of improving quality through audit. When team or organisational responsibility and accountability are added to this process of assuring and improving quality, the term 'governance' is used. Clinical governance links quality assurance with group responsibility. Individuals, departments and organisations should all be able and willing to demonstrate the mechanisms by which quality is being assured. This may be CPD for individual professionals seeking revalidation, or clinical governance for teams and organisations seeking reaccreditation.

COLLABORATIVE CARE: COLLABORATIVE LEARNING

Belbin's famous comment that people are rarely perfect, only teams can be[20], is highly relevant to the way we keep up to date in diabetes. The management of people with diabetes is a multidisciplinary endeavour[21]. Professional development of the team involves appreciating expert knowledge of each person, not forgetting that the most important member of the team is the person with diabetes[22]. Learning is an integral and fundamental part of the care process: sharing the care should mean sharing the learning[23]; between people (e.g. professional/professional or professional/patient) or between teams (e.g. primary and secondary care[24] or both.

RESEARCH EVIDENCE AND QUALITY OF CARE

Research is centrally concerned with better understanding the world around us. The methods and results need to be valid, understandable and relevant. However, research is not a pure affair with an objective beginning or end. Although much research is valid (if not generalisable), the fact that much important research has not even been done (and the research that has been done is not always published or available) means that the availability of research (or lack of it) is, in itself, a significant source of bias. The choice of research commissioned, the methods used and the research that becomes published and available is to a large extent, the product of the prevailing world view. Consequently we should distinguish between evidence of absence (good research showed no relationship . . .) and absence of evidence (the research has not been done . . .). In addition, it is important to remember that the outcomes defined by researchers may be different to those considered important by other people.

THE DIMENSIONS OF QUALITY

Because this book is designed to cater for the needs of wide variety of people who must communicate well, the authors take the definition of words seriously. 'Quality' is a word whose meaning has various interpretations. One practical way to consider quality is to make sure we are doing as well as we possibly can within the constraints of evidence and resources. The shortfall in reaching this potential is sometimes referred to as 'Achievable Benefit Not Achieved'. People who take quality seriously constantly ask themselves (and others) 'How can we improve?'

When deconstructed, quality can have many dimensions, some of which have to be pursued at the expense of others. Donabedian provides us with a useful taxonomy[25]. Perhaps the most important dimension or value of the information that underpins decision making is not effectiveness, efficiency, equity, appropriateness or acceptability, but *explicitness*. No information is value-free – it is important that the assumptions, values and evidence (of any kind) used to make decisions are made explicit.

STRENGTH OF EVIDENCE – METHODS, VALIDITY AND RELEVANCE

Evidence that influences decision making comes from many directions, people and methods. In order to judge the relative value of evidence, we need first to grade it hierarchically against criteria of likely validity. The important issues here include the clarity of the question being addressed, the selection of the correct method to address this question, and the correct execution of this method ('right question, correct method, method done correctly').

There are many scales, the most commonly used of which can be found in Chapter 1. People will always debate the value of large randomised controlled trials (RCTs) compared to even larger systematic reviews. Equally important is the tension between quantitative research (e.g. does something cause something else and by how much?) and qualitative research (how do we think, why do we behave, or what do we value?). Quantitative research usually gives us answers to questions. Qualitative research tends to suggest the questions to answer. Many professionals are historically exposed to the former and hence value research that contains numbers, and specific answers to focused questions (i.e. quantitative research) at the expense of qualitative research. Sadly, this bias means we deny ourselves the benefit of research which takes 'a holistic perspective which preserves the complexities of human behaviour'[26].

The second issue concerns the strength of evidence that is relevant. This will depend on the local situation and the degree to which the research evidence is generalisable. Is the local situation, population or person so different from the population on which the research was done that no useful inferences can be made?

THE VALUE-LADEN NATURE OF RESEARCH – WHOSE OUTCOMES?

When designing, conducting or appraising quantitative research on, for instance, the effectiveness of an intervention in managing diabetes, the three important elements of the design are the population, the intervention and the outcome. Unfortunately, although the population and the intervention are often undisputed, the outcomes chosen by the researchers can differ from those that might be chosen by people with diabetes. This is often understandable: the two groups may be pursuing different objectives (e.g. causation versus quality of life, respectively). However, in chronic and complex conditions such as diabetes, quality of life can be an overlooked outcome. Researchers, like clinicians, need always to consider the values, wishes and aspirations of the patient.

ASSESSING LEARNING NEEDS

Keeping up to date is strongly influenced by context, need, motivation and methods. An important place to start is to assess your own educational needs. There are many tools for doing this, but the most pragmatic approach is via reflection (e.g. stimulated by questionnaire[24]). The disadvantage of this approach is that there is no evidence that proves what we *think* we need to learn is what we *do* need to learn. We do not relish straying outside our comfort zones, preferring instead to learn about things with which we are already moderately confident. Specialisation within our comfort zone is more attractive than addressing broader needs outside it. This leads to the paradox that, as professionals, we usually spend time learning in areas where we are already reasonably competent, rather than addressing areas where our knowledge and skills might be weak. In addition, we tend to be biased towards developing our practice skills (e.g. retinal examination[27]) at the expense of our skills at keeping up to date. Learning to appreciate values and beliefs (e.g. who should be the primary decision maker in diabetes care[15]) is rarely considered systematically. It is not clear how these domains are related, but true adult learning needs to change more than just skills. True education challenges and changes our belief systems.

FINDING KNOWLEDGE TO IMPROVE PRACTICE

In order to keep up to date, a willingness to search for evidence and incorporate it into practice must be matched by the necessary facilities and opportunities.

DATABASES

The most commonly used electronic database is Medline. The paper version, still available in many libraries, is called Index Medicus. This database of structured details of research papers (titles, authors, etc., and sometimes abstracts) contains details of approximately 10 million articles from approximately 3800 journals. It is important to remember that not all journals are listed in Medline, so relying on this source alone will inevitably miss many sources of evidence immediately. A complementary database is Excerpta Medica (Embase), the nearest European equivalent to Medline. It is very similar with a substantial overlap but has less of a North American flavour and tends to be stronger on pharmaceutical evidence. No matter how frequently one uses these databases, it is important to get good quality training, preferably from a medical librarian. Good introductory books on searching databases are available which lead one through real-life situations[17].

Other important databases include the Cochrane Library, the product of the International Cochrane Collaboration[28]. For many people, such databases of secondary research evidence (where the unit of analysis is other research rather than human subjects, for example) are a good source of reliable evidence if one has faith in those who have searched and appraised on your behalf. The most important criterion of quality here is the explicitness and quality of the methods used to perform the research, be it primary research with people or secondary research by distilling and concentrating the fruits of other research. More details of these databases are available in local libraries. It is important to be familiar with primary research databases: (Medline, Excerpta Medica, etc.) as well as with secondary research databases (Cochrane Library, Journal of Evidence Based Medicine on CD) and local specialist databases on diabetes available locally.

Other important source of secondary evidence include journals of secondary publication such as *Drugs and Therapeutics Bulletin*, published by the Consumers' Association (one of the few journals in the world to grade the references on methodology and potential bias), the *Journal of Evidence Based Medicine*, and *Bandolier* (www.ebandolier.com).

THE USE OF THE INTERNET

The use of the Internet in keeping up to date is becoming essential. There are two main uses of the Internet. First, as a source of information to be read or downloaded. Second, the Internet's interactive nature makes it an ideal mechanism for discussion groups and mutual support for professionals and the public[29,30].

Information regarding health, especially chronic health issues, is one of the most common reasons for people to access the Internet. People living with diabetes often develop a very active involvement in research and support mechanisms, and hence find the Internet invaluable but frustrating. High-quality research from electronic journals, the National Institutes of Health, diabetic associations and forums, proceedings of conferences and official publications are often found on the Internet[19]. However, it is vitally important to check the credibility and validity of information, as quality control is highly variable. Few tools exist at present to allow people to check the credibility of the information available. Similarly, critical appraisal tools for the Internet are still, at the time of writing, in their infancy. The Internet is good for getting the first word on a subject, but poor at the last word. It is best used for discussion groups and for airing opinions rather than promulgating research of a dubious nature.

The Internet is particularly attractive to people living and working in poorer countries. Access is far cheaper than building and maintaining a library. Journals are increasingly available in some form over the Internet. Furthermore, professionals can stay in daily contact with colleagues with similar specialist interests in diabetes regardless of where they are in the world. This virtual community of professionals will find international borders and relative poverty less restrictive in their ability to stay up to date with the latest evidence. Poorer countries have an even greater incentive to make the best of the limited financial resources available, both in terms of formal care and in promoting collaborative and self-care. The Internet can be a useful tool to gain this information, especially through co-operating with professionals and institutions from wealthier countries.

PROFESSIONAL ORGANISATIONS

BMJ's Clinical Evidence, a compendium of the best available research findings on common and important clinical questions, is updated and expanded every six months. The first issue was published in book format in January 1999. More details are available via http://www.clinicalevidence.org.

INSTITUTES

There are learning institutes around the world where lifelong learning and evidence-based practice are so much a part of the culture that they sometimes even find their way into the place name. These places include McMaster University in Hamilton, Canada, Newcastle University in Australia, and the Centre for Evidence Based Medicine in Oxford, the UK.

The natural centres of evidence should be libraries, but too many libraries sadly resemble their ancestors as neatly hushed repositories of data and text. In contrast, other libraries have developed into bustling nodes in the information jungle where assistance is almost always on tap to help individuals develop the confidence and skills to cope with the knowledge explosion. Clinicians spend useful time turning problems into questions and questions into answers, either in their surgeries, in their clinics or in their libraries.

Other institutions have a role in collating, appraising and disseminating secondary research evidence. These institutes can be international centres, or function at a national level such as the UK's NHS Centre for Reviews and Dissemination whose role is to address issues of more pressing national concern (www.york.ac.uk/inst/crd/).

PATIENT/DISEASE SUPPORT GROUPS

The Internet is becoming an extremely powerful resource for support groups for people living with diabetes. This is likely to become more important as more people become connected. Chronic disease self-management has been revolutionised through the creation of extended support and electronically accessible support groups.

MANAGING THE KNOWLEDGE

Knowledge management is likely to be a common phrase of the twenty-first century. The essential steps are searching, appraising, storing, communicating and implementing knowledge.

SEARCHING

There are two types of searching: passive browsing and specific searching. We all browse; it serves the important function of keeping us interested and aware of some of the developments (albeit unsystematically). What browsing does not do is to keep us systematically up to date with the best research evidence. In fact, due to the volume of knowledge and its variable quality, there is simply not the time to keep broadly and systematically up to date through browsing, not matter how specialist we are.

Active searching always involves being very clear about the nature of the issue being addressed. The specific skill of turning problems into answerable questions needs to be developed. There are good texts that address this[16,18]. Like all good research, the actual steps being taken should be repeatable: that is, using the same methods should derive the same results. It is therefore important to be explicit about the methods. Good-quality searching needs access to libraries and electronic databases. The strengths and weaknesses of all the databases need to be taken into account when searching. Large databases such as Medline are notorious for imbuing a falsely high sense of completeness.

APPRAISING

There are many guides to systematically appraising the literature available on the Internet (e.g. www.phru.org.uk/~casp/). The fundamental steps are:

- Why was the research done?
- How was the research done?
- What was found?
- What does it mean for me/us?

In more detail:

1. Does this paper address the issue I am interested in (especially in terms of population and outcome)?

2. Does it use appropriate methods and are the methods used correctly?

3. What are the results, including a quantification of certainty (e.g. confidence interval/limits)?

4. How relevant are the results to me?

COMMUNICATING INFORMATION

It is not enough just to be able to understand research findings. One must be able to communicate them to many audiences in any ways depending on the context[31]. For instance, as discussed in Chapter 1, using relative risk as a measure of effectiveness may be important for someone interested in the strength of possible causative mechanisms and pathways. Absolute risk may be of more interest to a public heath professional who is trying to quantify the disease burden and the likely effect of intervention in a population. Calculating the numbers needed to treat may be of more use in a clinical consultation when an individual's chance of additional benefit may be of prime concern.

STORING

Lifelong learning is only of real value when there is individual or institutional memory. Storing evidence is best done on a computer rather than in a shoebox. Electronic data have many advantages:

- it is much easy to search large quantities of electronic data;
- it is more convenient to manipulate, incorporate, analyse and move electronic data;
- electronic data are much more amenable to being overwritten, thus destroying less valid (and potentially dangerous) research data.

Invest in a personal or departmental electronic database to store *and retrieve* research in the form of citations (e.g. Reference Manager, Endnote, etc...).

PUTTING NEW THEORY INTO PRACTICE

CHANGING PERSONAL PRACTICE

Adopting some of the techniques of evidence-based practice and lifelong learning can fundamentally change the quality of care. It can also help professionals deal positively and constructively with uncertainty, which in turn makes learning an exciting challenge rather than a necessary chore.

The most important feature of lifelong learning is that it legitimises uncertainty. The only price to pay for this is the undertaking to address uncertainty and ignorance openly, honestly and explicitly.

CHANGING DEPARTMENTAL POLICY: A JOURNAL CLUB –AN EXAMPLE OF EVIDENCE BASED PRACTICE IN ACTION

An example of this transition from a solution-based approach to learning 'just in case' to a problem-based approach 'just in time' is the tradition of running a journal club – a task that comes to most of us at some time. Journal clubs, probably more accurately termed 'learning clubs', have, for many of us, been associated with a poorly run, variably attended meeting with little systematic learning. Guidance on how to run an effective journal club is available, however[16]. They can be one of the most useful and effective forms of team learning if they are well organised. More importantly, such clubs can encourage the culture necessary to legitimise uncertainty and deal with it constructively.

The most common mistake with such events is to start with papers that may be unrelated to current everyday problems and practice. It is much more important to begin with real problems on the ward or in the clinic or surgery. Journal clubs, as a way of keeping up to date and run in the way outlined below, have the dual advantage of being highly relevant (an important principle of adult learning) as well as varied (no session within the journal club runs for more than about 20 minutes). A method employed at McMaster Medical School, Canada is represented in Figure 34.3.

DEVELOPING COUNTRIES

With the increasing globalisation of research activity and the relative poverty of many countries, it is important to acknowledge the different strategies for keeping up to date depending on worldwide location. Two points:

2 weeks ago	last week	This week
Identify an important practical problem that needs addressing A	Identify an important practical problem that needs addressing B	Identify an important practical problem that needs addressing C
	Quickly sort all the different pieces of evidence for validity and relevance and choose the best A	Quickly sort all the different pieces of evidence for validity and relevance and choose the best B
Refereence: Sackett, Richardson et al[16]		Detailed discussion of the critical appraisal of the evidence and implications for practice A

Figure 34.3. How journal clubs can operate[16].

1. Traditional repositories of text and data in the form of libraries with expensive book and journal subscriptions are not the most cost-effective infrastructure to help professionals and the public keep up to date. The infrastructure facilities are more likely to consist of access to databases and other electronic media, and the skills are those of searching and appraising the appropriate evidence in order to make better and more explicit decisions.

2. Good research is not confined to industrialised nations. High-quality research is done in poorer countries. Restricting one's search of evidence to richer countries or to the English-speaking world introduces significant bias.

CHANGING PROFESSIONAL BEHAVIOUR

There is good evidence, not only of wide variation in professional practice for a particular condition, but of effective interventions not implemented. Despite the known benefit conferred by early thrombolysis[32], the median proportion of eligible patients receiving such treatment in 11 European countries in 1996 was 36%[33]. Why is this? The problem with most methods for changing professional practice (i.e. getting research into practice) is that the traditional ways of doing this bear little relation to how professionals actually change their own practice. Simple distribution of written materials rarely meets the needs or working style of decision makers. Effective dissemination needs, at least, to be:

- consistent
- co-ordinated
- contextualised.

The information then needs to be actively debated and incorporated into practice, not received passively not delivered didactically.

Systematic reviews of randomised controlled trials on interventions to promote change in clinical practice can provide us with some answers as to which method we should use to be most effective in influencing our colleagues (see Box 34.1)[34].

THE BARRIERS TO CHANGING PROFESSIONAL PRACTICE

Barriers to changing professional practice can be classified into those inherent to the professional and those associated with their working environment.

Professional

Professionals may fail to appreciate there may be a better way of managing particular groups of patients. Appreciating the possibility of improvement is the first step in achieving it.

Box 34.1. Interventions to promote behavioural change among health
professionals (adapted from Bero *et al.*[34]). Reproduced with permission.

Consistently effective interventions

- Educational outreach visits
- Reminders
- Multifaceted interventions
- Interactive educational meetings

Interventions of variable effectiveness

- Audit and feedback
- The use of local opinion leaders
- Local consensus processes
- Patient mediated interventions

Interventions that have little or no effect

- Educational materials
- Didactic educational meetings

In practice, human beings are not good at systematically handling multiple
information sources and competing pressures and priorities in a short space of
time[35].

Environmental

One of the most important barriers to practice improvement is the poor communication of research findings. Rarely is the presentation of data and conclusions made relevant to decision makers, be they professionals or members
of the public[36,37].

It is fruitless exhorting professionals to stay up to date with latest research
evidence if the necessary infrastructure (e.g. a dependable and user-friendly
information system) is not available on the wards or in the clinics[36] or if
insufficient training is available.

In many hospitals and primary care settings, there can still be a lack of peer
group agreed criteria and standards for quality of care. This is the most
important starting point to develop a system of clinical governance[38].

Both of the above

Quite simply, there may be insufficient incentives (of any nature) to encourage
change.

HOW CAN PROFESSIONAL CHANGE BE ACHIEVED?

Although the evidence on which clinical practice is based is increasingly
scrutinised, the evidence on how best we should help people improve their

clinical practice is given less attention. Professionals probably change practice much more on the basis of belief than rigorous evidence[39]. A 'Review Group' of the Cochrane Collaboration is devoted to this area: the Cochrane Effective Practice and Organisation of Care Group (EPOC); see www.abdn.ac.uk/ hsru/
There are four broad approaches to changing professional practice.

1. Make the information and proposed changes *understandable* (interactive education, active dissemination).
2. Make changes *easy to implement* by:
   - providing infrastructure (information systems, contextualised prompts).
   - providing peer support (research-aware environment, local consensus and opinion leaders).
3. Make it *rewarding* (incentives – CME/CPD points, money, airmiles).
4. Make it *obligatory* (regulation).

Because single interventions appear to have little effect on practice and therefore negligible effect on outcome (e.g. patient/population health), the most effective methods combine these approaches. Non-interactive education and passive dissemination appear to be largely ineffective[33]. Evidence of professional change only starts to become apparent when simple education is supplemented by a genuinely evaluative culture (e.g. the routine and systematic use of audit), local consensus conferences and the active involvement of opinion leaders[41]. The following steps and interventions should be considered:

1. *Contextual analysis*. Just as we need a diagnosis before we start treating a patient, so we need a contextual or diagnostic analysis before we start to implement change. Spend a bit of time at the start identifying what the barriers and levers for change will be. Talk to relevant clinicians and managers to understand what will help and what will hinder implementation. Assess the educational needs and objectives of the implementation programme.

2. *Awareness raising*. Try to involve as many people as possible in commenting on draft guidelines or new practices, so that there is early ownership. Publicise developments and changes though local newsletters in the hospital or in primary care. Simple postal dissemination does not seem to be effective in promoting change; however, it may promote recognition and awareness that can then be built upon.

3. *Identify local 'opinion leaders'*. These are local health professionals who are considered to be influential in educating other staff about the clinical topic. They are likely to be listened to and their clinical opinion respected and adopted. They should be used to lead or support the educational and training events as part of the guideline implementation process. These opinion leaders usually have the enthusiasm to promote their messages, but may be limited by time, and some thought should go into how to use their time most efficiently.

4. *Use existing educational events* such as postgraduate lectures or clinical governance meetings (for hospital departments or primary care groups) to promote best practice to hospital staff and general practitioners. Didactic lectures are of dubious effectiveness, but are still the mainstay of medical education. Interactive and participatory sessions are more likely to promote change and subsequent guideline adoption. Involve your audience, listen to what they want to learn and provide concrete examples for them to learn with.

5. *Arrange educational outreach visits* by relevant medical and nursing specialists – taking the message out to the clinicians. These visits take place in the practice setting, for example general practitioners' surgeries, or individual departments, and so tend to be more interactive and less formal. This is a strategy commonly used by the pharmaceutical industry and one that appears to be effective, yet one that the health service has been slow to adopt. The main reason for this inertia has been the lack of time and resources to send someone out to train other staff. However, it may be the only way to influence doctors who would not otherwise attend existing educational events. Such a targeted strategy may be valuable in changing the practice of those who deviate from recommended practice the most – a 10-minute discussion may prevent many time-consuming, inappropriate referrals.

6. *Prompts and reminders* can be very effective aids in getting timely access to the right information for clinical decision making. Posters for wards and stickers or markers in medical records can be simple methods of reminding staff of important matters, for example, prompting staff to check that all post-myo-cardial infarction patients are discharged on aspirin and beta-blockers. Desk-top calendars and computer versions which can be accessed via a local intranet are more sophisticated methods. Standards can also be incorporated into relevant referral forms to encourage compliance with referral requests, for example with radiology requests. Recommendations can also be incorporated into reports (such as laboratory reports or investigations) or referral letters to reinforce desired practice. Computerised decision support will become an increasingly powerful reminder method as it allows prompts to be made at the same time as clinical decision making.

7. *Audit and feedback* allow individual wards and departments to see how their own clinical practice matches up with recommended standards and subsequently, to monitor change. This information on performance can be important to demonstrate weaknesses in practice that justify the need for local change. This can be used in educational and training events to link key messages with evidence about current practice. It can also provide the basis for evaluation of the implementation and the sustainability of changes in clinical practice.

8. *Patients themselves* can be influential in encouraging health professionals to make the right decisions. Well-informed patients will know what treatments

they should be taking and what standards of care should be provided. This is particularly true of patients with chronic diseases and younger, more empowered patients. It is worth considering strategies that target patients themselves, such as posters in waiting areas, messages in the local press or discussions with local patient organisations.

Different mechanisms will work for different individuals so local approaches should be tailored accordingly. Implementation should be systematic and planned rather than haphazard and opportunistic, and adopting a stepwise approach may allow the best use of limited resources.

The final stage of implementation should be to evaluate the process of change and learn any lessons from it. Has there been the desired change? If so, what worked? If not, what were the barriers and how can they be overcome? Changing practice is an ongoing process that must be reflective and adaptable if it is to succeed. Evaluation can be through audit of guideline standards or more qualitative techniques of interviews with guideline users and developers.

THE FUTURE

There is no doubt that many of the changes we are currently witnessing regarding the volume and variability of information available will not only increase, but will accelerate. This has profound consequences for the provision of health care[42,43].

Keeping up to date will take a leap forward with two emerging technologies. First, as digital television incorporates the Internet, the amount of information available through broad band conduits will be huge. Second, this technology allows us to tune the information coming into our homes and surgeries in the form of preselected 'channels' to search the areas in which we are interested; a change from 'push' technology to 'pull' technology. Such volumes of knowledge do not always equate with empowerment; it is as likely to cause bewilderment and confusion. The most likely consequence is that we will all have to live with greater degrees of uncertainty.

The biggest challenge for the professional of the twenty-first century is to evolve from being considered as a primary source of knowledge, to becoming a facilitator of the methods of finding, appraising and using that knowledge in partnership with patients. This ultimately involves the skill of being more transparent with uncertainty whilst maintaining a professional credibility.

The most important attribute for lifelong learning professionals will remain a questioning and open attitude to the knowledge and values that underpin decision-making at every level. This includes a willingness to be open with uncertainty whilst maintaining a positive and therapeutic relationship with people and families living with diabetes.

ACKNOWLEDGEMENTS

With special thanks to Andrea Trigg-Jones and Dave Sackett. We are indebted to Professor Jeremy Grimshaw for guiding our thoughts regarding the science and art of changing professional behaviour.

NOTE

All websites in this chapter were correct when this book went to press.

REFERENCES

1. Sibley JC, Sackett DL, Neufeld V et al. (1982) A randomised trial of continuing medical education. *N. Engl. J. Med.* **306**: 511–15.
2. Medicine-based evidence: a prerequisite for evidence-based medicine. *BMJ* **315**: 1109–10.
3. Popay J, Williams G (1998) Qualitative research and evidence-based healthcare. *J. R. Soc. Med.* **91(Suppl. 35)**: 32–37.
4. Rosser J, Watt IS, Entwistle V (1996) Informed Choice Initiative: an example of reaching users with evidence based information. *J. Clin. Effect.* **1**: 143–145.
5. Gray JAM (1998) Hallmarks for quality of information. *BMJ* **317**: 1500.
6. Headrick LA, Wilcock PM, Batalden PB (1998) Interprofessional working and continuing medical education. *BMJ* **316**: 771–4.
7. Antman E, Chalmers TC, Lau J, Kupelnick B. A (1992) Comparison of results of meta-analyses of randomized control trials and recommendations of clinical experts. *JAMA* **268**: 240–248.
8. Haynes RB, Davis DA, McKibbon A, Tugwell P (1984) A critical appraisal of the efficacy of continuing medical education. *JAMA* **251**: 61–64.
9. Davis DA, Thomson MA, Oxman AD, Haynes RB (1995) Changing physician performance. A systematic review of the effect of continuing medical education strategies. *JAMA* **274**: 700–705.
10. Bashook PG (1986) Future directions in continuing education. *Diab. Educator* **12**(Suppl.): 215–218.
11. Weinberger M, Cohen SJ, Mazzuca SA (1984) The roles of physicians' attitudes in effective diabetes management. *Soc. Sci. Med.* **19**: 965–969.
12. Mazzuca SA (1986) The role of the clinical environment in the translation of research into practice. *Diab. Educator* **12**(Suppl.): 219–224.
13. Sackett DL, Rosenberg WM, Gray JAM, Haynes RB, Richardson WS (1996) Evidence-based medicine: what it is and what it isn't. *BMJ* **312**: 71–72.
14. Smith R (1999) (Editor's Choice) 'I don't know': the three most important words in education. *BMJ* **318**: 7193.
15. Anderson RM, Donnelly MB, Davis WK (1992) Controversial beliefs about diabetes and its care. *Diab. Care* **15**: 859–863.
16. Sackett DL, Richardson WS, Rosenberg W, Haynes RB (1997) Evidence-based Medicine – How to Practice and Teach EBM. Churchill Livingstone.
17. Greenhalgh T (1997) How to read a paper – The basics of evidence based medicine. London: *BMJ*.

18. Sackett DL, Haynes RB, Guyatt G, Tugwell P (1991) *Clinical Epidemiology; A Basic Science for Clinical Medicine.* : Boston: Little, Brown.
19. LaPorte RE, Akazawa S, Drash A, et al. (1995) Diabetes and the Internet. *Diab. Care* **18**: 890–95
20. Belbin RM (1991) Management Teams: Why they succeed or fail. Butterworth-Heinemann.
21. Apfel J, Coles C, Crace C, et al. (1996) Training and professional development in diabetes care. *Diab. Medicine* **13(Suppl. 4)**: S65–76.
22. Siddons H, McAughey D (1992) Professional development brings specialist knowledge. The role of the diabetes specialist nurse: the Manchester model. *Prof. Nurse* **7**: 5.321–24.
23. Rainwater NG, Giordano BP (1986) Professional education – fostering a team approach? *Diab. Educator* **12(Suppl.)**: 240.
24. Marsden P, Grant J (1990) The learning needs in diabetes of general practitioners. *Diab. Medicine* **7**: 1.69–73.
25. Donabedian A (1980) The definition of quality: a conceptual exploration. In *Explorations in Quality Assessment and Monitoring. Volume 1: The Definition of Quality and Approaches in its Assessment.* Ann Arbor, MI: Health Administration Press.
26. Black N (1994) Why we need qualitative research. *J. Epidem. Comm. Hlth.* **48**: 5.425–26.
27. Stead JW, Dudbridge SB, Hall MS, Pereira Gray DJ (1991) The Exeter Diabetic Project: an acceptable district-wide education programme for general practitioners. *Diab. Medicine* **8**: 9.866–69.
28. Godlee F (1994) The Cochrane collaboration. *BMJ* **309**: 6960.969–70.
29. McKay HG, Feil EG, Glasgow RE, Brown JE (1998) Feasibility and use of an Internet support service for diabetes self-management. *Diab. Educator* **24**: 2.174–79.
30. Lewis D, Komondor K (1950) Diabetes on the Internet: a useful resource for educators. *Diab. Educator* **22**: 5.503–4.
31. Fahey T, Griffiths S, Peters TJ (1995) Evidence based purchasing: understanding results of clinical trials and systematic reviews. *BMJ* **311**: 1056–60.
32. Baigent C, Collins R, Appleby P, Parish S, Sleight P, Peto R (1998) ISIS-2: 10-year survival among patients with suspected acute myocardial infarction in randomised comparison of intravenous streptokinase, oral aspirin, both, or neither. The ISIS-2 (Second International Study of Infarct Survival) Collaborative Group. *BMJ* **316**: 7141.1337–43.
33. European Secondary Prevention Study Group (1996) Translation of clinical trials into practice: a European population-based study of the use of thrombolysis for acute myocardial infarction. European Secondary Prevention Study Group. *Lancet* **347**: 9010.1203–1207
34. Bero LA, Grilli R, Grimshaw JM, Harvey E, Oxman AD, Thomson MA (1998) Closing the gap between research and practice: an overview of systematic reviews of interventions to promote the implementation of research findings. *BMJ* **317**: 465–8.
35. McDonald CJ (1976) Protocol-based computer reminders, the quality of care and the non-perfectability of man. *N. Engl. J. Med.* **295**: 24.1351–55.
36. Haynes RB, Sackett DL, Tugwell P (1983) Problems in the handling of clinical and research evidence by medical practitioners. *Arch. Int. Med.* **143**: 10.1971–75.
37. Haynes RB, Mulrow C, Huth E, Altman D, Gardner M (1990) More informative abstracts revisited. *Ann. Intern. Med.* **113**: 69–76.
38. Donaldson LJ (1998) Clinical governance: a statutory duty for quality improvement. *J Epidemiol. Comm. Hlth.* **52**: 73–74.

39. Grol R (1997) Personal paper. Beliefs and evidence in changing clinical practice. *BMJ* **315**: 7105.418–421

40. Freemantle N, Harvey EL, Wolf F, Grimshaw JM, Grilli R, Bero LA (1999) Printed educational materials to improve the behaviour of health care professionals and patient outcomes (Cochrane Review). The Cochrane Library, Oxford, Update Software Issue 1.

41. Thomson MA, Oxman AD, Davis DA, Haynes RB, Freemantle N, Harvey EL (1999) Audit and feedback to improve health professional practice and health care outcomes (Parts I and II) (Cochrane Review). The Cochrane Library, Oxford, Update Software Issue 1.

42. Coiera E (1996) The Internet's challenge to health care provision. *BMJ* **312**: 7022.3–4

43. Berwick DM (1998) The NHS's 50 anniversary. Looking forward. The NHS: feeling well and thriving at 75. *BMJ* **317**: 57–61.

Index

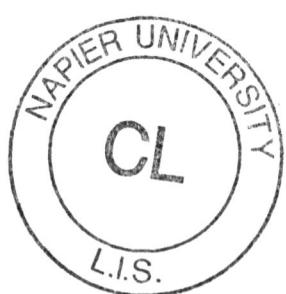